Encyclopedia of Pestilence, Pandemics, and Plagues

Encyclopedia of Pestilence, Pandemics, and Plagues

Volume 2, N–Z

Edited by
JOSEPH P. BYRNE

Foreword by
Anthony S. Fauci, M.D.

GREENWOOD PRESS
Westport, Connecticut • London

Library of Congress Cataloging-in-Publication Data

Encyclopedia of pestilence, pandemics, and plagues / edited by Joseph P. Byrne ; foreword by
Anthony S. Fauci.
   p. cm.
  Includes bibliographical references and index.
  ISBN: 978-0-313-34101-4 (set : alk. paper)
  ISBN: 978-0-313-34102-1 (v. 1 : alk. paper)
  ISBN: 978-0-313-34103-8 (v. 2 : alk. paper)
  1. Epidemics—Encyclopedias. 2. Communicable diseases—Encyclopedias. I. Byrne, Joseph
Patrick.
  [DNLM: 1. Disease Outbreaks—Encyclopedias—English. 2. Communicable Diseases—
Encyclopedias—English. WA 13 E564 2008]
RA652.E535   2008
614.4003—dc2   2008019487

British Library Cataloguing in Publication Data is available.

Library of Congress Catalog Card Number: 2008019487
ISBN: 978–0–313–34101–4 (set)
       978–0–313–34102–1 (vol. 1)
       978–0–313–34103–8 (vol. 2)

First published in 2008

Greenwood Press, 88 Post Road West, Westport, CT 06881
An imprint of Greenwood Publishing Group, Inc.
www.greenwood.com

Printed in the United States of America

∞™

The paper used in this book complies with the
Permanent Paper Standard issued by the National
Information Standards Organization (Z39.48-1984).

10 9 8 7 6 5 4 3 2 1

Contents

List of Entries

Guide to Related Topics

Biological, Physiological, and Medical Theories

Air and Epidemic Diseases
Astrology and Medicine
Ayurvedic Disease Theory and Medicine
Chinese Disease Theory and Medicine
Contagion Theory of Disease
Disease in the Pre-Columbian Americas
Disease, Social Construction of
Folk Medicine
Germ Theory of Disease
Greco-Roman Medical Theories
    and Practices
Humoral Theory
Islamic Disease Theory and Medicine
Magic and Healing
Malthusianism
Panspermia Theory
Paracelsianism

Biomedical Research into Disease Causes, Prevention, and Treatment

Animal Research
Antibiotics
Avicenna (Ibn Sina)
Behring, Emil von
Drug Resistance in Microorganisms
Ehrlich, Paul
Enders, John Franklin
Fernel, Jean
Fracastoro, Girolamo
Galen
Haffkine, Waldemar Mordechai
Hansen, Gerhard Armauer
Henderson, Donald Ainslie
Hippocrates and the Hippocratic Corpus
Human Subjects Research
Jenner, Edward
Kitasato, Shibasaburo
Koch, Robert
Laveran, Charles Louis Alphonse
Leeuwenhoek, Antony van
Manson, Patrick
Microscope
Nicolle, Charles Jules Henri
Paracelsus
Pasteur, Louis
Pettenkofer, Max Josef von
Poliomyelitis, Campaign Against
Reed, Walter

Rhazes
Rush, Benjamin
Ross, Ronald
Sabin, Albert
Salk, Jonas E.
Schaudin, Fritz Richard
Scientific Revolution and Epidemic
    Disease
Semmelweis, Ignaz
Simond, Paul-Louis
Simpson, William John Ritchie
Sydenham, Thomas
Theiler, Max
Wu Lien Teh
Yellow Fever Commission, U.S.
Yersin, Alexandre

Biological Causes of Disease

Bacterium/Bacteria
Ectoparasites
Insects, Other Arthropods, and
    Epidemic Disease
Protozoon, –zoa
Virus

Colonial Experience and Disease

Colonialism and Epidemic Disease
Latin America, Colonial: Effects of
    Imported Diseases
Leprosy, Societal Reactions to
Measles in the Colonial Americas
Slavery and Disease
Smallpox in Colonial Latin America
Smallpox in Colonial North America
Smallpox in Europe's Non-American
    Colonies
Yellow Fever in Colonial Latin America
    and the Caribbean

Cultural and Societal Effects of Epidemic Disease

AIDS, Literature, and the Arts in the
    United States

Black Death and Late Medieval
    Christianity
Black Death, Economic and
    Demographic Effects of
Black Death, Flagellants, and Jews
Black Death: Literature and Art
Cinema and Epidemic Disease
Corpses and Epidemic Disease
Disease, Social Construction of
Flight
Latin America, Colonial: Effects of
    Imported Diseases
Leprosy, Societal Reactions to
Literature, Disease in Modern
Personal Liberty and Public Health
Plague Literature and Art, Early Modern
Plague Memorials
Poison Libels and Epidemic Disease
Poliomyelitis and American Popular
    Culture
Popular Media and Epidemic Disease:
    Recent Trends
Scapegoats and Epidemic Disease
Tuberculosis and Romanticism
Venereal Disease and Social Reform in
    Progressive-Era America

Diseases

Animal Diseases and Epidemics
Babesiosis
Bartonella Diseases
Bubonic Plague
Cholera
Conjunctivitis
Diphtheria
Disease in the Pre-Columbian Americas
Dysentery
Early Humans, Infectious Diseases in
Encephalitis
Enteric Fevers
Ergotism
Gonorrhea
Hemorrhagic Fevers
Hepatitis
Human Immunodeficiency Virus
    (HIV)/AIDS

Human Papilloma Virus and
    Cervical Cancer
Influenza
Legionnaires' Disease
Leprosy
Lyme Disease
Malaria
Measles
Meningitis
Pneumonic and Septicemic Plague
Poliomyelitis
Relapsing Fever
St. Vitus's Dance
Schistosomiasis
Severe Acute Respiratory Syndrome
    (SARS)
Sleeping Sickness
Smallpox
Social Psychological Epidemics
Sweating Sickness
Syphilis
Tuberculosis
Typhus
West Nile Fever
Whooping Cough
Yellow Fever

Drugs and Pharmaceuticals

Antibiotics
Penicillin
Pharmaceutical Industry
Sulfa Drugs
Vaccination and Inoculation

Epidemics and Other Historical
Disease Outbreaks

AIDS in Africa
AIDS in the United States
Armstrong, Richard
Biblical Plagues
Black Death (1347–1352)
Black Death: Modern Medical Debate
Bubonic Plague: Third Pandemic in
    East Asia

Bubonic Plague: Third Pandemic in India
    and Oceania
Bubonic Plague in the United States
    to 2000
Cholera: First through Third Pandemics,
    1816–1861
Cholera: Fourth through Sixth
    Pandemics, 1863–1947
Cholera: Seventh Pandemic, 1961–Present
Diagnosis of Historical Diseases
Encephalitis, Epidemic Outbreaks in the
    Twentieth Century
Gorgas, William Crawford
Hemorrhagic Fevers in Modern Africa
Historical Epidemiology
Influenza Pandemic, 1889–1890
Influenza Pandemic, 1918–1919
Insect Infestations
Irish Potato Famine and Epidemic
    Diseases, 1845–1850
Leprosy in the Premodern World
Leprosy in the United States
London, Great Plague of (1665–1666)
Malaria in Africa
Mather, Increase and Cotton
Measles Epidemic in Fiji (1875)
    and Eugenics
Measles in the Colonial Americas
Plague: End of the Second Pandemic
Plague in Africa: Third Pandemic
Plague in Britain (1500–1647)
Plague in China
Plague in East Asia: Third Pandemic
Plague in Europe, 1500–1770s
Plague in India and Oceania:
    Third Pandemic
Plague in Medieval Europe, 1360–1500
Plague in San Francisco, 1900–1905
Plague in the Contemporary World
Plague in the Islamic World, 1360–1500
Plague in the Islamic World, 1500–1850
Plague of Athens
Plague of Justinian, First Pandemic
Plagues of the Roman Empire
Plagues of the Roman Republic
Pneumonic Plague in Surat, Gujarat,
    India, 1994

Epidemiology

Factors in Disease Outbreaks

Institutions

Medical Personnel

N

NAPOLEONIC WARS. Between 1796 and 1815, the French general, and later Emperor, Napoleon Bonaparte (1769–1821) led or sent millions of French soldiers and their allies on sweeping campaigns of conquest that stretched from the Caribbean, to Moscow and Danzig on the Baltic, to the Pyramids of Egypt. As was the case with every premodern army, disease was a constant companion, and disease epidemics punctuated the two decades of turmoil. These took countless lives among Napoleon's men, those who opposed him, and the luckless civilians encountered along the way.

Conditions of eighteenth-century **warfare** lent themselves readily to the spread of disease. Continental armies, especially those of the French Revolutionary period of the 1790s and Napoleon's time, were enormous and drew in recruits with little concern for their general health. In barracks and camps, sanitation and **personal hygiene** were of minimal concern—though Napoleon himself emphasized both—which gave rise to many food-, water-, and parasite-borne diseases. Crowded quarters, minimal health care, unbalanced **diets**, and the stress of military regimen weakened resistance to disease, leaving diarrheal and respiratory infections virtually endemic. Finally, venereal diseases such as **syphilis** and **gonorrhea**, spread largely by prostitution and rape, also accompanied the era's armies. Though Napoleon wished to have prostitutes banned from his camps, he was careful to have them registered and medically treated.

Exposure of an army to novel **environments** also exposed them to new pathogens. From 1794 to 1797, the British forces that garrisoned and fought the French in Haiti encountered the ravages of the tropical **yellow fever**, which had recently been imported by their colleagues from nearby Martinique. Of 20,000 troops who served, over 60 percent fell ill, and over 3,500 died, most in the swampy, filthy staging areas around Port-au-Prince in the summers of 1794 and 1795. In 1797 the command decided to abandon the island. In 1802, after François Dominique Toussaint L'Ouverture (1743–1803) took control of much of the island with his successful slave revolt, Napoleon sent 25,000 French troops to quell the rebellion. Yellow fever struck the French this time, killing more than a hundred soldiers and sailors per day during the summer months from May to September. New arrivals were most vulnerable and died most readily, and by early 1803 some 40,000 Frenchmen of the 50,000 who served are believed to have succumbed to yellow fever and **malaria**. Toussaint held on with British help and watched the French evacuate later in 1803.

On the Continent, the typical culprit was louse-borne **typhus**. During Napoleon's successful campaign in Italy in 1796, **epidemic** typhus broke out in Mantua, spreading quickly among both French and Austrian armies, and from them to civilian populations as far south as Sicily. In 1799 Austrian and Russian troops defeated the French in the Piedmont region of northwest Italy. Typhus again broke out as the French retreated out of Italy. About a third of the French army fell to the disease, the city of Nice suffered thousands of civilian deaths, and, as the disease spread southward through Liguria, Genoa lost nearly 14,000 residents.

Meanwhile, Napoleon himself was in Egypt, battling the British for control of the eastern Mediterranean. Here his army suffered defeat at the Battle of the Pyramids and encountered endemic **bubonic plague**, which became epidemic in December 1798. The very terror of plague demoralized his men, and Napoleon went so far as to hug one of the victims to show his disbelief in its contagious nature. He stressed cleanliness in the French camps and insisted that company surgeons treat plague victims as well as they could. Blocked by the British navy, the French moved counterclockwise from Alexandria north to Jaffa in Syria, but plague hounded them. While unsuccessfully besieging Acre (Acco), Napoleon lost over 600 men per day. The shrinking French force left Jaffa, abandoning 50 plague victims after giving them opium to drink as a poison, lest they be captured and tortured by the Turks. Many vomited it up and lived to meet their captors. While his army retired to Cairo, where they lost between 30 and 40 men per day, Napoleon returned to France. The army's commanders eventually surrendered to the British, beaten as much by the plague as by the rival Empire.

Napoleon's successful campaign against the Austrians in 1805 resulted in his capture of the Habsburg capital of Vienna into whose hospitals he placed his multitude of wounded and disease ridden. As usual, typhus was the most common ailment, and it spread rapidly in the overcrowded and filthy conditions of even the grandest facility. After the Battle of Austerlitz on December 2, Napoleon used the city of Brno to house his own and his allies' 48,000 wounded. Crammed into houses, churches, monasteries, barns, and stables, the troops were soon suffering from typhus. It swept through like a scythe, leaving 12,000 soldiers and over 10,000 civilians dead. Time and again typhus plagued the day's armies: in March and April 1807 the Prussian defenders of the Baltic port city of Danzig (Gdansk) held out until typhus broke their resistance and forced the garrison to surrender to a French force that was little stronger for having suffered the disease as well.

In the summer of 1809, with Napoleon off fighting in central Europe, the British army launched its largest expeditionary force to date. Planners hoped that by taking the Dutch port of Antwerp they could crack the hold that the French had on most of western Europe. Some 40,000 incompetently led British troops landed in the Scheldt River estuary in July. Despite early successes, Antwerp proved unassailable. In late August an epidemic struck the British troops, who were campaigning in the marshy, low-lying area of Walcheren that seemed to produce the miasmas that then-current medical theory blamed for the fevers, and that in fact hosted the mosquitoes that did cause them. "Walcheren fever" has been identified as a mix of malaria, typhus, **typhoid**, and **dysentery**. Despite the campaign's failure, the army remained in place until late winter 1810, by which time

16,000 men had sickened, and 60 officers and 3,900 soldiers had died. Deaths caused by battle wounds or injuries were about 100. This disaster prompted a Parliamentary inquiry and major changes at the Army Medical Board.

The main British effort to thwart "Boney" was in Spain and Portugal, during the Peninsular Campaigns. The usual diseases dogged both sides, and even yellow fever played its part in 1810. Late in the year, after unsuccessfully testing British Gibraltar, the French laid siege to Cadiz, which was filled with refugees from the surrounding countryside. Soon the fever broke out in the city, sickening thousands and killing 2,788. Had it been during the warmer months, the effect would have been far deadlier. Including the famous victory at Waterloo in 1815, in the quarter century of wars against the French, British armed forces lost about 240,000 men. Of these, roughly 30,000 died as a result of battle and 210,000 succumbed to disease.

Napoleon's greatest assault, and his greatest defeat, was his invasion of Russia in the summer of 1812. Perhaps as many as 600,000 French, Polish, and other allied troops marched across Russian Poland and toward Moscow. The conditions in the Russian Polish territories were dreadful, and the men contracted any number of diseases including typhus. What supply line there was was hampered by the Russians, and their practice of "scorching the earth" left little in the way of food and other necessities. One estimate has 10 percent of the French force dead or fallen along the way before the enemy was engaged. Napoleon's victory at Borodino was won with fewer than half of the remaining French force able to fight, thanks to exhaustion and disease. After the short French occupation of Moscow in September and October, the grueling winter retreat to western Europe reduced the force tremendously. Pneumonia, typhus, trench fever (caused by louse-carried *Bartonella quintana*), and starvation all took their toll. Perhaps only 30,000 men, or 5 percent of the original force remained alive by spring. Many of these, as well as the Russian troops who pursued them (who lost around 60,000 men to disease in the process), brought typhus with them into what is now Germany, from Danzig in the north—where a Russian siege from January to May 1813 resulted in 11,400 French military and 5,592 civilian deaths from typhus—to Bavaria in the south, which wisely established **cordons sanitaires** and **quarantined** the retreating French.

Retreating ahead of his army, Napoleon returned to Paris, raised a new army of half a million men by early summer 1813, and unleashed an unsuccessful campaign in Central Europe. 105,000 of these men would die in battle, and another 219,000 of disease. After their defeat at Leipzig in October, the French left over 100,000 wounded and sick in and around the town of Freiburg, whose normal population was closer to 9,000. Typhus was rampant, and the impact on the civilian population incalculable. As a result of the French retreat from Moscow, the 1813 French offensive, and the Allies' push back to Paris that ended in 1814, somewhere between 200,000 and 300,000 Germans lost their lives to the diseases disseminated by Europe's armies. *See also* Colonialism and Epidemic Disease; Historical Epidemiology; Malaria in Medieval and Early Modern Europe; Plague in the Islamic World, 1500–1850; Thirty Years' War; Typhus and War; War, the Military, and Epidemic Disease.

Further Reading

Palmer, Alan. *Napoleon in Russia.* Emeryville, CA: Carroll and Graf, 2003.

Peterson, Robert K. D. "Insects, Disease, and Military History: The Napoleonic Campaigns and Historical Perception." *American Entomologist* 41 (1995): 147–160. http://entomology.montana.edu/historybug/napoleon/napoleon.htm

Prinzing, Friedrich. *Epidemics Resulting from Wars*. Oxford: Clarendon Press, 1916.

Raoult, Didier. "Evidence for Louse-Transmitted Diseases in Soldiers of Napoleon's Grand Army in Vilnius." *Journal of Infectious Diseases* 193 (2006): 112–120. http://www.journals.uchicago.edu/doi/full/10.1086/498534?cookieSet=1

JOSEPH P. BYRNE

NEOLITHIC REVOLUTION AND EPIDEMIC DISEASE. In the Paleolithic period (Old Stone Age), from approximately 30,000 to 7000 BCE, individual small groups of hunters and gatherers led a nomadic existence rather than living in larger groups with other people. This lifestyle and the absence of domesticated **animals** such as horses and cows limited the spread of disease. Most infections in this period occurred as a result of one of several distinct factors: trauma (causing osteomyelitis); zoonotic diseases, animal diseases that spread to humans; or infections acquired by eating, being injured by, or having contact with wild animals and their excreta. In addition, some diseases would have been contracted from the soil, such as anaerobic **bacteria** that penetrate the skin, and tapeworms.

The Neolithic Period (or New Stone Age) in human history occurred in Europe and the Near East from approximately 7000 to 3500 BCE. It was a revolution in both economic and social terms. Primary food sources changed from wild plants and animals, birds and fish, to cultivated plants, such as early wheat, barley, olives, the vine, and domesticated animals, such as pigs and goats. Some animals, particularly bovines, became domesticated for other uses, such as transport.

The development of agriculture fostered, and was dependent upon, the cooperation of large numbers of families who lived in close proximity to each other. There were other consequences such as population growth, craft specialization, and formation of social hierarchies created by a more predictable food supply and its control by elites. The development of agriculture also resulted in poorer, carbohydrate-rich diets and consequent undernutrition that led to less individual resistance to infection.

Disease.   Disease began to play an important part in Neolithic society soon after the establishment of the earliest settlements between the eighth and third millennia BCE. Although they were scattered rather thinly and the population lived in relatively small hamlets, within a relatively short period after the start of the growing of the first food crops and the start of the domestication of animals and pastoralism, human population would have grown quite dramatically, compared to the previous hunter-gatherer communities living within the same region.

The early development of pastoralism brought with it significant dangers to the human population. Most, if not all, infectious diseases of civilization have spread to humans from the animal population. In prehistory, contacts were closest with domesticated animals, and it is therefore not surprising that many of the infectious diseases common to humans are also recognizable in animals. For example, of what we call the sporadic zoonotic diseases, **smallpox** is almost certainly connected with cowpox, and **influenza** is shared with pigs and birds; other zoonotic diseases include **measles** and mumps. These new pathogens, however, did not appear to spread at once. Some of these sporadic zoonoses transmitted from domesticated animals remained occasional and dormant until proto-**urbanization** created the conditions for them to spread and sustain crowd **transmission**. However, survivors of **epidemics** began to acquire sophisticated immune systems, and tolerance was developed to parasitic worms. However, as people moved around, it became a disaster for any newly exposed population.

The change from hunting and gathering to primitive farming was not entirely detrimental to health, as a number of factors became firmly balanced. With the beginning of farming, some stabilization of general health likely occurred, with the return of female longevity back to the norm that existed during the earlier hunter-gatherer period. This eventually created an excess of survivals over deaths in the very young, and a population increase ensued. The ending of a nomadic existence meant less stress on women during pregnancy, and postnatal adjustment and genetic adaptation of each population to endemic infections would have occurred. Most of the pathological conditions that existed in these periods would have been related to the creation of more stable communities and the formation of permanent villages. Their establishment meant that people began to live in poor conditions and in very close proximity, so that hygiene suffered and individuals were exposed to an increasing number of disease organisms.

Early forms of Neolithic social organization may have created dietary and sanitary codes, some of which might be recognizable today, that would have reduced risk of infection, but it was not just worms and other parasites that flourished in the favorable conditions created by agriculture for their spread among the human population. Protozoan, bacterial, and viral infections also had an expanded field as the human population, together with their flocks and herds, grew. However, it is only when communities become large enough, where encounters with other individuals become frequent enough, and when people lived in close proximity in poor, unhygienic conditions, that the infections brought about by these microorganisms spread. Many diseases need relatively high population densities in order to thrive and were quite insignificant to hunter-gatherer bands in early prehistory, becoming significant only with the development of permanent settlement, farming, and subsequent population nucleation. In fact, the earliest forms of settlement in small agricultural communities involved new risks of parasitic invasion. Increased contact with human excrement that accumulated in proximity to living quarters allowed for a variety of intestinal parasites to thrive.

Urban centers that first developed toward the end of the Neolithic period and then spread into the ensuing Bronze Age, made few if any arrangements for sanitation. The inhabitants would, as a rule, have used the streets and open squares and areas alongside walls for urination and defecation. The consequences of this would have been not only an increase in contagious ova, worms, and other pernicious parasites, carriers of any number of diseases, but also the contamination of supplies of public drinking **water**, such as streams, wells, and cisterns, which would thus have put public health in jeopardy. Other microorganisms would also have contaminated water supplies, particularly where a community had to rely permanently on one source. Plowing soils increased the risk of fungal disease. Stored food was often infected with **insects**, bacteria, and fungal toxins. Also, the existence of closed rural endogamous societies would have had a profound epidemiological effect, as various inherited diseases and disabilities that such inbreeding often produces would have been present.

In some parts of the Eastern Mediterranean and the Near East, for example, irrigation for farming recreated the favorable conditions for the transmission of disease parasites that prevailed in the tropical rain forests from which many of the diseases originally emerged—particularly warm shallow water, in which potential human hosts would provide a more than suitable medium for disease. Amongst them was infection by the parasitical blood fluke that pierced the skin, *Schistoma* sp., which produces **schistosomiasis** or bilharzia. Amongst the most virulent and prevalent of diseases in the period was **malaria**, particularly infection by the *Plasmodium falciparum*, spread by the female *Anopheles* mosquito. More recent evidence points to the spread of malaria to Europe and the Near East from North Africa as early as 8000 BCE.

The Evidence.   The evidence for disease in the Neolithic period, although not plentiful, can be found in the human skeletal remains from excavated cemeteries of the period. Although modern **paleopathology** can only determine incidence of chronic disease, recent work in the field of human ancient DNA (aDNA) may in the future be able to identify or infer other Neolithic disease patterns. At the same time, an understanding of the virulence and prevalence of disease may be achieved through studies of the ancient environment, through the determination of, for example, climate change and land use.

Although the understanding of changes in disease patterns brought on as the result of the Neolithic Revolution is often restricted mainly to Europe, North Africa, and the Near East, many of the societies that existed in other parts of the world such as South Asia and China would have undergone many similar experiences, and many of the diseases that emerged as a result may have become endemic and eventually become many of the pandemics that affected the ancient world in later millennia. *See also* Animal Diseases (Zoonoses) and Epidemic Disease; Diagnosis of Historical Diseases; Disease in the Pre-Columbian Americas; Early Humans, Infectious Diseases in; Environment, Ecology, and Epidemic Disease; Folk Medicine; Human Immunity and Resistance to Disease; Insect Infestations; Smallpox in the Ancient World.

Further Reading

Arnott, Robert. "Disease and the Prehistory of the Aegean." In *Health in Antiquity*, edited by Helen King (London: Routledge, 2005), pp. 12–31.

Cohen, Mark Nathan, and G. J. Armelagos, eds. *Paleopathology and the Origins of Agriculture.* Orlando, FL: Academic Press, 1984.

Groube, Les. "The Impact of Diseases upon the Emergence of Agriculture." In *The Origins and Spread of Agriculture and Pastoralism in Eurasia*, edited by David R. Harris, pp. 101–129. London: University College of London Press, 1996.

Scarre, Chris. "The World Transformed: From Foragers and Farmers to States and Empires." In *The Human Past: World Prehistory and the Development of Human Societies*, edited by Chris Scarre, pp. 176–199. London: Thames and Hudson, 2005.

ROBERT ARNOTT

NEWS MEDIA AND EPIDEMIC DISEASE.   Freedom of the press is embedded in the First Amendment to the U.S. Constitution and has since been one of the keystones of the liberal Western ideal. Americans expect their news media to be free from interference by government or other interests, to be unbiased, and to be accurate. However true this might be for major contemporary news outlets in the United States (still defined as daily newspapers and broadcast and cable television), it has hardly been the norm in other times and places. Political parties, churches, governments, and other social and political groups have traditionally published newspapers, and even in free nations like Britain the government-affiliated British Broadcasting Corporation (BBC) long had a monopoly on radio and television. Cable news television, the Internet, and talk radio have opened news reportage to a far wider field than ever before.

The news media could be said to have been born with the printing press in the mid-1450s. In most European countries censorship by the church and/or state was the norm.

In the sixteenth and seventeenth centuries, printers produced cheap handbills and broadsides (posters) warning of **bubonic plague** or providing information about it and about official actions of public note. Prayers and advertisements for patent medicines often accompanied lurid images of dancing skeletons or funeral processions. In England and some other countries, printers produced and sold weekly bills of mortality, which listed plague deaths and other fatalities by parish. The dissemination of this government data was vital in a commercial center like London, its trends dictating business as usual or upper-class flight and economic depression. Cheap almanacs, too, played a role in shaping public response to disease by predicting threatening celestial configurations or weather patterns. As commercial ventures in a crowded market, these contained advertisements and recipes for plague cures and other medicines that were often sold at the same shops where the almanacs were. In England, a markedly political press developed alongside political parties during the civil turmoil of the seventeenth century. The party in power had its newspapers defending plans, personnel, and policies, whereas the opposition sniped and criticized in the pages of its organs.

Newspapers came to America during this period, but without the political tension to sustain a reasonably free—let alone an opposition—press. Boston's *Publick Occurances*, the earliest English language newspaper in America, reported on a **smallpox** outbreak in the colonies in 1690. Fearing public panic, the Massachusetts governor forced the paper to suspend its reports. Three decades later Boston's popular religious leader **Cotton Mather** sparred with the editors of the *New England Courant* over their coverage of another outbreak of smallpox. A reasonably free press has to keep a steady balance between fact and speculation, and between the public's "right to know" and the potential for panic and social disruption.

Governments shape this balance by withholding or releasing definitive information on disease: during the early stages of plague epidemics in Marseilles, France, in 1720, and in Moscow in 1770, the respective governments downplayed or even denied reports of plague through the press, lest foreign countries suspend trade, and residents flee. Newspapers debated the merits of war and peace, of various public policies for dealing with **cholera**, of contagionism and **miasma** theory, of **germ theory**, and the merits of **vaccination**.

America's newspapers in the nineteenth century were usually tied either to political parties ("Republican" and "Democrat" are still in the names of some newspapers, whereas "Tribune" denoted the people's protector and advocate) or commercial interests. Papers shaped their coverage of **epidemics** of **yellow fever** and cholera with these interests in mind, often sensationalizing their reporting with lurid details and ethnic stereotyping to build circulation. William Randolph Hearst's (1863–1951) "yellow journalism" that beat the drum for war with Spain in the mid-1890s was as much about emphasizing the threat of yellow fever as it was about the early cartoon "Yellow Kid." When plague hit San Francisco in 1900, the local press followed the lead of the California governor, denying the presence of plague and openly undermining public health officials' efforts to contain the spread of the disease. At the same time, the press in New Orleans stood foursquare behind its city's claims of plague and anti-plague efforts; this support resulted in a much shorter and less deadly outbreak. The difference between reactions may lie in the older and more mature New Orleans's previous experience with yellow fever and other infectious diseases.

With the professionalization of journalism in the late nineteenth and early twentieth century, and its key role in the muckraking campaigns of the Progressive Era, journalists tended to gravitate in favor of government reform and scientific and technological advance. In the wake of general acceptance of germ theory, popular media from magazines to movies to advertisements emphasized the threat of germs and the need to sanitize the home and workplace. **Personal hygiene** products to cleanse the body, refrigerators to preserve food safely, and window and door screens to keep insects out were the mark of the modern family. Coverage of the **influenza pandemic of 1918–1919** had its own local logic, but by and large the government received support for its efforts and thus felt justified in releasing the gruesome details. By the 1920s the *New York Times* set the national tone for what at least appeared to be the objective reporting of verified facts, a far cry from its jingoistic war-mongering of two decades earlier.

Broadcast journalism began with radio, a medium that featured news as a small though important part of its content. In totalitarian states like Nazi Germany and the USSR, the ruling party controlled the radio waves and filtered all news through its own propagandizing lens. In the United States, the large commercial networks—RCA, NBC, and CBS—controlled the dissemination of news over the airwaves. Ironically, it was a fictionalized broadcast, Orson Welles's (1915–1985) 1938 *War of the Worlds*, that demonstrated the medium's potential for creating mass hysteria. Radio brought the terrors of the London Blitz (1940) and the subsequent American involvement in World War II (1939–1945) into American living rooms. Even more intimate were the images that television delivered, beginning in the mid-1940s. Voices and faces carried more weight than mere bylines, and when reporter and gossip columnist Walter Winchell (1897–1972) decided to oppose publicly the **Salk** polio vaccine in the early 1950s, he brought a great many Americans with him. The major problem with broadcast journalism was its necessarily shallow and narrow coverage of the issues of the day. Like radio, television was essentially an entertainment medium, in which even during an hour of news, major health stories competed with local color, sports, and weather. Newspapers and magazines like *Time*, *Newsweek*, and *U.S. News and World Report* were natural media for deeper and more serious discussions of such topics as vaccine successes and failures or outbreaks of new diseases in Africa.

A new wave of important innovations has changed the landscape from the late 1980s. The founding of Cable News Network (CNN) introduced America to the 24-hour news cycle, while satellite linkups could flood the world's televisions with on-the-spot reporting as events unfolded, unmediated by editing. At the same time, the Internet established equally unmediated platforms for news and opinion with no links to "mainstream" media, and talk radio, long relegated to late-night time slots, emerged with its largely populist, libertarian, and conservative slant. Late-night talk radio has long been dominated by Art Bell (b. 1945) and his successors and their attention to news of the weird—which has included emergent and reemergent diseases and other health threats, real and imagined. For more serious students of world health issues, the Internet provides a host of resources, most reliably the reports of the **World Health Organization** (WHO) and the U.S. **Centers for Diseases Control and Prevention** (CDC).

Emerging or reemerging diseases established themselves in Western media in 1994. **Pneumonic plague in India**, the **hantavirus** scare in America's Southwest, reports of flesh-eating **bacteria**, and magazine cover stories on infectious diseases converged with popular films featuring pestilence. **Drug-resistant** pathogens, **Ebola** fever, global warming, and the notion that a **pandemic** is only a jet airplane ride away fueled anxieties that have remained heated to this day.

In the midst of this cacophony, the traditional print media have found themselves drawn to unwarrantedly deep coverage, as was the case with the 2002–2003 **Severe Acute Respiratory Syndrome** (SARS) outbreak. Media critic Michael Fumento reported in mid-2003 that the disease to that point had killed 801 people and affected about 10 times that number worldwide. Malaria kills over 800 people every two and a half hours, he noted, and tuberculosis more than 800 people every three hours, yet neither disease received even the smallest fraction of articles the *New York Times* devoted to SARS: over 250. The Robarts Centre for Canadian Studies conducted a systematic study of U.S. and Canadian press coverage of SARS, its threat, and its effects. It revealed that the *Toronto Star* led with 556 articles over 91 days, while the *Star*, the *Globe and Mail*, the *National Post*, *New York Times*, and *USA Today* published 1,600 articles on SARS over the period, as many as 25 per day collectively. Fumento blames this "excessive" coverage in part on the hype provided by the WHO and CDC. This coverage sparked incidents of "hate speech" and property crime in Toronto, and analysts estimated that China, where SARS originated, lost some US $50 billion in reduced trade and tourism. On the other hand, an unprecedented range of voices were recorded, from the "man in the street" to victims, health professionals, economists, businesswomen, and members of advocacy groups.

In developing countries where large portions of the population are susceptible to a range of infectious diseases, the role of the media in informing and educating the people is crucial. Here the radio, **public health posters**, and billboards are often far more important than the Internet or television, and messages need to be tailored to groups differentiated by ethnic identities, languages, **religions**, political alignments, and levels of literacy. Media campaigns urging vaccinations, condom use, or disease screening are often lost to contradictory government assurances or cultural resistance. *See also* AIDS in Africa; AIDS in America; Bioterrorism; Bubonic Plague in the United States; Cinema and Epidemic Disease; Geopolitics, International Relations, and Epidemic Disease; Hemorrhagic Fevers in Modern Africa; Measles, Efforts to Eradicate; Plague in San Francisco, 1900–1908; Poliomyelitis and American Popular Culture; Poliomyelitis, Campaign Against; Popular Media and Epidemic Disease: Recent Trends; Sexuality, Gender, and Epidemic Disease; Smallpox Eradication; Social Psychological Epidemics; Tuberculosis in the Contemporary World; War, the Military, and Epidemic Disease.

Further Reading

Atkin, C., and Lawrence Wallack, eds. *Mass Communication and Public Health*. Newbury Park, CA: Sage, 1990.

Blakely, Debra E. Menconi. *Mass Mediated Disease: A Case Study Analysis of Three Flu Pandemics and Public Health Policy*. Lanham, MD: Lexington Books, 2006.

Burkett, William. *News Reporting: Science, Medicine, and High Technology*. Ames: Iowa State University Press, 1986.

Copeland, David A. *Debating the Issues in Colonial Newspapers: Primary Documents on Events of the Period*. Westport: Greenwood Press, 2000.

Davidson, A. E., and L. Wallack. "A Content Analysis of Sexually Transmitted Diseases in the Print News Media." *Journal of Health Communication* 9 (2004): 111–117.

Davis, Julia. *Evolution of an Epidemic: 25 Years of HIV/AIDS Media Campaigns in the United States*. Menlo Park, CA: Henry J. Kaiser Family Foundation, 2006.

Drache, Daniel, and Seth Feldman. "Media Coverage of the 2003 Toronto SARS Outbreak: A Report on the Role of the Press in a Public Crisis." Robards Centre for Canadian Studies, York University, Toronto, Canada. http://www.yorku.ca/drache/academic/papers/gcf_sars.pdf

Garrett, Laurie. "Understanding Media's Response to Epidemics." Public Health Reports 116 (Suppl 2) (2001): 87–91.

Moeller, Susan D. *Compassion Fatigue: How the Media Sell Disease, Famine, War and Death.* New York: Routledge, 1999.

Pratt, C. B., et al. "Setting the Public Health Agenda on Major Diseases in Sub-Saharan Africa: African Popular Magazines and Medical Journals, 1981–1997." *Journal of Communication* 52 (2002): 889–904.

Tomes, Nancy. "The Making of a Germ Panic, Then and Now." *American Journal of Public Health* 90 (2000): 191–198.

Wang, Xiao. "For the Good of Public Health or for Political Propaganda: People's Daily's Coverage of the Severe Acute Respiratory Syndrome Epidemic." *China Media Research* 3 (2007): 25–32.

Watney, Simon. *Policing Desire: Pornography, AIDS, and the Media.* Minneapolis: University of Minnesota, 1997.

Ziporyn, Terra. *Disease in the Popular American Press: The Case of Diphtheria, Typhoid Fever, and Syphilis, 1870–1920.* Westport, CT: Greenwood Press, 1988.

JOSEPH P. BYRNE

NICOLLE, CHARLES JULES HENRI (1866–1936). Charles Nicolle established his place among "plague-hunters" not only with his Nobel Prize-winning demonstration of the louse transmission of **typhus**, but also with his pioneering exploration of the then-novel concept that infectious diseases—like human civilizations—were "born," "grew," and "died." "There will be new diseases," he warned. "This is a fatal fact . . . . By the time we become aware of their existence, they will already be . . . adults. They will appear as did Athena, fully armed, from Zeus's brow."

Born to a **physician** and his wife in Rouen, France, Nicolle completed medical school but followed brother Maurice to the recently created **Pasteur** Institute in Paris after growing deafness disrupted his plan to follow his father's path. In 1893 he returned to his hometown in Normandy, leading the local effort to integrate the new science of microbiology into medical practice. In 1902 he was called to direct the Pasteur Institute in Tunisia, then a French protectorate. He held this position until his death in 1936. While in Tunis, Nicolle made important discoveries about the cause, nature, and transmission of diseases from **relapsing fever** and **pandemic influenza** to trachoma and leishmaniasis. He also developed a convalescent serum for measles and a method of improving vaccine manufacture.

Nicolle is best remembered for his work on typhus—a disease long feared, but today largely controlled. By the start of the twentieth century, bacteriology had uncovered the microscopic causes and transmission routes of many diseases. It had not, however, shed much light on typhus. The disease seemed to disappear between epidemics and could not be cultivated in animals. Moreover, it rarely struck Western countries any longer, making its study difficult. Posted in North Africa, near yet outside "the West," Nicolle encountered typhus. During a particularly severe **epidemic** in 1909, he discovered animals (chimpanzees, monkeys, and later guinea pigs) capable of preserving the disease for intra-epidemic study. He used his colleagues' careful epidemiological investigations to single out the louse as the disease's probable vector. Further tests confirmed this hypothesis. In 1928 Nicolle was awarded the Nobel Prize for his typhus research.

Typhus had long been associated with **war, poverty**, and famine. The louse was the material link between the disease and its preferred conditions of existence. His discovery, Nicolle noted, explained typhus's disappearance in the West: cleanliness, good **diet**, and relative peace (World War I would challenge, and ultimately support, his argument) held the disease at bay. Similarly, the continued presence of typhus in Tunisia reflected the extent to which "civilization" had yet to take hold there. Disease, Nicolle concluded, was its own civilization, existing in delicate balance with human civilization. Where humanity's civilization fell, disease rose. Moreover, disease evolved; consequently, new disease civilizations would emerge—often in the niches humans created. Here, Nicolle set in motion the very "one microbe causes one disease" specificity that became the hallmark of bacteriology. His ideas on the enduring place of plagues in human existence helped shape future thinking on disease ecology. *See also* Bacterium/Bacteria; Influenza Pandemic, 1918–1919; Typhus and Poverty in the Modern World; Typhus and War.

Further Reading

Pelis, Kim. *Charles Nicolle, Pasteur's Imperial Missionary: Typhus & Tunisia*. Rochester, NY: University of Rochester Press, 2006.

KIM PELIS

NON-GOVERNMENTAL ORGANIZATIONS (NGOs) AND EPIDEMIC DISEASE. The containment of **epidemics** is often seen as one of the primary public health responsibilities of governments. However, this role of the state becomes severely crippled during sudden natural disasters, civil strife, and **wars**. Even in times of relative stability, the disinclinations or inabilities of governments to address public health problems adequately have left entire populations more vulnerable to epidemics. Under these circumstances, the roles of non-governmental organizations (NGOs) are made more prominent. Historically, members of community bodies like parishes, guilds, and charities, as well as philanthropists and folk medical practitioners, have been the frontline in providing localized relief to the victims of epidemic outbreaks.

By the late nineteenth century, these groups had taken up geographically and functionally broader profiles. Health-based movements in the West had not only developed a greater awareness of the global dimensions of diseases, but they were also increasingly able to project their works beyond their local confines. Along with emergency relief efforts and provision of the latest curative health care, the main emphasis of these groups lay in heightening the urgency in tackling diseases that had become endemic, and therefore less noticeable than sudden epidemic outbreaks. The Rockefeller Foundation—established in 1913 from John D. Rockefeller's (1839–1937) Standard Oil, the first generation of modern multinational corporations—embarked on a global effort to eradicate **pandemic** hookworm disease as one of its main ideals. Other NGOs with public health-related activities included the **sanitation movements** in their worldwide campaigns for sexual health against **syphilis** from the late nineteenth century until the Second World War. Like the directors of the Rockefeller Foundation, these activists were eager to present **sexually transmitted diseases** as a global pandemic that required urgent and sustained public health responses.

Globally oriented NGOs such as the International Red Cross and the Red Crescent Society and their national counterparts have also been responsible for monitoring public health situations in war zones, where they have especially monitored for any potential epidemics. Humanitarian organizations like the Mèdecins Sans Frontiers (Doctors without Borders) and Oxfam have been providing emergency mass **vaccination** services as well as medical assistance and temporary freshwater supplies to war-torn and disaster-stricken areas, the populations of which are more vulnerable to epidemics like **cholera, measles, and meningitis**. The growing concerns from the late twentieth century over emerging and reemerging diseases are also increasingly reflected in the initiatives of prominent philanthropies with the global **eradication** of **AIDS** being the core aim of the Bill and Melinda Gates Foundation, and the improvement of effectiveness of responses to pandemics being one of the latest goals of the Rockefeller Foundation.

NGOs are also increasingly involved in supporting health communication, monitoring, and advocacy. A crucial function assumed by the non-state sector in dealing with epidemics is in the area of dissemination of information and updates on epidemiological trends. The popular media, in particular, made its mark during the **Influenza Pandemic of 1918–1919** in reporting news about the spread and public health responses to the virus. On the contrary, in light of heightened censorship as well as severe limitations of resources during the First World War, information being disseminated by official channels about the pandemic was not forthcoming. This function remains crucial in the contemporary era regarding epidemics like **Avian Flu**. Recognizing their influences, governments have even deployed print and broadcast media networks as partners against epidemics. In Southeast Asia, the newspapers and radio programs have been one of the principal portals in spreading preventive health methods against mosquito breeding during periodic outbreaks of **Dengue fever**.

Benefiting from the greater diffusion in knowledge and resources regarding medical matters, NGOs are also playing an increasing part in the field of advocacy in epidemic control and prevention. The principal agendas of these organizations are those of obtaining official recognition of the enormity and extent of the **contagion** and securing greater investment and commitment to improving access to medical treatment for victims. In this respect, AIDS has become the flagship disease for concerned groups. Being an epidemic that affects more vulnerable social and sexual minorities, health-based NGOs are also forming alliances with other interest groups and welfare organizations to amplify further the social relevance of their causes. In Kenya, these coalitions have even been institutionalized on a national basis in the Kenya Aids NGOs Consortium (KANCO), which consists of a wide network of civil society groups. The increasing recognition of AIDS as a regional and international issue is also seen in the establishment of groups like African Council of Aids Service Organization, International Council of Aids Services Organisations, as well as the Global Health Advocates (devoted to reduction of **tuberculosis, malaria**, and AIDS).

Although advocacy groups have frequently been either ignored or given official lip service commitments by governments, no one could dismiss the evolving watchdog function of the **World Health Organization** (WHO). Known before 1945 as the League of Nations Health Services, one of the primary duties of WHO is to monitor the spread of infectious diseases. Its importance was heightened during the **Severe Acute Respiratory Syndrome** (SARS) pandemic in 2003. Suspicious of the attempts of national governments to downplay the severity of the spread of the disease, countries and societies relied upon WHO inspectors for the final word. In turn, the latter's official position became crucial for governments in restoring political stability and investment confidence shaken by the SARS outbreak.

Given current trends, it is likely in the near future that the presence of NGOs will prove to be crucial simultaneously at the local, regional, and global levels in dealing with epidemics. *See also* AIDS in Africa; Bioterrorism; Capitalism and Epidemic Disease;

Colonialism and Epidemic Disease; Human Papilloma Virus and Cervical Cancer; Irish Potato Famine and Epidemic Disease, 1845–1850; Malaria in Africa; Measles, Efforts to Eradicate; Medical Ethics and Epidemic Disease; Pharmaceutical Industry; Poliomyelitis and American Popular Culture; Poliomyelitis, Campaign Against; Religion and Epidemic Disease.

Further Reading

Farley, John. *To Cast Out Disease: A History of the International Health Division of Rockefeller Foundation (1913–1951)*. New York: Oxford University Press, 2003.

Global Health Advocates. http://www.ghadvocates.org/

Hewa, Soma, and Philo Hove, eds. *Philanthropy and Cultural Context: Western Philanthropy in South, East and South East Asia in the 20th Century*. Lanham, MD: University Press of America, 1997.

Hunt, Alan. *Governing Morals: A Social History of Moral Regulation*. New York: Cambridge University Press, 1999.

International Council of Aids Service Organisations. http://www.icaso.org/

Kenya Aids NGOs Consortium (KANCO). http://www.kanco.org

Liew Kai Khiun. "'Terribly Severe though Mercifully Short:' The Episode of the 1918 Influenza in Malaya." *Modern Asian Studies* 41 (2007): 221–252.

Lipschutz, Ronnie, ed. *Civil Societies and Social Movements: Domestic, Transnational, Global*. Aldershot: Ashgate, 2006.

Weindling, Paul, ed. *International Health Organizations and Movements, 1918–1939*. New York: Cambridge University Press, 1995.

World Health Organization. *SARS: How a Global Epidemic Was Stopped*. Geneva: World Health Organization, Western Pacific Region, 2006.

LIEW KAI KHIUN

NURSES AND NURSING.   Today, nursing is the largest health-care profession, and it accounts for the greatest proportion of direct care during sickness. Good nursing care is especially important during **epidemics**. A nursing tradition developed during the early years of Christianity when the Church established a benevolent function of tending the sick. At this time, deaconesses cared for the sick poor, particularly during epidemics. Another account of nursing comes during the third century when a religious group of men called the *parabolani* brotherhood cared for victims of the **Plague of Cyprian** in the Mediterranean area. The religious ethos of charity continued with the rapid outgrowth of monastic orders in the fifth and sixth centuries and extended into the Middle Ages, when **typhus** and **bubonic plague** were particularly lethal. Monasteries added hospital wards, where "to nurse" meant to give comfort and spiritual sustenance. Religious nursing orders, such as the Knights of St. Lazarus in Jerusalem who cared for victims of **leprosy**, often established specialty hospitals for the sick. Historically, men have had important roles in nursing and predominated in medieval nursing in both Western and Eastern institutions. It was not until the seventeenth century when the French priest St. Vincent de Paul (1580–1660) challenged this model that religious orders of women became more prevalent. After the Reformation, secular nurses replaced religious women as nurses in Protestant countries such as England.

The epidemic-stricken cities of the mid-nineteenth century in the United States needed hospitals and nurses immediately. During the **cholera** epidemics, however, nurses were especially hard to find. Cholera nursing was dirty and dangerous, and religious congregations of women often filled the gap. Private and religious benevolent societies also developed a system of caring.

Times of **war** historically have been associated with epidemics such as cholera, **measles**, and **influenza**. The Crimean War was particularly influential on modern nursing when, in 1854, Englishwoman Florence Nightingale (1820–1910) and 38 nurses went to hospitals in Turkey and Crimea, where soldiers were sick from cholera and typhus. Nightingale established a record-keeping system, a series of sanitary reforms, and a nursing model that emphasized ritual, discipline, and skill that led to improvements in both military and civic hospitals. During the American Civil **War**, more soldiers died of disease than in battle. Lay women and religious sisters worked in military hospitals, on hospital ships, and on the battlefield. Their influence as nurses in reducing mortality was a critical event in changing public perceptions of nursing. During the Spanish American War, a third of the U.S. soldiers in army camps became ill with **malaria, typhoid fever, dysentery**, and diarrhea. Whereas male army nurses initially cared for the sick, during the Spanish American War a large cadre of female graduate nurses served. This war benefited from the nurse training school movement modeled after the Nightingale system that had begun in the United States after the Civil War.

Reform in nursing education during the early twentieth century focused on discipline and special skills. Nurses caring for victims of epidemics took temperatures, pulses, and respirations; provided skin care; used ice baths for fevers; provided comfort measures; and assisted with feeding. They bathed patients, changed linen, gave medications, and prepared and administered food for special diets. They kept the sick room clean and well ventilated and prepared **corpses**. Visiting nursing originated at the end of the nineteenth century in the United States, and typhoid fever was a common condition. Because of the potential for complications, including sudden death, care demanded the whole range of nursing knowledge, including treatment of delirium and management of emergencies such as hemorrhage. Visiting nurses were also an integral part of the public health crusade against **tuberculosis**. They provided physical care; carried out isolation procedures; and instructed patients and families about rest, sanitary measures, the control of sputum, and prevention of the spread of disease. They had to nurse across barriers of class, **race**, and language, and their work was hard and risky.

Beginning in the twentieth century, nurses were at the center of epidemic response teams. During **Walter Reed's yellow fever** experiments in Cuba, American nurse Clara Maass (1876–1901) died after she volunteered to be bitten by an infected mosquito. Through the Red Cross, nurses responded to the Armenian massacre in 1915 and led antityphus campaigns across Siberia in 1918. One of nurses' greatest challenges came during the **influenza pandemic of 1918–1919**. In an era before **antibiotics, physicians** could do little with their therapeutic regimens, but nursing care could provide hydration, warmth, good nutrition, and fever reduction. Chinese Red Cross nurses worked in army camps during World War II and played key roles in the Chinese National Health Administration's anti-epidemic units. Then, in 1948, the **World Health Organization** was established as the United Nations' public health agency. Its work includes combating epidemics, with nurses playing key roles in controlling cholera, tuberculosis, plague, and other diseases.

By 1965 nurses not only taught individuals about preventive measures, but they also screened populations for disease, participated in surveys and registrations, and performed health histories. After 1970 old and new diseases represented a continuing challenge. New strains of tuberculosis developed, and nurses carried out new infection control

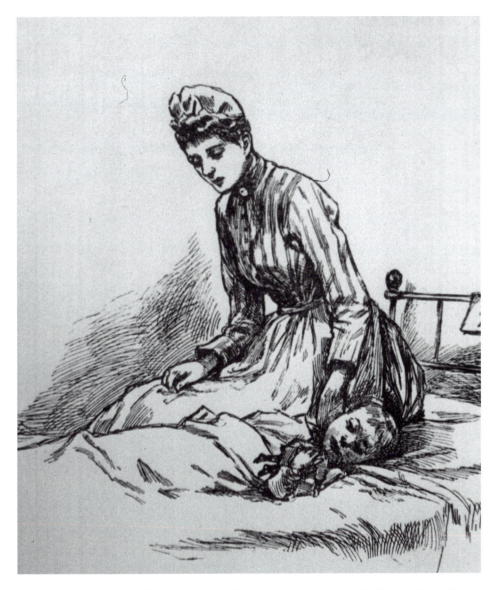

Nurse with a child in a hospital, 1870. Courtesy of the National Library of Medicine.

measures while also relying on the standard therapeutic regimens of rest, nutrition, and isolation. All over the world, increasing numbers of nurses are caring for victims of **AIDS**. Through close patient monitoring, mastering new technologies, and translating research into practice, they continue to provide life-saving care. When medical care appears unable to cure AIDS, nurses remind patients and the public that they remain at the center of patient care. *See also* Hospitals and Medical Education in Britain and the United States; Hospitals in the West to 1900; Hospitals since 1900; Leprosarium; Pest Houses and Lazarettos; Religion and Epidemic Disease; Sanatorium; Typhus and War.

Further Reading

Buhler-Wilkerson, Karen. *No Place Like Home: A History of Nursing and Home Care in the United States*. Baltimore: Johns Hopkins University Press, 2001.

Byerly, Carol. *Fever of War: The Influenza Epidemic in the U.S. Army during World War I*. New York: New York University Press, 2005.

Harvard University Library. *Contagion*. http://ocp.hul.harvard.edu/contagion/nightingale.html

Kalisch, Philip A., and Beatrice J. Kalisch. *American Nursing: A History*. Philadelphia: Lippincott, Williams, and Wilkins, 2004.

Warren, Mame. *Our Shared Legacy: Nursing Education at Johns Hopkins, 1889–2006*. Baltimore: Johns Hopkins University Press, 2006.

BARBRA MANN WALL

P

PALEOPATHOLOGY.   The term paleopathology derives from the Greek words *paleos* (ancient), *pathos* (suffering), and *logos* (study) and is defined as the scientific study of disease in ancient human and **animal** populations preserved predominantly as skeletons or mummified remains. In the present context, the focus will be on human remains and the evidence for infectious diseases as they are the primary, and often sole, source for knowledge of the health of our predecessors.

History and Scope of Paleopathology.   Paleopathology as a scientific study was made more widely known by Sir Armand Ruffer (1859–1917), a British **surgeon** working in early twentieth-century Egypt, but the origins of the discipline go back to the Renaissance period of the fifteenth and sixteenth centuries. Self-trained naturalists studied skeletons of extinct animals found in caves and quarries and described the observed pathological lesions and signs of trauma. However, these studies of the strange and curious were largely seen as entertainment. Only with the nineteenth-century advances in medicine and scientific techniques for the investigation of human individuals were their diseases regarded as valuable medical science. Although these early researchers concentrated on interesting individual cases, a shift toward population-based studies was seen during the twentieth century advocated by, for example, the German pathologist **Rudolf Virchow**, and today a more multidisciplinary biocultural approach is the norm, using all available information to reconstruct past population health.

Methodology and Techniques.   The **diagnosis** of a specific disease relies primarily on visual macroscopic observations of what is recognized as abnormal or pathological and is based on the knowledge of how diseases affect the human skeleton and other tissues in a modern clinical context. In recent years techniques such as ancient DNA analysis to detect a pathogen's DNA, and histology to observe changes on a microscopic level have enhanced the understanding of our ancestors' sufferings. Radiology is another useful tool, and it has been extensively, but not exclusively, used to study mummified remains, as it is a nondestructive technique. Key to a potentially correct diagnosis is the careful description of all pathological changes seen in an individual skeleton, as well as a description of the distribution pattern of these changes within the preserved bones. It is important to consider all possible diseases that could have led to the observed changes and distribution patterns (differential diagnosis).

Limitations.   Skeletal elements can only react in a limited way to disease by either forming or destroying bone, or a mixture of both. It takes several weeks for the skeletal system to respond to any pathogen infiltration. This means that any acute disease will not be visible in bone because the person died before any bone changes could occur, and the bioarcheologist is usually left with evidence for chronic disease only. In the exceptional case of soft tissue preservation in mummified remains, but also in skeletons, acute diseases such as **smallpox** or **bubonic** and **pneumonic plague** may be observable through the detection of the causative agent's own DNA. Nevertheless, this technique is destructive and cannot at present be applied to study large numbers of individuals. We are therefore largely restricted to macroscopic observations of specific chronic infectious diseases such as **tuberculosis** (TB), treponemal disease (venereal and endemic **syphilis**, bejel, and pinta) and **leprosy**, as well as the so-called nonspecific infectious responses of periostitis, osteomyelitis, and osteitis. These terms refer to the origin within a bone from which the infection derives, whether the periost (tissue covering the outer surface of bone) or a more internal bone structure such as hard cortical (surface) bone or the medullary cavity, where yellow marrow is stored. Different pathogens—for example, staphylococci or streptococci—may cause identical bone changes, hence the name nonspecific infectious disease.

Infectious Diseases and Paleopathology.   Tuberculosis, also known as scrofula and phthisis, is probably one of the oldest infectious diseases affecting both humans and animals, and human skeletal evidence for TB in the Old World goes back as far as the fifth millennium before present. TB has affected humans since the beginning of animal domestication, although skeletal manifestations of the disease in archeological populations are rare. It is a disease of civilization, and the increase in TB infections worldwide has been associated with crowded living conditions, poor levels of **personal hygiene**, and **poverty**. Typical bone changes associated with TB are Pott's disease, or abnormal bending of the spinal column as a result of the destruction of vertebra, and destructive joint lesions affecting the large joints such as the hip and knee. Less diagnostic are bone changes to the visceral surface of ribs as these can also occur in nontubercular lung diseases.

However, only 3 to 5 percent of individuals suffering from TB will develop bone changes, and this might be the reason why relatively few cases of the disease have been reported in archeological populations. On the other hand, people may have died before they developed visible bone changes. New diagnostic techniques such as ancient DNA analysis can help to identify individuals with TB even in the absence of bone changes, and in the future more accurate prevalence rates can be expected.

Treponemal disease, or treponematoses, comprises a group of four syndromes: venereal syphilis, endemic syphilis (bejel), yaws, and pinta. Bone changes are absent in pinta, but prolific new bone formation on long bones can be found in the other syndromes. As a result of their similarity in appearance differentiation among the three diseases is difficult, especially in partially preserved archeological skeletons. In historical times venereal syphilis had the most devastating impact on society of the treponematoses because of its ultimately lethal course, and skeletal changes of the tertiary form of the disease can be seen as stellate (star-shaped) scars on the skull (*caries sicca*), especially on the frontal bone. Again, similar to TB, only 5 to 15 percent of people infected with venereal syphilis will develop bone changes, and a significant proportion of archeological individuals will remain undiagnosed in the absence of any skeletal indicators. It currently remains controversial whether ancient DNA analysis can extract the pathogen's molecular structure.

Equally, the origin of venereal syphilis has been a point of controversy for decades with the Columbian theory favoring the New World as the cradle of the disease, and its dissemination into the Old World resulting from Columbus's travels. However, skeletal remains with evidence for venereal syphilis from the Old World have been dated to the pre-Columbian period. It appears that the disease was present worldwide even before its devastating effects on war-torn late fifteenth- and sixteenth-century Europe where it went hand-in-hand with deprivation, poverty, and prostitution.

Similarly to venereal syphilis, leprosy has provoked strong negative reactions in the noninfected: during the medieval period, people suffering from the disabling disease were largely confined to leprosy hospitals or **leprosaria** and stripped of their worldly possessions. Skeletal changes resulting from leprosy have only been studied since the mid-twentieth century, and the geographical source of the disease still remains somewhat unclear, but is likely to have originated from the Indian subcontinent. The currently oldest unequivocal skeletal evidence for leprosy comes from individuals found in Egypt dating to the second millennium BCE, but not until the medieval period do the numbers of skeletons with evidence for the disease increase. However, only 5 percent of individuals suffering from leprosy will show bone changes, and because the diagnosis is based largely on the distribution pattern of bone lesions, the disease might be missed in incompletely preserved archeological skeletons. Furthermore, leprosy is a disease that progresses slowly, and individuals might have died before bone changes could develop.

Nonspecific infections have been observed in skeletons worldwide, and population-based studies demonstrate an increase in chronic infectious diseases during the **Neolithic Revolution**, with the onset of agriculture and a sedentary lifestyle and subsequent increasing population numbers. For example, chronic maxillary sinusitis, visible as new bone formation on the inside of the maxillary sinuses, became more prevalent in societies with high rates of air pollution and crowded living conditions, where cross-infection could easily occur.

Although paleopathology is unable directly to diagnose acute infectious disease in skeletal remains, demographic studies may reveal periods of increased mortality. For example, mass burials discovered in the city of London and dated to the years of bubonic plague epidemics in the fourteenth century show a specific demographic profile. Here members of society were present indiscriminately, and not only the most vulnerable such as young children and elderly adults. *See also* Black Death: Modern Medical Debate; Diagnosis of Historical Diseases; Disease in the Pre-Columbian Americas; Early Humans, Disease in; Historical Epidemiology; Syphilis in Sixteenth-Century Europe; Urbanization and Epidemic Disease.

Further Reading

Aufderheide, Arthur C., and Conrado Rodríguez-Martín. *The Cambridge Encyclopedia of Human Paleopathology*. Cambridge: Cambridge University Press, 1998.

Larsen, Clark S. *Bioarchaeology: Interpreting Behavior from the Human Skeleton.* New York: Cambridge University Press, 1997.

Ortner, Donald J. *Identification of Pathological Conditions in Human Skeletal Remains,* 2nd edition. New York: Academic Press, 2003.

Powell, Mary L., and Della C. Cook. *The Myth of Syphilis: The Natural History of Treponematosis in North America.* Gainesville, FL: University Press of Florida, 2005.

Roberts, Charlotte A., and Jane E. Buikstra. *The Bioarchaeology of Tuberculosis: A Global View on a Reemerging Disease.* Gainesville, FL: University Press of Florida, 2003.

Roberts, Charlotte A., and Keith Manchester. *The Archaeology of Disease,* 3rd edition. Stroud: Sutton Publishing, 2005.

TINA JAKOB

PAN AMERICAN HEALTH ORGANIZATION.   *See* International Health Agencies and Conventions.

PANDEMIC.   *See* Epidemic.

PANSPERMIA THEORY.   Panspermia is the theory that the origins of life on Earth are extraterrestrial. Proponents of panspermia believe that the seeds of life, in the form of spores, microbes, or pre-biotic compounds (life's building blocks), exist in space and, once introduced into the planet's atmosphere, developed into terrestrial life. Some modern-day advocates of the theory further contend that the bombardment of earth by organisms from space continues and is sometimes responsible for outbreaks of disease.

Panspermia, a Greek word that literally means "seeds everywhere," was coined in the fifth century BCE by the philosopher Anaxagoras (c. 500–428), who claimed that the universe was filled with *spermata* (seeds) that blossomed into life when they reached the earth. Modern proponents of the extraterrestrial origin of life, also known as exogenesis, have included Lord Kelvin (1824–1907), Svante Arrhenius (1859–1927), and Sir Francis Crick (1916–2004), co-discoverer of the DNA's double helix structure. The most active modern champions of panspermia have been two astrophysicists, Sir Fred Hoyle (1915–2001), founder of the Institute of Astronomy at Cambridge University, and his student, Dr. Chandra Wickramasinghe (b. 1939), director of Cardiff University's Centre for Astrobiology in Wales.

Concerning the great **influenza pandemic of 1918–1919**, Hoyle and Wickramasinghe noted that the outbreak seemed to have multiple points of origin and that remote regions such as small Alaskan fishing villages were struck despite their isolation. Persuaded that human contact alone could not account for the extremely rapid and unusually extensive spread of the disease around the world, they argued that the **pandemic** was caused by **viruses** that had originated in interstellar space, entered the earth's atmosphere as cometary dust, and later rained down from the stratosphere, a view almost universally dismissed by experts on the pandemic. More generally, they charted a correlation between influenza epidemics and increases in sunspot activity, hypothesizing that increased solar activity results in increased levels of cosmic dust containing flu viruses entering earth's atmosphere. The two have also attributed specific outbreaks of **Legionnaires' disease, polio,** and mad cow disease to extraterrestrial pathogens.

Supporters of panspermia have sought to link the development of new diseases to microbes from space, as when Dr. Hoyle proposed that **AIDS** was introduced from outer space. In 2003 Dr. Wickramasinghe and two colleagues published a letter in the prestigious British medical journal, *The Lancet,* suggesting that the corona virus responsible for the **SARS** epidemic in China was extraterrestrial in origin. They cited the high altitude of the location of the initial outbreaks of the disease and the frequency of meteor showers in that region, and predicted, incorrectly, imminent independent outbreaks of SARS as more of the virus made its way from the stratosphere to the surface. Like other claims linking terrestrial disease to extraterrestrial pathogens, this proposal was rejected by the greater research community.

Further Reading

Hoyle, Fred, and Chandra Wickramasinghe. *Diseases from Space*. London: J. M. Dent, 1979.
Hoyle, Fred, Chandra Wickramisinghe, and John Watkins. *Viruses from Space*. Cardiff: University College Cardiff Press, 1986.
Ponce de Leon, Samuel, Antonio Lazcano, Eske Willerslev, et al. "Panspermia—true or false?" *The Lancet* 362 (2003): 407–408.

TERESA LESLIE

PARACELSIANISM.   Paracelsianism is a historical movement or system of ideas and practices that takes its name from texts ascribed to the sixteenth-century German doctor Theophrastus Bombastus von Hohenheim, called **Paracelsus**. Few were printed during his lifetime, but he left a wealth of unfinished manuscripts behind him as he traversed Europe. Publication of these began in earnest during the 1560s, and by the end of the century, most of his medical and philosophical treatises were in print, as were a number of spurious alchemical and magical books published under his name, making identification of Paracelsus's real voice problematic. Few of his religious treatises were published before the twentieth century, but these circulated widely as manuscripts and fed the growing desire for further reformation espoused by the Rosicrucians and pietistic religious groups inspired by Paracelsus's medical and religious ideas.

Paracelsians viewed the cosmos as having been created by the Judeo-Christian God as described in the first book of the Bible, *Genesis*, which they interpreted as a series of chemical separations of specific kinds from chaotic primeval matter. All subsequent natural causes and effects were likewise chemical, from the actions of planets on the organs of the body to the operations of drugs and diseases. The use of chemically prepared, sometimes highly toxic medicines was widely associated with Paracelsians in the sixteenth century, but soon adherents of other medical theories also began to use chemical drugs, rendering the simple association of "chemical" with "Paracelsian" problematic. In practice, even Paracelsian **physicians** were eclectic, drawing on whatever therapeutic methods they, their mentors, and their patients believed effective.

Although not oriented particularly toward epidemic diseases, Paracelsian medicine found favor against dangerous and intractable diseases such as **leprosy, epilepsy, bubonic plague**, and other "fevers," a broad classification that encompassed many infectious and acute diseases. Chemically concentrated toxic metal salts, which act quickly to provoke the desired vomiting, urination, and cleansing of the bowels were readily adopted by physicians and patients as an alternative to drawn out dosing with unconcentrated herbal remedies, depleting diets, and bloodletting.

Paracelsian philosophical, therapeutic, and religious ideas ran contrary to the basic tenets of university teaching at a fundamental level, discouraging the adoption of Paraceslian medicine in the medical schools and the guilds or colleges of physicians. As a result, Paracelsians were most visible as itinerant healers, **surgeons**, and physicians serving as personal physicians to Europe's kings and princely courts. Consequently, they attained a visibility and cultural influence beyond their numerical strength and precipitated a hostile reaction by traditional academic physicians and theologians, who saw in Paracelsus's writings the seeds of social discord and medical malpractice. Many Paracelsians were Protestants, some with radical and pietistic sympathies that brought them into political conflict with the Catholic Church and universities. Similarly, as Protestant orthodoxies hardened, Paracelsians found themselves increasingly labeled heterodox within Lutheran and Reformed regions. The name Paracelsus remained controversial until it was rendered impotent with the passage of time and the introduction of yet newer physical, medical, and metaphysical principles in the Enlightenment. *See also* Apothecary/Pharmacist; Empiric; Humoral Theory; Medical Education in the West, 1500–1900; Scientific Revolution and Epidemic Disease.

Further Reading

Debus, Allen G. *The Chemical Philosophy: Paracelsian Science and Medicine in the Sixteenth and Seventeenth Centuries.* New York: Science History Publications, 1997.

Grell, Ole, ed. *Paracelsus: The Man and His Reputation, His Ideas and Their Transformation.* Leiden: Brill, 1998.

Trevor-Roper, Hugh. "The Paracelsian Movement." In *Renaissance Essays*, edited by Hugh Trevor-Roper, pp. 149–99. Chicago: University of Chicago Press, 1985.

JOLE SHACKELFORD

PARACELSUS (THEOPHRASTUS BOMBAST VON HOHENHEIM; 1493–1541). Paracelsus, perhaps best known as an alchemist and seeker of the mythical Philosopher's Stone (which was supposed to turn lead into gold and cure all diseases), was also an early contributor to several modern sciences, including chemistry, biochemistry, pharmacology, and toxicology. Though a firm believer in **astrology** and **magic**, Paracelsus was one of the first Renaissance **physicians** to reject openly the Galenic **humoral theory** and to recognize the usefulness of chemical compounds in treating disease, thereby raising the status of alchemy and encouraging its transition into chemistry and its medical application, iatrochemistry.

Paracelsus probably took his classical nickname ("Greater than Celsus" the Roman medical writer; a common practice among Renaissance scholars) while studying medicine at the University of Ferrara around 1515. Although not a true humanist himself, Paracelsus embraced the humanist philosophy of learning directly from experience and seeking knowledge from the world around him. Whereas university-trained physicians in sixteenth-century Europe generally relied on classical authorities for their knowledge of medicine, Paracelsus rejected their texts out-of-hand, teaching his students and readers that all useful medical knowledge should be gained through the experience of treating patients and traveling.

Paracelsus's constant wanderings helped spread his reputation across Europe and the Middle East as both a miraculous healer and a conjuror of demons. Although not the most infamous alchemist of the sixteenth century—a German named Johann Faust (c. 1480–1540) claims that title—Paracelsus nonetheless made his name by discovering "occult" (hidden) knowledge previously considered off-limits. He gained much of this knowledge by separating, isolating, and recombining chemical elements and compounds, primarily in an effort to identify remedies for specific diseases. As Paracelsus held that illness was caused by faulty alchemical processes within the body—rather than by an imbalance of Galenic humors—he reasoned that a physician could compensate with an appropriate dose of an accurately prepared chemical remedy.

One of the best diseases to which Paracelsus could apply his theory was the newly emergent **syphilis**, for which classical texts like Galen's provided neither explanation nor treatment. Aside from periodic recurrences of the **bubonic plague**, syphilis was one of the most virulent public health threats of the sixteenth century, and the disease generated many innovative cures. Paracelsus championed the use of a mercury compound (*essentia mercuralis*), despite its often lethal consequences, while denouncing as **quacks** the proponents of the ineffective but popular and less deadly guaiac, an extract of a New World tree.

In 1529 Paracelsus wrote two works in 11 volumes on the "French disease" (syphilis) in an attempt to revolutionize medical practice in the context of this terrible **epidemic**. Although these works (like the rest of his books) proved too ambitious, idiosyncratic, and combative to achieve this goal in his lifetime, Paracelsian treatment of disease through chemistry was to find many adherents in subsequent generations. *See also* Medical Education in the West, 1100–1500; Medical Education in the West, 1500–1900; Paracelsianism.

Further Reading

Ball, Philip. *The Devil's Doctor: Paracelsus and the World of Renaissance Magic and Science*. London: William Heinemann, 2006.

Pagel, Walter. *Paracelsus: An Introduction to Philosophical Medicine in the Era of the Renaissance*, 2nd edition, revised. Basel: Karger, 1982.

Weeks, Andrew. *Paracelsus: Speculative Theory and the Crisis of the Early Reformation*. Albany: State University of New York Press, 1997.

CHRISTOPHER RYLAND

PASTEUR, LOUIS (1822–1895). The French microbiologist and chemist Louis Pasteur is, with German biologist **Robert Koch**, one of the founders of bacteriology and **immunology**. Pasteur was born in Dôle, France, and studied in Paris at the École Normale Supérieure, where he showed promise as an artist but soon turned to science. In 1849 he was appointed acting professor of chemistry at the University of Strasbourg. From 1854 to 1857 he was professor of chemistry and dean of sciences at the University of Lille, eventually returning to the École Normale Supérieure as administrator and director of scientific studies. In 1867 the Sorbonne appointed him professor of chemistry. His own microbiological research center, The Pasteur Institute, was inaugurated in Paris in 1888.

From his early work on crystals, such as those of tartaric acid, a product in the fermentation of grapes, Pasteur proceeded to examine the process of fermentation itself, a topic that would provide him with important background information and methods for his later research on contagious diseases. Yeast had been thought to be a chemical structure that served as a catalyst in the conversion of sugar into alcohol, but Pasteur discovered that yeast was organic matter, feeding on sugar and thus producing alcohol. When wine soured, it simply indicated the presence of the "wrong" kind of microorganisms. Pasteur conducted numerous experiments to prove his point, also examining the souring of milk. In 1857 he discussed this latter problem in his famous report on lactic acid fermentation.

Pasteur's discoveries raised the question of how these microorganisms entered the fluids. There existed at the time a belief in "spontaneous generation," which meant that microorganisms could come into existence without parental organisms. Pasteur proved, however, that nothing would happen with a fermentable fluid when surrounded by sterile **air**. As soon as "regular" air was brought in contact with the substance, microorganisms began to develop. Hence, he concluded that air contains spores of microbes.

The next step for Pasteur was to examine the problem of contagious diseases that seemed to spread through direct or indirect contact. Could microorganisms possibly cause these as well? There had been **germ theories of disease** for a long time, yet they could not be proven until Pasteur's day. Pasteur was aware of these theories and in 1857 became convinced that microorganisms might also be responsible for infectious diseases. Though at first it was only a theoretical concept, in the mid-1860s Pasteur began to work on an actual problem: he was asked to examine a deadly disease of the silkworm, which threatened to ruin the silk industry in France. By the late 1860s Pasteur had identified two different silkworm diseases and the microbes that were responsible for them. Even though in the middle of his investigation Pasteur suffered a stroke that left the left half of his body permanently paralyzed, he continued to work. Indeed, already as a young student he had been convinced that it "means a great deal . . . to have will power; for deeds and work always follow the will."

But his findings did not have an immediate effect, as many physicians did not think that a link existed between the ailments of the silkworm and those of human beings. In 1876 and 1877, however, Pasteur showed that microorganisms were the cause for a disease in higher animals and human beings: anthrax. At about the same time, Robert Koch came to the same conclusion. In 1877 Pasteur published a study on anthrax, a paper that became a significant document in supporting the germ theory of disease.

Pasteur applied the methods he had used in his experiments with fermentation to prove that anthrax **bacteria** spread the disease. These experiments showed that no matter how often an infected substance was passed from animal to animal, anthrax bacteria continued to multiply and thus remained potentially as deadly as in the blood of the first infected animal.

Once he had established these facts, Pasteur wondered what could be done to protect human beings and higher animals from those often-deadly diseases. He thus became interested in the concept of **vaccination** that had first been applied by the English physician **Edward Jenner**. Pasteur realized that a germ can change and consequently can actually be used as a vaccine. He first experimented with the problem of fowl **cholera** in chickens and found that some cultures of microorganisms did not cause the disease and instead made chickens resistant against virulent cultures in the future. Pasteur became convinced that it would be possible to produce vaccine in the laboratory. He proceeded to create a vaccine against anthrax, the effectiveness of which he demonstrated in a well-publicized demonstration in 1881. However, his anti-rabies treatment is usually cited as Pasteur's greatest triumph. In July 1885 he successfully treated the first human being, Joseph Meister, a boy suffering from rabid dog bites.

If Pasteur were alive today, he might be worried that we depend on techniques directed against microorganisms above all. Indeed, Pasteur taught that many other factors might have an effect on the course of an illness, such as the hereditary constitution of a patient, his/her nutritional state, his/her emotional equilibrium, the season of the year, and the climate.

Even before the opening of The Pasteur Institute, Pasteur had many students who would make important contributions to microbiology. Today The Pasteur Institute is a private nonprofit foundation with about 20 establishments on five different continents. Research is focused on fighting infectious viral, bacterial, and parasitic diseases such as

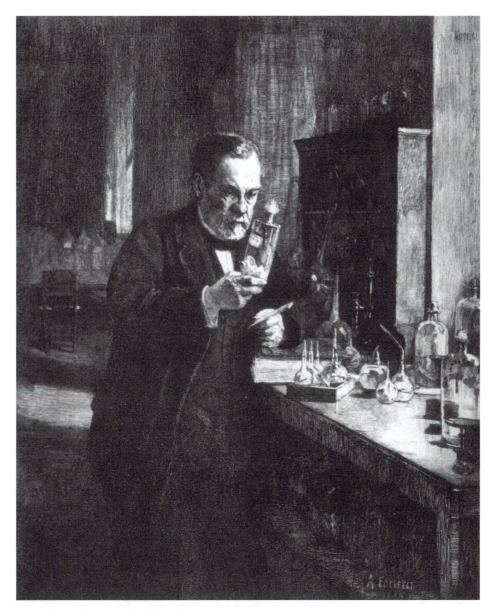

Dr. Louis Pasteur. Courtesy of the National Library of Medicine.

AIDS. It has produced eight recipients of the Nobel Prize; its distinguished alumni include **Alexandre Yersin**, a French doctor of Swiss extraction who discovered the bacterium that causes **bubonic plague**, *Yersinia pestis*, which was named after him. *See also* Contagion Theory of Disease, Premodern; Microscope.

Further Reading

Debré, Patrice. *Louis Pasteur*. Translated by Elborg Forster. Baltimore: Johns Hopkins University Press, 1998.

Dubos, René. *Pasteur and Modern Science*, new first edition. Madison, WI: Science Tech Publishers, 1988.

Geison, Gerald L. *The Private Science of Louis Pasteur*. Princeton: Princeton University Press, 1995.

ANJA BECKER

PENICILLIN.   Penicillin was the first to be discovered of the important class of drugs called **antibiotics**, which are chemical substances produced by microorganisms (or sometimes now synthetically) that destroy or inhibit the growth of other microorganisms. Penicillin acts by interfering with the synthesis of cell walls in **bacteria**, causing them to rupture. Because **animal** cells are enclosed by membranes rather than walls, they are not affected by this process.

British scientist Alexander Fleming (1881–1955) discovered penicillin almost accidentally at St. Mary's Hospital in London. While investigating the staphylococci bacteria in 1928, he noticed that one of the culture plates on which he was growing the microorganism was inadvertently contaminated by a *Penicillium* mold and that no bacterial colonies were growing in the area immediately surrounding the mold. Fleming reasoned that the mold was excreting a substance that inhibited the growth of the staphylococci. He then cultured the mold on the surface of a broth in a flask and filtered off the mold. The broth, which he called "penicillin," exhibited an ability to inhibit the growth of a variety of bacteria, including some that caused serious diseases. Fleming published his results in 1929, suggesting that penicillin might prove useful as a topical antiseptic for humans that could be applied locally to wounds or infected areas. He did not propose its use as an internal therapeutic agent to combat infectious diseases in the body. Fleming and others attempted to isolate pure penicillin from the broth, but these efforts proved unsuccessful.

The introduction of penicillin as an effective therapeutic agent was accomplished at Oxford University. While researching the literature on the enzyme lysozyme, also a discovery of Fleming's, Ernst Chain (1906–1979), working in Howard Florey's (1898–1968) laboratory in 1939, read Fleming's paper on penicillin. The Oxford workers became interested in penicillin and eventually isolated it in a purer form. Toxicity tests revealed that penicillin was not harmful to experimental animals. In 1940 the Oxford group showed that mice injected with a deadly strain of streptococci bacteria survived if treated with penicillin. Clinical trials with humans in 1941 also yielded results indicating that penicillin promised effectiveness in the treatment of a number of infectious diseases.

Substantial amounts of penicillin would be needed for the extensive clinical trials required to confirm the promise of the early results and to provide adequate supplies of the drug for therapeutic use if it proved effective. In 1941 Florey tried to interest Americans in large-scale production of penicillin. Recognizing that penicillin could play a vital role during the **war**, the U.S. government eventually coordinated federal research laboratories, academic institutions, and pharmaceutical companies to increase production of the drug. Penicillin production began to increase dramatically by early 1944, jumping in the United States from 21 billion units in 1943 to 1,663 billion units in 1944. The American government eventually removed all restrictions on its availability, and by March 15, 1945, penicillin was available to the consumer at the corner pharmacy.

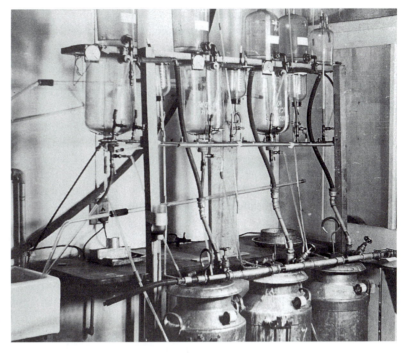

Equipment used for making early forms of penicillin; glass flasks and leads into tops of milk-churns. Wellcome Library, London.

Penicillin was a true wonder drug, much more potent against infectious diseases than any previously discovered chemical substance. In 1945, Fleming, Florey, and Chain shared the Nobel Prize in Medicine or Physiology for their discovery. The drug also opened up the door to the "era of antibiotics." Penicillin and its variations remain important substances in today's pharmaceutical arsenal against disease. *See also* Antibiotics; Pharmaceutical Industry.

Further Reading

Brown, Kevin. *Penicillin Man: Alexander Fleming and the Antibiotic Revolution*. Stroud, UK: Sutton, 2004.

Hobby, Gladys. *Penicillin: Meeting the Challenge*. New Haven: Yale University Press, 1985.

Williams, Trevor. *Howard Florey: Penicillin and After*. New York: Oxford University Press, 1984.

JOHN PARASCANDOLA

PERSONAL HYGIENE AND EPIDEMIC DISEASE.   Until the eighteenth century, hygiene, Greek for "health," was concerned with the preservation of health and prevention of illness through personal attention to lifestyle. The theoretical basis of hygiene changed when **epidemic** disease ceased to be assigned to individual susceptibility or the supernatural and became associated with dirt and germs.

Classical Hygiene Transformed.   In the Classical tradition, individuals could protect themselves against epidemic disease through attention to their **environment, diet,** sleep, exercise, evacuations, sexual activity, and peace of mind. Hygiene manuals such as the *Tacuinum Sanitatis* (fourteenth/fifteenth centuries) offered advice on what constituted good **air**, food, and **water**, when to undergo purging or bloodletting, and how to recognize pestilential localities. There were debates as to whether epidemics were spread by **contagion** (physical contact) or miasma (foul air). People, where possible, tried to avoid both. Nevertheless, within this "clean living" philosophy, domestic and bodily cleanliness played little part. In Europe, public bathing declined from the Middle Ages as it became associated with prostitution, while private bathing was considered dangerous because it opened the pores to pestilential air. Clothing was brushed or sponged rather than washed, infestation with lice and parasites was common, and there were varying standards of waste disposal. When Charles II (r. 1660–1685) and his court fled from London to Oxford during the plague of 1665, for example, their excrement was left under the carpets. Other cultures' practices contrasted with those of Europe. Dutch travelers of the seventeenth century were amazed to witness Africans of the Guinea coast washing their bodies, wiping themselves after defecating, and burning their excrement. By the nineteenth century, however, westerners perceived themselves as clean and the rest of the world as dirty. In the wake of the great **cholera** epidemics, Edward Morse (1838–1925), an American writer, saw the filth of the Orient as a menace to Europe.

The new emphasis on personal cleanliness from the eighteenth century had social as well as medical origins. French nobility, in particular, adopted cleansing rituals as a move toward civilized manners. This Old World gentrification quickly spread to the New World. In the nineteenth century, bathtubs, washbasins, and flush toilets were given their own room in wealthy homes, and cleanliness became a sign of good breeding. The unclean, namely the poor, were deemed socially unacceptable. William Buchan (1729–1805), a Scots physician, was among the first to associate the poor with dirt, disease, and danger to others. In *Domestic Medicine* (1769), he suggested that putrid fevers were caused by uncleanliness amongst the inhabitants of overcrowded houses who breathed bad air and wore filthy clothes. It was insufficient, he claimed, to be clean oneself, if dirty neighbors spread infections afar. An editorial of 1777 in *The Pennsylvania Packet*, edited by Benjamin Franklin (1706–1790), warned of infectious miasmas arising from perspiration-soaked linen. In England, a Commission for Enquiring into the State of Large Towns (1844) reported that dirt and epidemic disease were inseparable. Furthermore, epidemics caused **poverty** because they killed male breadwinners.

Better Health through Cleanliness.   With **germ theory** and the discovery of **bacteria** by **Louis Pasteur** and others in the later nineteenth century, dirt became the visible manifestation of the hidden agents of epidemic disease, and cleanliness the first line of defense in preventing infection. City authorities built public baths, and immigrant groups added their own, such as Russian Vapor Baths and Turkish Baths. In London, by 1912, there were over 3 million annual visits to public baths and washhouses even though many health reformers maintained that the poor "liked dirt." Homemade soaps prepared from lye or "potash" and fat, or natural soap from plants such as soapwort (*Saponaria officinalis*), were replaced by commercial products. Pears' soap, created in the 1790s by London barber Andrew Pears (b. 1770), was fiercely marketed in the United States by Thomas Barratt (1841–1914). In the north of England, William Lever (1851–1925) built a "hygienic" town, Port Sunlight, on the proceeds of selling Sunlight

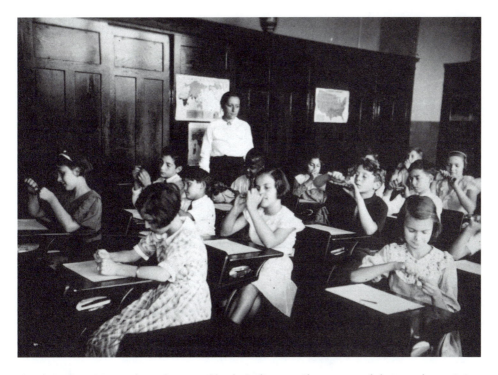

Teacher showing students how to file their fingernails as part of the regular training in personal hygiene in Miss Kniberg's class at the Avon Avenue School, Newark, New Jersey. Courtesy of the National Library of Medicine.

soap. Lever Brothers exploited new fears of germ-spreading to promote their Lifebuoy **"disinfectant"** soap. An American advertisement for Lifebuoy urged "Daddy" to wash off "dangerous city dirt" before touching his loved ones. From 1919, all soldiers in the U.S. Army were compelled to use Lifebuoy. The work of Sir Joseph Lister (1827–1912) on antisepsis and the emphasis on **hospital** cleanliness were powerful examples for personal and domestic hygiene. The British household bleach Domestos claimed to kill all known germs. The use of dentifrice, toothbrushes, and mouthwashes such as Listerine (named after Lister) spread through western society. Toilet paper was marketed in the 1880s, and cotton underclothes largely replaced the infrequently laundered woolen and flannel garments.

From 1882, pupils in French schools were taught how to wash and use the toilet. In the United States, schools and health officials conducted crusades against diseases like **tuberculosis** by emphasizing the preventative power of personal hygiene. Children earned badges for completing health chores and took home instructions in cleanliness. After about 1910, public health campaigns in the United States switched their emphasis from public sanitation to personal hygiene, particularly in areas of high immigration. Metropolitan Insurance, for example, ran an immigrant campaign with the slogan "A bath a day keeps sickness away." In 1927 big soap manufacturers including Lever Brothers,

Palmolive, and Colgate founded the Cleanliness Institute with headquarters in New York City. The Institute produced pamphlets such as *Better Health through Cleanliness*, aimed at health and social workers, and *The Cleanliness Journal*, which advised on presenting the cleanliness message. Twentieth-century handbooks of personal hygiene (now defined as the science of preserving and *improving* health) prioritized soap and water in the prevention of epidemic disease.

Epidemic diseases began to decline before the advent of effective vaccines and **antibiotics**, largely because of improvements in personal and public hygiene. Today, in countries with limited hygiene resources, diarrheal diseases cause 1.5 million deaths a year. In 2007 the *British Medical Journal* conducted an international survey to determine the greatest medical breakthrough of the past 160 years. Sanitation, the handmaiden of hygiene, was the undisputed winner. *See also* Children and Childhood Epidemic Diseases; Early Humans, Disease in; Ectoparasites; Greco-Roman Medical Theory and Practice; Insects, Other Arthropods, and Epidemic Disease; Leprosy, Societal Reactions to; Plague and Developments in Public Health, 1348–1600; Public Health Agencies in Britain since 1800; Public Health Agencies, U.S. Federal; Sanitation Movement of the Nineteenth Century; War, the Military, and Epidemic Disease.

Further Reading

Smith, Virginia. *Clean: A History of Personal Hygiene and Purity*. New York: Palgrave Macmillan, 2007.

Tomes, Nancy. *The Gospel of Germs: Men, Women, and the Microbe in American Life*. Cambridge, MA: Harvard University Press, 1998.

Varron, A. G. "Personal Hygiene during the Middle Ages." *Ciba Symposium* 1 (1939–1940): 215–223.

Vinikas, Vincent. *Soft Soap, Hard Sell: American Hygiene in an Age of Advertisement*. Ames: Iowa State University Press, 1992.

CAROLE REEVES

PERSONAL LIBERTIES AND EPIDEMIC DISEASE.   As long as disease was seen as a product of nature (**miasma**) or the supernatural (planetary conjunctions or divine will), the individual played a minor role (perhaps angering God by sinning) in disease causation or **transmission**. Once **physicians** suspected human agency—however unwitting—societies quickly took measures to eliminate or at least reduce the threat of the individual to the social fabric. Such measures often, if not always, encroached upon personal liberties. Over time they ranged from requiring a health pass for travelers to burning a victim's goods to locking one up in a pest house or exiling one to a leper colony. A society facing an epidemic must strike a balance between traditional societal freedoms (however vague or limited) and reasonable public activities to lessen the threats posed by disease. The restrictions on the few have long been thought to safeguard the health of the many.

Loss of personal liberty is clearest when one who has, or is suspected of having, a disease is forcibly removed from the stream of everyday life. Those who suffered from **leprosy** (Hansen's Disease) were often set apart from larger society. From Ancient Israel to contemporary Japan and China, societal authorities have ostracized these disease victims. Depending on the place and time period, lepers were driven from villages, provided a life in local **leprosaria** and care for their disabilities, or sent across country to leper colonies, where names were changed and past identities shed. During the **Black Death** and subsequent plague **epidemics**, one of the Latin West's coping mechanisms was to isolate plague victims, often shutting them inside their own houses along with healthy family members. Though supported with food and other supplies from charity or the public coffers, no one could leave until the victim had recovered or had been dead a fixed time, and all others had a clean bill of health. The family's residence would then be scrubbed down, and goods and furnishings suspected of harboring plague would be fumigated or destroyed. Though medieval and early modern societies had a clear understanding of neither germs nor **contagion**, they acted very much as though they did.

Plague hospitals and **pest houses** were alternatives to shutting in. Though the victims were still forcibly isolated, family members were either left alone or temporarily quarantined to determine the state of their health. During epidemics such facilities were notoriously overcrowded, understaffed, and unbelievably filthy. Though many inmates in fact survived, condemnation to a pest house was tantamount to a death sentence. Even with more modern and sanitary conditions, the issues of forced institutionalization remained; the life of "Typhoid" **Mary Mallon** is an excellent case in point. Although **sanatoria** for people with **tuberculosis** had first developed as voluntary hotels for the well off, during America's Progressive Era in the early twentieth century, sanatoria were increasingly controlled by the state, and victims of TB underwent mandatory institutionalization.

From the last third of the fourteenth century, authorities in port cities and other vulnerable points along frontiers established facilities at which suspect people and cargoes would be forcibly detained for set periods of **quarantine**. Goods were often fumigated or otherwise disinfected, whereas the people were observed for signs of disease. Though developed during plague time, both the isolation hospital and quarantine became common tools in the fight against epidemic disease. Each, of course, also restricted or violated generally accepted rights to live and travel freely. Nonetheless, in the age of **cholera** pandemics during the nineteenth century, few ports administered by Western nations did not have quarantine facilities. Even returning soldiers found their voyages home delayed by mandated quarantine.

Other travel restrictions included closed city gates, ***cordons sanitaires*** along national borders or within cities, and mandatory health passes, which proclaimed the good health of the bearer. Again, plague prompted these measures, and they constitute some of the earliest provisions for international cooperation on public health matters. Today, nations reserve the right to deny entry to those suffering from, or believed to be suffering, from certain infectious diseases, and the questionable practice of "profiling," or giving special scrutiny to people from certain countries or with certain backgrounds, is used as a means of screening. Unrestricted access to the United States across its borders, especially that with Mexico, has long invited immigration by people who have not been screened for infectious diseases. Fears of violating immigrants' supposed human rights have hindered efforts to identify and screen these people, many of whom find themselves in the food services industries. The perceived threat of global bioterrorism has also heightened the sense of insecurity and increased levels of restrictions on passengers and cargo.

With the development of prophylactic vaccines, humankind took a huge step toward effective control of infectious diseases. Early epidemiologists understood that for vaccines to protect a population, a certain threshold percentage (always less than 100) of that population had to receive the vaccine to induce effective "herd immunity." Mandatory **vaccination** was the best way to insure high compliance rates, but over the past two centuries, many population groups balked at being forcibly immunized. Does accepted understanding of personal rights include that to refuse to allow infective material to be injected into one's body? Anti-vaccination campaigns developed around state efforts to control **smallpox, polio, measles**, and in the mid-2000s, the vaccine to prevent **cervical cancer**. The state argues that public safety warrants enforced immunizations, and that after suspension of required immunizations, the diseases in question quickly rebounded dramatically. Critics usually question the effectiveness and safety of the drugs or refuse on biblical or other religious grounds or on the grounds of one's right to one's own person. Ironically, staunch British opposition to mass vaccinations in the 1890s led to a policy of surveillance, containment of outbreaks, and targeted vaccinations, the very model used by the **World Health Organization** in successfully eradicating smallpox in the 1960s and 1970s.

One source of opposition to mandated medical procedures is the experience with unscrupulous or **human subjects** testing. Blacks in America hold a righteous grudge against medical researchers for their roles in the infamous Tuskegee syphilis studies from the 1930s. Some Black activists have voiced concerns that **AIDS** was planted in their communities by the CIA and that drug testing was really part of the plot. The use of disease patients for uninformed drug testing is clearly unethical, but it was carried out under totalitarian regimes. Prisoners, too, though protected by international conventions, have been forced to undergo medical experiments with more or less legitimate goals. In European colonies, native sufferers from such diseases as **sleeping sickness** and leprosy became test subjects for numerous drugs and other treatments, the power differential between native and colonial doctor providing wide latitude. Historians have also looked critically at the attempts by Christian medical aid workers to convert stricken animists or Muslims under their care. In the tight confines of medical facilities where does the right to proselytize cross the patient's right to be comforted rather than threatened with eternal torments or enticed with eternal life? On a larger scale, rights to conduct religious practices unmolested have been suspended many times in the face of public health threats. European plague laws restricted gatherings for liturgies and processions, including funerals. Colonial laws tried to regulate Indian rituals in sacred rivers and control the spread of disease during **pilgrimages**.

Finally, sexually transmitted diseases (STDs) have presented important challenges to the balance of civil rights and public health. In general, one has a right to privacy regarding his or her health, medical treatment, or medication. If one presents a threat of exposure of an infectious disease to a community, then investigators may very well ascertain past contacts in order to warn them of possible exposure. When an STD is the issue, then the contacts will have been sexual contacts, the identification and contact of whom present major issues of confidentiality. Because these might include cases of adultery, underage sexual contact, or homosexuality, officials tend to treat these with the greatest concern for privacy. Because of its association with homosexuality, AIDS advocates traditionally resisted standard reporting of the cases. Around the outbreak of AIDS in America there also swirled other controversies, not least of which was that of the gay bathhouses in cities like New York and San Francisco. These facilities played a unique role in urban homosexual community life, yet the contacts made there could be life-threatening. Some shut down voluntarily; others were closed by order of the authorities. AIDS activists saw this not only as a violation of property rights, but also of the right of free association. Protests led to the reopening of many of these bathhouses, which many consider to be a contributing factor to the resurgence of AIDS among American homosexuals from the mid-2000s.

The history of the relationship of public health and personal freedom is riddled with examples of resistance and rebellion. History tells of inmates of pest houses in Italy, France, and Russia who rose up and fled their noxious setting, terrorizing the healthy countryside beyond. In Manila, The Philippines, in 1937 hundreds of lepers broke out of San Lazaro leprosarium and marched on the Presidential Palace for better living conditions. In the same year, 1,100 Japanese lepers in an island colony rebelled, beating their guards and going on hunger strike for better conditions. Irate neighbors burned down plague hospitals, and a Russian mob rioted at the removal of religious images during the last of Moscow's plague epidemics. *See also* AIDS in Africa; AIDS in America; Black Death, Flagellants, and Jews; Colonialism and Epidemic Disease; Human Subjects Research; Irish Potato Famine and Epidemic Disease, 1845–1850; Leprosy in America; Leprosy, Societal Reactions to; Medical Ethics and Epidemic Disease; Poison Libels and Epidemic Disease; Poliomyelitis and American Popular Culture; Public Health Agencies, U.S. Federal; Race, Ethnicity, and Epidemic Disease; Religion and Epidemic Disease; Sexual Revolution; Trade, Travel, and Epidemic Disease; Tuberculosis in the Contemporary World; Venereal Disease and Social Reform in Progressive-Era America.

Further Reading

Alexander, John T. *Bubonic Plague in Early Modern Russia: Public Health and Urban Disaster*. Baltimore: Johns Hopkins University Press, 1980.

Bray, R. S. *Armies of Pestilence: The Effects of Pandemics on History*. Cambridge, UK: Lutterworth Press, 1998.

Byrne, Joseph P. *Daily Life during the Black Death*. Westport, CT: Greenwood Press, 2006.

Colgrove, James. *State of Immunity: The Politics of Vaccination in Twentieth-Century America*. Berkeley: University of California Presss, 2006.

Colgrove, James, and Ronald Bayer. "Manifold Restraints: Liberty, Public Health, and the Legacy of *Jacobson v Massachusetts*." *American Journal of Public Health* 95 (2005): 571–576.

Fairchild, Amy L, Ronald Bayer, and James Colgrove. *Searching Eyes: Privacy, the State, and Disease Surveillance in America*. Berkeley: University of California Press, 2007.

Farmer, Paul. *Pathologies of Power: Health, Human Rights and the New War on the Poor*. Berkeley: University of California Press, 2005.

Knobler, Stacey, et al., eds. *The Impact of Globalization on Infectious Disease Emergence and Control: Exploring the Consequences and Opportunities*. Washington, DC: National Academies Press, 2006.

McBride, David. *From TB to AIDS: Epidemics Among Urban Blacks Since 1900*. New York: State University of New York Press, 1991.

Selin, Helaine, and Hugh Shapiro, eds. *Medicine across Cultures: History and Practice of Medicine in Non-Western Cultures*. Dordrecht: Kluwer, 2003.

Treadwell, Perry. *God's Judgment? Syphilis and AIDS: Comparing the History and Prevention Attempts of Two Epidemics*. Lincoln, NE: Writer's Club Press, 2001.

Watts, Sheldon. *Epidemics and History: Disease, Power and Imperialism*. New Haven, CT: Yale University Press, 1997.

JOSEPH P. BYRNE

PERTUSSIS. *See* Whooping Cough.

PEST HOUSES AND LAZARETTOS. Before the development of **germ theory**, the **contagion theory of disease** had a vague but powerful hold on Western notions of public health. It certainly seemed that people developed the same diseases as those with whom they had come into contact. Isolating the sick from the healthy seemed a reasonable response, especially when a plague or other widespread outbreak of disease was in the neighborhood. Long-term isolation of those suffering from Hansen's disease (**leprosy**) in monastery-like **leprosaria** or lazarettos had been practiced for centuries before the fourteenth century. The **Black Death** prompted shorter-term accommodations for those suffering through the plague (*peste* or a variation in most European languages). Rather than spending years under medical supervision, as in well-run leprosaria or later **sanatoria** for long-term respiratory disease patients, the resident of the pest house (*Pesthaus, pesthuis*) or lazaretto (*lazaret, lazzaretto*, lazar house; the term was appropriated from that for a leprosarium) was expected to die or (less likely) recover from the disease within a week or two. Unlike a **quarantine** facility, which housed for a set period of days those suspected of having a disease, the pest house warehoused the obviously sick and dying.

During late medieval and early modern plague epidemics, isolating the sick from family and neighbors could mean running them out of town, shutting them up in their own houses, or providing isolation quarters—pest houses or plague hospitals—at public expense. Besides being unbearably inhumane, chasing the sick out of town only threatened the countryside. Shutting up the sick may have been what saved Milan from the ravages of 1348, and it was systematically practiced by Duke Gian Galeazzo Visconti (1351–1402) in that city-state in the 1390s. Generally the entire family was thus enclosed with its sick members, and public funds provided food and guards until either all died or the survivors had lasted an expected period of time. Almost always an option of the wealthy and powerful, critics noted the hardships this practice placed on the less well-off family. In *Journal of the Plague Year* (1722) English novelist Daniel Defoe (c. 1660–1731) has his protagonist rail against the monstrous cruelty of shutting in, in favor of well-run and plentiful pest houses.

Hospitals were features of most European cityscapes, and in times of epidemics, they could serve to isolate and care for the stricken. In most cases, other residents were removed during the crisis. Monasteries, too, were appropriated by local governments or donated by religious orders as plague facilities, as was the case in seventeenth-century Barcelona, Spain, and Prato, Italy. Invariably, the demand for space outstripped its supply, and otherwise clean, sanitary quarters devolved into chambers of horror. Contemporary visitors recorded the sights, sounds, and smells that assaulted their senses. The emotional numbness of the caregivers and the corpse-haulers made them seem demonic to some observers, who noted that this was a foretaste of hell itself. During heavy outbreaks, in the precincts of hospitals developed shantytowns of shacks and even simple lean-tos in which the suffering were placed.

Pest houses proper eventually supplemented or replaced ad hoc arrangements as part of more or less concerted attempts at protecting public health. One of the earliest known dates to the late 1300s and was at the Venetian Adriatic colony of Ragusa (Dubrovnik), on the island of Mljet in an abandoned convent. In 1429 the Venetian government supplemented it with a purpose-built pest house at Supetar. The Venetians had their own temporary structure in 1403, which they replaced with a permanent lazaretto in 1424. This also served as a maritime quarantine facility. In plague time this *Lazaretto Vecchio* (Old) quickly filled, so the *Lazaretto Nuovo* (New) appeared in 1468. Even so, in the winter of 1576 carpenters had quickly to build 1,200 huts in the Arsenal shipyard to accommodate the flood of sufferers. Like a leprosarium, a proper pest house or plague hospital might be spacious and laid out like a church; in Catholic areas an altar would be located at the crossing so all could see. Milan's San Gregorio Lazaretto, completed in 1524, consisted of a porticoed square of 288 connected 15 by 15 foot rooms around a huge open space in the center of which was a raised altar for services. The horrors of human misery met with even in such a large and well-planned facility were described by visitors and famously by Italian novelist Alessandro Manzoni (1785–1837) in *I promessi sposi* (1825–1827).

A well-planned facility would include a graveyard, quarters for personnel, and separate quarters to serve survivors who were past the acute stage and recovering (convalescing). By the seventeenth century, a typical small pest house would be provided with at least a surgeon or two, a physician when possible, and some female caregivers and male body-carriers. Their salaries were provided by the public treasury, as were food and medicines. They were usually isolated at the site and died in great numbers. To some lazarettos patients had to bring their own bedding, though charity and administrators' ingenuity usually served to provide such necessities. In some places, officials provided patients upon release a fresh suit of clothing and a small bit of cash, because their clothing and household belongings would have been incinerated in their absence.

When **bubonic plague** subsided in the eighteenth century, the pest house remained to isolate the sufferers from other acute and contagious or supposedly contagious diseases such as **smallpox, yellow fever**, and **cholera**. American "pest houses" were often both quarantine facilities and isolation quarters for those with infectious diseases. Philadelphia had a famous pest house at Lazaretto Station, built in response to an outbreak of yellow fever in 1799. The site served as a cargo and passenger inspection site and quarantine station, and one estimate claims that one-third of all Americans' ancestors arrived through this facility. New York City's residents established their first pest house with funds dedicated to it and a medical school that would eventually become Columbia University's School of Medicine. To deflect the stigma attached to leprosy, New Orleans's nineteenth-century leprosarium was known as "the pest house." Across North America and England, one still finds place names linked with "Pest" or "Lazaretto," and many local historians know of old or demolished buildings that once served to isolate sufferers of cholera, smallpox, or **influenza**. *See also* Disinfection and Fumigation; Hospitals in the West to 1900; Leprosy, Societal Reactions to; London, Great Plague of (1665–1666); Personal Liberties and Epidemic Disease; Plague and Developments in Public Health, 1348–1600; Plague in Europe, 1500–1770s; Plague Literature and Art, Early Modern European; Public Health Boards in the West before 1900.

Further Reading

Byrne, Joseph P. *Daily Life during the Black Death*. Westport, CT: Greenwood Press, 2006.

Cipolla, Carlo. *Faith, Reason and the Plague in Seventeenth-century Tuscany*. New York: Norton, 1979.

Slack, Paul. "Responses to Plague in Early Modern England." In *Famine, Disease, and the Social Order in Early Modern England*, edited by Walter R. Schofield, pp. 167–187. New York: Cambridge University Press, 1989.

JOSEPH P. BYRNE

PESTICIDES.   Pesticides are substances or mixtures of substances that are intended to kill, prevent, or repel arthropods or other pest organisms such as rodents. Humans have been using pesticides developed using herbal remedies since antiquity. For example, it is believed that ancient Egyptians used specific herbs to kill the aquatic snail hosts of human **schistosomiasis**.

Because pesticides are designed to kill or repel living organisms, there is always the risk of harm to humans, animals, and the environment. Any pesticide can be harmful if used improperly. In the United States, pesticide use is strictly regulated by the Environmental Protection Agency and various state agencies. Pesticides benefit humans by killing organisms that can transmit diseases to humans and animals or damage food or fiber crops. Pesticides such as rodenticides are beneficial because they target hosts in the life cycle of human pathogens (e.g., rats with oriental rat fleas that transmit **bubonic plague**). However, the overuse of pesticides can cause populations of target organisms to develop resistance because all individuals surviving the application of a pesticide will produce offspring that are all resistant to the pesticide and to other pesticides in the same chemical family.

Pesticides can be classified as either natural or synthetic. Natural pyrethrum, derived from finely ground chrysanthemum flowers, has been used as a pesticide for at least 2,000 years, though a synthetic version is now available. Pesticides are also classified on the basis of their chemical structure. Inorganic pesticides, which contain no carbon atoms, include arsenicals like calcium arsenate. Most of these have been removed from the market because of their high toxicity in mammals. Silicon dioxide powders that abrade the connective tissues of arthropods, causing them to dehydrate and die, are still in use. The organic pesticides, which contain carbon atoms, are mostly synthetic pesticides. The chemical structure of many modern pesticides was derived from phosphorus-containing organic compounds (organophosphates) developed from chemical warfare agents during World War I (1914–1918) such as mustard gas. Organophosphates disrupt the chemical mechanism by which nerves transfer messages to organs. Some are quite poisonous, but most do not persist in the environment. Carbamates are organic pesticides that also target the nervous system of pests. Most carbamates kill a broad range of pests and have a low toxicity for mammals. Organochlorine pesticides were commonly used in the past, but many have been removed from the market because of their detrimental effects upon human health and their persistence in the environment (e.g., DDT). Rachel Carson's 1962 book *Silent Spring* alerted the American public to the dangers associated with organochlorines. Interestingly, DDT dust is still approved for application to rodent burrows beneath buildings in the southwestern United States where bubonic plague remains endemic. Pyrethroid pesticides were developed as a synthetic version of the naturally occurring pesticide pyrethrin found in chrysanthemum seed coats. Some synthetic pyrethroids are toxic to the mammalian nervous system.

Another way that pesticides can be classified is by their target organisms. Examples include insecticides, herbicides, fungicides, rodenticides, molluscicides (target snails and slugs), acaricides (kill mites), nematicides (target small worms called nematodes), and repellents that repel pests at low concentrations and kill them at higher concentrations.

Over the past century, pesticides have played extremely important roles in controlling epidemic and epizootic diseases that have pests for vectors, including mosquito-borne malaria, yellow fever, and various encephalitis viruses; lice, tick, and flea-borne typhus;

tick-borne Lyme disease; tsetse fly-borne sleeping sickness; and kissing bug-borne Chagas' disease. Though promising new biological control methods have been introduced, pesticides will continue to play an important role in controlling pests for the foreseeable future. *See also* Animal Diseases (Zoonoses) and Epidemic Disease; Ectoparasites; Insect Infestations; Insects, Other Arthropods, and Epidemic Disease.

Further Reading

Evans, Howard Ensign. "The Tactics of Insect Pest Management." In *Insect Biology*, edited by John L. Capinera, pp. 390–412. (Reading, MA: Addison-Wesley Publishing Company, 1984.

Hemingway, Janet, and Hilary Ranson. "Chemical Control of Vectors and Mechanisms of Resistance." In *Biology of Disease Vectors*, 2nd edition, edited by William H. Marquardt, pp. 627–638. New York: Academic Press, 2004.

McWilliams, James. *American Pests: The Losing War on Insects from Colonial Times to DDT*. New York: Columbia University Press, 2008.

Russell, Edmund. *War and Nature: Fighting Humans and Insects with Chemicals from World War I to Silent Spring*. New York: Cambridge University Press, 2001.

Tren, Richard, et al. *Malaria & the DDT Story*. London: Institute of Economic Affairs, 2001.

STEVE MURPHREE

PETTENKOFER, MAX JOSEF VON (1818–1901). Max Josef von Pettenkofer was born on December 3, 1818, in the Bavarian town of Lichtenheim, the son of an impecunious peat bog farmer. With the support of his uncle, court **apothecary** to Ludwig I of Bavaria (1786–1868), Pettenkofer entered the University of Munich in 1837, specializing in science. Having excelled in his studies and taken additional courses in medical chemistry, Pettenkofer obtained a position in the Royal Mint in 1845. He researched, among other things, the separation of metals, human metabolic processes, the ventilation of buildings, and the insulating properties of fabrics.

Pettenkofer achieved fame for his work on the **epidemiology** of **cholera** and kindred intestinal diseases. He was by no means the first to apply epidemiological methods to understanding **epidemics**, but his methods were ingenious and exact. He began to study cholera in 1854 when **germ theory** was merely an adventurous speculation. During an epidemic in Bavaria, he compiled a spot-map with which to identify environmental correlates of the disease and to work out whether cholera could be passed directly from person to person. One finding particularly interested him: moist, low-lying areas were most frequently and severely hit.

Pettenkofer measured the level of soil moistness in different parts of Munich and produced graphs showing often tight correlations between high levels of groundwater and cholera morbidity. An 1873 study of an epidemic at the Royal Bavarian prison was widely considered a model for epidemiological research. Such analyses led Pettenkofer to conclude that cholera is caused by a microorganism, called "x," which was a necessary but insufficient cause of the disease. The germ caused sickness only when it produced a dangerous substance, or "z," which required it first to mature in a suitable medium, or "y." The perfect medium was moist soil containing rotting organic matter. A cholera germ could infect a new host only having spent time in damp ground. It did not spread directly from person to person, Pettenkofer concluded.

Pettenkofer's theory brought him into conflict with the leading bacteriologist **Robert Koch**. In 1883 Koch correctly claimed to have identified a specific bacillus in the stools and intestines of cholera victims in Egypt. He then went to Calcutta, India, where he claimed to have proven that this bacterium was responsible for the disease and that it spread from person to person via contaminated drinking **water**. For decades, Pettenkofer and his supporters (especially in British India) argued against Koch's position on epidemiological grounds; he and several students even ingested solutions of the putative cholera bacillus in an attempt to refute Koch's germ theory (they survived after short bouts of diarrhea).

For his opposition to Koch, history has not been kind to Pettenkofer. But in fact he made a very sound attempt at explaining an epidemiologically complex picture. Nor was he entirely incorrect: bacteria might not need to ripen in moist soil, but a correlation with high levels of groundwater is often real and important. Moreover, he helped highlight the insufficiency of Koch's near-exclusive emphasis on the germ: a later generation of scientists, including his student Elie Metchnikoff (1845–1916), would reveal that the germ is only part of the story. Perhaps most significantly, Pettenkofer's arguments about the dangers of drinking water coming into contact with foul soil led to major, life-saving sanitary improvements in Munich.

Feeling sidelined by the imperial German government and devastated by the deaths of his wife and three of his five children, on February 10, 1901, Pettenkofer tragically took his own life. *See also* Cholera: First through Third Pandemics, 1816–1861; Cholera: Fourth through Sixth Pandemics, 1862–1947; Contagion and Transmission; Demographic Data Collection and Analysis, History of; Environment, Ecology, and Epidemic Disease; Sanitation Movement of the Nineteenth Century.

Further Reading

Evans, Richard. *Death in Hamburg: Society and Politics in the Cholera Years, 1830–1910*. New York: Oxford University Press, 1987.

Hume, Edgar Erskine. *Max von Pettenkofer: His Theory of the Etiology of Cholera, Typhoid Fever and Other Intestinal Diseases*. New York: P.B. Hoeber, 1927.

Waller, John. *Leaps in the Dark*. New York: Oxford University Press, 2004.

JOHN WALLER

PHARMACEUTICAL INDUSTRY.   For most of human history, medicines were simple preparations of plant drugs (e.g., infusions [teas], hand-rolled pills, or poultices). Healers gathered the drugs locally or bought them from traders in spices and other exotic goods. By the late Middle Ages, the profession of specialized preparers and sellers of medicines—**apothecaries**—appeared in the West from the Islamic world. Medicine making, however, remained a small-scale affair until the early 1600s. At that time a number of influences inspired change. The discoveries of New World drugs stimulated trade and new thinking concerning therapy. **Paracelsus** and his followers advocated the use of chemicals as medicines in the sixteenth century, a departure from the traditional plants prescribed by the classical Roman **Galen**. Alchemists, who originally sought the "elixir of life" and other substances of transcendental powers, turned to more mundane applications of their techniques opening up the new field of chemistry. Others working with mining and metals added to laboratory technology. Most important of all, apothecaries picked up on the new developments and began to apply methods in the backrooms of their shops.

In the 1620s, the Society of Apothecaries of London (incorporated 1617) started to produce both galenical (plant-based) and chemical preparations. By 1703 the Society gained the monopoly of providing drugs and medicines to the Royal Navy. In France one of the first great manufacturers was Antoine Baumé (1728–1804). By 1775 his catalog included over 2,000 items and about 400 chemical preparations. In the North American colonies, wholesale druggists usually obtained their drugs from England through London import houses. When the Revolutionary War broke out, the colonists were forced to begin manufacturing medicinal chemicals and preparations to replace those from Britain. Although many of these small manufactories closed after the Treaty of Paris, a few specializing in fine chemicals continued on and formed the basis for the American chemical and pharmaceutical industries. In 1813 J. B. Trommsdorff (1770–1837), founder of the first journal dedicated to scientific pharmacy and industrial chemistry, established an early German factory for drug preparations. Well into the 1800s, however, pharmaceutical manufacturing remained largely a small to medium sized industry. With the exception of milling, machine power (steam engine) did not apply well to most aspects of medicine making, which involved precise hand operations.

A major contributor to the growth of the pharmaceutical enterprise in the eighteenth and nineteenth centuries was the making and selling of secret nostrums, the so-called "patent medicines." A direct descendent of the panaceas and "cure-alls" of **quacks**, mountebanks, and traveling medicine peddlers, these preparations usually contained harsh laxatives or potent narcotics often in a highly alcoholic vehicle. In an age when trained **physicians** were few and costly, many common folk turned to these remedies for treatment of minor as well as serious ailments. As printing technology improved and the popular press grew, so did advertising for patent medicines, which became a staple of newspapers and magazines. These advertisements in turn helped create a larger demand for medicines that further stimulated the young pharmaceutical industry as a whole.

The development of alkaloidal chemistry in the early 1800s by pharmacists Friedrich Wilhelm Adam Sertuerner (1783–1841), Pierre Joseph Pelletier (1788–1842), Joseph Bienaimé Caventou (1795–1877), Friedrich Ferdinand Runge (1795–1867), and Pierre Jean Robiquet (1780–1840) provided an early incentive to manufacturers. Sertuerner's discovery of how to extract morphine from opium allowed the marketing of pure constituents from plant drugs in concentrated form. Because the alkaloids were very potent, they required careful standardization, which spurred further scientific inquiries and inspired manufacturers to establish testing laboratories and boast about the purity of their products. By the middle of the nineteenth century, synthetic organic chemistry, stimulated by the making of coal-tar dyes, began to yield new drugs such as salicylic acid (1874), eventually leading to the invention of acetylsalicylic acid (aspirin) in 1898. By the end of the 1800s, manufacturers started to design complex machines that could produce end dosage forms such as sugarcoated pills and filled gelatin capsules in large quantities. Even more importantly, pharmaceutical companies in the late 1800s turned to the production of biologicals such as **diphtheria** antitoxin. The work of **Louis Pasteur, Emil von Behring,** and **Robert Koch** captured the imagination of the public who came to see science as not just a tool to explore the nature of the physical universe but as a weapon against disease. By the end of the nineteenth century, the applications of discoveries in biology and chemistry by German drug manufacturers catapulted that nation into the forefront of medicine production.

The dominance of the German pharmaceutical industry continued from the 1880s until the outbreak of World War I (1914–1918). Up to that time western nations imported large quantities of drugs from Germany that were protected by patents and trademarks. However, after their entry into the **war**, countries opposed to Germany, like the United States, seized patents and other rights for distribution to their own national firms. In the United States, the greatest prize was the right to sell acetylsalicylic acid under the trade name Bayer Aspirin, which was acquired by Sterling Products in 1918. With the patents in hand, Great Britain, France, and the United States greatly expanded their production of drugs such as procaine, barbital, arsphenamine, and aspirin.

After World War I, Germany's leadership in chemistry helped reestablish its prominence in pharmaceutical manufacturing. In 1932 Gerhard Domagk (1895–1964) discovered the antimicrobial powers of sulfonamide, which inspired the world's pharmaceutical companies to synthesize and test hundreds of related chemicals. This effort led eventually to the discovery of a number of new drug classes (sulfonylureas and thiazide diuretics) that helped expand the international market for pharmaceuticals.

World War II (1939–1945) was a key event in the maturation of the modern pharmaceutical industry. In the United States the Office of Scientific Research and Development fostered programs to find new antimalarials, blood products, steroids, and anti-infective agents. **Penicillin**, initially discovered and tested in Britain, was produced on a massive scale in the United States for the Allies. After the war, the penicillin example drove companies for the first time to spend huge amounts of money on drug research and development. New firms that made related products (baby food, vitamins, **pesticides**) entered the pharmaceutical fields hoping to reap the expected profits.

During the 1950s, the United States became the leader in the international pharmaceutical enterprise. Laboratories poured out new drugs such as tranquilizers, antidepressants, radioactive isotopes, and antihypertensives. Emphasis remained on drugs to combat infectious disease. **Polio** vaccine, introduced in 1955, demonstrated to the public the power of pharmaceutical research and its promise for the future. Modern management methods replaced the old model of family ownership. Large capital investment came into the industry, as did vertical integration.

The reputation and future of the pharmaceutical industry came into question in the early 1960s with the thalidomide disaster. Thousands of mainly European children were born with birth defects caused by their mothers' ingestion of the drug. (The United States was spared by the efforts of the FDA's Frances Kelsey [b. 1914], who held back the drug's approval.) The regulation of drugs changed internationally because of the disaster with new stringent rules about safety and efficacy adopted in many nations. Research in the industry shifted from battling infection to tackling the maladies of the populations of wealthy nations (e.g., anxiety, high blood pressure, diabetes, and arthritis). Moreover, pharmaceutical companies began selling potent drugs (oral contraceptives and hormone replacement therapies) to prevent or treat naturally occurring conditions (pregnancy and menopause). Profits grew dramatically as the demographics of the West shifted to older populations with greater needs for medicines.

In the 1980s, firms applied the emerging tools of biotechnology to develop new drugs. The first successful product was human insulin (Humalin) produced by Lilly in 1982. The massive success of highly advertised therapies such as Tagamet (cimetidine) for stomach problems encouraged the pursuit of "blockbuster" drugs (i.e., those with sales of over $500 million internationally). In order to market their products widely, pharmaceutical companies led the movement toward economic globalization. International mergers and acquisitions occurred at a fever pitch during the 1990s as much of the world's medicine production came into the hands of a dozen or so major firms. Conventional drug discovery and development has slowed with fewer innovative products appearing each year. The hope for the future of the drug industry is pharmacogenomics (i.e., adapting therapies to the specific genetic make-up of the patient). If and when this advancement occurs, the nature of the pharmaceutical industry will change dramatically. *See also* Antibiotics; Capitalism and Epidemic Disease; Drug Resistance in Microorganisms; Germ Theory of Disease; Human Immunodeficiency Virus/Acquired Immune Deficiency Syndrome (HIV/AIDS); Human Subjects Research; Humoral Theory; Industrial Revolution; Popular Media and Epidemic Disease: Recent Trends; Poverty, Wealth, and Epidemic Disease; Smallpox Eradication; Sulfa Drugs.

Further Reading

Anderson, Stuart, ed. *Making Medicines: A Brief History of Pharmacy and Pharmaceuticals.* Oxford, MS: Pharmaceutical Products Press, 2005.

Boussel, Patrice, Henri Bonnemain, and Frank J. Bové, *History of Pharmacy and the Pharmaceutical Industry.* Paris: Asklepios Press, 1983.

Liebenau, Jonathan, Gregory J. Higby, and Elaine C. Stroud, eds. *Pill Peddlers: Essays on the History of the Pharmaceutical Industry.* Madison, WI: American Institute of the History of Pharmacy, 1990.

Sonnedecker, Glenn. "The Rise of Drug Manufacture in America." *Emory University Quarterly* 21 (1965): 73–87.

Worthen, Dennis. "Pharmaceutical Industry." In *American Pharmacy: A Collection of Historical Essays,* edited by Gregory J. Higby and Elaine Stroud (Madison, WI: American Institute of the History of Pharmacy, 2005) pp. 55–73.

GREGORY J. HIGBY

PHARMACIST. *See* Apothecary/Pharmacist.

PHTHISIS. *See* Tuberculosis.

PHYSICIAN. There is **paleopathological** evidence that during human prehistory, humans assisted their fellows who were injured or disabled. The bones of some prehistoric humans indicate injuries that would have totally incapacitated the individual, but nonetheless display evidence that they healed, with the person living for years following the injury. This could only have occurred with the assistance of others. In even the most primitive society, tribe, or social group, there is usually one individual who is the healer. Before the professionalization of the physician, healers over the eons have been known by many names and titles: shaman, medicine man, wise man, sorcerer, physician, doctor. For our purposes the label physician will be applied broadly at first and later in the narrower sense of one who is a formally educated and professionally accepted medical healer.

Prehistoric Physician. The earliest known depiction of a physician, "The Shaman," can be found in the cave of Trois Frères in France dating back 17,000 to 20,000 years ago. He is depicted wearing a deer face mask and has attributes of other animals. Animal masks were probably worn to scare away the demons and evil spirits believed to be responsible for causing illness. They also served to impress the patient with the power of the physician.

Ancient Egyptian Physicians. Medicine, **magic**, and **religion** were inseparable in ancient Egypt. The oldest description of medical practices can be found in the medical papyri from ancient Egypt. The most detailed of these papyri were named after Egyptologists Georg Ebers (1837–1898) and Edwin Smith (1822–1906) and were written circa 1550 BCE. They contain medical texts believed to date back to the Old Kingdom (3300–2360 BCE) and describe hundreds of medications, incantations, and magical and religious rituals. The Ebers Papyrus deals primarily with infections and medical conditions, whereas the Smith Papyrus contains case histories of surgery and battle injuries. These were essentially the medical textbooks of the time. Modern physicians are amazed at the advanced stage of medical treatments described in these documents, including many medical treatments that remain valid to this day. Of course, the ancient Egyptian physician/priest/magician could not separate these from spiritual elements, because they were tightly interwoven into their belief system. In a sense, these early physicians had discovered the concept of holistic (mind-body-spirit) medicine. Imhotep, a physician, priest, scribe, magician, architect, and vizier (second only to Pharaoh), is the best-known Egyptian physician and might be called the "Grandfather of Modern Medicine."

Asian Traditions. **Chinese medicine** developed independently of, but at approximately the same time as, ancient Egyptian medicine. Under the influence of Confucianism (Confucius, 551–479 BCE), medical training, testing, and practice were regularized, and physicians became members of the official bureaucracy. Herbs and acupuncture were integral elements of Chinese medical treatment, and the use of both was developed to a high degree. Further west, Mesopotamian and Persian physicians believed that when the god of death (Nergal) visited humankind, he was accompanied by the plague demon (Nasutat) who had a whole host of lesser demons that caused specific diseases such as jaundice and **tuberculosis**. Treatments and medications were recorded on clay tablets, and many of these tablets have survived into modern times. Sumerian and Persian **surgeons** were hampered by the eighteenth-century BCE Code of Hammurabi: they were well rewarded if they were successful, but if they failed the punishment was severe. For example, if the surgeon performed a successful eye operation he commanded a high fee, but if the patient lost his eye or died, the surgeon's hands were cut off.

Among the Greeks and Romans. Greek physicians from the fifth century BCE generally followed western medicine originated by the Egyptians, but they continued to improve on medical practices. **Hippocrates**, the "Father of Modern Medicine," combined his era's rationalized natural philosophy with medical theory and practice. Hippocrates focused entirely on the treatment of the sick person and completely ignored the healthy one. He devised a method of **diagnostic** investigation based on observation and reason, but his followers' medical practice relied on the rudiments of **humoral theory**.

Galen, educated in second-century CE Alexandria, Egypt, was physician to two Roman Emperors and treated wounded gladiators. He wrote over 400 essays on medicine, most of which were destroyed by fire, but his surviving works had a profound effect on medical theory and physicians' practice in the West for some 1,500 years. His championing and development of humoral theory ended up retarding the development of medical science and practice until modern times. Unlike Hippocrates, Galen felt that a physician should first maintain the health of his patient and treat the illness if good health could not be maintained. Though he lived through the Antonine Plague, Galen wrote little that survives on infectious or epidemic diseases.

Celsus (second century CE), a famous Roman medical author, wrote *On Medicine* (*De re medica*), which is the earliest scientific medical text in Latin. Much of what is known about Roman medicine today comes from this work. Dedicated to empirical observation like Galen, Celsus described the four signs of inflammation: rubor (redness), calor (heat), dolor (pain), and tumor (swelling). These signs of inflammation are still taught in medical schools today.

One of the major factors in the fall of the Roman Empire in the West was a series of plagues and **epidemics**. To Roman physicians, the myriad symptoms were confusing, and as a consequence most forms of infectious diseases were categorized as "plague." It is believed that the diseases of **smallpox, bubonic plague, typhus, diphtheria,** scarlet fever, and **cholera** were all included under the diagnoses of plague. Roman physicians were ineffective when faced with these virulent diseases: their medicines and therapies were powerless. In part because of their inability to fight these plagues, the people of the late classical period (300–600 CE) lost faith in physicians and turned away from medicine and science.

Medieval and Early Modern Physicians in the West.   The medieval West saw the decline of classical rationalism and scientific thinking and the rise of institutionalized religion (Islam, Roman Catholicism, Eastern Orthodoxy) with its emphasis on the supernatural rather than the natural world. Even so, the sense of charity in Christian and Muslim societies dictated that both religions support the practice of medicine. Galenic medicine all but disappeared in the Latin West, with medical ministration left in the hands of **folk** healers and monastic *infirmarii*. The classical tradition of professional physicians remained alive in Byzantium, and Islamic cultures adopted Galenic professionalism from the Greeks and adapted it to their own traditions. Throughout the great pandemic of the **Plague of Justinian**, Byzantine and Muslim physicians displayed their inability to prevent the spread of the disease or heal its effects. This seems to have stirred especially Muslim physicians to study and advance Greco-Roman medical knowledge and practice, recording their new observations and techniques in treatises such as **Avicenna's** tenth-century *Canon*. Byzantine and Muslim physicians practiced in **hospitals** and **bimaristan**, respectively, supported by the wealthy, and availed themselves for what we might call private practice. Muslim physicians taught and studied in educational centers in cities such as Baghdad, Cairo, and Cordoba (Spain), whereas Constantinople's secular educational institutions and hospitals trained Byzantium's medical professionals.

Only in the eleventh century did the Latin West again begin producing physicians in the Greco-Roman mold. The first medical school appeared in southern Italy, at Salerno, where Catholic, Byzantine, and Muslim cultural traditions mixed. Within two centuries Church-controlled schools in many cities of western Europe were churning out physicians trained in Galenic humoral theory as transmitted through translations of Arabic texts. While many physicians exclusively served important people such as kings, nobles, and the pope, in towns physicians formed guilds to protect the integrity of their practice and limit competition. What a modern observer would call internal medicine was professionalized in the medical schools and guilds, and with the exclusion of **empirics, quacks,** and even **surgeons** from their ranks. Nonetheless, physicians were helpless in the face of the **Black Death** and succeeding waves of plague; nor could they successfully treat conditions such as **leprosy, smallpox,** or **syphilis,** the last of which emerged in the sixteenth century. Nor, until quite late, were physicians generally allowed to serve as public health officials on urban health boards or magistracies, though well-reputed physicians were often asked for advice during times of plague or the threat of plague.

Physicians of the Nineteenth and Twentieth Centuries.   Despite the **Scientific Revolution** and the Enlightenment, and the earlier challenge of the medical ideas of **Paracelsus,** Galenism continued to be the dominant medical paradigm until well into the nineteenth century. The first medical school in colonial North America was founded in 1765. At the beginning of the nineteenth century, most medical practitioners in America had never seen the inside of a medical school. They received only tutoring as an apprentice to an older and equally unqualified practitioner. With the rise of industrialization, diseases and plagues were rampant. Epidemics of **cholera,** tuberculosis, **influenza, typhus, meningitis,** and scarlet fever took many lives, and physicians were unable to fight them adequately. An epidemic of cholera broke out in Europe and caused 52,000 deaths in Britain alone before spreading to America, where it ran unchecked from 1831 until 1833. Around the middle of the nineteenth century, medical advances began to sweep across Western medicine, revolutionizing the medical care that physicians could provide. Names such as **Louis Pasteur** and **Robert Koch** (germ theory), Joseph Lister (1827–1912; sterilization), **Ignaz Semmelweis** (infection control), and Wilhelm Conrad Roentgen (1845–1923; x-ray) became household names and placed medicine on a recognizably scientific pathway. Developments in anatomy, physiology, histology, materia medica (pharmacy), biochemistry, and microbiology enhanced **medical education** and helped create a new breed of scientifically trained physicians. Increasingly, Western physicians were also given extensive training in hospitals to complement their classroom and laboratory experiences. One by one, infectious diseases came to be understood by medical researchers, themselves often physicians. Physicians could now distinguish and diagnose diseases as never before and apply appropriate treatments—or recommend public health measures—that were derived from medical research. Physicians often served as medical missionaries, bringing increasingly effective Western medicine to outposts in European colonies and establishing clinics, hospitals, and eventually training facilities.

As the twentieth century dawned, medical education and the means of successful treatment were making great strides, but with a new century came new challenges. Just as the First World War was coming to a close, the great **influenza pandemic of 1918–1919** descended. During the worldwide flu pandemic, there were an estimated 650,000 deaths related to flu in the United States alone. Physicians were ineffective in stemming the tide of this ravenous disease with their still-meager array of medications. There was, however, a small group of uniquely trained physicians who knew how to use their hands to bolster the body's immune response to fight the virus. DOs (Doctors of Osteopathy), using manipulative therapy and minimal medications, had a rate of effective treatment well above that of physicians using primarily pre-**antibiotic** pharmaceutical medications.

One of the most important developments in the medical profession was its tendency to specialization. Focused curricula and apprentice-like residencies in hospitals allowed medical students and young physicians to acquire true expertise in a wide and still expanding range of specialties such as pediatrics, obstetrics/gynecology, cardiology, oncology, and tropical and infectious diseases. Spurring this was a growing list of new technologies for diagnosing and treating patients, and an even longer and faster growing list of pharmaceuticals. Professionalization of **nursing** (begun in the nineteenth century) and public health services helped create more stable and predictable working environments for physicians in both developed and developing regions of the world. This has proven to be especially important in areas where infectious diseases are endemic, and social disruptions such as wars and famine create conditions conducive to epidemics and detrimental to regularized health care.

Twenty-First-Century Physicians.   As remarkable as the advances in medical science have been over the last 150 years, the twenty-first century promises to dwarf those achievements. Yet there is another worldwide pandemic (**Bird Flu**) looming on the horizon. Medical science has predicted the pandemic, and for the first time in the history of the world, physicians and health authorities from around the globe are amassing the forces of medical science to do battle against this impending pestilence. **Vaccines** and other medications are being stockpiled. Educational programs for the public are being developed, and worldwide communications are available. The battle against epidemic disease may never be won, but medical science and physicians continue working to improve the odds. *See also* Air and Epidemic Diseases; Apothecary/Pharmacist; Ayurvedic Disease Theory and Medicine; Colonialism and Epidemic Disease; Early Humans, Disease in; Hospitals and Medical Education in Britain and the United States; Hospitals in the West since 1900; Medical Ethics and Epidemic Disease; Non-Governmental Organizations (NGOs) and Epidemic Disease; Plague and Developments in Public Health, 1348–1600; Public Health Boards in the West before 1900; Public Health in the Islamic World, 1000–1600; Rush, Benjamin; Sydenham, Thomas.

Further Reading

Bates, Don. *Knowledge and the Scholarly Medical Traditions.* New York: Cambridge University Press, 1995.

Bynum, W. F. *Science and the Practice of Medicine in the Nineteenth Century.* New York: Cambridge University Press, 1994.

Bynum, W. F., et al. *The Western Medical Tradition 1800 to 2000.* New York: Cambridge University Press, 2006.

Campbell, Sheila, et al., eds. *Health, Disease and Healing in Medieval Culture.* Toronto: University of Toronto Press, 1992.

Conrad, Lawrence, et al. *The Western Medical Tradition 800 BC to AD 1800.* New York: Cambridge University Press, 1995.

Ferroul, Yves. "The Doctor and Death in the Middle Ages and Renaissance." In *Death and Dying in the Middle Ages,* edited by Edelgard DuBruck and Barbara I. Gusick, pp. 31–50. New York: Peter Lang, 1999.

Fissell, Mary E. *Medicine before Science: The Business of Medicine from the Middle Ages to the Enlightenment.* New York: Cambridge University Press, 2003.

Garcia-Ballester, et al., eds. *Practical Medicine from Salerno to the Black Death.* New York: Cambridge University Press, 1994.

Gevitz, Norman, *The DOs: Osteopathic Medicine in America,* 2nd edition. Baltimore: Johns Hopkins University Press, 2004.

Gottfried, Robert S. *Doctors and Medicine in Medieval England, 1340–1530.* Princeton: Princeton University Press, 1986.

Hymes, Robert P. "Not Quite Gentlemen? Doctors in Sung and Yüan." *Chinese Science* 8 (1987): 9–76.

Lindemann, Mary. *Medicine and Society in Early Modern Europe.* New York: Cambridge University Press, 1999.

Lloyd, Geoffrey, and Nathan Sivin. *The Way and the Word: Science and Medicine in Early China and Greece.* New Haven: Yale University Press, 2002.

Nutton, Vivian. *Ancient Medicine.* New York: Routledge, 2004.

Pelling, Margaret. *The Common Lot: Sickness, Medical Occupations and the Urban Poor in Early Modern England.* New York: Longman, 1998.

Pormann, Peter E., and Emily Savage-Smith. *Medieval Islamic Medicine.* Washington, DC: Georgetown University Press, 2007.

Russell, Andrew W., ed. *The Town and State Physician in Europe from the Middle Ages to the Enlightenment.* Wolfenbüttel: Herzog August Bibliothek,1981.

Unschuld, Paul. *Chinese Medicine.* Brookline, MA: Paradigm, 1998.

THOMAS QUINN WITH JOSEPH P. BYRNE

PILGRIMAGE AND EPIDEMIC DISEASE.   According to the medieval English poet Geoffrey Chaucer (c. 1343–1400), in the Middle Ages spring was the season when people longed to go on pilgrimage; but as it turned out, people liked to go on pilgrimage in all seasons and in all times. Indeed, like farming and building, pilgrimage—the act of traveling to a special place for religious reasons—has developed in every society we know of, from the most primitive to the most sophisticated. Nor has modernity damped this longing. In fact, modern communication and transportation has encouraged it; every year many millions of people set out on pilgrimage to destinations all over the world, and most return.

Pilgrims are, hence, travelers and subject to the same medical issues as all travelers; because of the peculiar nature of pilgrimage, however, they also run additional risks. Although traveling is essentially *individual*, pilgrimage is more often a *mass* movement— to a fixed and predetermined place, with route and mode of travel often an integral part of the experience. It is this *mass* element, with thousands or even millions of people journeying to the same place, often at the same time of year, and staying for days or even weeks in crowded conditions, that amplifies especially the epidemic risks of traveling.

A good example comes from Islam. In the last month of the Muslim year, 2 million pilgrims from every continent travel to Mecca, Saudi Arabia. There, they spend weeks in a crowded city and then return home, often together, in packed ships and airplanes. In Varanasi, India, more than 70,000 Hindu pilgrims bathe every day in the holy Ganges River, so running a documented 66 percent risk of contracting and spreading some kind of infectious disease.

Much of the specific effect of the mass movement of pilgrimage on the spread of epidemic disease has to do with the intrinsic health and **personal hygiene** of the pilgrims themselves and with the nature of the pilgrimage sites to which they travel. Much also has to do with the kinds of diseases endemic to their place of departure, to their place of arrival, and to their modes of transportation.

For instance, the classic medieval pilgrimages to Compostella in Spain, to Rome, and to Jerusalem do not seem to have brought epidemics back to northern Europe. One reason was that the way was long, slow, and covered mainly on foot or horseback, thus excluding the most vulnerable; next, the medieval European population was relatively well fed; finally, the most common infectious diseases were not very transmissible. Thus, though leprosy was indeed brought to Europe by returning Crusaders and pilgrims, its long latency period and relative lack of contagiousness meant that it never amounted to an epidemic. Likewise, although medieval pilgrims did die of **malaria** in Rome, its mode of transmission via mosquitoes did not allow it to flourish in the inhospitable climate (from the point of view of the mosquito) of northern Europe, and no epidemics of malaria related to pilgrimage are recorded.

On the other hand, certain microbes *do* take to a pilgrim lifestyle, especially those that are easily transmissible from person to person. **Cholera** provides a good example. Centuries ago, Indian pilgrims initially carried it with them to Mecca, where it thrived. Later, it migrated to Palestine with returning pilgrims, and there were recurrent cholera epidemics between 1831 and 1918. Similarly, the disastrous cholera epidemics of nineteenth-century England are also thought to have followed a pilgrim route. More recently, from 1984 to 1986, cholera epidemics were documented in Mecca itself, and in 1994 *Vibrio cholera* took its return journey from Mecca back to Southeast Asia, from whence it had originated.

Smallpox, too, which is easily transmitted by fomites, is another classic disease of pilgrimage. In the 1930s, an outbreak in Africa was traced to pilgrims, and the last major epidemic in Europe was carried to Yugoslavia by a pilgrim who had contracted it in Mecca. Meningococcal **meningitis**, which is not only highly contagious but also provokes a carrier rate as high as 11 percent, has been carried to America, Africa, and Asia by returning pilgrims.

Less contagious diseases such as **tuberculosis**, **Dengue**, and **poliomyelitis** have also had documented mini-epidemics traced to the gathering and then dispersal of pilgrims. Upper respiratory illnesses are particularly efficiently spread in this way. For instance, while in Mecca, 40 percent of pilgrims get some sort of viral upper respiratory illness, and pilgrims to Rome have spread **Legionnaires' disease**. Gastroenteritis is also common; in 2003 Norwalk **virus** was spread from Lourdes to nursing homes in France and Switzerland by returning Christian pilgrims.

Yet it is not the case that pilgrimage *must* lead to epidemics. For example, although millions of pilgrims visited Rome during the Jubilee Year of 2000, no epidemics occurred. Why not? Because healthy, well-fed pilgrims, with sophisticated hygiene and appropriate immunizations, are not efficient vectors. This observation suggests that the epidemic risk of pilgrimage could be limited by appropriate public health measures. Thus Saudi Arabia now requires pilgrims to Mecca to show proof of **vaccination** against **yellow fever**, meningitis, and polio. In addition, as a preventative against meningitis, each arriving pilgrim is given a prophylactic dose of ciprofloxacin. Furthermore, to minimize foodborne epidemics, pilgrims are not permitted to bring food with them from outside the country; to minimize respiratory infections, face-masks are recommended. Education on hygiene, toiletry, and spitting, and the provision of adequate housing and nutrition, has also been instituted.

With similar efforts on the part of all cities and states that belong to pilgrimage routes, it is possible to envision a reversal of the ancient linkage between pilgrimage and epidemics. Pilgrims would return home not sicker but healthier than when they left, with a new knowledge of hygiene and immunization. And instead of being a vehicle for epidemics and public illness, pilgrimage would become a vehicle for public health. *See also* Black Death, Flagellants, and Jews; Cholera: Fourth through Sixth Pandemics, 1862–1947; Cholera: Seventh Pandemic, 1961–Present; Religion and Epidemic Disease.

Further Reading

Omar, W. "The Mecca Pilgrimage." *World Health Organization Chronicles* 11 (1957): 337–342.
Risse, Guenter B. *Mending Bodies, Saving Souls: A History of Hospitals.* New York: Oxford University Press, 1999.

VICTORIA SWEET

PILGRIMS. *See* Pilgrimage.

PINK EYE. *See* Conjunctivitis.

PLAGUE AND DEVELOPMENTS IN PUBLIC HEALTH, 1348–1600. The development of public health, defined as the implementation of specific policies aimed at controlling the outbreak or spread of disease, is generally acknowledged to have begun during the **second plague pandemic** (1348–1772). Europeans' experiences with plague in the fourteenth and fifteenth centuries led them to believe that the disease was passed from infected to healthy persons. Thus, although public health measures across Europe had traditionally included a wide range of sanitation and cleansing efforts, plague also prompted the development of new approaches that aimed to curtail contact between sick and healthy. These included the use of **quarantine**, **pest houses** and convalescent homes, and limitations on the movement of people and **trade** goods.

Fourteenth-century Western medicine was based upon **humoral theory**, which attributed disease to an internal imbalance of bodily humors. In the case of an **epidemic** like the **Black Death**, corrupt or "miasmatic" air created by filth was blamed for inducing such an imbalance, or for poisoning the body. Thus, alongside religious appeals for mercy from God, the earliest responses to plague included efforts to ward off disease through the cleaning and **disinfection** by fumigation of public spaces. Large bonfires burning aromatic herbs such as rosemary were used to purify the air, while renewed mandates on street cleaning and restrictions on dumping trash or offal aimed at reducing potential threats. The practice of trades, such as tanning, that produced noxious odors was banned or restricted to certain parts of town or times of day. As **corpses** accumulated faster than burial traditions could accommodate, concern with miasmas led to legislation dictating how the dead bodies should be collected and buried.

Italy holds a place of prominence in the history of public health, particularly in relation to plague, as municipal officials in a number of city-states, including Venice, Milan, and Florence, developed the earliest administrative bodies specifically charged with overseeing and enforcing public health measures. Over time, these officials helped create the "Italian model" of plague legislation, a variety of public health measures based on emerging notions of contagion designed to protect the healthy by removing or isolating the sick.

As early as 1348, both Venice and Florence had appointed small ad hoc groups of men to oversee health issues, thus establishing the first temporary health boards. These men were principally concerned with internal matters including sanitation and prevention of resale of clothing or bedding owned by the infected. By 1486 Venice made such boards permanent, renewed yearly. In the next century, health boards became permanent fixtures in other cities, including Florence and Milan, creating one of the hallmarks of modern public health.

Outside of Italy, city governments responded to plague outbreaks by creating temporary health committees, often by simply delegating their own members to oversee health measures. In such cases, officials were advised by medical authorities and relied heavily upon the cooperation of both medical practitioners—**physicians**, **surgeons**, and **apothecaries**—and residents to report cases of illness to the proper authorities. Whether a city relied on temporary or permanent officials to oversee public health, however, the overall approach to plague epidemics was the same.

Among the policies implemented by Italian health boards and later adopted by other municipal officials were the use of quarantines, restrictions on the movements of individuals, the revival of isolation hospitals, and the creation of convalescent homes. In 1374 both Genoa and Venice monitored ships' ports of origin and turned away any coming from infected areas. In 1377 Venice's trading colony Ragusa (Dubrovnik) instigated a maritime quarantine, requiring all arriving ships to anchor outside the harbor for 30 days so that authorities could verify that crew and cargo posed no health threat. Later expanded to 40 (*quaranta*) days, perhaps based on the Hippocratic belief that the 40th day distinguished acute diseases from chronic, this quarantine proved successful, and the practice later spread to other port cities. Similar quarantines were subsequently also used by landlocked cities, as travelers and their goods were required to remain outside the gates for up to 40 days to prove their health. This sort of preventive measure was accompanied in many areas by the use of a reactive quarantine—the restriction of infected persons and their families (and often anyone they had been in contact with) to their homes as a means of preventing further spread of disease. Authorities marked the doors of infected homes by various means (a wreath, bundle of straw, horseshoe, or other symbol) and municipal authorities often appointed individuals to act as both guards and provisioners for the shut-ins. In many cities, however, such restrictions were not absolute, as individuals were permitted outside the house either during prescribed hours (when fewer people were in the streets) or with identifying markers, such as a white stick. At the end of the period, a home would have to be cleaned and disinfected or fumigated.

The alternative to confining the infected to their homes was the use of isolation hospitals. Used first by Europeans during the Middle Ages in response to **leprosy**, these institutions, known as **pest houses** or lazarettos, gained new favor in the plague era. Whereas some areas relied upon the use of existing buildings outside city walls, others built new structures, some meant to accommodate thousands of people. At the same time, governments established convalescent homes as a means of continuing the isolation of those no longer in the acute stages of the disease, yet still not considered sufficiently healthy to be released.

In times of plague authorities also implemented further restrictions on the movements of individuals. Principally, this meant shutting some city gates and posting guards at those that remained open. These guards monitored traffic into and out of the city, questioning travelers and often requiring them to carry official papers (a sort of health passport) declaring their place of residence and testifying to their good health. Such travelers, and their goods, were often quarantined outside of city walls for a variable number of days to ensure they posed no direct threat. Beginning with the Duchy of Milan in the late fourteenth century, officials in Italian city-states expanded their control over movement by monitoring traffic not just at city gates, but also along roads, and by setting up information networks to share news of any suspected outbreaks. Here again, Italy was foremost in the creation of communication networks among separate governments (in this case the various city-states), a practice that carried over later into the rest of Europe.

Despite the existence of increasingly centralized monarchies in much of Europe, public health issues continued to be handled primarily by municipal officials. Although England is often noted for having lagged behind Italy in adopting plague measures based on contagion theory, English monarchs were the earliest in their attempts to legislate national plague policies. The first attempt appeared in 1518, during the reign of Henry VIII (r. 1509–1547). The next set of royal orders did not appear until 1578, a lengthy interval that allowed individual cities in England to devise their own emerging programs of public health. The plague orders of 1578, set forth by the Privy Council under Elizabeth I (r. 1558–1603), provided a standard of response for the local justices of the peace, though one not always easily enforced. The English legislation included the harshest terms of shutting in, which gave confined families no chance for respite or outside contact, and which subsequently engendered strong resistance.

By the sixteenth century, popular reaction to plague restrictions varied with the strength of how tightly they were enforced. In Italy, where the health boards gained a great deal of power, efforts to control the movements of individuals by limiting or canceling festivals, processions, and other cultural traditions that brought large numbers of residents into close proximity were met with strong resistance from the people. In these city-states, public health regulations easily shifted to become social control measures, aimed particularly at the poor, at beggars, and at prostitutes. Similarly, England's strict confinement laws raised objections, especially from victims and physicians. In other areas of Europe, however, there is evidence of greater cooperation between residents and officials. In Seville, for example, though municipal officials utilized many of the same restrictions as elsewhere, they also allowed residents the opportunity to gain exemptions from restrictions under controlled circumstances. In this way, officials were often able to diffuse resentment or tensions caused by public health controls. *See also* Contagion Theory of Disease, Premodern; Cordon Sanitaire; Environment, Ecology, and Epidemic Disease; Leprosarium; Personal Liberties and Epidemic Disease; Plague in Europe, 1500–1770s; Plague in Medieval Europe, 1360–1500; Public Health Boards in the West before 1900; Public Health in the Islamic World, 1000–1600.

Further Reading

Bowers, Kristy Wilson. "Balancing Individual and Communal Needs: Plague and Public Health in Early Modern Seville." *Bulletin of the History of Medicine* 81 (2007): at press.

Byrne, Joseph P. *Daily Life during the Black Death*. Westport, CT: Greenwood Press, 2006.

Carmichael, Ann G. *Plague and the Poor in Renaissance Florence*. New York: Cambridge University Press, 1986.

Cipolla, Carlo. *Public Health and the Medical Profession in the Renaissance*. New York: Cambridge University Press, 1976.

Porter, Dorothy. *Health, Civilization and the State: A History of Public Health from Ancient to Modern Times*. New York: Routledge, 1999.

Slack, Paul. *The Impact of Plague in Tudor and Stuart England*. Boston: Routledge & Kegan Paul, 1985.

KRISTY WILSON BOWERS

PLAGUE: END OF THE SECOND PANDEMIC. The **Second Plague Pandemic** began with the **Black Death** (1347–1352) and is widely believed to have initiated a cycle of recurring **epidemic** disease in Europe that lasted for the next 400 years. In both Europe and the Middle East, the recurring epidemics were frequent to the point that every year since the beginnings of the **pandemic**, plague was raging somewhere. The sudden disappearance of plague from northwestern Europe after about 1650 is therefore extremely puzzling for historians and has led to a number of different theories based upon the nature of the disease itself, public health measures, and historical developments.

During the period between the sixteenth and mid-nineteenth centuries, a cooling period known as the Little Ice Age began. **Bubonic plague**, widely accepted as the cause of the recurring plagues of the Second Pandemic, is a bacterial disease that occurs naturally in rodents and thrives among black rat (*Rattus rattus*) populations. The inception of the Little Ice Age may have been enough to decrease the presence of the black rat in Europe, and perhaps affect its fleas (*Xenopsylla cheopis*), which transmit the plague **bacterium** from rats to humans. Supporting this theory is the relative lack of plague activity during the 1640s, which was the coldest period of the Second Pandemic. Throughout the Second Pandemic, plague was generally less active during winter months so it seems likely that cooler global temperatures could have contributed to the end of plague. However, because temperatures have always been frosty in northern Europe, which was no less plague ravaged than any other region, this theory is debatable.

If rats were the carriers of the plagues of the Second Pandemic, then the most likely culprit is the black rat because it lives in close proximity to humans, travels frequently by stowing away on ships and other transportation, and was most likely present in large numbers in Europe and the Middle East during times of plague. It has been suggested, however, that black rat populations dwindled prior to the disappearance of plague. One theory is that the brown rat (*Rattus norvegicus*) was introduced to Europe in the eighteenth century and gradually became the dominant species, edging out its less robust cousin. Because the brown rat does not live in close proximity to humans as the black rat does, the likelihood of transmission of infected fleas is less likely, thus decreasing the chance of human plague. However, since the introduction of the brown rat seems to have occurred after the disappearance of plague from Western Europe, and the two species seem to coexist quite happily, this theory has been largely discredited.

Another suggestion is that improved housing left the black rat homeless. For instance the reconstruction of London after the Great Fire (1666), which occurred a year after the ravages of the **Great Plague of London** (1665–1666), may have robbed rats of their former homes within the city, which were replaced by new, less habitable structures. This theory is weak, however, because housing improvements were not universal throughout early modern Europe, and only London was purged by fire.

On a wider scale, the rat population may have been culled by the increasing use of arsenic as rat poison in the late early modern period, as suggested by contemporary historian Kari Konkola. However, because it is quite difficult to control rats effectively by poison, and because other rat poisons had been available before arsenic, it is unclear whether such a method could explain the complete disappearance of plague.

Historian A. B. Appleby proposes that acquired immunity to bubonic plague developed among rats. In this case, infected fleas would not transmit the disease to humans, since their hosts no longer died of plague. Evidence suggests, however, that immunity in rats does not persist long, often less than a decade, which is not substantial enough to explain the plague's sudden disappearance.

A human resistance theory is plausible if the disease that caused the plagues of the second pandemic was a disease transmitted strictly person to person, allowing the gradual build-up of human resistance through recurring exposure. However, if the people of Europe were gradually building up immunity to plague, then it seems likely that the disease would have subsided gradually but noticeably over time. Because the plague disappeared suddenly, this explanation seems unlikely.

Diseases themselves are known to change over time. For example, recently there has been great trepidation at the prospect of the Bird Flu virus mutating into a lethal human pandemic. An entirely plausible explanation for the disappearance of plague is that the germ (pathogen) itself may have evolved, in this case mutating into a less deadly form. If mutating to a less deadly version increases the chance of survival in a pathogen, then it is likely to occur, because the disease itself is dependent upon the survival of the hosts. The main problem with this theory, however, is that it is impossible to prove, and all indications are that such evolution did not occur.

More credibility has been afforded the role of human agency in the disappearance of plague. Plague **quarantine** and isolation measures evolved throughout the Second Pandemic. Isolation of the sick or suspected carriers was the basic principle, whether this meant closing off a whole town with a *cordon sanitaire* in the case of serious, uncontrollable epidemics or setting up **pest houses** within towns in which the sick could convalesce during minor or anticipated outbreaks. If plague was known to be active in another country, plague-free cities, and eventually nation-states, usually forbade entry to travelers from that region. Maritime trade and travel were similarly restricted with the implementation of quarantine stations for sailors and the closing of harbors to foreign ships, because it was noted that plague often arrived by sea. The gradual acceptance and implementation of these measures in Europe throughout the early modern period may have hindered the reintroduction of plague and consequently led to its disappearance. This is especially true along the great cordon erected by Austria along its border with the Ottoman Empire.

The gradual disappearance of plague specifically from northern Europe in the seventeenth and eighteenth centuries may also be attributed to nations such as England, France, and the Netherlands shifting their maritime commerce away from the Mediterranean basin, thereby cutting themselves off from the critical hub of the plague's reintroductions into Greater Europe. However, despite this shift, trade still continued on various levels between Northern European countries and the Mediterranean basin. The flourishing commerce between England and Turkey during the eighteenth century for example, did not spark a reintroduction of plague into northern Europe.

Generally, the disappearance of plague has also been associated with improvements in **diet**, nutrition, and sanitation in early modern Europe. Nutrition, however, does not seem to affect resistance to or contraction of bubonic plague, and several famines occurred in the latter part of the early modern period indicating that any dietary improvements were not universal. Public sanitation procedures included burning or disinfecting the possessions of the sick, habitual fumigations—because a commonly held belief was that plague was spread by noxious vapors in the air (**miasma** theory)—and in some cities, waste disposal regulations were enforced. Numerous north Italian cities, such as Florence, instituted public health boards to enforce plague-time sanitary regulations. On the whole, however, it seems unlikely that there were universal improvements in the cleanliness of cities or personal hygiene in Europe to the extent needed to end plague for good. For centuries, Islamic peoples practiced far better personal hygiene and cleanliness than Europeans, yet plague persisted much longer in the Middle East.

Responses to plague in the Middle East were limited by lucrative maritime trade and multicultural policy that encouraged human movement rather than limiting it. Additionally, Islamic belief held that human intervention was futile because God sent the plague, and it was customary for Muslims to visit and care for their sick rather than abandon them as Europeans were prone to doing. It was not until the early nineteenth century that plague controls began to be implemented in the Middle East by the Ottoman Viceroy of Egypt, Muhammad Ali (1769–1848). Ignoring the public outcry it caused, he enforced a merciless combination of European quarantine and sanitation methods advised by foreign plague doctors and enforced by the armed forces to stamp out the disease by 1844. Egypt was free from plague for the next three generations, which seems to serve as testimony to the efficacy of these measures.

Plague's disappearance is most likely the result of a combination of the aforementioned explanations, though the validity of each theory rests primarily on uncertain factors such as the nature of the plague pathogen itself and the degree of mutation that occurred over the course of the Second Pandemic. The issue is still very much a matter of historical debate. *See also* Black Death: Modern Medical Debate; Diagnosis of Historical Diseases; Human Immunity and Resistance to Disease; Insects, Other Arthropods, and Epidemic Disease.

Further Reading

Appleby, A. B. "The Disappearance of Plague: A Continuing Puzzle." *The Economic History Review* 33 (1980): 161–173.

Galvani, A. P., and M. Slatkin. "Evaluating Plague and Smallpox as Historic Selective Pressures for the CCR5-Delta 32 HIV-resistance Allele." *Proceedings of the National Academy of Sciences* 25 (2003): 15,276–15,279.

Konkola, Kari. "More than a Coincidence? The Arrival of Arsenic and the Disappearance of Plague in Early Modern Europe." *Journal of the History of Medicine and Allied Sciences* 47 (1992): 186–209.

Rothenberg, Gunther. "The Austrian Sanitary Cordon and the Control of Bubonic Plague: 1710–1871." *Journal of the History of Medicine and Allied Sciences* 28 (1973): 15–23.

Scott, Susan, and Christopher J. Duncan. *Biology of Plagues: Evidence from Historical Populations.* New York: Cambridge University Press, 2001.

Slack, Paul. "The Disappearance of Plague: An Alternative View." *The Economic History Review* 34 (1981): 469–476.

Watts, Sheldon. "The Human Response to Plague." In *Epidemics and History: Disease, Power and Imperialism*, edited by Sheldon Watts, pp. 1–25. Redwood, CA: Wiltshire, 1997.

KARL BIRKELBACH

PLAGUE IN AFRICA: THIRD PANDEMIC. In the mid-nineteenth century, a third **bubonic plague pandemic** began to sweep the globe, arousing terrible collective memories of the **Black Death**, the second plague pandemic that had begun 500 years earlier. By the time it ended around 1950, this new pandemic had produced a highly variable death toll. Most of the roughly 15 million lives it ended prematurely were impoverished inhabitants of India, China, Burma, and Indonesia. Perhaps the worst single outbreak was a dreadful **pneumonic plague epidemic** during 1910–1911, during which an estimated 60,000 perished. In Africa and adjacent Indian Ocean islands, worst hit were Mauritius, the French colonies of Senegal and Madagascar, and some areas of East and Central Africa.

Bubonic plague is usually a disease of wild rodents. This zoonosis now exists in a series of permanent reservoirs from its origins in the Himalayan foothills, to Indonesia, the

Rocky Mountain foothills of the southwestern United States, South Africa, and Argentina. Only accidentally does it cross over to humans. The pathogen is the bacillus *Yersinia pestis*, and the most efficient flea vector is the biting rat flea, *Xenopsylla cheopis*. For all their historical severity, bubonic plague outbreaks develop only when humans come within the range of an infected rat flea. In the Northern Hemisphere today, the odds of this happening would be astronomically small. A century ago, the risk was greater, especially for the urban poor who lived in overcrowded, unsanitary, and rat-infested housing. Also at risk were tradesmen or workers employed around bakeries, grain storage units, cargo ships, and other places where rats gravitated.

Despite breakthroughs in turn-of-the-century bacteriology and **immunology**, current plague control practices such as the burning of "infected" houses and personal effects derived in part from older European public health measures, but were also products of Orientalist and racist images of colonized subjects. Two new procedures, however, seemed more promising: rat control by means of trapping and poisoning, and mass **inoculation** with an anti-plague vaccine. These control techniques gave mixed results. Rodent kills eliminated millions annually but had little impact on the fecundity of rodents. Rat control through better building construction did succeed, especially in Western maritime cities, which might otherwise have been vulnerable to plague importation. Finding an effective and safe vaccine also proved elusive right to the present day, although effective **antibiotic** therapy has made the quest moot.

Origins and Spread.   Emerging from its wild rodent reservoir in the Himalayan borderlands soon after 1855, and traveling this time not west but east, the third pandemic infected the densely populated provinces of south China before attacking Canton and then the British colonial port of Hong Kong in 1894. There it rekindled international fears, especially when it reached Macao and Fuzhou a year later, and struck Singapore and Bombay in 1896. Transported rapidly by British steam ships throughout the empire and beyond, bubonic plague took only a few years to reach every continent.

From the moment bubonic plague resurfaced in Hong Kong, international concerns arose that this old scourge would emulate **cholera** as a global menace. Though not alone, France was especially vocal in blaming lax British sanitary controls. Whereas earlier meetings of the International Sanitary Convention (founded 1851) had been preoccupied with the global cholera pandemics; the Venice Conference of 1897 was the first to deal exclusively with what the Europeans perceived as "Asiatic plague." Delegates could not agree on binding measures, but they did erect **quarantine** and inspection barriers at the Suez Canal, facilities already in place against cholera, to guard Europe against plague. They also agreed to establish specific quarantine measures applicable to passengers and the crews of ships sailing from infected ports.

In Colonial Africa, European health officials, in an effort to mobilize the population for plague control, sometimes showed excessive enthusiasm. The British, for example, paid such generous bounties for rat-tails during and after epidemics in Malawi and Uganda that the premiums actually had an impact on the local economy. But mobilizing the entire population to control potentially infected rodents placed civilians at risk of infection. Intrusive French officials in Senegal and Madagascar attempted residential urban segregation ostensibly to control plague and generated political opposition to other, more beneficial, health measures.

Bubonic plague was rare or unknown in Sub-Saharan Africa before 1900, but it certainly had been no stranger to North Africa and Egypt. Both the **Plague of Justinian** (first pandemic) and the second pandemic (1347 to the early nineteenth century) had wreaked havoc in the region. Plague in fact did not recede from the southern shores of the Mediterranean until after 1844. Although modernization coincided with plague's departure, commercial expansion had also introduced cholera from India. Still, when bubonic plague returned to Alexandria as part of the third pandemic in 1899, Egypt had not experienced a major epidemic of any kind for almost 20 years.

Alexandria's and Egypt's experience with the third plague pandemic was exceptionally mild in comparison with earlier experiences, and it challenged medical experts, religious and political leaders, and the general public to put forward plausible explanations. Apart from older ones based upon God's unknowable will, three basic points stood out. First, sanitary reforms had transformed the disease **environment** of Alexandria; second, the city's health officials had efficiently implemented modern plague control measures with a high degree of support from most Alexandrines; and third, Alexandria's peculiar cosmopolitan mix of foreign minorities and Egyptian nationals had somehow combined to produce cooperation rather than confrontation between the general public and health authorities assigned the task of controlling the plague epidemic.

Yet Alexandria's victory over Y. pestis was only partial. Although its residents had every reason to rejoice over its attenuated impact in 1899, sporadic and light outbreaks of bubonic plague returned to the city annually over the next 30 years. Worse, although Alexandria had been the only plague site in all of Egypt in 1899, soon after the disease spread to Port Suez and towns throughout the Nile Delta. From there, plague traveled far south, sparing Cairo but visiting Upper (southern) Egypt every year. There it became mildly endemic, taking roughly 10,000 lives by the time it finally burned itself out in the 1930s.

Alexandria represented perhaps the best possible result public health authorities could have hoped for from a bubonic plague epidemic at the beginning of the twentieth century. Instead of blaming victims, health officers made them as comfortable as could be expected. Egyptian health assistants were permitted to participate in plague control efforts. Isolation for patients and "suspects" was compulsory, but Muslim victims received *halal* food (that met Muslim purity requirements), and laborers were paid compensation for work days lost. Such sensitivity gave the public confidence that plague control operations served the wider interest. In too many other urban jurisdictions, interest groups worked at cross-purposes, so that political and social tensions became magnified under the plague **microscope**.

Cape Town suffered its first laboratory-confirmed case of bubonic plague in January 1901, probably imported from Argentina in a shipment of fodder for horses during the South African **War**. The vast majority of African cases and deaths occurred in the initial stages of the plague outbreak, through March 15, 1901. Thereafter, health officials forcibly evicted most Africans from the port and city center, where the infected rats and fleas were concentrated, and dispatched them to Ndabeni, a new location outside the city. The last plague case recorded for Cape Town occurred on November 9. The final tally was 389 dead among 807 reported cases.

According to local health officials, a series of factors made Cape Town vulnerable to plague. The list included wartime concentrations of troops constantly moving in and out of town; refugees pouring into an already overcrowded city; a mixed population with what observers called "filthy habits"; antiquated sewers that served as a convenient transportation network for the extraordinary number of rats; and large quantities of forage and other stores for their food supply.

Missing from the mix was a global ecological insight into plague epidemiology, which only a few far-seeing observers were beginning to grasp. The third pandemic was gaining hold in southern Africa because the region provided an excellent natural environment for bubonic plague. Y. *pestis* thrived in a temperature range from 15 to 28 degrees Celsius with moderate humidity, and the X. *cheopis* flea multiplied fastest in a range from 20 to 28 degrees. Not only did Cape Town and most other cities of southern Africa maintain such temperatures much of the year, but X. *cheopis* proved to be commonly found in the countryside as well. Given such an attractive combination of human and natural factors, bubonic plague spread rapidly beyond Cape Town. In mid-April 1901, while plague was still gripping Cape Town, an epidemic broke out at Port Elizabeth in the eastern Cape. There, too, whites forced black Africans into a designated residential location called New Brighton, and urban Africans responded with a determined and partially successful resistance to relocation. Plague persisted on and off in Port Elizabeth until 1905, and remained in East London between 1903 and 1905. Moderate outbreaks occurred in Durban in 1902, where white panic was rampant, and in Johannesburg, where authorities burned down African slums within a few hours of discovering bubonic plague in 1904. Y. *pestis* continued its exploration of the South African hinterland, especially in southwestern Transvaal and northwestern Orange Free State, where it established a permanent reservoir among gerbils and other *veldt* rodents. Even today, the large permanent reservoir of enzootic plague poses a major threat to rural South Africans, especially those without affordable access to early diagnosis and antibiotic treatment.

Bubonic plague was the most persistent and dramatic infectious disease to strike Senegal in the twentieth century, even if chronic diseases such as **malaria** and **dysentery** killed more people. From the time it first appeared in 1914 until its final departure in 1945, scarcely a year went by without a recorded outbreak in either rural or urban areas. Recorded Senegalese deaths from plague exceeded 35,000 over 32 years, but this figure represents an unknown fraction of the real toll. Senegal may have suffered the highest case rates per 10,000 population in Africa, and worldwide second only to India.

Another scene of recurring plague is the island of Madagascar, which was heavily victimized earlier in the third pandemic but had very few cases after the late 1930s. Beginning in 1989, however, human plague again became a major health problem, especially in the capital of Antananarivo, the highlands just to the south, and at the northwestern port of Mahajanga. In 1997 alone, close to 2,000 cases were recorded, and for the decade, approximately 6,000, with case fatality rates of 20 percent. This new visitation of plague has been difficult to control for a number of suggested reasons. A permanent reservoir of Y. *pestis* persists among sylvatic rodents; three new variants of Y. *pestis* have recently emerged and may be acquiring selective advantages; most ominously, the first naturally occurring antibiotic-resistant strain of Y. *pestis* was recently isolated in Madagascar. To underscore the dangers represented in India and Madagascar, the **World Health Organization** in 1996 reclassified plague as a "reemerging" rather than a dormant disease. *See also* Colonialism and Epidemic Disease; International Health Agencies and Conventions; Personal Liberties and Epidemic Disease; Plague in East Asia: Third Pandemic; Plague in India and Oceania: Third Pandemic; Plague in the Contemporary World; Race, Ethnicity, and Epidemic Disease; Travel, Trade, and Epidemic Disease; Yersin, Alexandre.

Further Reading

Echenberg, Myron. *Black Death, White Medicine: Bubonic Plague and the Politics of Public Health in Colonial Senegal, 1914–1945*. Portsmouth, NH: Heinemann, 2002.

———. *Plague Ports: The Global Urban Impact of Bubonic Plague, 1894–1901*. New York: New York University Press, 2007.

Kirk, Joyce F. *Making a Voice: African Resistance to Segregation in South Africa*. Boulder, CO: Westview Press, 1998.

Van Heyningen, Elizabeth. "Cape Town and the Plague of 1901." In *Studies in the History of Cape Town*, Vol. 4, edited by Christopher Saunders, Howard Phillips, and Elizabeth van Heyningen, pp. 66–107. Cape Town: University of Cape Town, 1981.

MYRON ECHENBERG

PLAGUE IN BRITAIN, 1500–1647.   From 1500 to 1666, the plague was a constitutive force within British culture, affecting all aspects of lived experience from the way people prepared food to the content of their prayers and the terms of their labor. It halted trade, sent the wealthy in **flight** to the country, closed theaters, and killed thousands. Visitations were most frequent in larger cities in the southeast, with Ireland and Scotland experiencing relatively few. The worst visitations in England paralyzed portions of the nation with fear, bringing some to near standstill in 1498, 1504–1505, 1509, 1511–1521, 1523, 1535, 1543, 1563–1564, 1578, 1592–1593, 1603–1612, 1625–1626, 1636–1639, 1641, and 1643–1647. **London's Great Plague**, England's final plague **epidemic** and an outbreak second in impact only to the **Black Death** of 1349, struck in 1665. In every decade on average from 1500 to 1647, plague struck major ports and cities before traveling by less obvious patterns into the suburbs and then north and east into smaller towns and villages.

Some speculate that in this period the plague was not only epizootic, infecting entire rat populations, but also enzootic to the island. The fact that plague did visit London and other southeastern cities more frequently, suggests that even if it had been endemic in England, new carriers crossed the channel and increased its virulence. The primary vector was the flea, carried on rats. This has led to speculation that the rats came across the channel on ships, but it is also possible that clothing and bedding provided a suitable, temporary habitat for the fleas.

Few scholars attribute regular visitations to human-to-human transmission. The relatively slow speed at which plague spread and the fact that old and young, men and women, alike were susceptible supports the consensus that humans most often contracted the disease from fleas, not from each other. In addition, although plague visited London and other large cities more frequently than villages, it often killed a larger percentage of the population in rural communities—as many as 1 in 10 according to the historical record. This is a low number compared to the mortality rates reported from the first pandemic in the fourteenth century, but it was enough to threaten national, parish, and familial stability on a regular basis.

Records of burials in parish registers, wills proved, and London's bills of mortality are the primary sources for determining the years in which plague caused dramatic increases in mortality rates. The number of dead listed on a weekly bill, for example, should correspond with the number of burials. These published bills are particularly useful, because from them we can establish the number of dead for a given parish each week, increases and decreases in weekly mortality rates over time, and comparative mortality rates by region. At the time, the bills were the primary means by which people learned that plague was increasing or decreasing in virulence. The bills helped citizens determine when to close up shop and flee from the city, hunker down, or initiate thankful celebration.

Yet, there are many variables that make it difficult to rely upon these documents. Only London published bills of mortality, some parish records have not survived, and it was often the case that parish officials underreported the numbers of plague dead in order to avoid panic or intervention from the national government. Prior to the mid-sixteenth century, records of all kinds are spotty, and even in towns that paid "searchers" to enumerate the dead, the information collected never included case-specific correlation between the number that the dead person represented on the bill and the symptoms he or she had. What this means is that, if anything, the numbers we have are inaccurate because they are low. Nevertheless, the triangulation of data (wills, burials, and bills) allows us to identify useful patterns: higher rates of death from plague in poorer parishes than in wealthier ones, in late summer and early autumn than in winter, and in parishes closer to ports than in those further away, but a roughly uniform number of plague deaths with respect to victim age and gender.

Just what constituted "plague," however, was and still is difficult to determine with absolute certainty. Men and women in Britain at the time could not have known that **bubonic plague** was caused by the plague bacillus *Yersinia pestis* that was transmitted when the rat flea (*Xenopsylla cheopis*) jumped from the black rat (*Rattus rattus*) to a human and bit. Yet, we can use their accounts of basic symptoms (fever, overly swollen lymph glands, and small skin lesions), of a two to six day incubation period, of fatality rates from 50 to 80 percent, and of the plague's seasonal schedule, to confirm that bubonic plague was the primary contributor to deaths in these years. Although they did not have the technology we do now, people of the period were able to distinguish between bubonic plague and lesser diseases that had lower mortality rates, different symptoms, and/or longer incubation periods, such as the **sweating sickness, smallpox,** and **syphilis.** Although it is possible that **pneumonic plague** also contributed to high mortality rates, the symptoms, incubation rate, and mortality rate for pneumonic plague do not coincide closely enough with historical accounts of the plague in Britain to allow for consensus.

The primary source of plague was the bubonic form, and the primary vector was the rat flea, not humans. Mortality rates for people dropped when plague had run its course in the animal population and killed off the majority of the rat and flea population. One reason that 1666 marks the end of plague in Britain may be that the fire of London not only killed rats, but it also consumed many of the oldest thatched-roof buildings, which had made ideal homes for the black rat. Although there were a few reported cases of plague after 1666, there was never another major visitation in Britain.

Because they realized that a distinct threat was upon them, English monarchs and their advisory councils took action to deal with this particular scourge. King Henry VIII of England (1491–1547) had seen his own father, King Henry VII (1457–1509), grapple with the disease, and Henry VIII had spent many months in flight from the plague and away from the nation's capital in London. During these times, his primary advisor, Thomas Cardinal Wolsey (c. 1473–1530) remained behind to ensure that government affairs remained on course. In 1518, nine years into the reign of Henry VIII, Wolsey created a set of plague orders that were based on those used on the continent; however, they were never employed nationwide or even in London. Instead, Henry VIII sent Thomas More (1478–1535) to Oxford to enforce the plague orders there. A lawyer by trade who had written *The Utopia*

(1516), who would become Lord Chancellor of England, and whom Henry VIII would execute for refusing to support his divorce from Catharine of Aragon (1485–1536), Thomas More went to Oxford to guarantee that all plague victims were quarantined within their homes so that the king could pass through the city in safety.

The success of these single-city plague orders was small compared to the nationwide standards for plague orders employed on the continent. Italian territorial states led the way, with other nations following. It would take six decades before England saw its first nationwide plague orders in place. Before this, Henry VIII's daughter Queen Elizabeth I (1533–1603) called the nation to attention through church-directed worship. In 1563, the first serious plague year of her reign, Elizabeth I and her advisory committee charged Matthew Parker, Archbishop of Canterbury (1504–1575), and Bishop Grindal (1519–1583) of London with formulating the first nationwide schedule of prayer and fasting for the prevention of disease. Prior to this, **flight** alone served to secure the nation's head. With the issue of this document, Elizabeth I broke tradition with her forebears, prescribing actions to be taken by all citizens, not only by leaders.

In 1578, the next major plague year in her reign, Elizabeth I and her council created a secular version of the nationwide prayer orders. It consisted of seventeen separate orders to the justices of the peace in all parishes in the nation. It was modeled upon continental orders similar to those followed by Thomas More to secure Oxford in 1518. These orders depended upon the shutting up of victims in their homes, collection of taxes to assist the poor, and orderly reporting by justices of the peace. These orders were thorough and flexible enough to gain them reissue in every major visitation through 1666, when they were finally revised.

When he assumed the throne after Elizabeth I's death in 1603, James I of England (1566–1625) reissued Elizabeth I's orders unchanged, but within a year, he had issued an act that increased the penalties for people who attempted to escape from sealed houses. In "An Act for the charitable relief and ordering of persons infected with the Plague," James I decreed that infected persons who attempted to escape would be forcibly returned to them, and any who ran would face death. This act was not only more severe in its pronouncements upon plague victims but it also carried more weight than Elizabeth I's orders because it was ratified by Parliament. There are no records showing that anyone was ever tried for this crime, and there were no additional changes to plague policy in the period, but writers increasingly registered their concerns regarding the inhumane practice of shutting in victims and their families.

With the printing press came the opportunity for medical practitioners, social satirists, and clergymen to hawk their written wares. The latest diagnosis and remedy for plague accompanied exclamations against bad **air**, the uncharitable nobility, and sin. The number of medical treatises printed in English in the period number nearly 200, and of these, more than four dozen were exclusively about the plague. Writers also took the opportunity to cry out in sorrow and anger over the conditions they witnessed, and they did so by publishing short pamphlets that circulated widely. One common theme was the city versus the country. As London's citizens fled in large numbers to the country, those who dwelt in the villages aimed to turn them away, for fear of infection. Flight, in fact, did more to disable economies and civil administration than the literal disease, and it damaged relationships both within cities and between city and country. In other pamphlets, authors told tales of odd and amusing behavior in plague-time in order to alleviate suffering through laughter. In sermons, the themes were never intended to provoke mirth but rather to encourage repentance. Clergymen compared London to the biblical Sodom and Gomorrah but also to Nineveh, a city that God threatened to strike with plague but then chose to spare when the king and his subjects all prayed for forgiveness.

Records of playhouse and fair closings also illustrate the social and economic impact of plague. When plague visited London, the monarch would issue a stay against plays and order the closing of markets in order to prevent these large public gatherings from becoming sites of increased infection. Actors and vendors forced to close shop had to seek alternative forms of income. This is one reason why William Shakespeare (1564–1616) wrote his narrative poems *Venus and Adonis* and *The Rape of Lucrece*. Playhouses were closed in 1593–1594, so he turned to narrative poetry and hoped that his patrons would pay him well enough to get him to the next season. Actors and others also opted in some cases to take their shows and their wares on the road, performing and selling in neighboring towns that were not infected. Many, however, were trapped within infected regions without the means to escape. They witnessed the cessation of all commerce and the upturning of life as they knew it. In his famous *Journal of the Plague Year* (1722), Daniel Defoe's (c. 1660–1731) protagonist lives through such a crisis in 1665.

The plague left its mark on individual bodies but also on cities, nations, and their products. Some have claimed that were it not for plague we would not have Thomas More's *Utopia*, William Shakespeare's plays and poetry, or the genre of the novel, with its origins in the work of Daniel Defoe. Others, like theorist Michel Foucault (1926–1984), tell us that in the early plague orders we find the birth of the modern police state. The plague legislation from this period was certainly as far-reaching as its literature, which to this day can make us tremble with threat of "A plague o' both your houses!" (*Romeo and Juliet*). *See also* Black Death: Modern Medical Debate; Demographic Data Collection and Analysis, History of; Diagnosis of Historical Diseases; Pest Houses and Lazarettos; Plague and Developments in Public Health, 1348–1600; Plague in Europe, 1500–1770s; Plague Literature and Art, Early Modern European.

Further Reading

Barroll, John Leeds. *Politics, Plague, and Shakespeare's Theater: The Stuart Years*. Ithaca: Cornell University Press, 1991.

Byrne, Joseph P. *Daily Life during the Black Death*. Westport, CT: Greenwood Press, 2006.

Champion, Justin A. I., ed. *Epidemic Disease in London*. London: Centre for Metropolitan History Working Papers Series 1, 1993.

Dobson, Mary J. 1997. *Contours of Death and Disease in Early Modern England*. New York: Cambridge University Press, 1997.

Dyer, Alan. "The Influence of Bubonic Plague in England 1500–1667." *Medical History* 22 (1978): 308–326.

Healy, Margaret. *Fictions of Disease in Early Modern England: Bodies, Plagues and Politics*. New York: Palgrave, 2002.

Lee, Christopher. *1603: The Death of Queen Elizabeth I, the Return of the Black Plague, the Rise of Shakespeare, Piracy, Witchcraft, and the Birth of the Stuart Era*. New York: St. Martin's Press, 2004.

Porter, Stephen. *Lord Have Mercy upon Us: London's Plague Years*. Stroud, UK: Tempus, 2005.

Shrewsbury, J. F. D. *A History of Bubonic Plague in the British Isles*. New York: Cambridge University Press, 1970.

Slack, Paul. *The Impact of Plague in Tudor and Stuart England*. Oxford: Oxford University Press, 1985.

Totaro, Rebecca. *Suffering in Paradise: The Bubonic Plague in English Literature from More to Milton.* Pittsburgh: Duquesne University Press, 2005.

Wilson, F. P. *Plague in Shakespeare's London.* New York: Oxford University Press, 1999.

REBECCA TOTARO

PLAGUE IN CHINA.   Because European plague **epidemics** have often been described as "coming from the East," it is assumed that China has been the source of all plague and pestilence. The historical record documenting epidemics in China is far from clear on these origins.

Traditional Chinese sources contain lists of epidemics noted in the dynastic histories and other sources that start in 243 BCE during the Qin dynasty; William McNeill (b. 1917) summarized these in the Appendix to his *Plagues and Peoples.* Based, as they are, on fragmentary and often now unavailable sources, such lists are problematic. In a careful review of historical evidence for epidemics that can be reliably considered as plague (caused by *Yersinia pestis*), Carol Benedict in *Bubonic Plague in Nineteenth Century China* presents credible historical evidence that plague existed in Yunnan Province in Southwest China as early as 1772. Its association with rats is clearly described in a poem by Shi Daonan (1765–1792) entitled "Death of Rats." The telling line reads: "A few days following the death of the rats,/ Men pass away like falling walls." Clearly the association of the epizootic in rats and human disease was known in China by the late eighteenth century.

The frequent local epidemics of plague in Yunnan, then Guangxi province, and finally in Guangdong province are well documented by Benedict. She shows how both the lucrative opium **trade** and the **ecology** of the indigenous host of the rat flea, the yellow-chested rat (*Rattus flavipectus*), contributed to and explained this spread.

Since the development of **germ theories** of disease in the late nineteenth century, two epidemics of plague in China have been of major significance. By 1894–1895, plague had spread outward from its initial endemic focus in Yunnan Province and had a major impact in Hong Kong, along the South China coast, and in Taiwan, soon spreading to South Africa, San Francisco, and some of the Japanese islands, becoming the third worldwide plague pandemic after the **plague of Justinian** in the sixth century and the **Black Death**, which began in the fourteenth century. The second major epidemic of plague in China occurred in the winter of 1910–1911 in the northeastern provinces of China. This epidemic took the form of **pneumonic plague**, but it did not spread beyond North China to become a dispersed pandemic. Both of these epidemics, the first in Hong Kong and the second in Manchuria, however, presented opportunities for the study of plague with the new tools and concepts of bacteriology, and both epidemics led to major advances in understanding of both the causes and spread of plague.

Plague in Hong Kong occurred at such a time and place that both bacteriology and **colonialism** were in full play. British colonial policy extended to matters of public health, both to protect the colonizers and to protect colonial investment. The Chinese resistance to Western public health measures was as much resistance to unwanted state interference in their lives as it was to the real lack of effective measures against disease in most cases. Civic activism by the British as well as the Chinese gentry was at work in Hong Kong in 1894 when the plague arrived. Medical science had just begun to unravel the role of rats and fleas in the transmission of this dread disease, though the microbe responsible for plague had not yet been identified. The proper measures to combat the plague in Hong

Kong were debated; Western medicine had to rely on accounts of plague epidemics from centuries earlier; **Chinese disease theory and medicine** relied on remedies and prophylactics not well understood by the Western authorities.

The opportunity to study an epidemic of plague in a city with a Western administrative structure and a semblance of a Western medical establishment drew two research teams to Hong Kong. The Pasteur Institute sent a skilled and experienced bacteriologist, **Alexandre Yersin**, to study the plague, and **Shibasaburo Kitasato** arrived from the Institute for Study of Infectious Diseases in Tokyo. Both soon isolated strains of **bacteria** associated with cases of the plague, but because of difference in techniques they found different organisms. Kitasato found a Gram-stain-positive organism in the blood of plague patients, whereas Yersin found a Gram-stain-negative organism in the buboes and other affected tissues of plague patients. This controversy was quietly resolved when Kitasato repeated Yersin's work and he subsequently agreed that Yersin's Gram-stain negative organism was the true cause of plague; his isolate appears to have been a spurious commensal organism. Surprisingly, to this day, this confusion over the "credit" for discovery of the plague bacillus exists in many textbooks and historical accounts.

The index case of plague in the Manchurian epidemic, as best determined by contemporary investigation, was a migrant trapper who died in Manchouli on the Chinese-Russian border in mid-October 1910. At that time, aided by the expanding railroads, Chinese hunters from the south would travel to Manchuria to trap the Siberian marmot or tarbagan (*Marmota sibirica*) for its fur. Plague was already known to be endemic among these common burrowing rodents. At the end of the trapping season, these migrant trappers would return to their homes in the south. Plague spread rapidly among the poor and crowded camps of these migrants and was carried south along the railway, initially, in this case, the Russian-controlled Chinese Eastern Railway. Plague reached Harbin on October 27, 1910; Changchun, the northern terminus of the Japanese-controlled South Manchuria Railway, on January 2, 1911; and Peking (Beijing) on January 12, 1911. When people could not get on the trains, they fled south by road and spread the disease into the countryside. Although the Russian and Japanese authorities were implementing local measures, only the central Chinese government could officially act on a broad scale. In a move to respond to both Chinese and foreign pressure, the Manchu Court through the Ministry of Foreign Affairs sent **Wu Lien Teh**, a Malaysian Chinese physician, educated at Cambridge and working for the Chinese government as Vice Dean at Peiyang Medical School, to Harbin to investigate the plague on its behalf. In late December 1910, Wu and a senior medical student named Lin arrived in Harbin. Lin was particularly valuable because Wu, as an "overseas Chinese," was not fluent in Chinese, especially the local dialects.

On his third day in Harbin, Wu managed to do a limited postmortem examination on a woman who had just died, and he observed massive infection of lung, heart, spleen, and liver with bacteria with the morphology and staining characteristics of Yersin's plague bacillus. As an astute clinician with the most up-to-date education, he made the clinical diagnosis of **pneumonic plague**, while the local Russian doctors in Harbin suspected **bubonic plague** and continued to examine patients without respiratory precautions. A senior French physician, Girard Mesny (d. 1910), sent to Harbin a little later, refused to accept Wu's evaluation and failed to take precautions. He died six days later.

Mesny's death may have been a turning point, because in January 1911 the Chinese government sent troops and police to Manchuria in an attempt to control population movements and to enforce **quarantines**. A new plague hospital was hastily set up and the old one burned down. With the ground frozen, it was impossible to bury the dead. At one point Wu reported seeing 2,000 coffins in rows with more dead on the ground because of a shortage of coffins. Worried that rats might become infected by eating the **corpses**, Wu was able to enlist the support of some local officials, and then following the traditional Chinese approach, he wrote a memorial to the throne. Three days later he received an Imperial Edict allowing mass cremation of the dead bodies.

The rigid quarantines, cold weather, and strict isolation of the sick led to control of this epidemic, which ended in mid-March 1911. One outcome of this epidemic in which an estimated 60,000 people died, was an International Plague Conference, hosted by the Chinese government in Mukden (Shenyang) in April 1911. This conference was the first scientific conference held in China, and its proceedings became a standard reference on contemporary understanding of plague. China established the North Manchurian Plague Prevention Service under Dr. Wu in Harbin, the first official recognition of western public health by the Chinese government. Subsequent work by Wu and his colleagues on both cholera and plague in China led to the expansion of this service to become the National Quarantine Service, the first organization for public health in China up until the invasion by Japan in 1936. *See also* Animal Diseases (Zoonoses) and Epidemic Disease; Plague in East Asia: Third Pandemic; Plague in India and Oceania: Third Pandemic.

Further Reading

Benedict, Carol. *Bubonic Plague in Nineteenth-century China*. Stanford: Stanford University Press, 1996.

Gamsu, Mark. "The Epidemic of Pneumonic Plague in Manchuria, 1910–1911." *Past & Present* 190 (2006): 147–83.

McNeill, William H. *Plagues and Peoples*. New York: Anchor Books, 1989.

Wu, Lien-Teh. *Plague Fighter: The Autobiography of a Modern Chinese Physician*. Cambridge: W. Heffer, 1959.

WILLIAM C. SUMMERS

PLAGUE IN EAST ASIA: THIRD PANDEMIC.   From the 1860s to 1960, plague caused by the bacillus Y*ersinia pestis* swept around the world with several major **epidemics** in East Asia, most notably in China, Hong Kong, and Manchuria in the 1890s, 1910–1911, 1917, and 1920–1921. Although **bubonic plague** was the major killer during this **pandemic, pneumonic plague** also was present, particularly in the Manchurian epidemics. In working to combat the plague outbreak in Hong Kong in 1894, **Alexandre Yersin** and **Shibasaburo Kitasato** isolated for the first time the **bacterium** Y. *pestis* as the agent of the disease. Biovar orientalis, the type responsible for the third pandemic, most likely evolved from sylvatic (wild) biovar antiqua sometime in the past. Small epidemics began to be noticed in Yunnan province in southwestern China in the late eighteenth century. These early epidemics involved rural areas with low population densities, so the disease spread slowly.

Bubonic plague is a vector-borne disease with fleas serving as the vectors. Several varieties of fleas are capable of carrying Y. *pestis*, most notably *Xenopsylla cheopis*, the rat flea. Rats are the most common host for plague-carrying fleas, although other animals such as marmots and susliks often served as hosts in China and Russia. Rats are highly mobile and often stow away on ships and other conveyances carrying grain, making it easy to spread plague over great distances.

Bubonic Plague in China.   There were small epidemics in western Yunnan from the 1770s onward, but the disease remained confined to the western part of the province well into the nineteenth century. The first major modern plague epidemic in China came in 1866 when refugees from social and political unrest brought the disease to K'unming, the capital of the province of Yunnan. From there the disease spread slowly across south China reaching the seaport of Canton in 1892. This slow progress of the disease was not characteristic of earlier plague pandemics and has led to questions about the validity of the plague diagnosis for earlier epidemics. Once established in the seaports of China, it was an easy step for plague to spread to nearby Hong Kong in 1894. From the Chinese port cities, the disease spread readily worldwide, reaching first Bombay in 1896 and then Calcutta in 1898. After that few countries remained untouched as the disease spread from China to the United States in 1900. Plague-infected rats stowed away on ships leaving Chinese harbors, spreading the disease worldwide. The epidemic had turned into a pandemic by the early twentieth century. The third plague pandemic originated in China as a new biovar, and readily available transportation and international commerce made it possible for Y. *pestis* to have a worldwide reach and establish itself as endemic in several new regions such as the Americas.

Plague remained endemic in China well into the twentieth century, spreading throughout the country, though it was more common in the southwest than elsewhere. After the first major epidemic in the 1890s, the number of plague cases declined after 1920, but the disease continued to produce a steady death rate characteristic of an endemic infection.

The British authorities in Hong Kong acted quickly once the disease reached the city, setting up three plague hospitals to try to control the disease. Word of the outbreak led medical authorities elsewhere to send aid. One team, led by Dr. Shibasaburo Kitasato, arrived from Japan in early June 1894. Kitasato, trained in Germany by **Robert Koch**, set up shop at Kennedy Town hospital and quickly began to conduct autopsies to try to determine the agent of disease. Shortly thereafter Dr. Alexandre E. J. Yersin arrived from French Indochina. The idealistic Yersin had trained in **Louis Pasteur's** laboratory in Paris. Initially denied access to any corpses, he set up operations in a straw hut and eventually gained access to the bodies of some of the suspected plague victims. Both men eventually identified bacteria they claimed to be the agent of disease. Yersin's identification was the more concrete, clearly indicating it was a Gram-negative organism, and thus a likely human pathogen. Both men claimed to be the discoverers of the plague bacillus, but over time the scientific community (and Kitasato himself) recognized Yersin's work, and the bacteria Y*ersinia pestis* was named in his honor in 1970 (it had previously been named *Pasteurella pestis*).

The outbreak of plague in Canton and Hong Kong illustrated the conflict between Western "scientific" medicine and **Chinese disease theory and medicine**. The **germ theory** of disease had come to be accepted in the West although not yet throughout Asia. By the late nineteenth century, the European mode for dealing with infectious disease was rigorous isolation of infected victims coupled with massive sanitation campaigns all controlled by the state. The Chinese model for dealing with infectious disease often involved care of the infected victims by their families and voluntary efforts at infection control. Europeans in Canton were critical of the performance of the local governments in dealing with the plague epidemic. In Hong Kong the Chinese merchant elite had sponsored the charitable Donghua Hospital, which quickly worked to take charge of plague treatment in 1894. The Donghua Hospital Directorate often did not isolate plague victims from their families and often tried to assist the sick and dying to return to China. The British colonial authorities responded to the plague outbreak by isolating plague patients through forced hospitalization and rigorous efforts at enforcing sanitation. Such an approach often tore families apart as plague victims were isolated from their relatives. In the early 1890s the connection had not yet been made between fleas and the spread of the disease, and plague was still often seen as a contagious disease caused by dirty conditions. Although there is some basis in fact for relating unsanitary conditions to the spread of the plague, the British response in the 1890s was also conditioned by a presumed European superiority to all things Asian. The weight of the colonial government was brought to bear in enforcing European standards for plague treatment, arousing intense resentment by Chinese in Hong Kong and mainland China. In essence, colonialist state medicine took control from civic activism in confronting the plague.

The gradual spread of bubonic plague across China in the early stages of the pandemic led to several million deaths, but it did not cause panic or the massive mortality rates of the **Black Death**. Even in Hong Kong, where 50,000 to 100,000 people are estimated to have died in 1894, the outbreak was finally contained. The British authorities in Hong Kong often underreported the total of plague deaths, as deaths in the native population often went uncounted. Nonetheless, the death rate in Hong Kong, for example, from 1894 to 1923, was low, usually less than 5 deaths per 1,000. On the other hand, the case fatality rate (the ratio of plague deaths to plague cases) was quite high, generally exceeding 90 percent during most years of the period. Plague did not infect all of China in any one year, and so different regions of the country were often free of the disease for several years at a time.

Plague returned to southern China with another epidemic in 1917–1918. The death toll was lower than before, but several thousand people died nonetheless. The Chinese government was better prepared to confront the outbreak, so the pockets of infection were usually controlled, and the epidemic did not spread throughout the country. In essence the Chinese government had adopted the western model of **quarantine** and government control to fight the disease.

Plague Elsewhere in East Asia.   The plague also spread to the Chinese island of Taiwan (Formosa), with the first case occurring in 1897. Until 1917 plague would be a regular visitor to the island. The death rate on the island was quite low, generally less than 1 per 1,000 with a case fatality rate generally in the 80–90 percent range. Here the disease was imported from the mainland and tended to be concentrated in periodic epidemics when the disease gained a foothold from a ship.

As bubonic plague spread beyond the borders of China, several other Asian countries developed epidemics or continued to experience unusually high numbers of cases. Early in the twentieth century, the disease spread to the French colony of Vietnam, where it was more concentrated in the south than the north. Even in 1910, the worst year for plague cases, the number of cases was far below that of the late 1960s, which arose from the disruptions caused by American military efforts in South Vietnam. Plague would remain endemic in Vietnam until the early 1950s when it appeared to be eradicated. Thailand, too, fell victim to the plague with 586 cases in 1917 of which 580 were fatal. The Dutch colony of Java remained free from the disease until November 1910 when a ship carrying rice from Burma also brought rats carrying plague-infected fleas to the island. The disease spread gradually from east to west. The first wave from 1910 to 1914 affected the eastern part of the island. After a period of remission from 1915 to 1919 the plague began to spread across the rest of the island, and from 1920 to 1927 there were over 8,000 fatal cases per year, primarily in central Java. A third phase occurred from 1930 to 1934 with most of the deaths in the eastern part of the island. Nonetheless, the mortality rate throughout the period remained quite low in the Dutch colony. After 1934, plague erad-ication efforts by the government—mainly the destruction of older houses and the construction of brick houses that were less amenable to flea infestation—helped to bring the epidemic to a close. In both the French and Dutch colonies, a conflict existed between European and native medical practices that was similar to that which had occurred earlier in Hong Kong.

For the most part, Japan remained plague-free in the early twentieth century. Japanese officials enforced rigorous inspection standards on ships entering Japanese ports from infected Chinese ports. Even though a few cases developed, the disease never made inroads into the native rat population, so no disease reservoir developed on the islands. Japanese medical and military authorities watched with interest the course of the disease in China, and some ultimately turned to the development of plague as a biological weapon during World War II (1939–1945).

Manchuria and an Old Plague Reservoir.   The third bubonic plague pandemic developed in southwestern China, but there was another plague reservoir in Mongolia and parts of Asiatic Russia. The Mongolian plague was probably the older biovar medevalis rather than the biovar orientalis. Plague was endemic in Mongolia with marmots, or tarabagons as Russians called them, serving as the primary host for Y. Pestis-carrying fleas.

Rural Mongolian and Manchurian folk legends long warned against coming into contact with marmots that appeared to be sick. As fur prices increased in the early twentieth century, new, less careful trappers began trapping marmots. In 1910 an epizootic occurred leading to massive deaths of marmots in Manchuria. Trappers who came into contact with the infected animals soon became infected with the plague. The initial cases appear to have been bubonic plague. However, secondary pneumonic plague infections often ensued and soon the disease had developed as primary **pneumonic plague**. Unlike bubonic plague, which tends to be a disease of summer, pneumonic plague is often a disease of winter as close human contact helps to spread the disease. Railway workers in several northern Manchurian cities who lived in close proximity to each other soon became infected in large numbers during the winter of 1910–1911 as the disease spread along the rail line south from Manzhouli to Harbin. As was generally the case with pneumonic plague, the case fatality rate approached 100 percent, so the disease burned itself out once there was no longer a susceptible population to become infected.

The Chinese government, eager to avoid foreign criticism and to prevent the Russians from exercising control of the situation, sent the young Cambridge-trained Dr. **Wu Lien Teh** to the area to take charge of fighting the disease. Thoroughly imbued with a European approach to medicine and unable to speak Chinese, Dr. Wu imposed quarantines to limit the spread of the disease and tried to provide what palliative care that he could for those infected with the plague. The combination of quarantine and the disease burning itself out led to the control of the plague, but not before 60,000 Manchurians had died. Local authorities did not always welcome Wu's efforts, as resentment against Western methods for disease control often aroused hostility among many people, and the Western explanation for the spread of pneumonic plague confounded Chinese traditional medicine. In response to this outbreak, the Chinese government established the Manchurian Plague Prevention Service at Dr. Wu's instigation, which continued in operation until the Japanese invasion in 1931.

Manchuria was struck again by plague in 1920–1921. Like the earlier outbreak, this epidemic had a large number of primary pneumonic plague cases and originated from the Mongolian-Manchurian reservoir. The Manchurian Plague Prevention Service was able to curtail the impact of this epidemic as it had done with an epidemic in southern China in 1917–1918.

The End of the Third Pandemic.   Plague continued to be recorded throughout East Asia after the mid-1920s but in declining numbers, as only small, easily contained epidemics occurred. Even the disruptions caused by World War II did not lead to a major plague outbreak. Worldwide, the aggregate number of plague cases continued to be around 5,000 annually until 1953. During the 1950s, the number of cases declined sharply, numbering slightly more than 200 in 1959. Health authorities concluded that the third pandemic was over by 1960.

Reasons for the end of the third pandemic are hard to pinpoint. During the 1950s, several forces came to bear that helped to diminish the impact of plague. Improved sanitation and **pesticides** helped to reduce rat habitat. **Antibiotic** treatment, if started early enough, was often effective in treating bubonic plague, so death rates continued to drop. However, environmental disruption increased during the 1950s, so humans came into contact more often with environments in which sylvatic plague existed. Plague continued to be endemic in parts of Mongolia and Manchuria in 1960, but elsewhere the disease appeared to be eradicated or severely limited. *See also* Animal Diseases (Zoonoses) and Epidemic Disease; Bubonic Plague in the United States; Colonialism and Epidemic Disease; Environment, Ecology, and Epidemic Disease; Haffkine, Waldemar Mordechai; Plague in China; Plague in India and Oceania: Third Pandemic; Plague in San Francisco, 1900–1908; Plague in the Contemporary World; Simond, Paul-Louis; Trade, Travel, and Epidemic Disease.

Further Reading

Benedict, Carol. *Bubonic Plague in Nineteenth-Century China.* Stanford: Stanford University Press, 1996.

Echenberg, Myron. "Pestis Redux: The Initial Years of the Third Bubonic Plague Pandemic, 1894–1901." *Journal of World History* 13 (2002): 429–449.

Gamsu, Mark. "The Epidemic of Pneumonic Plague in Manchuria, 1910–1911." *Past & Present* 190 (2006): 147–183.

Gregg, Charles T. *Plague: An Ancient Disease in the Twentieth Century,* revised first edition. Albuquerque: University of New Mexico Press, 1985.

Hull, Terence. "Plague in Java." In *Death and Disease in Southeast Asia,* edited by Norman Owen, pp. 210–234. Singapore: Oxford University Press, 1987.

Nathan, Carl F. *Plague Prevention and Politics in Manchuria, 1910–1931.* Boston: East Asian Research Center, 1967.

Orent, Wendy. *Plague.* New York: Free Press, 2004.

Pollitzer, Robert. *Plague.* Geneva: World Health Organization, 1954.

Wu Lien-Teh. *Plague Fighter.* New York: W. Heffer and Sons, 1959.

JOHN M. THEILMANN

PLAGUE IN EUROPE, 1500–1770s. By 1500 Europe was experiencing a period of intense change: the European "Renaissance" blossomed, and the European economy boomed as a result of **trade**. Maritime and overland commerce, which had finally recovered from the fourteenth century's catastrophic plague outbreaks, produced wealth on an unprecedented scale, but at the same time, contact with the plague-devastated Near East made sure that the **Black Death** remained a very real part of European life. Europe suffered numerous outbreaks of the plague between 1500 and the 1770s. Although these were not as widespread as the first **epidemics** of 1347–1352, they continued to kill tens of thousands of people. Cities like Florence were ravaged in the sixteenth century; towns like Montelupo in Tuscany and much larger cities like Barcelona, Amsterdam, and London were hit in the seventeenth; and Marseilles and Moscow were hit with plague in the eighteenth century. By relying on detailed period records left behind by bureaucrats, who inherited the Renaissance humanists' attention to detail, and on chronicles left by an increasing number of literate artisans and middle class people, scholars are able to reconstruct the plague's movements. Such records and accounts also help contemporary scholars to quantify mortality rates for the various epidemics that struck Europe in an attempt to understand its effects and European responses to it.

Although these records allow scholars to reconstruct the plague's effects and movements, there is some debate over the causes of plague's continued presence in Europe from 1500 to the 1770s. Scholars propose two theories to explain why the plague remained a part of European life for such a long time: the "plague reservoir" theory and the "trade" theory, espoused above. Those who support the "reservoir" theory argue that the plague remained ever-present in Europe, in pockets or "reservoirs" from which it spread—quite likely from one urban area, or town, to another through interregional and international contact. The "trade" theory suggests that the plague receded or even left Europe altogether after the initial epidemics of the fourteenth century only to be reintroduced

---

THE CITY COUNCIL OF BARCELONA, SPAIN, ON THE PLAGUE OF 1651

For many days now eight or ten carts have traveled throughout Barcelona with the sole purpose of removing corpses from houses, which are often thrown from the windows into the street and then carried off in the carts by the grave diggers, who go about playing their guitars, tambourines, and other instruments in order to forget such grave afflictions, the memory alone of which is enough to want to be done with this wretched life, which seems to be worth nothing. These grave diggers stop their carts at a street corner and cry out for everyone to bring the dead from their houses, sometimes taking two from one house, four from another, and often six from another, and after filling their carts they would take the bodies to be buried in a field near the monastery of Jesus called the "bean-field." Apart from these [carts] some forty or fifty stretchers were used to carry those bodies which didn't fit in the carts, and it often happened that the grave diggers would carry dead babies or other children gravely ill with the plague on their backs. The entire city is now in such a lamentable and wretched state that men cannot even remember themselves nor can they imagine the travails they suffer. . . . Priests and confessors were missing in almost all the parishes, some having died and others being absent from the city, and as a result monks administered the sacraments in the churches and especially in certain parishes. The need was so pressing that often the priest left the church with the Holy Sacrament (may it be praised) [the Eucharist or Communion] and returned only after having given last rites to fifty or sixty or more persons, and it was beyond the strength of any one person to do so much.

From *A Journal of the Plague Year: The Diary of the Barcelona Tanner Miquel Parets, 1651,* edited by James S. Amelang (New York: Oxford University Press, 1991) pp. 106–7.

through trade contact with the Near East after 1500. Both theories provide plausible explanations for the presence of the plague in towns and urban centers throughout Europe. The fact that the plague outbreaks of the sixteenth through eighteenth centuries were mostly urban provides a stark contrast to earlier epidemics which struck city and countryside alike. There is no scholarly consensus over what caused the Black Death to become an urban epidemic as opposed to a more geographically diverse plague, and scholars are especially divided over what caused it to disappear from the European continent. The examples of plague outbreaks that follow focus on the plague in urban Europe.

In the High Renaissance, Florence, Italy, was hit with plague nine times between 1509 and 1531. During those outbreaks, Florence lost several thousand inhabitants. Combining religious practice, increasingly good medical advice, and a strong centralized government, Florence, and many other Italian cities, developed a multifaceted response to the Black Death. For example, the Florentine government set up **quarantines** and built **pest houses** to sequester the sick and dying, but it also allowed Florentine citizens to conduct religious ceremonies in order to deal with the spiritual and psychological effects of the plague. Also, the Florentine government provided assurances that its authority would remain constant: a bulwark of stability in the face of nature's uncertainties. This potent concoction of religion, practical medicine, and civic strength proved to be a recipe for public order. The Florentine example of blending of civic and religious response to outbreaks of the plague is mirrored throughout Italy. Even as the Renaissance gave way to the **Scientific Revolution** and the Enlightenment, the average Italian faced the new challenges to religion brought about by intellectual and scientific advancements in a remarkably static fashion.

One might be tempted to think, anachronistically, that the dawn of the Scientific Revolution brought an end to the importance of religion in civic attempts to deal with the plague. The small Tuscan town of Montelupo provides startling evidence to the contrary. There, during a plague outbreak of 1630–1631, local officials sought to restrict religious processions in order to halt the spread of the plague. Townspeople "revolted" against authority and sound medical advice, holding their procession as planned. People from the surrounding towns declared their support by joining the Montelupese in their procession. Strangely, as historian Carlo Cipolla noted, the townspeople's devout stubbornness, contrary to reason, seems to have had no effect on the spread of the plague in Tuscany. In fact, in broader terms, by the 1660s the plague had all but disappeared from peninsular Italy.

Throughout the seventeenth and eighteenth centuries, religion remained an important part of Italian life, but outside of Italy, the strength of the church was increasingly challenged by the emergence of centralized, national governments, including those of Spain and France. However, all of these national governments, and their local representatives, still remained remarkably similar to the Italian cities in their approaches to dealing with the plague. The difference between the Italian city-states and the emerging nation-states was primarily one of scale.

As in Italy, pest houses were one of the first methods utilized by European national, regional, and local governments to deal with the plague. Those infected with the plague were sequestered with others who had the plague in an attempt to stop the disease from spreading. There, they were given medical and spiritual attention. Many of the doctors and priests who attended sick patients became infected with plague and died. Some historians claim, however, that because plague victims were isolated in pest houses, the pestilence did not spread as quickly or as virulently.

In cases in which a plague outbreak was confined to one locale or part of a city, governmental officials often set up *cordons sanitaires*, which meant that no one was allowed in or out of an infected area. This was a cruel but probably effective method of stopping the plague's spread. Finally, often on a national level, governments instituted restrictions on trade with areas known to be infected with plague. These were meant to prohibit all types of traffic between a region infected with plague and one that remained untouched by the disease. Eighteenth-century Austria, for example, set up a *cordon sanitaire* between itself and the Ottoman East, where the plague was a constant threat.

During the 1651 outbreak of the pestilence in Barcelona, tens of thousands of people died from the disease. A tanner, Miquel Parets, left a first-hand account of the plague year that details his personal loss and his anger at local officials for shunning their duties. He argued that the social and governmental elite of the city, rather than caring for the sick and seeking to prevent the spread of the plague, neglected all of their civic and religious duties, instead fleeing to the countryside to avoid death. Parets, echoing the sentiment of fourteenth-century plague chroniclers, noted that the plague destroyed the basis of Barcelona's social structure, the family. He knew this intimately, as he lost his wife and three children to the plague. Eventually, the local government set up quarantines, pest houses, and rigorous attempts to rid the city of "infected" clothing and the dead. Barcelona experienced only one more, relatively minor, plague outbreak in 1653. The initial and rather inept manner in which the plague outbreak was handled in Barcelona is characteristic of plague outbreaks throughout Europe in the seventeenth and even eighteenth centuries. Once governmental officials, in Barcelona and elsewhere, rigorously implemented plague preventatives, the outbreak nearly always ended.

The French city of Marseilles suffered a plague epidemic in 1720 and 1721 that took the lives of over 40,000 victims. Records indicate that the Marseillaise officials initially dealt with the outbreak much like their counterparts in Barcelona. However, the outbreak at Marseilles could have been dealt with more efficiently. Early on, local doctors knew that Marseilles was experiencing a virulent outbreak of plague, but governmental officials refused to act on their **diagnosis** and advice. In fact, the government even rejected local doctors' pleas to isolate plague victims and quarantine those under suspicion. When the officials finally decided to take action, it was too late; the plague had already killed thousands. But, once measures were put in place to deal with the plague, including quarantines, pesthouses, and a *cordon sanitaire*, the plague subsided and disappeared. By 1722 the last major plague outbreak in western Europe, which killed half of Marseilles's population and a sizable number of Provence's residents, was over. From there, the plague retreated to Russia where it was greeted in the Marseillaise fashion. The Tsarist government in Russia denied that the plague was affecting its chief city, Moscow, until it became obvious to Muscovites and foreigners alike that they were indeed dealing with a virulent plague outbreak.

The refusal by the Russian government to deal with the plague outbreak, let alone to provide for precautionary measures against it, led to a large number of deaths. Eventually, as with Marseilles, Muscovite governmental officials realized that they had to implement measures to stop the plague. They ordered large sections of the city to be cordoned off and burned to get rid of plague victims, their homes, and everything associated with the outbreak. The vast majority of those who died from the plague were urban (and rural) poor, and as the deaths mounted, so too did their frustration. They did not want the government to destroy their homes, nor did they want to die from plague. Riots broke out throughout

Moscow and the surrounding districts, and the Russian government responded with heavy-handed tactics. Protestors and rioters alike were mowed down with cannon balls and musket volleys. The rioters were subdued, and "slums" were burned or cleansed. It is quite likely that 50,000 to 70,000 Russians died between the years 1770 and 1772. This outbreak in Russia represented the last major occurrence of plague in Europe, ending a long and deadly relationship.

There are a number of theories that attempt to explain the disappearance of the Black Death from Europe in the 1770s. These theories are as varied as mutation of the disease into a less virulent strain or perhaps changes in climate that made Europe an unsuitable environment for the disease. Although scholars continue to debate the nature and type of disease that killed millions in Europe over a 300-year period, one contributing factor that most agree led to the plague's disappearance seems to have been human intervention. Even though it often took governmental officials too long to respond to outbreaks of plague in their municipalities, once decisive action was taken, cases of the plague became increasingly infrequent. At first, the plague was eradicated on a local level, but by the 1770s, through intervention and prevention programs, the Black Death had disappeared from Europe. *See also* Apothecary/Pharmacist; Black Death, Economic and Demographic Effects of; Black Death: Modern Medical Debate; Bubonic Plague; Contagion Theory of Disease, Premodern; Corpses and Epidemic Disease; Diagnosis of Historical Diseases; Disinfection and Fumigation; Flight; Historical Epidemiology; Hospitals

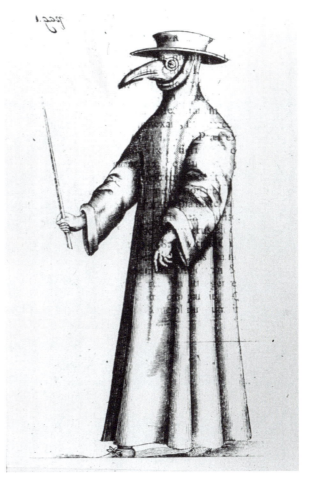

Plague doctor. The hat, mask suggestive of a bird beak, goggles or glasses, and long gown identify the person as a "plague doctor" and are intended as protection. Descriptions indicate that the gown was made from heavy fabric or leather and was usually waxed. The beak contained pungent herbs or perfumes, thought to purify the air and relieve the stench. The pointer or rod was intended to keep patients at a distance. Courtesy of the National Library of Medicine.

in the West to 1900; Humoral Theory; London, Great Plague of (1665–1666); Medical Education in the West, 1500–1900; Paracelsianism; Plague and Developments in Public Health, 1348–1600; Plague: End of the Second Pandemic; Plague in Britain, 1500–1647; Plague in Medieval Europe, 1360–1500; Plague in the Islamic World, 1500–1850; Plague Literature and Art, Early Modern European; Plague Memorials; Pneumonic and Septicemic

Plague; Public Health Boards in the West before 1900; Religion and Epidemic Disease; Thirty Years' War; Urbanization and Epidemic Disease.

Further Reading

Alexander, John T. *Bubonic Plague in Early Modern Russia: Public Health and Urban Disaster.* Baltimore: Johns Hopkins University Press, 1980.

Ansari, B. M. "An Account of Bubonic Plague in Seventeenth-Century India in an Autobiography of a Mughal Emperor." *Journal of Infection* 29 (1994): 351–352.

Bertrand, Jean Baptiste. *A Historical Relation of the Plague at Marseilles in the Year 1720.* New York: McGraw-Hill, 1973.

Byrne, Joseph P. *Daily Life during the Black Death.* Westport, CT: Greenwood Press, 2006.

Cipolla, Carlo M. *Faith Reason and the Plague in Seventeenth-Century Tuscany.* New York: W. W. Norton, 1981.

Cohn, Samuel K. *The Black Death Transformed: Disease and Culture in Early Renaissance Europe.* London: Hodder Arnold, 2003.

De Mertens, Charles. *Account of the Plague Which Raged at Moscow 1771.* Newtonville, MA: Oriental Research Partners, 1977.

Kostis, K. P. "In Search of the Plague. The Greek Peninsula Faces the Black Death, 14th to 19th Centuries." *Dynamis* 18 (1998): 465–478.

Martin, A. Lynn. *Plague?: Jesuit Accounts of Epidemic Disease in the 16th Century.* Kirksville, MO: Truman State University Press, 1996.

Naphy, William G., and Andrew Spicer. *The Black Death and the History of Plagues, 1345–1730.* Stroud, UK: Tempus, 2001.

Parets, Miquel. *A Journal of the Plague Year: The Diary of the Barcelona Tanner Miquel Parets.* Translated and edited by James S. Amelang. New York: Oxford University Press, 2001.

Velimirovic, Boris, and Helga. "Plague in Vienna." *Review of Infectious Diseases* 2 (1989): 808–830.

WILLIAM LANDON

PLAGUE IN INDIA AND OCEANIA: THIRD PANDEMIC. In the last decade of the nineteenth century, **bubonic plague** traveled from China to Hong Kong, and thence to Bombay. From this metropolis, India's "first city," plague spread to other parts of the country within four years. By 1930, 12 million persons had succumbed to the disease.

The priority in British colonial medical policy, hitherto, had been to preserve the health of the Europeans and keep **epidemics** from spreading to their quarters in towns and cities, from the areas inhabited by Indians. Rural regions were beyond the concern of the imperial power. The British attributed epidemic diseases, which they considered endemic to India, initially to the **environment** and then to the "habits" of their subjects. When plague struck Bombay, in September 1896, the authorities knew nothing of its etiology, nor how to treat the disease. It had struck at a premier port and administrative center of British India. The fear was that Bombay, with such extensive commercial intercourse with Europe, would threaten the whole world with a revival of the frightful scourge of earlier times. It was not long before it spread by land and by sea to other parts of the province— to Ahmedabad in September, and Karachi and Poona by December—along the lines of communication. Until 1900 plague was an urban phenomenon, but as each of the more populous towns became a focus for disseminating infection into the surrounding areas, it spread from city to village and from village to village.

The colonial government consequently resorted to drastic controls to prevent its spread and empowered itself with the Epidemic Diseases Act of 1897 to enforce them. The first measure to be implemented was mass **disinfection**, on an unprecedented scale, with potassium permanganate, phenyl, lime chloride, sulfur fumigation, with the pouring of carbolic acid down drains, and even with the burning of fires to rid the air of plague germs. This was in keeping with the **miasmic** theory of the cause of disease, then prevalent. The other steps taken included the inspection of houses in which plague victims resided, the opening up of the roofs of houses, marking them "UHH" (unfit for human habitation) and sometimes even burning them down. The afflicted were subjected to medical examination, and their clothing and bedding were destroyed. Those exposed to the infection were segregated in health camps, and the plague victims hospitalized. Restrictions were imposed on road and rail **travel** within the country, and passengers were subjected to examination at railway stations and to detention at **quarantine** camps. The British authorities also prohibited fairs and **pilgrimages**, which they saw as breeding grounds of disease. As for foreign travel, quarantine was imposed against Bombay's port and, with the outbreak in Karachi, against all Indian ports. The Haj to Mecca by Muslim Indians was also prohibited for some time. When quarantine was lifted, all outbound vessels were inspected, their holds cleaned with lime wash, the crews medically examined, and their clothing disinfected.

This intervention was unparalleled: never before had the medical establishment wielded such power. The British ascribed the plague to the conditions in which they perceived Indians to be living: filthy, with poor ventilation, open drains, and overcrowding in the growing cities. The other causative factor, according to the British perspective, was Indian customs, prejudices, and the "native" remedies to which the people resorted. The real culprit was said to be the Indians' poor stamina, lack of **immunity**, and **poverty**, whereas it was observed that the European was surprisingly immune. There was the usual blame game within the establishment; the sanitary commissioner of India blamed the government of Bombay for ignoring his suggestions. On the other hand, the Indians' perception was ambivalent: some regarded plague as a judgment from God, whereas a practitioner of **ayurveda** ascribed it to the consumption of acids, salts, and bitter, in excess, and to the inhaling of damp **air**. The local **press**, publishing in the regional languages, held the municipal authorities squarely responsible, for neglecting drainage in the city of Bombay.

The anti-plague operations were more intense in the cities and towns than in the rural areas, and hence the resistance was also urban-based. The population of Bombay halved, as people fled in panic. The draconian steps met with vigorous opposition from Indians, who perceived them as culture and gender insensitive. The inspection of homes by soldiers was considered an invasion of domestic privacy, whereas the enforced segregation went against the local traditions of relatives' caring for patients. Hospitalization was looked upon as polluting: hospitals were places where caste, religious and *purdah* observances, and food and drink prescriptions were violated. It was generally believed that people went there to die. Furthermore, it was rumored that the hearts of plague patients would be taken out to be sent to Queen Victoria (1819–1901), who had been angered by the disfigurement of her statue by protestors. The "body" was seen to have been violated with the examination of the arm pits of both men and women for the presence of buboes. In the case of the latter it was considered a dishonor that male doctors performed the examination. The extracts from contemporary newspapers show the extent of opposition, despair, and anger. One example plaintively stated that it seemed the "body" belonged to the master (meaning the colonial power) and not to the slave. Inspections were evaded, and the infectious diseases hospital raided. This opposition is also to be seen in the background of a rising national consciousness against British rule, and thus the enforcement of measures was perceived as one more instance of the colonial state's high-handedness and arrogance.

Yet Indian responses were not all negative and by no means uniform, even within communities. In fact, the great nationalist leader Lokamanya Tilak (1856–1920) endorsed segregation of the infected and alluded to the superstitious folly of those who regarded hospitals as chambers of death. The newspapers he was associated with, *Maratha* and *Kesari*, regularly reported the havoc caused by the enforcement of anti-plague steps in the city of Poona. It was against the manner in which the medical intervention was carried out that he protested. The plague commissioner of Poona, W. C. Rand, was so unpopular that he was assassinated. Among the Muslims in Bombay, there were contrary reactions: whereas some such as the Ismaili Khojas, led by the Aga Khan (1877–1957) were cooperative, others saw the closure of mosques and burial grounds as religious interference. Bodies of victims were sprinkled with disinfectants and cremated, contrary to the community's burial prescription. The political leader, Badruddin Tyabji (1844–1906) explained to his fellow Muslims, at a public meeting, why these measures had been adopted. Because people had been refusing medicine, food, and drink when they did go into hospitals, caste and community hospitals were opened in the cities of Bombay province. These were for the exclusive use of these groups and were founded at Indian initiative and with Indian funding.

Within months of the outbreak, **Waldemar Haffkine**, the Russian bacteriologist assigned by the government of India to investigate the causes and to devise a method to deal with this reemergent disease, developed a prophylactic in a Bombay laboratory. Though Haffkine faced the intrigues and hostility of the British Indian Medical Service officers, who had a monopoly in the medical establishment, he persevered in perfecting the vaccine. The Aga Khan endorsed it, and his community, the Ismaili Khojas, was among the first to accept the prophylactic, both in Bombay and in Karachi. Various leading medical practitioners including Bhalchandra Krishna Bhatvadekar (1852–1922), chairman of the standing committee of the Bombay municipal corporation, propagated it in newspapers, explaining its efficacy. Medical organizations such as the Bombay Medical Union and the Grant College Medical Society endorsed the vaccine. Haffkine was made director of the Plague Research Laboratory, (PRL) in 1899, and by 1901, 8,601,123 doses of the plague vaccine had been produced and sent out to different regions of India. However, a setback to its propagation occurred, when an accident took place in 1902, at Malkowal, a village in Punjab. Nineteen vaccinated persons died of tetanus. Although this incident cost Haffkine his job, he was later exonerated when the commission of inquiry found that the contamination of the vaccine had not happened in his laboratory. The accident diminished the demand for the vaccine in the Punjab for a while, but not elsewhere. Doctors were deputed to Bombay, from both British India and the princely states, to study inoculation at the PRL.

The vigorous opposition to anti-plague measures led to a change in colonial policy, and the enforcement of controls was abandoned from the 1900s. It was then decided to promote preventive steps, with the support of the people. Inoculation was propagated by voluntary organizations involved in health care, through lectures accompanied by magic lantern demonstrations (early forms of slide shows), and through the publication of pamphlets, and the harmlessness of the vaccine was explained at citizens' meetings. That inoculation was done by Indian doctors made it more acceptable, and its endorsement by leaders, such as Tilak and the other nationalist Gopal Krishna Gokhale (1866–1915), made it acceptable in the small towns and districts. Editors of regional-language newspapers were taken around the Bombay Bacteriological Laboratory, as the PRL was renamed in 1906, to see for themselves the method of the preparation of the vaccine. They then wrote papers explaining the procedures and discounting rumors. The Plague Research Commission, a body appointed by the government to determine the causes of the recurrent plague epidemics, showed in its 1908 report that the bubonic plague infection depended on the extent of the disease in the rat. Plague spread among rats and from rat to man through the rat flea *Xenopyslla cheopis*. Subsequently, rat destruction was adopted on a war footing, and the municipalities employed rat brigades.

Plague was never able to invade all of India. The most striking feature was its extremely uneven and irregular distribution: Assam and Eastern Bengal were immune. This was discovered to be the result of the plague flea, which breeds most freely and lives longest in the debris of cereals; thus, places with a link with the grain trade were affected. By the 1930s, some control had been achieved over the disease.

Plague also struck Sydney, Australia, in 1900, but there were only a total of 1,363 cases during the twentieth century, a huge contrast to India. An expert staff was trained in Sydney to search out plague rats, which were found in wharves, warehouses, shops, stables, and dilapidated cottages. The produce trade in hay, straw, chaff, and animal foodstuffs was found to be closely associated with plague rats. Plague, however, did not spread all over Sydney, thanks to the efforts of President of the Board of Health Dr. J. Ashburton Thompson (1846–1914), and investigations showed that it was confined to a very limited area. *See also* Colonialism and Epidemic Disease; Disease, Social Construction of; Flight; Plague in Africa: Third Pandemic; Plague in China; Plague in East Asia: Third Pandemic; Plague in the Contemporary World; Pneumonic Plague in Surat, Gujarat, India, 1994; Public Health Agencies in Britain since 1800; Trade, Travel, and Epidemic Disease; Vaccination and Inoculation.

Further Reading

Arnold, David. *Colonizing the Body: State Medicine and Epidemic Disease in Nineteenth Century India.* Berkeley: University of California Press, 1993.

Catanach, Ian. "Plague and the Tensions of Empire: India, 1896–1918." In *Imperial Medicine and Indigenous Societies,* edited by David Arnold, pp. 149–71. New York: Manchester University Press, 1988.

Chandavarkar, Raj. *Imperial Power and Popular Politics.* New York: Cambridge University Press, 1998.

Harrison, Mark. *Public Health in British India: Anglo-Indian Preventive Medicine, 1859–1914.* New York: Cambridge University Press, 1994.

Hirst, Fabian. *The Conquest of Plague: A Study of the Evolution of Epidemiology.* Oxford: The Clarendon Press, 1953.

Ramanna, Mridula. "Plague in Bombay: Responses to Colonial Authority Control Measures." *Wellcome History* 35 (Summer 2007): 2–4.

MRIDULA RAMANNA

PLAGUE IN MEDIEVAL EUROPE, 1360–1500. In 1360, a decade after the **Black Death**, the second wave of the second **bubonic plague pandemic** hit Europe, and major outbreaks recurred roughly every decade to 1500. The mortality rates of the 1360 plague and subsequent outbreaks were never as high as during the 1347–1352 plague years. As in the 1347–1352 plague years, later outbreaks killed people in all age groups, but they were particularly unsettling because they included a disproportionate number of infants, children, and adolescents. This disparity caused some modern scholars to question whether the "Black Death" was actually the bubonic plague or another disease or set of diseases. Whatever the cause, Europe's once populous countryside was nearly emptied, and city populations, too, were thinned from successive plague outbreaks, which kept Europe's population well below pre-plague levels. This depopulation initially crippled Europe's economy, but by 1500, it had recovered, far surpassing the pre-plague economy. Demographic and economic effects like these were accompanied by secular and religious responses to the Black Death; especially civic attempts to deal with the perceived causes of the plague and religious fervor that sought to remedy the spiritual effects of sin manifested by the plague.

The second wave of the plague appears to have killed mainly those Europeans who were born after the first outbreak of the Black Death. The traditional argument to explain the 1360 plague's focused mortality states that the generation that survived the first wave of plague may have developed at least some temporary immunity to it. So, when the plague reappeared in 1360, the adult population was often able to fend it off, but the young population was unable to cope. Others argue that the changes to the age structure of the European population as a result of the Black Death and the resulting natalism left a greater number of children and adolescents at risk when plague epidemics recurred.

The European economy, at first ravaged by the plague, eventually benefited from the dramatic decrease in the supply of laborers. For example, after the plague struck, arable land, which was at a premium, became more accessible in rural Europe after successive waves of plague. Economic historians argue that this abundance of land, combined with advances in agricultural technology, allowed fewer Europeans to produce surpluses of grain. This, in turn, meant a better-fed and healthier population as a whole. And, in the years following the 1360 plague outbreak, in real terms, urban wages increased dramatically which meant that the population that survived the plague had access to greater wealth. The rise in urban and rural wages is explained by "demand" which outstripped the supply of labor. After a brief period of inflation, by 1400 Europe's economy adjusted and expanded well beyond its pre-plague zenith. These direct effects of plague were accompanied by secular and religious responses to the epidemic.

In an attempt to deal with the "bad **air**" or "miasma" that was thought to contribute to spreading the plague, some European cities and towns focused on removing anything that produced a noxious smell, especially when plague had been reported in the neighborhood. Refuse was collected, streets were cleaned, tanners' shops and slaughterhouses were required to remove animal byproducts from city centers to outlying regions, and human waste was dealt with more promptly. City ordinances such as these were not based upon biological or epidemiological foundations. Rather, they were based upon medieval medical concepts that today seem quaint, but cleaner cities nevertheless meant less disease.

Religion also reacted to and changed with the plague. Although religious responses varied by region, nearly all of Europe accepted the plague as God's judgment. The 1360 epidemic seemed especially biblical in nature, visiting God's judgment on the second generation—those who were born after the Black Death struck in 1347. Continued outbreaks of plague led many Europeans to believe that Christ could not be their intercessor and their judge at the same time. So, as with artistic responses to the Black Death, many Europeans turned to pre-plague traditions that they modified to make sense of and remedy the plague. The cult of the Virgin and the cult of the saints, both of which existed before the plague, provided the spiritual balm that Europeans craved. The Virgin interceded on behalf of the faithful, and the saints, especially St. Sebastian, were thought to provide spiritual and physical protection from the plague. These "cults," linked with penance and processions provided comfort to Europeans in the uncertainty brought on by the Black Death.

Between the years 1360 and 1500, the Black Death killed hundreds of thousands of Europeans. Nearly every European was touched by the plague, and nearly everyone lost a friend or relative to it. Although the Black Death certainly affected medieval Europe demographically, it also brought about new economic, civic, and religious responses, which allowed Europe to begin a long period of recovery to which the Renaissance bears witness. *See also* Black Death and related articles; Contagion Theory of Disease, Premodern; Diagnosis of Historical Diseases; Flight; Historical Epidemiology; Human Immunity and Resistance to Disease; Medical Education in the West, 1100–1500; Pest Houses and Lazarettos; Plague and Developments in Public Health, 1348–1600; Plague in China; Plague in the Islamic World, 1360–1500; Quarantine.

Further Reading

Byrne, Joseph P. *Daily Life During the Black Death.* Westport, CT: Greenwood Press, 2006.

Cohn, Samuel K. *The Black Death Transformed: Disease and Culture in Early Renaissance Europe.* London: Arnold, 2002.

Herlihy, David. *The Black Death and the Transformation of the West.* Cambridge, MA: Harvard University Press, 1997.

WILLIAM LANDON

PLAGUE IN SAN FRANCISCO, 1900–1908. The San Francisco **epidemic** of **bubonic plague** comprised part of the **Third Pandemic** that had ravaged South and East Asia since the mid-nineteenth century. In 1894 **Alexandre Yersin** and **Shibasaburo Kitasato** had independently identified the *Yersinia pestis* bacterium responsible for plague's spread. In 1897 **Paul-Louis Simond** theorized the rat-to-flea-to-human transmission of plague. Many members of the United States medical community doubted this theory until later in the decade, however, and postulated other causes for its spread, including infection through contaminated dust, and racial susceptibility, particularly among Asians.

Bubonic plague arrived in Honolulu, Hawaii, in 1899, spread by ships that harbored rats infested with infected fleas. On January 2, 1900, the ship *Australia* landed at San Francisco's Angel Island **quarantine** station, bringing goods from Honolulu. After fumigation and quarantine, the *Australia* entered San Francisco's port. However, it unknowingly transported infected rats into the city.

On March 6, 1900, Wong Chut King (b. 1859) was discovered dead in the basement of a Chinatown Hotel. His death exacerbated existing prejudices toward Chinese civilians, who had long been perceived as threats to local whites. San Francisco officials responded with a total isolation of Chinatown. They repealed it, however, after three days, stating that there was no conclusive proof of plague. Joseph Kinyoun (1866–1919), a federal bacteriologist and quarantine officer for the U.S. Marine Hospital Service, forerunner of the U.S. Public Health Service, stationed at Angel Island, confirmed plague. Hoping to avoid panic and financial ruin, city officials demanded that he remain silent.

Despite official denials, plague continued to spread. On May 15, Kinyoun carried out orders from Surgeon General Walter Wyman (1848–1911) to cordon off suspected areas of Chinatown, inspect all Chinese houses, isolate suspected plague victims on Angel Island, and inoculate all Chinese residents with the **Haffkine** vaccine, a dangerous and unpopular treatment. However, Chinese community leaders challenged the orders. On May 28, Judge William Morrow ruled that the restrictions discriminated unfairly against Chinese civilians. The state of California instituted a second quarantine, but by mid-June the courts had again struck it down.

In August 1900, Kinyoun recorded the first reported cases of bubonic plague among white San Franciscans. By the end of 1900, however, there were only 22 officially documented cases, and many locals continued to deny plague.

By 1901 Kinyoun's public and discriminatory responses to plague had alienated both local leaders and the Chinese community. To settle the acrimony, Surgeon General Wyman appointed a panel of national experts to inspect San Francisco. In February 1901, this panel examined suspected cases and confirmed bubonic plague conclusively. Hoping to stifle their findings, California's Governor, Henry Gage (1852–1924), struck a deal with Surgeon General Wyman. Gage promised to work with federal officials in exchange for keeping the panel's report private.

In April 1901, Wyman replaced the maligned Kinyoun with Rupert Blue (1868–1948), another physician with the Marine Hospital Service. Blue worked more closely with Chinatown leaders and hired an interpreter and go-between to the Chinese community. Blue tried to relax suspicions among the Chinese community and rejected some of his predecessor's harsher measures. He also tested new theories that linked rats to the spread of plague. Blue's new approaches did not immediately stifle plague. Although new infections slowed in 1901, reported cases grew in summer 1902.

In October 1902, and again in January 1903, U.S. public health leaders met at national conferences and censured Governor Gage for suppressing evidence of the outbreak. At the second meeting, furious officials recommended a nationwide boycott of California unless the state ceded control over the plague campaign to federal officials. The newly elected governor, George Pardee (1857–1941), assented to these demands and allowed Blue free rein. Blue employed fumigation, rat eradication, and improvements of buildings to destroy rat breeding grounds. He also used anti-serum rather than **vaccinations**, a more expensive but much less risky form of therapy. With these measures in place, the last reported case appeared on February 19, 1904.

By fall 1904, city officials lobbied Wyman to lift federal intervention. Although Blue urged caution, Wyman withdrew him on April 4, 1905. Blue's concerns would be substantiated in 1907, when a second wave of bubonic plague struck San Francisco, just a year after the city's great earthquake. By then, however, San Franciscans were quick to call on the federal government for assistance. Blue returned to San Francisco, his com-

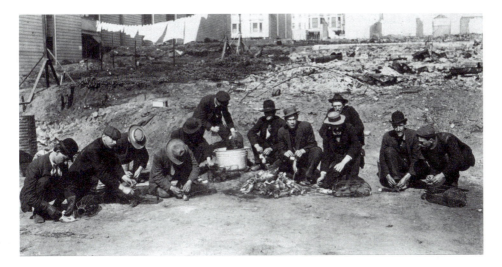

Tagging the morning's catch. Twelve rat-catchers attach tags to dead rats to identify where, when, and by whom they were collected. A man in the center dips a rat trap into a bucket of antiseptic solution. Photo taken between 1907 and 1909. Courtesy of the National Library of Medicine.

mitment to the theory of the rat flea vector reinforced by a 1906 confirmation of Simond's theory by the British plague commission in India. Supported by local groups like the Citizens' Health Commission, Blue's second campaign focused on exterminating rats and on early treatment. The last reported case of plague came in March 1908, bringing the final tally for both epidemics to 280 reported cases and 172 deaths.

As illustrated by city, state, and federal responses, political and economic imperatives initially took precedence over public health tactics. City and state leaders denied the existence of plague because they feared its impacts on commerce. Civic and public health officials **scapegoated** the city's Chinese community, whose members they considered racially susceptible to disease. Targeted quarantines, vaccinations, and cleanups of Chinatown resulted in significant Chinese distrust of the public health community and a failure to admit the existence of plague in other parts of the city. *See also* Bubonic Plague in the United States; Plague in China; Plague in East Asia: Third Pandemic; Plague in India and Oceania: Third Pandemic; Race, Ethnicity, and Epidemic Disease.

Further Reading

Chase, Marilyn. *The Barbary Plague: The Black Death in Victorian San Francisco*. New York: Random House, 2003.

Craddock, Susan. *City of Plagues: Disease, Poverty, and Deviance in San Francisco*. Minneapolis: University of Minnesota Press, 2000.

Shah, Nayan. *Contagious Divides: Epidemics and Race in San Francisco's Chinatown*. Berkeley: University of California Press, 2001.

JULIA F. IRWIN

PLAGUE IN THE CONTEMPORARY WORLD. After the end of the **third plague pandemic** around 1960, plague did not simply vanish, although it causes far fewer deaths in the early twenty-first century than such waterborne diseases as **cholera**. **Bubonic plague** remains endemic in central and east Asia, Africa, and North and South America with continued animal infections in areas such as Mongolia, China, the Democratic Republic of the Congo, Ecuador, and the four corners region of the American Southwest. There have continued to be episodic outbreaks since 1960, most notably in South Vietnam during the 1960s, and scattered outbreaks in diverse regions of the globe such as the Democratic Republic of the Congo, Madagascar, and Ecuador. In addition, **pneumonic plague** also remains a threat in various regions. The plague is still regarded as a major public health hazard, and the **World Health Organization** (WHO) requires immediate notification of national and international public health bodies when cases are diagnosed.

The *Yersinia pestis* **bacterium** has developed 76 strains of three biovars (biotypes), and all three biovars continue to be present in the wild. Biovar Orientalis is the most common and is endemic in North America, South America, Asia, and India, whereas biovar Medievalis is endemic in central Asia, and biovar Antiqua is endemic in Africa. Most scientists agree that biovar Orientalis has evolved from either biovar Antiqua (responsible for the **Plague of Justinian**) or biovar Medievalis (responsible for the **Black Death**), or both. There is now some indication that a fourth biovar, Microtus, may have evolved in China in the late twentieth century. Bubonic plague was introduced during the third plague pandemic into some regions where it is now endemic, such as the United States and Madagascar.

By 1959 the number of plague cases annually reported worldwide had declined to slightly more than 200, down from nearly 5,000 in 1953. **Pesticides** and rodenticides helped to produce the decline, killing both fleas and rats, the traditional hosts for the plague bacillus. Mortality rates also declined during the 1950s, reflecting the increased use of **antibiotics** and sulfa drugs as well as better patient care. Thereafter mortality rates continued to decline and hover between 4 and 10 percent. These figures are somewhat deceptive, however, because some outbreaks still produce mortality rates of 50 percent or higher. Generally the outbreaks of bubonic plague that produce high mortality rates are combined with cases of pneumonic plague, which still produces mortality rates of over 90 percent if not treated immediately. Plague vaccines continue to be developed and have proven widely effective in preventing plague outbreaks and limiting the mortality rate for those people infected.

Like many other disease-causing microorganisms, however, *Yersinia pestis* is developing resistance to antibiotics. During an outbreak of bubonic and pneumonic plague in Madagascar from 1996 to 1998, several cases displayed a resistance to treatment with chloramphenicol and ampicillin, two commonly used antibiotics. Plague in the early twenty-first century continues to display wide diversity in its ability to infect humans and in the mortality rate of those people infected. Most cases of bubonic plague have been treatable with antibiotics, as have cases of pneumonic plague, when the treatment is started almost immediately. Some cases are not always readily diagnosed, often leading to fatalities because treatment is started too late to be effective.

Another issue remains troubling. During World War II, the Japanese military began the development of biological weapons. Unit 731 went so far as to field test bubonic plague weapons in China. After the end of the war several countries continued to develop plague as a biological weapon. The Soviet Union developed the most extensive plague arsenal, although the Russian state—along with the United States and the United Kingdom—has renounced biological warfare. Plague is more difficult to deliver than anthrax, but its potential as a weapon for a rogue state or a terrorist group cannot be discounted.

Plague during the Vietnam War.   The outbreak of plague in Vietnam during the 1960s illustrates the impact of **environmental** factors on plague as well as an aggressive plague prevention campaign. *Yersinia pestis* was endemic in Southeast Asia but seemed to be under control until the Vietnam War broke out. Between 1965 and 1970, more than 25,000 cases of plague were officially reported in South Vietnam, although the actual total was many times higher. This outbreak was the first major epidemic to occur after the use of insecticides for killing fleas, which are the carrier of the *Yersinia pestis* bacteria, and antibiotics for treatment, suggesting that plague epidemics are still possible under the right set of circumstances.

As part of its strategy in the Vietnam War, the United States engaged in a major use of defoliants that helped to force the Vietnamese people off the land. South Vietnam had been a major rice exporter in 1964 but was a net importer the next year because of the damage caused by defoliation. As people moved into refugee camps, they entered surroundings that were ripe for epidemics because of overcrowding and poor sanitation. Once American troops began to withdraw in the early 1970s, the number of plague cases declined as the refugee camps were dispersed.

American troops were required to receive a series of anti-plague **vaccinations**, although cases were reported among U.S. troops, as among military support and civilian personnel, because they were not always up to date with their vaccinations. Almost all American troops infected by bubonic plague survived.

The South Vietnamese people were not so lucky. Many of the refugee camps had poor sanitation, and rats were common, although some efforts were made to apply insecticides. Plague once again infected Vietnamese cities such as Hue in 1965 even though the last reported case had been in that city in 1950. As a general rule, however, this epidemic struck rural areas more heavily than urban areas; otherwise, the mortality rate might have been higher. Although reported plague cases exceeded 5,000 late in the decade, mortality rates remained low. This was the result of both the relatively low virulence of the strain of plague in the country and the use of antibiotics in treating the disease. Charles Gregg indicates that there were between 100,000 and 250,000 plague cases in South Vietnam in the decade after 1964, probably more cases than occurred in Indochina during the Third Pandemic. In this case the environmental changes produced by war helped to lead to the outbreak of the plague epidemic in a country in which the disease was endemic.

United States.   Bubonic plague first came to the United States during the third pandemic and has remained endemic in some regions of the West ever since. Plague in the United States remains a western phenomenon, with almost all cases originating west of the 100th meridian. Generally, cases in the eastern United States, such as one in Greenville, South Carolina, in 1984, have originated in the West. Prairie dogs, ground squirrels, and rabbits, rather than rats, provide the most common hosts for the fleas carrying *Yersinia pestis* in the United States. As Americans increasingly enjoyed the open spaces of the West after 1970, they increasingly came into contact with animals infected with bubonic plague, and the number of diagnosed cases increased during the 1970s. Although disturbing, the number of U.S. cases is lower than that in Asia or Africa. WHO reported only two cases in the United States in 2002, one in 2003, and only 61 total from 1997–2003. The mortality rate in the United States ran slightly over 10 percent in the 1970s and 1980s, in part because of misdiagnoses that led to failure to treat the disease properly until it was already too late.

Plague around the World.   Natural plague foci exist in several regions of the world. Since 1980 most cases of the plague have been found in 20 countries worldwide, especially in the Democratic Republic of the Congo, Madagascar, Ecuador, and Peru with scattered cases elsewhere including the United States, India, Kazakstan, and Mongolia. In 1997, for example, WHO reported 5,519 cases (2,863 in Madagascar) with 274 fatalities. By 2003 the number had declined to 2,118 cases (181 fatalities). Although bubonic plague presents regional health hazards, secondary and primary pneumonic plague that result from an initial infection, coupled with the ease of travel, make it possible for plague to spread beyond regions where it is endemic. In 2003, 11 plague cases were diagnosed in Algeria, the first cases in 50 years. During 2006, 1,174 cases of pneumonic plague with 50 deaths occurred in the Congo, illustrating the impact of an existing plague reservoir combined with poor sanitation. There are too many natural plague reservoirs and too many different hosts for us to expect the eradication of the disease. Improved sanitation, public health facilities, and antibiotic treatment have reduced this threat. Nonetheless, severe ecological disruption in a natural focus region and the threat of bioterrorism continue to present the specter of another plague epidemic. *See also* Animal Diseases (Zoonoses) and Epidemic Disease; Biological Warfare; Bubonic Plague in the United States; Drug Resistance in Microorganisms; Plague in Africa: Third Pandemic; Public Health Agencies, U.S. Federal; War, the Military, and Epidemic Disease.

Further Reading

Dennis, David T., et al. *Plague Manual: Epidemiology, Distribution, Surveillance, and Control.* Geneva: World Health Organization, 1999; available at http:www.who.int.emc.

Gage, Kenneth L., and Michael Y. Kosoy. "Natural History of Plague: Perspectives from More than a Century of Research." *Annual Review of Entomology* 50 (2005): 505–528.

Gregg, Charles T. *Plague: An Ancient Disease in the Twentieth Century*, revised first edition. Albuquerque: University of New Mexico Press, 1985.

Orent, Wendy. *Plague.* New York: Free Press, 2004.

JOHN M. THEILMANN

PLAGUE IN THE ISLAMIC WORLD, 1360–1500.   The first fully recorded plague outbreak in the Middle East was the **pandemic** known as the **Plague of Justinian**, named after the sixth-century Byzantine emperor. For the next 200 years or so, plague recurred in the area at intervals that ranged from 9 to 13 years. Then, for reasons unknown, it disappeared, both from the Middle East and from Europe until 1347, when the **Black Death** pandemic ravaged both regions. Following this outbreak, plague continued to recur regularly in the Middle East and North Africa until its suppression in the late nineteenth century. At one time or another, these recurrences affected most Islamic communities in southwestern Asia, North Africa, and the Iberian Peninsula. During the medieval period, 1360 to1500, plague was recorded as far afield as Astrakhan (southeast Russia) in 1364; Astarabad (Iran, southeast of the Caspian Sea) in 1435; Herat (western Afghanistan) in 1435 and 1464; Yemen in 1438; and Tabriz (northwest Iran) in 1487.

Late medieval visitations of the plague were so idiosyncratic that neither Muslim nor Christian **physicians** and theologians could determine the etiology of the disease, and consequently no cure was found for it. **Islamic medical theory** attributed the disease to a **miasma**, whereas religious opinion regarded it as a divine mercy and martyrdom for Muslims. Viewing plague as an act of God, most Muslim physicians did not advise the avoidance of infected areas; the Prophet Muhammad (570–632) himself had denied the existence of **contagion** and enjoined his followers neither to enter nor flee an affected area. There were, however, those who disagreed: **Rhazes**, the renowned ninth-century Baghdad physician, advocated **flight**, and in Muslim Spain, Ibn al-Khatib (1313–1375), a fourteenth-century Arab physician from Granada (unjustly accused of heresy and put to death in 1375) spoke out openly against prevailing religious ideas on contagion. He recognized that plague outbreaks occurred after the arrival of people from infected areas, and noted that people who were not exposed to epidemics, such as those in prison or nomads in the desert, did not catch the disease. To prove his point, Ibn al-Khatib gave the example of a man in Sale (on the Atlantic coast of Morocco) who escaped the plague by confining himself and his household behind walls, with plenty of food and drink, and refusing to leave until the plague had disappeared.

In 1360 Islamic communities in the Middle East were still suffering from the effects of the Black Death, which had greatly reduced their numbers. However, it is the cumulative effect of later recurring epidemics that accelerated this reduction. In Upper and in Lower Egypt, plague epidemics were cited in 55 years during the 170 year period between the outbreak of the Black Death there in 1347 and the Ottoman conquest of Egypt and Syria in 1517; in Syria, outbreaks were cited in 51 years. There were apparently 20 major plague epidemics in Egypt during this period, occurring on an average of every eight to nine years; in Syria-Palestine, there were 18 major epidemics, occurring every nine-and-a-half years. Of greater demographic importance, however, is the nature of the outbreaks; **pneumonic plague** recurred regularly after the Black Death, a case of **bubonic plague**. Arabic sources clearly describe the expectoration of blood, the rapid rate of infection, and the appearance of plague in winter months.

The most virulent outbreak to occur between 1360 and 1500 was that of 1429–1430 in Egypt. This epidemic was well documented by contemporary historians because Egypt had the greatest urban concentration in the region and because the historians themselves lived there. The epidemic reached Cairo in December 1429 and spread to Upper Egypt until the middle of March 1430, when it started to decline rapidly. Two Arabic historians, al-Maqrizi (1364–1442) and Ibn Taghribirdi (fl. 1430–1450), lived through the 1429–1430 outbreak in Cairo: the latter called it the "Great Extinction" saying he had not known of anything like it in Egypt or Syria since the year 749 AH, that is, since the Black Death. Their writings not only give a vivid picture of this epidemic's effect on Egypt, but also provide us with an idea of the consequences of plague epidemics on Islamic communities in general.

The annalist Ibn Taghribirdi, born in Cairo, describes what he himself had witnessed in the plague epidemic of the years 1429–1430 and incorporates some of al-Maqrizi's impressions about the outbreak. He records that the disease had appeared in Syria-Palestine the year before, when it struck Gaza, Jerusalem, Safad (in Galilee), and Damascus. He notes that the appearance of the epidemic in winter was unusual, because the disease normally appeared in spring. Ibn Taghribirdi relates that fasting was declared in Cairo for three days, and that people went out in a procession to the desert to pray, their voices loud in supplication to God for an end to the calamitous scourge. He comments that the death toll on that particular day was even higher than on the one before. He goes on to say that dead fish and crocodiles were found floating on lakes and on the River Nile, and that large numbers of deer and wolves were found dead in the desert between Suez and Cairo. Plague spread rapidly: at its peak, the dead in Cairo and its suburbs numbered 2,100 in one day and, in certain villages, the daily death toll was 600. The stench from decomposed bodies became intense, despite the cold weather. The author's daughter caught the disease and died on the same day, but no coffin was found for her; seven members of his brothers' families died too. He recounts an incident that he describes as a "horrific curiosity": in the confusion of burying such large numbers, a child was mistakenly taken and buried by the wrong family. Demand for coffins increased, and people resorted to carrying their dead on "planks of wood, on boxes, or in their arms". On the streets, the continuous flow of coffins was "like caravans of camels." It was difficult to bury the countless dead: grave-diggers worked through the night while relatives waited in cemeteries. Prices of shrouds rocketed, as did those of items needed by patients, such as sugar, purslane seeds, and pears, although "few received medication, while some died within the hour." Prayers over the dead were stopped in mosques; instead, they were held outside, over 40 or 50 corpses at a time. People would count each other after Friday prayers, with the absolute certainty that their number would be greatly diminished the following Friday. Everyone thought he would be the next to go; they surrendered themselves to the idea of death, repented, and made their wills. Legacies passed in quick succession from one inheritor to the next, as each new inheritor passed away. Youths started carrying prayer beads and spent most of their time praying. Because of high mortality and the preoccupation of the living with the dead, **trade** in the marketplace stopped. In the final stages of the epidemic, it was noticed that the disease struck "the elite, the notables and eminent persons while, previously, it had affected children, slaves, foreigners and servants." The disease was also thought to infect animals.

The immediate consequence of plague epidemics was urban and rural depopulation. The reduced productivity of the countryside greatly affected the prosperity of urban areas. The densely populated cities themselves, centers of trade and communication, were particularly vulnerable; here the disease spread readily and caused massive mortality.

From the middle of the fourteenth century, there was a marked decline in the population of the Middle East so that by the early fifteenth century, it had fallen by more than a third of its highest previous level. Not until the end of the nineteenth century did the population of the Middle East and North Africa return to what it had been before the Justinianic Plague of the sixth century. Furthermore, the recovery was mainly urban: the rural countryside today is less populated and less cultivated than it was fifteen centuries ago. See also Avicenna (Ibn Sina); Bimaristan; Plague in the Islamic World, 1500–1850; Public Health in the Islamic World, 1000–1600.

Further Reading

Borsch, Stuart. *The Black Death in Egypt and England*. Austin: University of Texas Press, 2005.

Byrne, Joseph P. *Daily Life during the Black Death*. Westport, CT: Greenwood Press, 2006.

Dols, Michael W. *The Black Death in the Middle East*. Princeton: Princeton University Press, 1977.

———. "The Second Plague Pandemic and Its Recurrences: 1347–1894." *Journal of the Economic and Social History of the Orient* 22 (1979): 162–183.

SELMA TIBI-HARB

PLAGUE IN THE ISLAMIC WORLD, 1500–1850. Throughout the medieval and early modern periods up until the modern era, plague **epidemics** were a constant fact of life in every part of the Old World, including that dominated by Islam. At the turn of the sixteenth century, outbreaks of plague seem to have become a global phenomenon, even being carried to the New World. Because the areas infected by **bubonic plague** and its **septicemic** and **pneumonic** variations steadily expanded from the early sixteenth century onward, plague was present in at least one location in the Islamic world virtually every year between 1500 and 1850, sometimes as sporadic outbreaks affecting only a single region, and other times, as extensive episodes spread over multiple regions. From the sixteenth century onward, plagues began to break out even more frequently than before. Although major plague outbreaks occurred every 10 years on average in both the Islamic world and in Europe during the fourteenth and fifteen centuries, they began to recur every few years in the sixteenth century. By the end of the sixteenth century, plague outbreaks recurred almost every year, becoming even more of a routine/seasonal incident. After the frequent recurrences throughout the seventeenth century, plague outbreaks began to take place less regularly in the Islamic world during the eighteenth and nineteenth centuries, though with a tendency to reappear in every new generation.

During the sixteenth century, the Islamic world saw the emergence and expansion of major regional empires. The sixteenth-century Ottoman (Turkish), Safavid (Persian), and Moghul (Indian) empires added immensely to the globalization of plague pandemics in the Old World, by providing developed **trade** and communication networks through which plague could travel even more freely than before. The growth of imperial domains produced an increased level of communication, interaction, and mobility between regions brought together by conquest and subsequently bound within an administrative, military, and commercial system, which gave rise to increased, widespread, and persistent plague outbreaks.

Among these imperial bodies, the Ottoman Empire had the most important influence on the expansion of plague epidemics in the Islamic world, and this lasted into the nineteenth century. Because it consolidated at the intersection of trade routes connecting the Balkans, Caucasus and Central Asia, Asia Minor, the Arabian Peninsula, Iran, North Africa, and the eastern Mediterranean, the Ottoman Empire provided a new set of connections over which plague could spread extensively. With ongoing conquests during the sixteenth century, the size and population of the empire doubled, but new trade networks connecting the eastern Mediterranean ports and the Red Sea, as well as those of the Indian Ocean, were also integrated to the old ones. The integration of these networks had an immense impact on the spread of plague epidemics, which contributed to the disease's globalization.

The Safavid Empire, which emerged on the eastern frontier of the Ottoman Empire in the beginning of the sixteenth century, expanded over all of Persian lands and remained in power until the eighteenth century. Having control over the Persian Gulf, the Safavids engaged in maritime trade connections with several European states and undertook a series of infrastructural provisions for the development of trade, such as building roads, bridges, and caravanserais, and providing increased security for promoting international trade. As a result, several cities thrived in the Safavid period as trade centers, especially for the silk trade. However, increased circulation of goods and people resulted in a series of epidemics in Safavid lands. The major cities of the empire were struck by repeated outbreaks of plague throughout this period.

The Moghul Empire emerged on the eastern frontier of the Safavid Empire in the early sixteenth century and expanded over the entire Indian subcontinent, remaining in power until the mid-nineteenth century. With a centralized administration, the Moghul Empire had strong commercial relations with several European countries. In addition to already established sea routes through the Red Sea and the Persian Gulf, trade connections flourished with East Africa, East Asia, and overland caravan routes westward. Given abundant international trade contacts, Moghul lands were repeatedly struck by plague outbreaks throughout this period.

Plague epidemics were particularly severe in the early modern Islamic world during the sixteenth and seventeenth centuries. There were several major outbreaks during the sixteenth century, the more important ones taking place in 1520–1522, 1534–1535, 1544–1545, 1553–1556, 1561, and 1565–1566. Yet the most terrible outbreak of the sixteenth century started in the 1570s and continued more or less until the end of the sixteenth century. Being particularly strong in Istanbul, Anatolia, the Balkans, Egypt, North Africa, and in Safavid and Moghul lands, this vast pandemic affected almost all parts of the Islamic world, as well as Europe. The seventeenth century also witnessed several major outbreaks: 1603, 1611–1613, 1620–1624, 1627, 1636–1637, 1647–1649, 1653–1656, 1659–1666, 1671–1680, 1685–1695, and from 1697 until the early years of the eighteenth century. The outbreaks of the eighteenth century were reported as mostly minor outbreaks; the major ones took place in 1713, 1719, 1728–1729, 1739–1743, 1759–1765, 1784–1786, and 1791–1792. Plague epidemics gradually disappeared during the course of the nineteenth century. The major outbreaks of the nineteenth century took place in 1812–1819 and 1835–1838. It is commonly held that the disappearance of plague epidemics in the nineteenth century in the Islamic world was the result of the adoption of quarantine measures and their implementation in the Ottoman Empire from 1838 onward. Indeed, cases of plague seemed to decrease dramatically all over Anatolia, Egypt, and the eastern Mediterranean lands of the Ottoman Empire immediately after the implementation of the new health regulations. Nevertheless, plague epidemics continued to linger for several decades in North Africa and Iraq, until the end of the nineteenth century. Although the adoption of quarantine measures certainly helped the temporary elimination of plague epidemics in the Islamic world, it is still questionable to what extent it facilitated a process of decline for the plague, which had already started in the eighteenth century and continued during the first half of the nineteenth century.

During the recurrent waves of the second pandemic, plague almost always spread to the Islamic world from western European port cities, such as Venice or Ragusa (Dubrovnik), through commercial contact with eastern Mediterranean port cities, and proceeding from coasts to inland regions. This was especially prevalent during the late fifteenth and early sixteenth centuries, when the networks through which plague spread had not yet been well established. After the integration of Egypt, Syria, North Africa, and the western Arabian peninsula into the Ottoman realms in the sixteenth century, and especially after the gradual consolidation of new trade and communication networks into the existing ones and the subsequent globalization of plague, the spread of outbreaks followed a more complex pattern of expansion, which was not only limited to the Mediterranean basin, but also included the networks of the Black Sea region and its hinterlands, the Caucasus and Central Asia, the Red Sea, as well as those of the Indian Ocean. Alexandria, Cairo, Algiers, Aleppo, Damascus, Smyrna, Thessalonica, Istanbul, Trebizond, Erzurum, Tabriz, and several other cities in the Islamic world constantly suffered plague outbreaks, which could suggest the endemicity of plague in these lands. In fact, for the eighteenth and nine-teenth centuries, it has been suggested that plague was endemic in certain parts of the Near East, especially in Persian Kurdistan, the Libyan desert, and the Asir region between Yemen and Hejaz in the Arabian peninsula, which were natural centers of the plague, from which it spread to other regions by rodents forming temporary centers for plague, in Albania-Epirus, Moldavia-Walachia, Istanbul, Anatolia, and Egypt. It is, however, hard to prove the endemicity of plague in these regions in the absence of compelling research findings.

Because of the long experience of the Islamic world with the plague, the terminology used in the sources is very clear, having been employed since the early chronicles written during the first pandemic. Islamic sources distinguish between *wabā'*, which was used to refer to epidemic disease in general, and *tā'ūn* for plague specifically. By the time of the second pandemic, both the bubonic and pneumonic forms were very accurately described in historical sources. Not only the medical sources, but also other historical sources are clear and consistent on the terminology, which suggests an established general familiarity with the disease. There are references to plague in a vast array of sources in the Islamic world, including court registers, imperial decrees, collections of legal opinion, chronicles, diplomatic correspondence, poetry, biographical dictionaries, travelogues, tombstones, and plague treatises.

The attitude of the Islamic world toward the plague has usually been portrayed as pas-sive, a conclusion drawn largely from the Islamic plague treatises, which were generally written by legal scholars during and after the **Black Death (1347–1352)**. Islamic teach-ing prohibited **flight** from plague-stricken areas, and this literature sought to legitimize this prohibition by maintaining that plague was a blessing or mercy of God and a means of martyrdom for the believer. The response recommended to Muslims in times of plague was to be patient and not flee. In fact, many did flee plague outbreaks, and those who remained sought ways to protect themselves and cure the sick. Prevention was emphasized more than treatment, perhaps because no exact cure for plague was known, nor was its cause. The theories of putrefaction and **miasma** prompted specific precautionary meas-ures. Following **Greco-Roman medical theories**, during plague outbreaks physicians recommended living at high altitudes and in places facing north. The air was to be disin-fected of any putrefying matter and kept clean inside houses and in the city with vinegar, sandalwood, and rosewater, as well as through **fumigation**. Nevertheless, there was an ongoing search for remedies against plague throughout the Islamic world. Islamic plague treatises written in this period are full of various methods of treatment (including instructions for bleeding and purging) and recipes for ointments, syrups, electuaries, unguents, plasters, fumigations, and similar remedies, as well as for foods and beverages thought to be helpful in the treatment of the disease. The common recipes were mostly made up of vegetable matter but sometimes also included animal parts and minerals. As in Europe, the use of Armenian earth, Lemnian earth, theriac, and bezoar stone was also widely recommended. In fact, Europe and the Islamic world shared a common body of medical theory and knowledge about the plague and practiced similar preventive measures and treatment methods throughout the early modern period. In addition to medicine, people resorted to **astrology**, **religion**, and **magic** in the search for a cure. Prayers, magical remedies, amulets, and similar spiritual methods of treatment acquired great importance in plague literature and daily life.

From the fifteenth century onward, plague treatises written in the Ottoman Empire reflect a new legal viewpoint on proper conduct during outbreaks. In contrast to the legal opinions expressed in the earlier literature, these works recognized a form of contagion, granted legitimacy to the need to exit a plague-infested city in search of clean air, and legally authorized such practices. The recognition of contagion also paved the way for initiatives for a public health system in the Islamic world. From the sixteenth century onward, the early modern Ottoman Empire began to adopt preliminary measures to monitor, control, and fight plague epidemics, such as using occasional **quarantines**, keeping records of death tolls, controlling the burial of the dead, and maintaining urban hygiene.

In the absence of clear statistical data and census records, it is virtually impossible to make precise demographic estimates about the Islamic world in this period. However, the effects of recurrent outbreaks were cumulative and destructive in the long run. The demographic stagnation continued in the Islamic world until the mid-nineteenth century, whereas European population growth exploded from 1500 to 1850. Nevertheless, the mortality rates for major urban plague epidemics were much lower in the Islamic world than in European cities struck during the seventeenth and eighteenth centuries. *See also* Contagion Theory of Disease, Premodern; Cordon Sanitaire; Islamic Disease Theory and Medicine; Plague in Europe, 1500–1770s; Plague in the Islamic World, 1360–1500; Public Health in the Islamic World, 1000–1600.

Further Reading

Dols, Michael W. *The Black Death in the Middle East*. Princeton: Princeton University Press, 1977.
———. "The Second Plague Pandemic and its Recurrences in the Middle East: 1347–1894." *International Journal of Middle Eastern Studies* 22 (1979): 162–189.
Gallagher, Nancy Elizabeth. *Medicine and Power in Tunisia, 1780–1900*. New York: Cambridge University Press, 1983.

NÜKHET VARLIK

PLAGUE LITERATURE AND ART, EARLY MODERN EUROPEAN. The recurrence of **bubonic plague** throughout Europe in the early modern period meant that the disease continued to stimulate the production of art and literature. Even when outbreaks became less frequent and widespread, during the latter part of the seventeenth century, the specter of yet another **epidemic** remained vividly present. Plague literature and art refers to works that are specifically tied to the experience or anticipation of plague by their content and purpose; that is, they contain direct reference to the disease, visually or verbally, and are created for plague-related aims, whether commemorative, *ex voto*, prophetic, didactic, or prophylactic.

Some scholars have interpreted fourteenth- and fifteenth-century macabre imagery as a response to the ravages of plague by a pessimistic, fearful, and death-obsessed society. However, macabre themes in poetry and art, such as the meeting of the three living and the three dead, and the Triumph of Death, predate the **Black Death**. Along with later variations, such as the Dance of Death, Death and the maiden, and the crowned skeleton, or King Death, such themes are more plausibly interpreted as articulating long-held Christian beliefs regarding the inevitability of death, the wages of sin, and the necessity for penance. Moreover, such imagery should not be seen as purely pessimistic, but rather as hopeful and hortatory, designed to urge the readers or viewers to amend their ways while there is still time and secure their salvation.

Plague Tracts: Helpful Advice and "Warnings to Beware".   The dominant form of plague literature in this period is the **physician**-composed plague tract, circulating first in manuscript in the wake of the Black Death and pouring off the presses by the dozens by the end of the following century. Earlier texts were often republished, and new ones were continually being written. The invention of the printing press in the later fifteenth century allowed for rapid dissemination to a wide audience of literate consumers. Publication in both Latin and, ever more frequently, in all European vernaculars, meant that readership was not restricted to a learned elite but extended to artisans, merchants, householders, aristocrats, and all those concerned to find remedies for and advice on dealing with the plague.

Some tracts were written for the use and instruction of governing officials; others, which debated contentious medical issues of the day, such as whether plague was spread by miasma (poisoned **air**) or **contagion** (from person to person), seem addressed to a more specialized audience. Most, however, were intended for the general public, as readily available self-help manuals. John of Burgundy, author of one of the most popular fifteenth-century treatises, proclaimed that he wrote to ensure that "if someone lacks a physician, then each and everyone may be his own *physicus, praeservator, curator et rector*." Another anonymous fifteenth-century writer began his tract "sorrowing for the destruction of men and devoting myself to the common good and . . . wishing health for all." Two hundred years later, the same intentions were still generating new compositions: as a French writer advised in 1617, "The plague is a dangerous illness that brooks no delays. One doesn't always have time or means of using physicians in good time. However, you can always use me, night or day, early and late, by means of this volume."

The treatises usually followed a standard pattern, proceeding from an explanation of causes and signs to preventative and curative measures. Across the Catholic and Protestant divide, all writers identified the ultimate origins of epidemics in divine displeasure at human sin. Plague was both punitive and remedial, God's means of chastising his people into virtue. Writers often took the opportunity to castigate what they saw as the sins most offensive to God. Traditional catalogues of vices (greed, sloth, immorality) were given specifically local flavor by reference to contemporary religious, social, and political grievances. For seventeenth-century

English Protestants, for example, the fault lay variously with seditious local Catholics, the conspicuous greed of governing classes, or the doctrinal rigidity of new religious groups such as the Puritans.

A key rationale for the popularity of plague tracts was the way they gave readers a sense of control over events, by providing explanations that made sense according to the beliefs of the day. Following classical and contemporary medical theories, the specific cause of plague was often identified as maleficent planetary conjunctions. Unfavorable celestial events led to poisoning and putrefaction of the local atmosphere. Such astrological interpretations did not conflict with belief in divine origins, because it was God who had set the planets in motion in the first place. Throughout the early modern period, almanacs containing, among much else, history and prognosis of plagues based on celestial movements circulated widely.

The chief reason for the popularity of the texts was hope for preservation and cure, and the longest section was thus devoted to prophylaxis. Authors recommended a regimen of **personal hygiene** and health, based on **humoral theories** and aimed at maintaining the body's correct humoral balance. Moderation in all things was the key: a calm, cheerful mind and a life of sobriety and restraint. Characteristically for the Renaissance, when many looked to the classical past for guidance on how to live in the present, in his plague treatise of 1481, the Florentine classical scholar and philosopher Marsilio Ficino (1433–1499) proposed Socrates (470–399 BCE) as a model of how to survive the plague—a Socrates, it should be said, recast in Ficino's image, as a sober, chaste, moderate, and melancholic seeker of truth.

Flight was invariably identified as the most effective form of prevention, and the classical tag "flee fast, stay long, come back late" was repeatedly quoted. Advice was also given for those forced by duty or circumstance to reside in a plague-stricken area. Because the aim was to combat the pestilential corruption of the surrounding air, precautions included isolation and the use of aromatics, fires, **fumigations**, and disinfectants. A closing section on treatment and cure of those already stricken provided medical recipes and discussed various surgical practices such as bloodletting and lancing the buboes.

Shock Tactics: Plague Narratives.   Overlapping and infecting the plague tract, but also recognizably distinct by virtue of their drama and emotional affect, are descriptive accounts of particular epidemics. Vivid and terrifying narratives of the physical and social desolation wrought by plague have a long tradition in literature, reaching back to Thucydides' (460–400 BCE) famous account of the **Plague of Athens**—often repeated, translated, adapted, and versified in later centuries—and Florentine poet author Giovanni Boccaccio's (1313–1375) equally celebrated prologue to the *Decameron*, describing the horrors of the Black Death. Daniel Defoe's (1660–1731) *Journal of A Plague Year* (1722), a dramatic evocation of the Great Plague of London in 1665, is the most famous early modern example of this category.

With their shocking evocations of disaster and death, such texts are often interpreted as purely journalistic, accurate, and reliable eyewitness accounts of what actually occurred. Yet as scholars have come to recognize, they are in fact highly crafted, fictional creations, with deliberately rhetorical goals. Defoe's *Journal* is a case in point, being written many decades after the events it purports to describe, in response to news of plague in Marseilles, France. For Defoe, as for his predecessors, the ultimate aim of the brutal evocation of plague's horrors is to reverse them—behind the dramatic vignettes and grue-some details is an intense desire for restoration and wholeness, for reconciliation between heaven and earth. Like preachers who include vivid anecdotes of contemporary life to bring home the moral message of their sermon, plague writers (many of whom in England were clerics) used narrative drama for emotional impact. Aesthetic horror was deliber-ately manufactured, drawing on well-established literary conventions, in order to move the reader's soul and set in motion what Defoe called the necessary "Work of Repentance and Humiliation." Yet the *Journal* also breaks new ground by humanizing the genre as never before, drawing on new devices of contemporary fiction to generate a more intensely personal, subjective, and hence vastly more compelling account, which explains its enduring popularity.

Plague Images: Heavenly Causes and Heavenly Cures.   The same concerns at work in plague literature—to provide comprehensible explanatory models and sources of hope for prevention and cure—also motivated the creation of Catholic-inspired plague art. In the early modern period, as previously in the aftermath of the Black Death, most plague imagery was prophylactic, designed to enlist the aid of powerful heavenly protectors against the disease. Images were not created for detached aesthetic contemplation but were functioning cult objects, the focus of collective prayer and ritual in churches, chapels, and city streets, and of individual and family devotion in the home. By making images in honor of holy figures, worshippers were setting up a kind of two-way contract, characterized by mutual obligations and benefits: worshippers would honor and celebrate their holy patrons, but they expected a proper return on their investment, in the form of special favors and protection against disasters. Plague images thus provided a concrete sense of comfort and hope for those facing the continuing threat of plague, an aspect that has not always been sufficiently recognized in studies of the impact of plague on early modern populations.

Sources of Hope: A Multiplicity of Heavenly Protectors.   A characteristic feature of early modern plague imagery is the multiplicity of options available for obtaining heavenly pro-tection against the disease. Worshippers could pick and choose from a multitude of celes-tial defenders. Local patron saints were often the first line of supernatural defense for many communities, because they were bound to their city by special ties of affection and interest and could be relied upon to plead its cause with all the vigor and passion of a citizen on an urgent embassy to a foreign dignitary. Helpful saints like Christopher guarded against sudden death, a particularly relevant fear for plague victims, whereas others, such as Sebastian and Roch, were credited with specialist plague expertise. Often, the most popular solution was to petition a whole phalanx of saints together with the Virgin Mary, queen of heaven and powerful agent of mercy before her divine Son, who, it was widely believed, could never turn down a maternal request. Where one saint was powerful, many gathered together were virtually irresistible. This essentially confident, optimistic conviction in multiple means of accessing supernatural protection was funda-mental to early modern men and women's ability to cope with the ongoing presence of plague in their midst.

Destruction and Deliverance: Changing God's Mind.   Plague images usually visualized the onset of the disease as deadly arrows shot down from heaven. The arrow as a metaphor for sudden, unexpected death and disease was familiar to Western viewers from classical antiquity (Apollo the archer, god of pestilence) and, above all, from the Old

Testament. Many early modern images show an enraged deity—God the Father or Christ the Son—in the clouds hurling down wickedly barbed arrows and needle-sharp lances upon sinful humanity. Heaped piles of **corpses**, studded with the "deadly darts" like so many pincushions, vividly conveyed the sense of plague's indiscriminate reach, cutting down young and old alike, men and women, merchant and pauper. Angels often assist God in the task of chastising humanity, kneeling on clouds to take better aim. Sometimes the plague arrows are thrown down by grinning demons, heavenly subcontractors, as it were, in the job of punishing sinners. By the seventeenth century, the arrows disappear, but the heaps of dead and dying remain, often given special poignancy by commonly recycled artistic motifs, such as the infant suckling in vain from the breast of a dead mother. Like plague narratives, these descriptive evocations of the dead and dying are less direct reportage than artistic compositions configured for maximum emotional affect.

Yet despite the carnage, the message of these plague images is not universally gloomy. No matter how angry God might be, if approached in the correct way, he could be persuaded to change his mind. As the special "friends of God," saints could argue with the enraged deity, and even do battle with him, as one thirteenth-century Italian preacher enthusiastically declared, on behalf of their worshippers. The Virgin can sway her son to clemency or intervene directly by sheltering worshippers under her protective mantle, against which plague arrows would seek their targets in vain. And Christ himself would argue humanity's cause, demonstratively displaying his wounds to turn aside his father's just wrath.

Plague images brilliantly visualize this ability to change God's mind by combining both threatening and merciful elements within the one composition. The plague arrows might have been launched, but their flight could be arrested. In a late-fifteenth-century panel by Tuscan painter Bartolomeo della Gatta (1448–1502), for example, Christ and his angels send down arrows from the heavens to devastate the town of Arezzo. But all is not lost: the plague saint Roch kneels to plead the city's cause, and Christ, convinced, changes his mind and sends other angels to catch the arrows as they fall and break them in mid-flight. Other examples show Christ loosing arrows with one hand while blessing with the other, or an angry Christ flanked by twin angels of justice, with threateningly upraised sword, of mercy sheathing the sword as a sign of reconciliation between heaven and earth. An early sixteenth-century canvas banner paid for by governing officials of the Italian town of Perugia and designed to be carried at the head of penitential processions during epidemics, depicts the city in the grip of plague, its populace kneeling in prayer before the gathered heavenly hosts. Christ holds downward-pointing plague arrows and raises aloft the sword of justice, ready to smite, but, in the nick of time, the Virgin Mary leans forward and grasps his sword arm to prevent the downward stroke. Plague images thus constantly balance the threat of punishment with promise of deliverance.

Sebastian: The Hedgehog Saint.   The most popular and frequently petitioned saintly defender against the plague was the fourth-century CE Roman martyr St. Sebastian. Scholars continue to debate why and when he was selected as a plague saint, but the key reason seems to be the potent combination of martyrdom—believed to be the most perfect imitation of Christ—and arrow symbolism in his legend. A captain in the imperial guard, Sebastian has the unusual distinction of being martyred not once but twice. The first time, he was shot through with arrows "like a hedgehog," as his *Life* reports, before being left for dead. Importantly, this was believed to be a real death—but the saint was resurrected by divine power, and found miraculously alive by Christians coming to collect his body for burial. The second time around, and the one that proved permanent, he was beaten to death and his corpse thrown in a sewer (from whence it was subsequently retrieved and honorably buried).

Given the longstanding conception of plague as heaven-sent arrows, Sebastian came to be venerated as a plague martyr. Moreover, he both suffered death from plague-like arrows and was resurrected through divine fiat. Because of this, he was venerated as a Christ-like savior against the plague, voluntarily accepting the arrows of disease on behalf of sinful humanity—hence the ubiquity of his presence in early modern plague art, where he is customarily represented both martyred and alive, bearing the plague arrows in his near-naked flesh, usually with no apparent ill effects. Sebastian offers himself as a literal shield between an angry God and a sinful humanity, a lightning rod deflecting to himself the plague arrows intended for his worshippers, grounding them harmlessly in his own body. The powerful combination of youthful vitality and deadly, wounding arrows reassured devotees of his unlimited protective powers against the disease.

Medical Specificity: Roch and Plague Buboes. Toward the end of the fifteenth century, the French lay pilgrim, Roch, emerged as a second universal plague saint. The rapidity with which his cult spread across Europe was the result of the coincidence of his appearance with the invention of the printing press, so much so that he has recently been dubbed the first saint of the new media. For worshippers, his appeal lay in the close alignment of his life and miracles with their own lived experience. According to his earliest biography, composed and published in 1479, Roch healed plague victims, was himself stricken with the disease, endured it patiently, and was then divinely cured. Resuming his travels, he was imprisoned as a spy, was a model prisoner, and on his deathbed was rewarded by God with the power to preserve against the plague.

Recent research has demonstrated that Roch is a problematic figure, whose existence cannot be historically documented and whose biography is replete with hagiographical *topoi*, conventional episodes common to many saintly narratives. Some scholars have even suggested he is completely fictitious, created as a saintly double of an obscure French bishop of the same name, Rachus or Rochus of Autun. Yet such debates only highlight the extent to which Roch's cult met a deeply felt need among early modern worshippers for a saint of their own time, to offer hope of cure from a disease whose symptoms were by this date long familiar.

Images of Roch stress his dual role as both healer and victim of the plague. Narrative cycles show him curing the inmates of a plague hospice, or lazaretto (see figure). At a time when many communities built plague lazarettos, and even the smallest settlement contained at least one civic hospice, this episode would have resonated directly with viewers' own experiences. Carefully particularized details of setting and costume, such as beds neatly ranged along the wall, the white nightshirts and caps of the sick, and the sober gray robes of the warden, here holding a urine specimen and attempting to dissuade the young man from what he saw as a suicidal disregard for his own safety, give these healing scenes a veracity and immediacy which speaks directly to worshippers. Naturalistic devices climax in demonstrative displays of patients' buboes. Although not clinically accurate by modern standards, the buboes are immediately recognizable and rhetorically compelling, magnetizing the gaze as dreaded signs of inevitable death imprinted on the bodies of

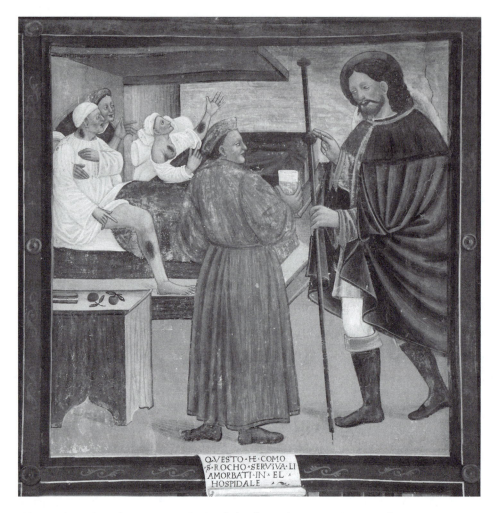

Giovanni Battista de Legnano, St. Roch healing plague victims in a hospice. Oratory of St. Roch, Santa Maria Maggiore, Piedmont, Italy, 1534. Courtesy of Louise Marshall.

otherwise healthy men, women, and children. The pathos of their bared and disfigured flesh calls upon the saint for cure and plays on contemporary fears to insist upon Roch's proven ability to heal the disease.

Yet the healer was not himself immune, and other images show Roch ostentatiously revealing the bubo on his own leg. Directed outward to contemporaries, the sight of Roch, scarred by the plague yet alive and well, must have been an emotionally charged image of promised cure. Here was tangible proof that one could survive the plague: a saint who had triumphed in his own flesh over the very disease threatening his worshippers. Moreover, like Sebastian, Roch too was venerated as a plague martyr, because, absent any opportunity of dying for the faith, the crown of martyrdom could also be won by physical suffering.

Such images create a charged dynamic between the morbidly disfigured bodies of plague victims, in image and in life, and the similarly marked body of the new saint, who welcomed the torments of the disease as a chance to imitate the sufferings of Christ, and was consequently endowed with the power to ward off such torments from his devotees.

Protestant Plague Imagery.   Though Protestants of all stripes accepted divine causation of plague and the efficacy of prayer and repentance, they denied any role to intervening saints and tended to avoid fanciful depictions of divine activity. Protestant plague-inspired art tended to focus less on the plague itself than on what was considered the proper response to it: stoical preparation for a "good death" in the bosom of one's family. Plague tracts, bills of mortality, and broadsides (cheap posters) often featured more generic symbols of death such as skulls with crossbones, flying skeletons, tombstones, and funeral processions.

Conclusion.   Both literature and art fulfilled vital roles in assisting early modern men and women to cope with the ongoing threat of plague. They provided explanations for the onset of the disease in terms that made sense to their readers and viewers, allowing some sense of understanding and control over events. Vivid verbal and visual evocations of plague's horrors were deliberately deployed to prick beholders' consciences, warning of the dangers of continued sinning and inspiring the necessary reformation of life. Among Catholics, plague images served as concretized prayers, offered up to a range of holy intercessors to invoke their protection against the disease. Both literature and art acknowledged the inevitability of sin, and hence of divine punishment through plague, but they also remained fundamentally optimistic that possibilities of protection and cure did exist and could be mobilized to secure the desired salvation from the disease at present or at least in the next life. *See also* AIDS, Literature, and the Arts in the United States; Astrology and Medicine; Biblical Plagues; Black Death and Late Medieval Christianity; Black Death: Literature and Art; Greco-Roman Medical Theory and Practice; Literature, Disease in Modern; London, Great Plague of (1665–1666); Plague and Developments in Public Health, 1348–1600; Plague in Britain, 1500–1647; Plague in Europe, 1500–1770s; Plague Memorials; Religion and Epidemic Disease.

Further Reading

Anselment, Raymond. *The Realms of Apollo: Literature and Healing in Seventeenth-Century England.* London: University of Delaware Press and Associated University Presses, 1995.

Bailey, Gauvin, et al., eds. *Hope and Healing: Painting in Italy in a Time of Plague, 1500–1800.* Worcester, MA: Worcester Art Museum, 2005.

Boeckl, Christine. *Images of Plague and Pestilence: Iconography and Iconology.* Kirksville, MO: Truman State University Press, 2001.

Crawford, Raymond. *Plague and Pestilence in Literature and Art.* Oxford: Clarendon Press, 1914.

Grigsby, Bryon. *Pestilence in Medieval and Early Modern English Literature.* New York: Routledge, 2004.

Harvard University Library. *Contagion.* http://ocp.hul.harvard.edu/contagion/pestilence.html

Healy, Margaret. "Defoe's *Journal* and the English Plague Writing Tradition." *Literature and Medicine* 22 (2003): 25–44.

———. *Fictions of Disease in Early Modern England: Bodies, Plagues, and Politics.* New York: Palgrave, 2002.

Jones, Colin. "Plague and its Metaphors in Early Modern France." *Representations* 53 (1996): 97–127.

Leavy, Barbara. *To Blight with Plague: Studies in a Literary Theme*. New York: New York University Press, 1992.

Marshall, Louise. "Confraternity and Community: Mobilizing the Sacred in Times of Plague." In *Confraternities and the Visual Arts in the Italian Renaissance: Ritual, Spectacle, Image*, edited by Barbara Wisch and Diane Cole Ahl, pp. 20–45. New York: Cambridge University Press, 2000.

———. "Manipulating the Sacred: Image and Plague in Renaissance Italy." *Renaissance Quarterly* 47 (1994): 485–532.

———. "Shaping the Sacred in Cycles of St. Roch: A New Plague Saint for Renaissance Italy." In *Crossing Cultures: Conflict, Migration, Convergence: Acts of the 32nd Congress of the International Committee of the History of Art*, edited by Jaynie Anderson, in press. Melbourne: Melbourne University Press, 2009.

Mormando, Francesco, and Thomas Worcester, eds. *Piety and Plague from Byzantium to the Baroque*. Kirksville, MO: Truman State Press, 2007.

LOUISE MARSHALL

PLAGUE MEMORIALS.   Plague memorials are commemorative monuments built for victims of plague throughout western Europe. In most cases, the erection of the monument fulfilled a vow that was made during a serious outbreak of the plague, often associated with a saint, the Virgin Mary, or the Trinity. The plague monuments also bear tangible witness to the communal impulse to honor the innumerable dead, whose resting-places were unmarked.

The first plague monuments were churches dedicated to the saints invoked during plague. Among the most important plague churches is St. Roch in Prague (1602), which was designed by Giovanni Battista Bussi for Emperor Rudolf II and is located on the grounds of Strahov monastery above Hradcany Castle. Others include the Mariensaule in Munich (1638), Rochuscapelle in Bingen (1666), and Karlskirche in Vienna (1715). In Venice, the most notable are the churches of San Giobe (1462), San Sebastiano (1506), and Santa Maria della Salute (1632). A vow from the Senate of Venice in 1576 to build a church dedicated to Christ the Redeemer resulted in the Festa del Redentore, which was celebrated on the third Sunday of July and during which the Doge publicly prayed to thank God for the end of the epidemic.

Other plague monuments include Baroque plague columns found in central and southern Europe. Influenced by the Brotherhood of the Holy Trinity (1652), the oldest of these monuments was a wooden structure built in Vienna in 1679, which represented the Trinity on a column. It was rebuilt in 1693. The new composition represented, below the Trinity figure, a cloud pyramid with angel sculptures and the praying figure of Emperor Leopold I (1640–1705).

The design of plague columns evolved to reflect Catholic ideals of the Counter-Reformation and the vision of the end of the plague as victory over sin. In addition to featuring at the base a number of plague saints, such as St. Roch, St. Sebastian, and Sts. Cosmos and Damian (as at Graz, 1679), designers emphasized the Virgin Mary. Whereas on the Leoben monument (1718) she appears halfway up the column, that at Zwett (1727) presents Mary at the foot of the memorial. In Horn (1724), the Virgin stands on the top of the column, whereas the Trinity is grouped at its foot. In Munich (1732), the Virgin stands alone. This model is also found in Nitra, Italy (1750), and Grad (1681). The column of Olomouc in the Czech Republic (1754) contains a chapel inside. These monuments were later transformed into secular victory columns by the ostentatious display of imperial dynastic emblems. The association between columns and the Habsburg monarchy led to the destruction of the Prague column at the end of World War I (1918).

An odd secular monument was the two horse heads in the Neumarkt of Cologne. They memorialized the miraculous healing of a woman whose husband swore he would see horses upstairs in his house before his wife could be healed, at which he turned and saw the animals leaning out of the window. More recent examples are the modern monument of Son Servera (Baleares), built to commemorate the plague of 1820, and the Cattle Plague Memorial in Mucclestone (Staffordshire, England), built after the epidemic of 1865. *See also* Black Death (1347–1352); Black Death: Literature and Art; London, Great Plague of (1665–1666); Plague in Britain, 1500–1647; Plague in Europe, 1500–1770s; Plague in Medieval Europe, 1360–1500; Religion and Epidemic Disease.

Further Reading

Avery, H. "Plague Churches, Monuments and Memorials." *Proceedings of the Royal Society of Medicine* 59 (1996): 110–116.

Boeckl, Christine M. "Giorgio Vasari's 'San Rocco Altarpiece': Tradition and Innovation in Plague Iconography." *Artibus et Historiae* 22 (2001): 29–40.

———. "Vienna's *Pestsäule:* The Analysis of a Seicento Plague Monument." *Wiener Jahrbuch für Kunstgeschichte* 49 (1996): 41–56.

ADRIANO DUQUE

PLAGUE OF ATHENS.   The so-called "Plague of Athens" lasted from 430 to 426 BCE in the early stages of the Peloponnesian War between Athens and Sparta in ancient Greece. It is the earliest well-described **epidemic** in European history and also one of the most controversial episodes in medical history. It illustrates very well the difficulties of retrospective diagnosis. Many different suggestions for its cause have been proposed, with no agreement whatsoever among the modern historians who have written over 200 articles about it. And so it remains, despite the availability of a lengthy contemporary description of the symptoms of the "plague" and its effects written by the Athenian historian Thucydides (c. 460–400 BCE), our main source of information on the plague. He recorded reports that the epidemic started in Ethiopia and Egypt before spreading through much of the Persian Empire and then reaching Greece. However, the only substantial information available to historians—his own account—relates solely to Athens and its port of Piraeus.

Thucydides wrote that he decided to record the symptoms so that it could be recognized should it ever recur in the future. The disease commenced with intense heat in the head; eye, throat, and tongue inflammation, with bad breath; sneezing and vomiting; upset stomach; cool skin with a rash of small blisters or ulcers; intense internal heat leading victims to throw themselves into water; sleeplessness; in the later stages ulceration of the bowels with diarrhea; gangrene of the extremities leading to loss of fingers, toes, genital organs, and eyes; and amnesia in some survivors. Modern suggestions for the cause of the disease include **typhus, smallpox, measles, bubonic plague,** a **hemorrhagic fever** like Ebola, **typhoid fever, influenza,** toxic shock syndrome, scarlet fever, anthrax, glanders, tularemia, Lassa fever, **ergotism,** and mycotoxins. The hypothesis that the epidemic was caused by a pathogen that cannot now be recognised because it has become extinct has also been proposed. Typhus and smallpox have attracted the most support, but there is no consensus. In 2006 an attempt was made to identify the pathogen in question by analysis of ancient DNA from skeletons from a burial pit in the Kerameikos, the cemetery of Athens, dating to about 430 BCE. It was suggested that DNA sequences from one skeleton point toward typhoid fever. However these DNA sequences are far from identical to the typhoid sequence. Moreover, the typhoid hypothesis has attracted little support from medical historians who have studied the text of Thucydides. Consequently, the identity of the pathogen responsible for the Plague of Athens remains uncertain.

Thucydides also describes the social, demographic, and political effects of the Plague of Athens. It clearly weakened Athens's military effectiveness in the war's early stages, and it took the life of Athens's most highly regarded civic leader, Pericles. *See also* Diagnosis of Historical Diseases; Greco-Roman Medical Theory and Practice; Hippocrates; Historical Epidemiology; Paleopathology; Smallpox in the Ancient World; War, the Military, and Epidemic Disease.

Further Reading

Cunha, Burke. "The Cause of the Plague of Athens: Plague, Typhoid, Typhus, Smallpox or Measles?" *Infectious Disease Clinics of North America* 18 (2004): 29–43.

Longrigg, James. "The Great Plague of Athens." *History of Science* 18 (1980): 209–225.

Morens, David M., and Robert J. Littman. "Epidemiology of the Plague of Athens." *Transactions of the American Philological Association* 122 (1992): 271–304.

Papagrigorakis, Manolis, et al. "DNA examination of ancient dental pulp incriminates typhoid fever as a probable cause of the Plague of Athens." *International Journal of Infectious Diseases* 10 (2006): 206–214; reply at 334–336.

Soupios, M. A. "Impact of the Plague in Ancient Greece." *Infectious Disease Clinics of North America* 18 (2004): 45–51.

Thucydides. *Peloponnesian War: A New Translation, Backgrounds, Interpretations.* Translated and edited by Walter Blanco and Jennifer Roberts. New York: Norton, 1998.

ROBERT SALLARES

PLAGUE OF CYPRIAN.   *See* Plagues of the Roman Empire.

PLAGUE OF JUSTINIAN; FIRST PANDEMIC.   This is the conventional name for a series of outbreaks of **bubonic plague** in the early middle ages, named for the Byzantine emperor Justinian I (r. 527–565) during whose rule the cycle began. Its first outbreak occurred in 541, and the **pandemic** returned in 18 waves until 750, on average every 11.6 years. It is highly probable that the pandemic originated in Africa. This was primarily a Mediterranean phenomenon: the Byzantine Empire, the Islamic world, and regions in southwestern Europe were hit more often than those in northern Europe, as the disease spread along trade routes, mostly through sea travel. As opposed to that of the late medieval **Black Death**, the identity of the **epidemic** disease as true bubonic plague has not been contested. The waves of the plague certainly caused large-scale mortality and—especially in important urban centers such as Constantinople—a sharp demographic decline, but it is still difficult to translate this into more specific demographic terms. Figures estimating the overall loss of life at 20 to 30 percent of the pre-plague population are often cited, but their accuracy and value are questionable. Certainly, labor became sparse and more expensive, more and better land was available, and manpower shortages limited military operations, whereas on a spiritual level the scourge encouraged the intensification of religious ritual and may have affected the initial spread of Islam.

There are abundant sources on the Plague of Justinian written in Greek, Syriac, Arabic, Latin, and Old Irish—mostly histories and chronicles and, to a lesser extent, narrations of saints' lives. Several sixth-century authors were eyewitnesses to the pandemic, such as the historians Procopius (d. 565), Agathias (c. 536–582), and Euagrius (c. 536–600) writing in Greek; John of Ephesus (c. 505–585), a bishop writing in Syriac; and the bishop and historian Gregory of Tours (538–593) writing in Latin. Arabic authors such as al-Madaini wrote in the late eighth and ninth centuries, as did some of the Greek and Latin authors such as Theophanes (758/60–817) and Paul the Deacon (c. 720–799), who referred to plague waves in the seventh and eighth centuries.

Several detailed descriptions of the disease enable us to identify it as bubonic plague. Procopius includes the longest account of the symptoms associated with the epidemic's first visitation in 542. Its onset was sudden and accompanied by fever. In a few days at the most, swellings developed mainly in the groin, but also inside the armpit, beside the ears, or on the thighs. Some of the infected fell into comas; others became delirious, whereas those who did not develop any of those symptoms died as a result of the mortification of the swellings. Furthermore, black pustules as large as lentils appeared in some of the patients, bringing about their death in less than one day. Others vomited blood. In those cases where the swellings became extremely large and the pus was discharged, the infected were sure to survive the disease, though sometimes with withered limbs or affected speech. Additional traits observed by other writers include patients with bloody eyes, a swelling that began in the face and spread down to the neck bringing about death, and diarrhea. John of Ephesus records the swelling in the groin, both in humans and animals. **Pneumonic plague** was probably not a prominent feature of this pandemic.

The disease was disseminated over large distances most probably through **trade** and **military** operations. Sources contemporary to the pandemic recognized this by observing that the disease spread from the ports inland. Accounts of the plague's **transmission** from human to human are contradictory: whereas some seem to affirm this, others point to the opposite, writing that **physicians** who attended plague patients were not infected by the disease.

Sources mention excessive mortality caused by the plague, often recording detailed numbers of fatalities: although these seem authoritative, they are usually rhetorical exaggerations. The closest we can come to calculating the plague-induced mortality is to do so for specific places during specific outbreaks. The total loss of life at Constantinople in 542 has been calculated at 20 percent of its population, 35 percent is suggested for Egypt in 744, and 25 percent is noted for Basrah in 749. Such figures can only illustrate the overall trends or patterns of plague-induced mortality in the period. Though the sources at our disposal focus on urban centers, there is ample evidence to suggest that mortality in the rural areas was equally high. This includes haunting images of the deserted and desolate countryside, of abandoned villages or those whose entire population had been snuffed out by disease.

As for the seasonality of the plague outbreaks, data point to an unquestionable peak in the months of April to August, with July exhibiting the highest incidence. In the Islamic world, there was a marked peak in April and a less pronounced one in August, with the period from March to August exhibiting the highest incidence of the disease throughout the year. Available data does not point toward any marked difference in the age or gender of the afflicted.

The first outbreak of the plague was the one recorded most comprehensively. Because contemporary sources place its entry point into the Byzantine Empire at Pelusium, at the

PLAGUE OUTBREAKS CONSTITUTING THE FIRST PLAGUE PANDEMIC (541–750)

1. 541: Pelusium (Egypt), Gaza, Negev, Alexandria; 542: Jerusalem and hinterland, Syria, Lycia, Constantinople, Asia Minor, North Africa, Sicily; 543: Italy, Western Balkans, Spain, Southern France; 544: Rome, Ireland; 547: Wales; 549: England, Ireland, Finland, Yemen.
2. 557–558: Amida (Syria); 558: Constantinople; 560–561: Cilicia (Asia Minor), Syria, Mesopotamia.
3. 571: Italy, Southern France; 573–574: Constantinople, Eastern Mediterranean; 576: Ireland.
4. 584: Spain, Southern France; 588: Spain, Southern France; 590: Rome, Southern France; 591–592: Western Italy, Istria, Antioch, Marseille.
5. 597: Thessalonica and hinterland; 598: Avar territory (European Turkey); 599: Constantinople, Western Asia Minor, Syria, Eastern Mediterranean; 599–600: North Africa, Italy, Southern France, Ravenna; 601: Verona.
6. 618–619: Constantinople, possibly Alexandria.
7. 626–627: Palestine; 627–628: Persia.
8. 639: Syria, Palestine, Iraq.
9. 664–666: Ireland, England; 669–670: Kufa (Iraq); 672–673: Egypt, Palestine, Kufa, Lichfield (England).
10. 680: Rome, possibly Ticinum (Pavia), Ely (England).
11. 684–687: England; 687: Syria; 689: Basrah (Iraq); 689–690: Egypt.
12. 693: Toledo, Spain; 694: Southern France; 698: Syria, Constantinople; 699–700: Iraq, Syria, Mesopotamia.
13. 704–706: Syria; 706: Iraq; 709–711: possibly Spain.
14. 713: Syria; 714–715: Egypt, possibly Crete.
15. 718–719: Iraq, Syria.
16. 724: Egypt; 725–726: Syria, Mesopotamia.
17. 732–735: Syria, Egypt, Palestine, Iraq; 735: Asia Minor.
18. 743–744: Egypt, North Africa; 744–745: Mesopotamia, Syria, Iraq; 735–746: Calabria, Sicily, possibly Rome, Continental Greece, Aegean; 747–748: Constantinople; 747–750: Iraq, Syria, Mesopotamia.

After this last visitation, the plague vanished until it resurfaced in the Second Pandemic, the Black Death.

Compiled by Dionysios Stathakopoulos

mouth of the extreme eastern branch of the Nile, scholars generally agree that the ultimate origin of the pandemic should be situated in central Africa, which remains a natural focus of sylvatic plague. From Pelusium it spread north to Alexandria, Gaza, and the Negev in 541, and the following year west across North Africa, east across the Levant, and north to Sicily, Asia Minor, and Constantinople. Plague appeared in Italy, the western Balkans, Spain, and southern France in 543, and it is mentioned in Rome and Ireland in 544. Sources record the pestilence in Wales in 547 and in 549 in England, Ireland, Finland, and Yemen. See the accompanying sidebar for information on later waves.

The immediate popular response to the plague outbreaks was often **flight**, practiced by both authorities and commoners. Imperial, civic, and religious authorities took measures to bury the large number of dead bodies in mass graves (very few of which have so far been discovered) and to restore normality. Religious leaders instigated religious responses to the disease by organizing litanies, fasts, prayers, and processions in both the Islamic and Christian worlds. The most famous of the last of these took place in Rome in 590 under Pope Gregory the Great (c. 540–604): a sevenfold litany that allegedly brought the scourge to a halt. Although plague victims consulted physicians, they offered little or no aid as they could neither understand nor manage the disease. Instead, people turned to holy men for help. The Christian cult of St. Sebastian as plague helper began in the course of the seventh century in Italy.

The demographic crisis caused by the plague is expressly mentioned in all sources and is also corroborated by other, indirect, evidence such as the number of shipwrecks (as indicators of overall ship numbers and frequency of maritime travel), which dropped about two-thirds between the sixth and seventh centuries. Humanpower shortages were manifested in the army; agrarian depopulation was evident in the Byzantine Empire, whereas after the last wave of the plague, transfers of population to rural areas and to its capital were necessary to revitalize their economic life. A shortage of laborers increased the value of labor, whereas more and better land was available to survivors. Egyptian data on land leases indicate a marked improvement in the security and duration of leases between the first and second halves of the sixth century. This suggests a shortage of human resources and, therefore, the willingness of landowners to lease out their land under positive conditions for the lessees. Estimates of the total population decline caused by the plague are pure guesswork and should not be taken at face value; nevertheless, one may safely assume that the loss of life was considerable and certainly weakened the Byzantine Empire and the new Islamic states. On the cultural level, the plague probably sparked an "intensification of devotion." Islam itself emerged in the midst of the pandemic, and in an unprecedented way both Christian and Muslim communities reacted with public acts of religious piety and humility such as litanies, fasts, and mass prayers. *See also* Diagnosis of Historical Diseases; Greco-Roman Medical Theory and Practice; Historical Epidemiology; Humoral Theory; Islamic Disease Theory and Medicine; Plagues of the Roman Empire; Religion and Epidemic Disease.

Further Reading

Conrad, Lawrence I. "TĀʿŪN and WABĀ': Conceptions of Plague and Pestilence in Early Islam." *Journal of the Economic and Social History of the Orient* 25 (1982): 268–307.

Dols, Michael W. "Plague in Early Islamic History." *Journal of the American Oriental Society* 94 (1974): 371–383.

Horden, Peregrine. "Mediterranean Plague in the Age of Justinian." In *The Cambridge Companion to the Age of Justinian*, edited by M. Maas, pp. 134–60. Cambridge: Cambridge University Press, 2005.

Little, Lester K., ed. *Plague and the End of Antiquity: The Pandemic of 541–750.* New York: Cambridge University Press, 2007.

Rosen, William. *Justinian's Flea: Plague, Empire, and the Birth of Europe.* New York: Viking, 2007.

Stathakopoulos, Dionysios. *Famine and Pestilence in the Late Roman and Early Byzantine Empire.* Aldershot: Ashgate, 2004.

Turner, David. "The Politics of Despair: The Plague of 746–747 and Iconoclasm in the Byzantine Empire." *Annual of the British School at Athens* 85 (1990): 419–434.

DIONYSIOS STATHAKOPOULOS

PLAGUES OF THE ROMAN EMPIRE.   Two major **pandemics** broke out in the Roman Empire prior to the **Plague of Justinian**: the Antonine Plague (166–190) and the Pestilence of Cyprian (251–270). In the first case the designation refers to the Roman emperor in whose reign the outbreak occurred—Marcus Aurelius Antoninus (121–180); in the second it refers to the author who recorded most of what we know about the specific visitation, Cyprian (d. 258), bishop of Carthage.

The Antonine Plague.   A number of Greek and Latin sources record the pandemic. The most celebrated **physician** of Antiquity, **Galen**, who was an eyewitness, provides some information, though in a scattered and not systematic manner. The contemporary historian Cassius Dio (c. 163–229) included information on its last outbreak. Documentary evidence from Egypt, written on papyrus, is extremely important for the quantification of the disease's impact and calculation of the loss of life it caused.

Scholars have identified the Antonine Plague as **smallpox** primarily based on Galen's descriptions, which amount to scattered references to specific patients rather than a complete description of the disease in one work. He recorded symptoms such as raging fever, upset stomach and bowels, diarrhea, black stools, occasional cough and catarrh, and chiefly a black exanthem that covered the entire body, a result of putrefied blood within the fever blisters. He added that it became scabby where there was no ulceration and fell away. Galen also mentioned cases of ulcerations inside the windpipe, infecting the larynx and ultimately damaging the voice. He gave the duration of the disease as 9 to 12 days. Neither he nor any source provided information on the disease's mode of transmission or its seasonality.

The **epidemic** broke out in Mesopotamia in 165 or early 166 CE, during the Roman-Parthian war, allegedly when a pestilential spirit was released from a golden casket in the Temple of Apollo. It spread first to Parthia (in present-day Iran), then to Smyrna (165), and was then disseminated with the Roman army back to the city of Rome (166), then more widely in Italy (Aquileia attested in 168–169), in Dacia (167), and to Egypt (attested in 168–169 and 179), the Rhine, and Gaul. Emperor Marcus Aurelius died of the epidemic in 180 either in Vienna or Sirmium (in present-day Serbia). The disease broke out again in 189, striking at least Rome and Italy. The sources record countless casualties in a language evoking rhetorical exaggeration. Cassius Dio writes that during the 189 outbreak, 2,000 people died each day in Rome. Papyrological data from Egypt (chiefly tax censuses) suggest a loss of life of about 20 percent as a result of the disease; overall the Antonine Plague caused a mortality of 7 to 10 percent, with armies and urban centers being hit the hardest (perhaps at 13 to 15 percent) producing a total number of deaths around 7 to 10 million over and above the normal mortality rate. Recent scholarship suggests that there were pockets of high incidence (where mortality would reach 25–30 percent) and others of low incidence, the mortality rates of which cannot be calculated.

Plague patients certainly consulted Galen, who claimed to have managed the disease in them. The emperor Marcus Aurelius and his son were among his clients. Apart from that, there is no other evidence on the employment of physicians during the outbreaks. **Flight** from affected areas is attested as a response to the disease. Authorities took measures to ensure the proper burials of the disease's casualties, erecting statues as **plague memorials** to honor victims among the nobility and paying for the burial of common people. When Marcus Aurelius was dying of the disease he reportedly sent his son and heir Commodus (161–192) away to protect him from contracting it.

The Antonine Plague was certainly a major phenomenon because of its duration and the high mortality it induced. It was a disruptive factor in the demographic landscape and in everyday life, but it seems that the Empire recovered quickly, as data on Egypt and building programs in Italy suggest.

The Pestilence of Cyprian.   A number of mostly Latin sources record the disease, most notably bishop Cyprian of Carthage, an eyewitness who devoted to it an entire oration, "On the Mortality." Additionally, there are mentions of the disease in some of his letters. Other sources include the letters of the eyewitness bishop Dionysius of Alexandria (late third century) and works of later historians such as the author of the *Historia Augusta* (late fourth century) and Zosimus (late fifth century). Cyprian is the only author to describe its symptoms: diarrhea, continual vomiting, raging fever, bloody eyes, loss of limbs as a result of putrefaction, affected gait, and/or hearing and/or eyesight. Some modern scholars have attempted to identify this disease with **measles**, but the evidence at hand is quite meager.

An eleventh-century Greek source places the origin of the pandemic in Ethiopia, but this may merely be an imitation of Thucydides' (460–400 BCE) account of the **Plague of Athens**. According to more securely dated information, the plague ravaged Egypt and Alexandria in 251 spreading in the same year to Rome, where it killed the emperor Hostilianus (d. 251). The disease may have been present in Italy as early as 248, but there is little evidence to allow more precise dating. In 252 it reached Carthage, flaring up again in the summer of 253, the same year in which, according to St. Jerome (c. 341–420), it ravaged Egypt and especially the great city of Alexandria; this may in fact be a reference to the outbreak in 251, but again a more precise dating is impossible. There is some evidence to suggest that there was an additional outbreak in Neokaisareia (northern Asia Minor) around 256. In 259 the disease decimated Roman troops in Syria, and in 262 it reached Italy, Greece, and Africa once again. Finally, the pestilence broke out among the troops in Sirmium in 270, killing the emperor Claudius II (c. 213–270).

The Pestilence of Cyprian occurred in a period of tensions between the Roman emperors and the emerging Christian community. The general persecution under emperor Decius (250–251) had set the tone. As a result, Christians were locally treated as **scapegoats** for any kind of natural disaster, including the pestilence. Cyprian, in a famous letter to the

---

BISHOP CYPRIAN OF CARTHAGE DESCRIBES THE SYMPTOMS OF THE PESTILENCE AND EXHORTS HIS FLOCK (252 CE)

This, in short, is the difference between us and others who know not God, that in misfortune they complain and murmur, while adversity does not call us away from the truth of virtue and faith, but strengthens us by its suffering. This trial, that now the bowels relaxed into a constant flux, discharge the bodily strength; that a fire originated in the marrow ferments into wounds of the fauces; that the intestines are shaken with a continual vomiting; that the eyes are on fire with the injected blood; that in some cases the feet or some parts of the limbs are taken off by the contagion of diseased putrefaction; that from the weakness arising from the maiming and loss of the body, either the gait is enfeebled, or the hearing is obstructed, or the sight darkened;—is profitable as a proof of faith. What a grandeur of spirit it is to struggle with all the powers of an unshaken mind against so many onsets of devastation and death! what sublimity to stand erect amid the desolation of the human race, and not to lie prostrate with those who have no hope in God; but rather to rejoice and to embrace the benefit of the occasion.

From Cyprian's "On the Mortality," in *Ante-Nicene Fathers*, Vol. 5 (Christian Literature Publishing Co., 1886).

governor of Africa, Demetrianus (third century), recorded such attitudes and countered them by writing that catastrophes in fact ensued not because Christians did not worship Roman gods, but because pagans did not worship the Christian God. Ecclesiastical authors of the period viewed the pestilence as a result of human sins and embedded it in an eschatological context. Plague is one of many signs and omens foretelling the end of the world; as such, Christians should endure it and view their suffering as a path to salvation almost equal to martyrdom. Though Roman rulers reportedly provided proper burials for all victims, Christian authors suggest that the pagan population largely abandoned the afflicted. To the contrary, Christians claimed to have not only tended their own brethren, but also to have extended their care toward anyone in need. From the pagan side, there is ample evidence to suggest a ritual response to the scourge taking the form of public religious rituals in city theaters and the consultation of oracular books. The sources are unanimous in their descriptions of mass mortality as a result of the outbreaks, but any given numbers—such as 5,000 victims in a single day—should be taken as rhetorical exaggeration. There is some evidence to suggest a disruptive effect caused by the outbreaks, but it impossible to quantify it, as the pestilence of Cyprian occurred in a period of extreme political, social, and military turmoil for the Roman Empire. *See also* Diagnosis of Historical Diseases; Greco-Roman Medical Theory and Practice; Historical Epidemiology; Plagues of the Roman Republic; Religion and Epidemic Disease.

Further Reading

Drinkwater, John. "Maximinus to Diocletian and the 'Crisis.'" In *The Cambridge Ancient History*, Vol. XII, *The Crisis of Empire A.D. 193–337*, 2nd edition, edited by A. K. Bowman, P. Garnsey, and A. Cameron, pp. 28–66. New York: Cambridge University Press, 2005.

Duncan-Jones, R. P. "The Impact of the Antonine Plague." *Journal of Roman Archaeology* 9 (1996): 108–136.

Gilliam, J. F. "The Plague under Marcus Aurelius." *American Journal of Philology* 82 (1961): 225–251.

Littman, R. J., and M. L. Littman. "Galen and the Antonine Plague." *American Journal of Philology* 94 (1973): 243–255.

DIONYSIOS STATHAKOPOULOS

PLAGUES OF THE ROMAN REPUBLIC.   Plagues and **epidemics** play a significant part in the history and literature of the Roman Republic (traditionally 509–31 BCE). References occur in a variety of sources, in which they are intertwined with **religion, morality,** and **war.** Early Roman descriptions of plagues and epidemics (known commonly as *pestis* in Latin) rarely focus on symptoms or etiology in ways that allow for **diagnosis.** This is, in part, because of a general disregard for medical theory, but also because the famous description of the **Plague of Athens** by Thucydides (460–400 BCE) became a standard trope and served as a literary model for Roman authors.

The evidence for the occurrence and effect of plagues on early Rome is sketchy. Romans would have recorded the occurrence of plagues in the schematic annual records kept by state and religious authorities (e.g., the *annales* and *fasti*). However, nearly all official records were destroyed in about 390 BCE when Celtic Gauls sacked Rome. Moreover, Roman history did not begin to be written until near the end of the third century BCE (Quintus Fabius Pictor [b. c. 254 BCE]) and did not really start to become a subject of

Roman interest until the mid-second century BCE, when Romans such as Marcus Porcius Cato (Cato the Elder; 234–249 BCE) began to address Roman history and culture. Most of these early works remain only in citations and fragments quoted by authors of the first century BCE. Consequently, although many descriptions by later historians such as Livy (59 BCE–17 CE; *From the Founding of the City*) and Dionysus of Halicarnassus (d. c. 8 BCE; *Roman Antiquities*) have proven to be reasonably accurate of even very early Rome, reports of plagues during the early and middle Republic are based on traditions that are rarely independently verifiable or supported by first-hand evidence.

For the Romans, themselves, the story of their remarkable rise to dominance was in large measure the result of aspects of their moral and religious character as a people, and early histories of Rome record plagues in ways that highlight these features. Livy (1.31) reports that Tullus Hostilius, one of Rome's early kings (r. 673–641 BCE) and a successful military leader, brought a plague on the city and on himself because of his neglect of the gods, rendering both it and him afraid and ineffective. A similar charge of bringing a plague on Rome as a result of religious impropriety was leveled at Scipio Aemelianus (censor in 142 BCE) by one of his rivals (Lucillus Fragment 394). As in many cultures, plague signaled to the Romans that their community was in some way out of favor with the gods, and that special consultation and communal action were required. Devastating plagues circa 436-33 BCE and circa 293 BCE induced the Romans to consult the Sibylline Books (a collection of mystic and prophetic writings attributed to oracular priestesses) and to take action through dedications to Apollo the Healer in 433 BCE (Macrobius [fourth and fifth centuries BCE], *Saturnalia* 1.17.14–16; Livy 4.21–25) and by bringing the cult of the healing god Asclepius to Rome and establishing it on Tibur island about 293 BCE (Livy, 10.47; Valerius Maximus [1st century] I.8.2; Ovid, *Metamorphoses* 15.622–744; Anonymous, *On Famous Men* 22.1–3). In both cases, these actions were said to have been immediately successful, and the stories provide us with important markers in Rome's religious development as well as insight into the archeological record.

Rome's story, however, is also one of nearly continual war, and numerous plagues and epidemic diseases played roles at different stages and at key moments in that story. Incidents often occurred (quite naturally) in situations involving siege, in which famine, poor **sanitation**, and crowded conditions contributed to both sides' vulnerability and, often, one side's defeat. As Rome battled Carthage in Sicily during the Second Punic War, a plague in 212 BCE struck both armies at the siege of Syracuse, but advantaged the besieging Romans (Livy 26.26). Returning from the east, Sulla's (138–78 BCE) successful siege of Rome in 87 BCE was aided by a devastating plague that weakened both armies but particularly Rome's defenders under Cinna (first century BCE; Plutarch, "Pompey"). Illness also began to play a role when Pompey was besieged by Julius Caesar (100–44 BCE) at Dyrrachium in 49–48 BCE (Caesar, *The Civil War* 3.48–49; Lucan, *Pharsalia* VI), shortly before the decisive battle of Pharsalus in which Caesar defeated the republican forces and took control of Rome. Besides siege, incidents of plague occur in the record with greater frequency after the second Punic War as Rome rapidly expanded its reach into new territories. This expansion created new vectors for disease and brought foreign populations into greater contact with each other through armed conflict and commerce throughout the Mediterranean basin. Significant plagues are reported in 187, 182–180, 176–175, 165, and 142 BCE (Livy 36.14, 37.1, 38.44.7, 40.19.3, 42.6; Julius Obsequens, *Book of Prodigies* 6 and 13).

In addition to accounts of historical plagues, plague became a kind of literary motif in Roman literature of the Golden Age (first century BCE through the reign of Augustus [27

BCE–14 CE]). Most authors (including Dionysus of Halicarnassus in his description of a Roman plague in 451 BCE) owe their descriptions and structure to the famous account of the Athenian plague (428–427 BCE) by the historian Thucydides (2.47–54). The Epicurean poet Lucretius (99–55 BCE), in his famous plague scene in *On the Nature of Things* (6.1138–1286), adapts this model with an Epicurean etiology of noxious particles in the air. The Augustan poet Virgil (70–19 BCE) in turn adapts Lucretius and Thucydides in his description of a plague in *Georgics* 3 that strikes animals in Noricum (somewhere between the Danube and Alps), and Ovid (43 BCE–17 CE; *Metamorphoses* 7.516–621) borrows from these accounts when he recounts how Juno struck Aegina (Greece) with a plague in retaliation for one of the god Jupiter's many affairs. In short, the extended descriptions of plagues and epidemics in Roman history and literature of the Republic are more literary than medical. *See also* Air and Epidemic Diseases; Disease, Social Construction of; Greco-Roman Medical Theory and Practice; Historical Epidemiology; Plagues of the Roman Empire.

Further Reading

Note: Accessible introductions and translations of Greek and Roman works can be found in the Penguin Classics series; original texts with translation can be found in the Loeb Classical Library series (Harvard University Press).

Nutton, Vivian. *Ancient Medicine.* New York: Routledge, 2004.
Sallares, Robert. *Malaria and Rome: A History of Malaria in Ancient Italy.* New York: Oxford University Press, 2002.

ERIC D. NELSON

PNEUMONIC AND SEPTICEMIC PLAGUE.   Infection of the human body with *Yersina pestis* is observed in two distinct forms: a blood and lymph borne infection that results in focal infection of the regional lymph nodes nearest the site of inoculation (usually a flea bite) and a pulmonary infection most often acquired by the respiratory route. The latter infection is known as the pneumonic form of plague, in contrast to the **bubonic** form of plague with its characteristic swollen lymph nodes. The causative organism, *Y. pestis*, is the same in both cases, the different pathologies being determined by the route of inoculation. When the victim's bloodstream and its defenses are overwhelmed with the bacteria so rapidly that the lymph nodes do not swell before death, the condition is said to be septicemic (blood-poisoning).

Pneumonic Plague.   In spite of the distinct clinical presentation of bubonic and pneumonic plague, early writers recognized the relationship of these two manifestations of the disease, perhaps on epidemiological grounds. French **physician** Guy de Chauliac (c. 1300–1368), writing on the plague of 1349 in his *Great Surgery* (*Chiurgia Magna,* 1363) noted:

> It was of two kinds: the first lasted two months, with continued fever and expectoration of blood. And they died of it in three days. The second was, all the rest of the time, also with continued fever and apostemes and carbuncles on the external parts, principally in the armpits and groin: and they died of it in five days.

It is thought that pneumonic plague accompanied many of the bubonic plague outbreaks of the **Black Death** and Second Pandemic (1347–1830s), accounting for death rates and other epidemiological factors not generally associated with plague.

The symptoms of pneumonic plague are distinctive and terrifying. The first sign of illness is stiffness, malaise, severe headache, nausea, vomiting, and general pain, with a temperature of 102 to 105°F, followed by cough with bloody sputum and acute respiratory distress. Without treatment, death from respiratory failure occurs in two to four days. In contrast, bubonic plague kills somewhat more slowly. The typical pathologic process involves coagulation necrosis in which the bacterial infection results in death of tissues with inflammation, bleeding into tissues, and then clot formation.

Because of the different mode of spread, the **epidemiology** of pneumonic plague is distinct from that of the vector (flea)-borne bubonic plague. The typical **epidemic** of pneumonic plague tends to occur in winter and early spring associated with indoor crowding and increased opportunities for person-to-person respiratory spread.

Pneumonic plague originates from cases of bubonic plague derived from the natural animal reservoirs of plague, usually flea-ridden rodents. A patient with the bubonic form of plague can develop a lung infection in the course of the bloodborne phase of the illness and may, through coughing, spitting, or other means of respiratory spread, infect others in close contact. Most often it is family members or medical personnel who are most at risk for such infection. Once the fulminant lung infection occurs, person-to-person spread becomes the rule, and a pneumonic outbreak can occur.

Prior to the introduction of **antibiotics**, there was little effective treatment for the pneumonic form of plague, and the mortality rate was close to 100 percent. Treatment with **sulfa drugs** (introduced in the late 1930s) and streptomycin (1940s) greatly diminished the mortality from pneumonic plague. Chloramphenicol and the tetracyclines further improved the treatment of plague in the 1950s and 1960s. Therapy with serum from animals inoculated with killed plague organisms was tried as early as the 1890s by French researcher **Alexandre Yersin** and his colleagues with some success at passive immunization. Active immunization of humans with various preparations of the plague bacillus, pioneered by **Waldemar Haffkine** in India, have been disappointing.

Because pneumonic plague results from human-to-human spread, simple isolation, **quarantine**, and sanitary precautions are effective in preventing or aborting outbreaks, so epidemics of pneumonic plague have not been observed since that of 1920–1921 in China, which resulted in 8,500 deaths. In 1994 there was an outbreak of **pneumonic plague in Surat, India**, and, although reported to be extensive, there appeared to have been fewer than 100 cases and 50 deaths.

Septicemic Plague.   Septicemia results when the *Y. pestis* enter the bloodstream and multiply with great rapidity. This may occur before involvement of the lymphatic system leads to the characteristic swelling known as buboes (primary septicemia), or it may result from complications attending bubonic—and thus be accompanied by buboes—or pneumonic plague. The symptoms of septicemic plague are more pronounced and violent than those of bubonic, with alternating high fever and chills, vomiting, diarrhea, and abdominal pain, often followed by bleeding from nose, mouth, and anus, as well as subdermal or internal hemorrhaging with accompanying gangrene. The untreated victim goes into shock, and these cases usually result in death. Very early treatment with the antibiotics streptomycin or gentamycin should lead to full recovery. Septicemic plague cannot be spread from one person to another without the flea vector or other means of introducing the infected blood into another's bloodstream. Many historians believe that, like pneumonic plague, septicemic plague accompanied many of the outbreaks of the Second Pandemic.

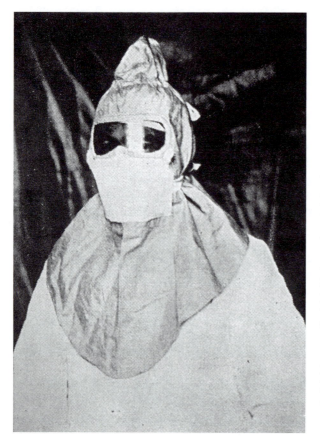

Protective mask used during the pneumonic plague epidemic in Manchuria, 1910–1911. Courtesy of the National Library of Medicine.

According to the **Centers for Disease Control and Prevention** (CDC), between 1990 and 2005, 107 cases of plague were reported in the United States; of these, 18 were primary septicemic, and 5 were primary pneumonic plague. The rapidity of death, high mortality of untreated pneumonic plague, and the relative ease of airborne distribution make Y. pestis of concern as a biological weapon. Because of the effectiveness of common antibiotics in treating plague, however, if a diagnosis is made promptly, the danger from weaponized plague can be mitigated. *See also* Animal Diseases (Zoonoses) and Epidemic Disease; Black Death: Modern Medical Debate; Bubonic Plague in the United States; Diagnosis of Historical Diseases; Human Body; Plague and Developments in Public Health, 1348–1600; Plague in Britain, 1500–1647; Plague in China; Plague in Europe, 1500–1770s; Plague in Medieval Europe, 1360–1500; Plague in the Contemporary World.

Further Reading

Gani, R., and S. Leach. "Epidemiologic Determinants for Modeling Pneumonic Plague Outbreaks." *Emerging Infectious Diseases* 10 (2004): 608–614.

Gregg, Charles T. *Plague: An Ancient Disease in the Twentieth Century*. Albuquerque: University of New Mexico Press, 1985.

Inglesby, Thomas V., et al. "Plague as a Biological Weapon: Medical and Public Health Management." *Journal of the American Medical Association* 283 (2000): 2281-2290.

Orent, Wendy. *Plague: The Mysterious Past and Terrifying Future of the World's Most Dangerous Disease*. New York: Free Press, 2004.

WILLIAM C. SUMMERS

PNEUMONIC PLAGUE IN SURAT, GUJARAT, INDIA, 1994. Pneumonic **plague** struck Surat, in western India, in September 1994. Because the disease is highly contagious, the outbreak caused panic and, within four days, one-quarter of the population of about 1.5 million chose **flight** and abandoned the city. This exodus caused anxiety elsewhere that plague might be spread by the Surat refugees.

The reemergence of plague, after many years, was ascribed to two factors: the condition of the slums and the occurrence of two natural disasters in the area. The city's population had tripled over the previous two decades without a simultaneous growth of infrastructure. Worsening the situation, an earthquake in the neighboring state of Maharashtra in the previous year had caused extensive damage. The disturbances and resettlement that followed brought wild rodents, which normally inhabited the forests neighboring Surat, into contact with the domestic rat population, which thrived in the **poverty**-ridden slums. Even though rats and fleas transmit **bubonic** rather than pneumonic plague, Surat's rat population is regarded as the original source of infection as the plague-infected rat population came into contact with the human population of Surat. The second disaster was the continuous monsoon rains and the flooding of the river Tapti, which had killed cattle whose rotting carcasses were scattered around the town and on which rodents fed.

Using the perspective of the political economy, Ghanshyam Shah has shown that plague was not just a biological phenomenon but the symptom of a sociopolitical disease. The local administration was corrupt and disinterested, serving only the interests of the rich and powerful at the expense of the poor and inarticulate; the municipal authorities did not ensure adequate garbage collection, water supply, or flood drainage; the private medical sector overprescribed modern medicines, and the public sector was inefficient and inadequate. Analysis of the social and demographic data of the victims showed that 80 percent were male blue-collar migrant workers, between the ages of 16 and 35, with little or no education, living and working in squalid conditions.

The outbreak was quickly diagnosed, and it did not have the impact originally feared. The fatality rate was 35 percent of the diagnosed cases, with around 80 people dying between September 18 and October 7, 1994. The most effective response came from the people who cleaned the streets and from junior doctors who worked tirelessly in public hospitals. Doctors of the New Civil Hospital rapidly administered antimicrobial therapy in the form of tetracycline and chloramphenicol, and the death rate dropped dramatically.

Under the dynamic leadership of the municipal commissioner, S. R. Rao, various public health and sanitation measures were undertaken in the post-plague period, making Surat among the cleanest cities in India. The corrective steps implemented included the decentralization of public health administration, the widening of roads, the demolition of illegal structures, and the instituting of sanitary improvements, including the installation of toilets and arrangements for garbage collection. The lesson Surat gave is that there is space within the system for remedial measures. *See also* Animal Diseases (Zoonoses) and Epidemic Disease; Antibiotics; Contagion and Transmission; Environment, Ecology, and Epidemic Disease; Plague in India and Oceania: Third Pandemic; Plague in the Contemporary World; Urbanization and Epidemic Disease.

Further Reading

Catanach, I. J. " Déjà vu? Indian 'Plague' 1896 and 1994." *History Now* 2 (1996): 1–6.

Ghosh, Archana, and Sami S. Ahmad. *Plague in Surat: Crisis in Urban Governance.* Delhi: Institute of Social Sciences, 1996.

Qadeer, Imrana, K. R. Nayar, and Rama V. Baru. "Contextualising Plague: A Reconstruction and an Analysis." *Economic and Political Weekly* (November 19, 1994): 2981–2989.

Shah, Ghanshyam. *Public Health and Urban Development: The Plague in Surat.* New York: Sage Publications, 1997.

MRIDULA RAMANNA

POISON LIBELS AND EPIDEMIC DISEASE.   Even the mere mention of poison or **epidemic** disease evokes a sense of mystery and danger. As both phenomena share associations with the hidden and the unknown, it is no surprise that people who have faced the frightening prospect of a mysterious illness have relied on the equally enigmatic but more concrete notion of poison as a direct causal agent. This has given rise to the phenomenon of the "poison libel," in which people who are trying to explain the origin and propagation of an epidemic disease have blamed individuals, or even entire social or religious groups, for deliberately using "poison" to spread disease.

Tracing the origin of disease to people spreading a poison reveals the natural tendency to relate an unknown and uncontrollable phenomenon, like epidemic disease, to one with a more obvious cause and effect, such as deliberate poisoning. Perhaps the most infamous poison libel comes from the time of the so-called **Black Death** in the mid-fourteenth century, when Jews were accused of poisoning the wells in order to spread plague to Christians. As a result, hundreds of Jews were either exiled or tried and executed (though the trials were hardly fair), and there are reports of mass suicides of Jewish communities to avoid the mistreatment that often followed the accusations. Similarly, the recurring episodes of **bubonic plague** and other epidemic diseases throughout sixteenth-century Italy encouraged many suggestions of plague-spreading conspiracies, in which nefarious individuals were thought to have smeared some kind of poison on the walls of a town to infect its inhabitants.

Just as libels usually offer little justification for their claims, the evidence offered in trials of plague-spreaders or well-poisoners was often flimsy at best and nonexistent at worst. It usually amounted to little more than a report of loitering or "suspicious" activity. Although many of the accused confessed to the charges of spreading poison and thus further fueled the possibility of its legitimacy, most confessed only under duress or threat of torture. Court documents lack any specificity in terms of what kind of poison was actually used, usually describing it as a powder or grease. The vagaries of the testimony, however, did not make poison spreading any less acceptable as a viable explanation. The seriousness in which the accusations were both made and acted upon demonstrates the urgency with which people tried to understand and control the disease at hand.

The notion that poison could be smeared on walls to cause epidemic disease sounds almost ludicrous to modern ears, yet the historical examples of "poison libels" must be understood in conjunction with the long-standing medical framework that linked poison and disease. The root of the association can be traced back to the earliest Western medical literature in which the cause of disease was linked to the concept of "**miasma**" or "bad air." The idea was that there was something foul, putrid, or even poisonous about the air itself that could bring illness, by virtue of its poisonous nature, to those who breathed it. Nor was direct contact required for someone to be poisoned. The belief that poison could act at a distance was virtually common knowledge, an idea embodied in the legend of the fabled basilisk—an animal reputedly able to poison through all five senses, including hearing and vision.

The relationship between poison and disease was considerably strengthened during the Black Death. At the outbreak of the plague, physicians struggled to understand its astonishing mortality, and in particular how it came to and moved across the whole of Europe. In response, doctors such as Gentile da Foligno (d. 1348) described this pestilential disease as some kind of poison in the environment, perhaps emanating from rotting corpses or putrid swamps, or a as a result of a poisonous exhalation from the ground after an earthquake. This poison could move around the environment and eventually find its way inside the human body, poisoning it. By association, the general notion of poison was imbued with the power to spread disease, and towns under a self-imposed isolation to prohibit the arrival of plague considered the spread of external poisons a very real threat indeed. Upon entering the city walls, travelers who were carrying any kind of ointment or potion were occasionally directed to consume them to prove to officials that they were not disease-causing poisons. The role of poison in disease was not merely a function of the plague, but in fact remained a much-discussed medical topic throughout sixteenth-century works on poison, such as those by Italian physicians Girolamo Cardano (1501–1576) and Girolamo Mercuriale (1530–1606).

Not only were poison libels an effort to identify a more tangible cause of a disease, but they were also, in many cases, an effort to associate a dangerous evil, such as poison, with marginal and often misunderstood social groups, who were themselves considered evil in some respects. Just as with the accusations against medieval Jews, whose different religious beliefs elicited scorn from the mainstream Christian majority, it was thought that those people spreading plague or poison were somehow in league with the devil. Associations with evil were especially common with respect to those people who were thought to practice some form of black magic and who could harness occult natural powers to bring ill-health to their targets. In this way, poison libels overlap to some extent with witch-hunts, though witchcraft (which could be used for good as well as evil) and poison conspiracies must not be thought of as the same thing. The way that poison libels target misunderstood social groups is also similar to the notion of "blood libels," accusations of using human blood in religious ceremonies. These, too, have historically been leveled against Jews, but they continue to be applied today, as case in the case of modern practitioners of Voodoo, who are often viewed as a peripheral community with bizarre and satanic rituals.

The general notion of poison as a cause of disease has persisted into the modern era as well. Because the line between medicine and poison can be very fine indeed, radically new drugs

> ## REPORT OF JEWISH "CONFESSIONS" TO POISONING WATER SOURCES IN SAVOY DURING THE BLACK DEATH (1348)
>
> On 19 September Balavigny confessed, without being put to the question [tortured], that three weeks after Pentecost Mussus the Jew of Villeneuve told him that he had put poison in the public drinking fountain of his own town, namely in the custom-house there, and that afterwards he did not drink its water, but only drank from the lake. He also confessed that Mussus had told him that he had likewise placed poison in the public drinking fountain at Chillon, namely in the custom-house under some stones. The spring was then investigated and some poison found. Some of it was given to a Jew, who died, thereby proving that it was poison. He said further that rabbis had instructed him and other Jews not to drink water for nine days after poison had been put in it, and he said that as soon as he had put poison in the spring he immediately warned other Jews.
>
> He confesses further that a good two months earlier he had been at Évian and, while talking the matter with a Jew called Jacob, had asked him, among other things, whether he had a letter and poison like the others; to which Jacob replied that he had. Afterward he asked him whether he had obeyed the instructions, to which Jacob replied that he had not placed the poison himself but had given it to Savetus the Jew who had put it into the spring *de Morer* at Évian. He urged on Balavigny the wisdom of dealing with the instructions in the same way.
>
> From the *Strassburg Urkundenbuch*; translated by Rosemary Horrox in her *The Black Death* (New York: Manchester University Press, 1994), p. 213.

or medical techniques have kindled fears of poison in the minds of wary medical consumers. Some early opponents of **vaccination**, for example, argued that it was tantamount to administering a poison and would be more harmful than the disease itself. Nor does the sentiment behind poison libels necessarily need to involve poison explicitly, but rather the more general notion that one group uses disease to control another. This is perhaps most clear when proponents of underrepresented groups accuse a real or perceived oppressor of "poisoning" them. The frighteningly fast spread of **Human Immunodeficiency Virus** in the late twentieth century brought suggestions that it was in fact a government-produced disease deliberately spread among the disproportionately affected minority groups, such as African Americans, homosexuals, and drug users. More recently, in 2003, skepticism of medical treatment led northern states of Nigeria to halt a Western-led effort to eradicate **poliomyelitis** after rumors circulated that the so-called vaccine was actually the AIDS **virus**.

The typical modern medical definition of poison that focuses on specific measurable variables, such as toxicity, somewhat obscures the complex and multilayered concept of poison as it has been employed throughout history. In the case of poison libels, poison has functioned in two major ways. First, it is a specific, discrete cause of disease that has made intuitive sense to those looking for an explanation. Second, poison has functioned as a convenient and medically acceptable way to assign direct human agency as a cause of disease. Although the relationship between poison and disease is no longer as medically rigorous as it once was, the sentiment of infection and corruption persists in the popular imagination and continues to influence the meaning of poison: we still speak of harmful ideas or ideologies spreading like poison and corrupting unsuspecting minds. Of course, poison libels are more about trying to make sense of the unknown than they are about poison, with the result being that they have at times constituted something of a "mob mentality" fueled by fear and ignorance. At the same time, these episodes richly provide both historical and contemporary insight for what they reveal about the confluence of both medical and social uncertainties. *See also* AIDS in America; Black Death, Flagellants, and Jews; Personal Liberties and Epidemic Disease; Poliomyelitis and American Popular Culture; Religion and Epidemic Disease; Scapegoats and Epidemic Disease; Vaccination and Inoculation.

Further Reading

Cantor, Norman F. *In the Wake of the Plague: The Black Death and the World It Made.* New York: The Free Press, 2001. (See especially pp. 147–68.)

Chase, Melissa P. "Fevers, Poisons, and Apostemes: Authority and Experience in Montpellier Plague Treatises." In *Science and Technology in Medieval Society*, edited by Pamela O. Long, pp. 153–169. New York: Annals of the New York Academy of Sciences, 1985.

Israeli, Raphael. *Poison: Modern Manifestations of a Blood Libel.* Lanham: Lexington Books, 2002.

Naphy, William. G. *Plagues, Poisons and Potions: Plague-Spreading Conspiracies in the Western Alps c. 1530–1640.* New York: Manchester University Press, 2002.

Stevenson, Lloyd G. *The Meaning of Poison.* Lawrence: University of Kansas Press, 1959.

FREDERICK W. GIBBS

POLIO. *See* Poliomyelitis.

POLIOMYELITIS.   Poliomyelitis (polio) was once the source of seasonal terror for parents. Beginning in the early twentieth century, polio was **epidemic** in developed nations, including the United States, during warm summer months. The fear of contracting the disease dictated many a family's summertime activities.

Biological Agent and Its Effects.   The infective agent for poliomyelitis is a single-stranded DNA **virus** in the picornavirus family, closely related to enterovirus and coxsackievirus. A virus cannot reproduce itself unless it enters a living human cell. Poliovirus has a natural affinity to human nervous system tissue, being specifically attracted to a type of nerve cell in the spinal cord and brainstem called an anterior horn cell. This cell, also known as the motor neuron, has as its function the control of muscular activity in the body. Infection of the motor neuron causes destruction of the cell, leading to weakness in the muscles controlled by that nerve cell. There are three major types of poliovirus and many variations within each type.

The virulence of the various types of poliovirus found across the world differs quite substantially. Type I was most common and most likely to cause limb paralysis in epidemics. Type II was milder and most likely to cause mild or asymptomatic cases. Type III was very rare but caused a severe form of polio termed bulbar polio. This form of the disease weakened the muscles that controlled the diaphragm. Weakness in these muscles caused respiratory failure and death.

There was known to be a broad spectrum of disease severity during any epidemic polio outbreak. Most who contracted the virus had either no symptoms at all or only very mild flu-like symptoms that resolved completely without specific treatment. About 10 percent of people experienced a minor illness consisting of fever, headache, and sore throat. Only 1 percent developed major illness characterized by viral **meningitis** and severe muscle aching lasting 5 to 10 days. One-third of the major illness cases developed the paralytic form of polio. Typically, these patients had a rapidly progressive weakness in one or more limbs. The severity of weakness was unpredictable and extremely variable from one patient to the next. The weakness could be temporary or permanent. Approximately 5 percent of patients with paralytic polio died of respiratory failure as a result of muscle weakness, despite devices such as the "iron lung" and the rocking bed. These contraptions assisted breathing for patients whose respiratory muscles were weakened by polio.

Transmission and Epidemiology.   Polio is spread through oral-fecal contact with the virus. This mode of transmission is typically exacerbated by poor sanitary conditions. Prior to routine **vaccination**, virtually everyone had been infected by poliovirus by adulthood, usually in early childhood. The majority of adults in countries with advanced sanitation infrastructure at the onset of the twentieth century had **immunity** to poliovirus. **Children** had a lower rate of immunity. In unsanitary conditions, however, children are more uniformly infected very early in life and are more likely to experience mild disease. It has been proposed that the late-nineteenth-century invention of modern plumbing and sewage containment led to the shift toward epidemic polio by preventing widespread infantile exposure to mild poliovirus. Once someone has been infected with poliovirus, lifelong immunity develops that prevents future reinfection. The prevention of common infantile polio subsequently allowed children to be infected with the more virulent strains later in life.

Epidemic polio, infantile paralysis, began in the early twentieth century. Historically, polio had been sporadic, but it had existed since ancient history. Paralytic poliomyelitis became epidemic in the United States and Europe during the early twentieth century.

Outbreaks of a few hundred or thousand cases were reported in Sweden in 1905 and in New York City in 1907 and 1916. Subsequently, the incidence gradually increased annually. There was an average of 5,000 to 10,000 reported cases per year in the United States until 1944. After 1944 there was a more dramatic yearly increase in incidence, peaking in 1954 with over 60,000 cases.

The introduction of the inactivated, "killed," polio vaccine (IPV) in 1955 led to an abrupt and precipitous decline in new polio cases. Within five years after introduction of IPV, the incidence of polio had declined 90 percent. The subsequent introduction of the oral, live, attenuated "Sabin" vaccine resulted in similar declines in Europe and Russia. Despite the development of effective vaccination, paralytic polio caused by naturally occurring, wild-type virus continues to affect Sub-Saharan Africa and the Indian subcontinent. In the past 25 years, over 90 percent of new cases have been in just four countries: India, Nigeria, Pakistan, and Afghanistan. Recent outbreaks in the 1990s around Nigeria and neighboring countries were the result of poor acceptance of vaccination efforts by the local populace. The **World Health Organization** leads an extensive vaccination campaign, but multiple conspiracy theories abounded in Nigeria regarding contamination of the oral Sabin vaccine, prompting widespread refusal of treatment. Vaccination rates below 50 percent resulted in outbreaks of polio affecting several hundred people a year, until the government was able to convince the population of the safety of the vaccines.

In the United States and Europe, polio has virtually been eradicated. Fewer than 10 cases per year have occurred in the United States. One minor outbreak occurred in a small, isolated religious community where childhood immunizations had been shunned.

Nearly all cases in the developed world are now traceable back to the live attenuated strain of poliovirus in the oral Sabin vaccine. It is estimated that one in 750,000 primary vaccines develop vaccine-related polio, although these cases are generally milder than wild-type polio. These cases are the result of mutation of the live attenuated vaccine back to a virulent form of virus. The oral Sabin vaccine has been commonly used for mass vaccination in the developing world. As wild-type polio approaches eradication in the whole world in the twenty-first century, widespread vaccination programs are beginning to transition exclusively to the killed Salk vaccine to eliminate all cases of polio.

Major Outbreaks with Public Health Responses.   The early twentieth-century public health response to polio focused on patient isolation. Historical reports suggest that public health officials and **physicians** patrolled neighborhoods where new cases were reported. The home was inspected for adherence to published hygiene and **quarantine** regulations. Patients, usually children, were often separated from the family and sent to **sanatoria** to recuperate away from unaffected children. There was a basic lack of understanding about the disease that made public health interventions ineffective and terrifying for the populace. The draconian measures employed did not halt or slow the seasonal outbreaks of disease. Specialized polio wards and hospitals were developed to care for the large number of acute and convalescing patients.

History of Research and Control of the Disease.   It was known as early as 1908 that polio was caused by a virus. In 1931 Sir Frank Macfarlane Burnet (1899–1985) discovered that more than one type of poliovirus existed, and that infection with one type did not prevent later infection with another type. Scientists described three types of polio in 1949 and discovered in 1952 that the poliovirus circulated in the bloodstream. The biologist **John Enders** reported in 1954 that he was able to grow poliovirus on non-nervous system tissue.

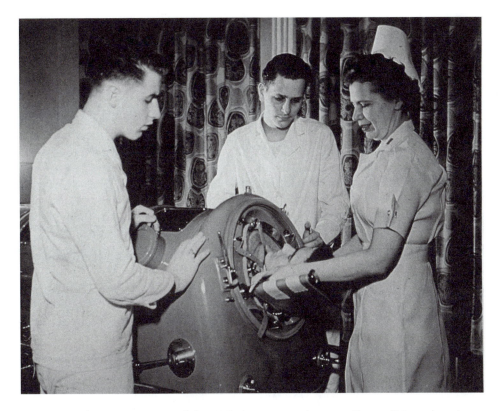

A nurse and two corpsmen of the U.S. Army attend to a poliomyelitis patient in an iron lung. Courtesy of the National Library of Medicine.

He used **antibiotics** to prevent **bacteria** from contaminating the viral cultures, thus producing pure virus for use in research. For their work Enders, Thomas Weller (1915–), and Frederick Robbins (1916–2003) received the Nobel Prize in 1954.

Early attempts to create a vaccine against polio were unfortunate failures. In 1954 two separate versions of a vaccine were widely tested. Both a killed and an attenuated live vaccine made on monkey nervous system tissue were developed. Neither addressed all three types of poliovirus. Both were unsuccessful and resulted in many healthy children contracting paralytic or fatal polio. In 1954 **Jonas Salk** was ready to test a killed virus vaccine (IPV) for effectiveness in inducing immunity to polio. When the results of the trial on nearly 2 million children were presented in 1955, it appeared that the vaccine was about 68 percent effective in preventing polio Type I, 100 percent effective against Type II, and 92 percent effective against Type III. This was an historical moment in medicine. The Salk vaccine is given as two injections spaced one month apart. A booster is needed every five years to maintain immunity. Because it is inactivated, the vaccine is safe for those with weak immune systems.

Albert Sabin developed a live attenuated poliovirus vaccine. This vaccine was also proven effective in a large trial conducted in Russia in 1956. Oral Sabin vaccine is given in three doses in the first two years of life, and a booster is given when the child starts school. The advantage of a live, attenuated vaccine is its long-lasting immunity. A disadvantage is that it cannot be used for patients with weakened immune systems, because it can cause active polio in these patients. Both Salk and Sabin vaccines are effective and have their advantages and disadvantages. The Sabin vaccine is nearly uniformly used in the United States at this time.

There is no medication to treat the poliovirus once active infection occurs. **Antibiotics** are ineffective against viruses, and no available antiviral medicine has any effect on the poliovirus. The focus of treatment is support for the afflicted patient through the illness and recuperation. Physical therapy is paramount. Long-term support of children in iron lungs confined children for long stretches of time. Modern ventilators now support respiratory failure if required. *See also* Animal Research; Environment, Ecology, and Epidemic Disease; Human Subjects Research; Medical Ethics and Epidemic Disease; Non-Governmental Organizations (NGOs) and Epidemic Disease; Personal Hygiene and Epidemic Disease; Poliomyelitis and American Popular Culture; Poliomyelitis, Campaign Against.

Further Reading

Blakeslee, Alton L. *Polio and the Salk Vaccine: What You Should Know about It.* New York: Grosset & Dunlop, 1956.

Centers for Disease Control and Prevention. *Polio (Poliomyelitis).* http://www.cdc.gov/doc.do/id/0900f3ec802286ba

Finger, Anne. *Elegy for a Disease: A Personal and Cultural History of Polio.* New York: St. Martin's, 2006.

Gould, Tony. *A Summer Plague: Polio and Its Survivors.* New Haven, CT: Yale University Press, 1997.

Kluger, Peter. *Splendid Solution: Jonas Salk and the Conquest of Polio.* New York: G. P. Putnam's Sons, 2004.

Mayo Clinic. *Polio.* http://www.mayoclinic.com/health/polio/DS00572

Oshinsky, David M. *Polio: An American Story: The Crusade that Mobilized the Nation against the Century's Most Feared Disease.* New York: Oxford University Press, 2005.

Seytre, Bernard, and Mary Shaffer. *The Death of a Disease.* New Brunswick, NJ: Rutgers University Press, 2005.

Shell, Marc. *Polio and Its Aftermath.* Cambridge, MA: Harvard University Press, 2005.

Silverstein, Alvin, Virginia Silverstein, and Laura Nunn. *Polio.* Berkeley Heights, NJ: Enslow, 2001.

World Health Organization. *Poliomyelitis.* http://www.who.int/immunization_monitoring/diseases/poliomyelitis/en/

LARA J. KUNSCHNER

POLIOMYELITIS AND AMERICAN POPULAR CULTURE.   Although people had suffered from **poliomyelitis** for thousands of years, few cases were reported in the United States until the latter half of the nineteenth century, and even then the isolated cases were rare. This changed, however, in the summer of 1916 when the first major polio **epidemic** hit the United States. By most accounts, the epidemic began in Brooklyn, New York, when a small number of children reported being unable to move their arms or legs. Terrified parents rushed their children to neighborhood and family doctors, who were initially baffled by the various symptoms. As the weeks passed, the number of cases continued to rise. Health professionals finally came to realize that they had an epidemic of infantile paralysis, or polio, on their hands, but they could offer no sufficient explanation for the outbreak, treat its symptoms, or prevent its spread. Polio eventually killed and crippled thousands of Americans and changed the national culture forever, as it became one of the world's most feared diseases.

Cultural Impact of Polio in the United States.   One immediate effect of the polio epidemic of 1916 was to shake the confidence of Americans who had come to believe that they lived in an enlightened period that included the gradual reduction of some infectious diseases, the spread of new and more effective techniques of sanitation, and the extension of life expectancy. The polio epidemic challenged their optimism and their confidence in science and technology as the medical profession seemed appallingly ignorant about the disease and impotent in the face of the growing human suffering it caused. As a result, the scientific community too often turned its attention to a frequent **scapegoat** in such situations, blaming the disease on the rapidly increasing numbers of foreign immigrants, as well as the dirty and often unhealthy slums in which they lived. This reaction drew directly on the new emphasis on public sanitation and **personal hygiene**, and scientists often explained the spread of polio to the upper classes as resulting from either direct contact with the poor or with family pets that had been similarly contaminated.

Ironically, targeting the poor turned out to be a significant mistake, as the disease was likely a byproduct of modern sanitation methods themselves. As public sewers were closed, infants found themselves less exposed to mild strains of polio, resulting in a loss of immunity in children and adults. Ultimately, then, polio struck people of all races and socioeconomic positions, whether urban or suburban, clean or dirty, rich or poor— although the young suffered the most. By December 1916, the polio epidemic had spread from New York to 27 states in the East, and eventually into the Midwest. Over 27,000 cases were reported in a seven-month period, and of those a full 6,000 perished, with most of the rest left paralyzed or deformed. To make it worse, following the initial epidemic in 1916, Americans experienced a terrifying recurrence of the disease each summer with parents every year fearing the beaches, swimming pools, water fountains, and fire hydrants that might spread the disease to their children.

Perhaps the greatest immediate effect of the polio epidemics on most Americans could be found in their experiences with the traditional public health measures used to combat the disease. The typical response was a combination of compulsory isolation, **quarantine**, and sanitation. Health officials often set timetables for exposure and determined whether patients could remain at home or had to be forcefully hospitalized by the "Sanitary Squads." In New York City thousands tried to flee the city by car, train, or ferry but were barred from leaving by quarantine guards who demanded written proof that the travelers were polio-free. At the same time, public health doctors monitored large groups of children in city parks, schools, and movie theaters, and theaters, schools, and amusement parks could be closed at the slightest hint of an outbreak. Many American children avoided these measures when their parents continued the isolation and quarantine policies on their own and without governmental insistence, because medical science seemed incapable of understanding and removing the polio threat. Sadly, none of these efforts accomplished much, and every spring American parents waited in dread for the summer months to arrive.

During the 50 years that polio terrorized millions of Americans, and even in the years following the development of effective and affordable vaccines, many critics argued that the threat of the disease had been consistently overstated. Other diseases and conditions were certainly more deadly, but attention had often been diverted from these to polio, leaving other problems under-addressed by government and medicine alike. Polio epidemics in the United States indeed killed thousands, and many rightly feared the disease for that reason alone. Still, many others were terrified of polio because it seemed to target the young as its most common victims, and because it typically left these children crippled, deformed, and isolated. Once the illness had been contracted, its victims were afforded no substantial medical treatment beyond physical therapy designed to assist their fight for survival. For example, in the 1940s, "rocking tables" were introduced to help patients avoid the buildup of fluids in the lungs, and, if the patient could not breathe, he or she would be confined to an "iron lung," which provided noninvasive assistance until the patient could once again breathe without help. Although these devices were helpful and saved the lives of many polio victims, they were also very expensive and cumbersome, and they became a visual representation of the horror of the disease. Even when not confined to an iron lung, patients often suffered for life, hobbling on crutches or being confined to a wheelchair, and the legions of victims continued to increase for decades until the 1950s, when there were more than 20,000 new polio patients each year.

Addressing the Polio Threat in America. In 1921 Franklin D. Roosevelt (1882–1945) contracted polio, suffering total paralysis from the waist down. As President, in 1938 Roosevelt helped found the National Foundation for Infantile Paralysis (known later as the March of Dimes) that raised millions of dollars for the rehabilitation of those who suffered from paralytic polio and later invested heavily in funding the research that led to effective polio vaccines. Exploiting the concerns and fears of ordinary Americans, the March of Dimes successfully initiated a new approach to fundraising when it sought small donations (only one dime at a time) from millions of individuals. The polio threat also led to a massive celebrity fundraising effort with endorsements and support offered by such cinema stars as Betty Grable (1916–1973), Humphrey Bogart (1899–1957), Jack Benny (1894–1974), and Veronica Lake (1922–1973) who raised public attention and massive contributions for the work of the March of Dimes. Even Mickey Mouse (b. 1928) raised money in movie theaters by singing "Hi Ho, Hi Ho, we'll lick that polio," before ushers passed around collection buckets to the patrons.

Finally, in 1946 the March of Dimes introduced another fundraising innovation, the "poster child." Rather than using photos of pathetic and pitiable children, the organization portrayed the child victims as happy, fresh-faced, and full of promise—except for that wheelchair or leg brace. These measures were successful, and by 1955, the March of Dimes had raised over $25 million for polio research, funding the efforts of both **Jonas Salk** and **Albert Sabin**, the 1954–1955 field trials of the vaccines, and later the provision of **vaccinations** free of charge for thousands of children. Once the Sabin and Salk vaccines were shown to be effective, the disease rapidly decreased in importance throughout most of the industrialized world, and the social impact of that success has been incalculable as few today fear the crutches, wheelchairs, and iron lungs of the recent past.

Only when millions of American school children stood in line waiting their turn to be vaccinated did the disease that had gripped several generations of Americans finally pass from the nightmares of parents and children alike. At the same time, the eradication of this last of the dreaded childhood diseases reinvigorated the faith of many Americans in the ability of medical science to find solutions to seemingly insolvable problems, and scientists once again earned the public's respect, admiration, and trust. Discovered during the height of the Cold War, the vaccines also inspired countless Americans, as the conquest of polio affirmed American technological and scientific prowess. *See also* Children and Childhood Epidemic Diseases; Poliomyelitis, Campaign Against.

Further Reading

Finger, Anne. *Elegy for a Disease: A Personal and Cultural History of Polio.* New York: St. Martin's Press, 2006.

Kluger, Jeffrey. *Splendid Solution: Jonas Salk and the Conquest of Polio.* New York: G. P. Putnam's & Sons, 2004.

National Museum of Health and Medicine. http://nmhm.washingtondc.museum/collections/archives/ agalleries/Polio/polio.html

Oshinsky, David M. *Polio: An American Story.* New York: Oxford University Press, 2006.

Shell, Marc. *Polio and Its Aftermath: The Paralysis of Culture.* Cambridge: Harvard University Press, 2005.

Wilson, Daniel J. *Living with Polio: The Epidemic and Its Survivors.* Chicago: University of Chicago Press, 2005.

BART DREDGE

POLIOMYELITIS, CAMPAIGN AGAINST.   It was not until the late nineteenth and early twentieth centuries that noticeable outbreaks of polio (**poliomyelitis**) began occurring. These were concentrated in areas, particularly the United States, where improved sanitation was reducing the incidence of other infectious diseases. Although the cause of this pattern is not certain, perhaps improvements in sanitation reduced infections of infants with less virulent forms of the disease, leaving them without the resistance that accompanies exposure.

Initial research blundered into blind alleys. A major change began with a tragedy. Franklin Roosevelt (1882–1945), a rising star in the Democratic Party, came down with adult-onset polio in 1921, almost completely losing the use of his legs. His political career seemed ruined, and he began a vain struggle to regain his physical mobility. One of his initiatives was to buy Warm Springs, a threadbare spa and resort in Georgia. He intended to turn Warm Springs into a combination vacation site and polio rehabilitation center. This plan failed because vacationers did not want to mix with patients who had been crippled by polio and who, some thought, were possibly still infectious. With the help of Basil O'Connor (1892–1972), his law partner, Roosevelt turned Warm Springs into a rehabilitation center and started the National Foundation for Infantile Paralysis (NFIP). The NFIP revolutionized philanthropic activities with the March of Dimes program that sought small contributions from everyday people.

The NFIP treated polio as horrible but conquerable. It was criticized for overstating the threat of a relatively rare disease, but its funds meant that no American victim of polio went without aid. When the idea of mixing racial groups at Warm Springs was resisted, the Foundation built a facility for African American patients at Tuskeegee, Alabama. Patients received help with the cost of medical care, physical rehabilitation, and, when necessary, iron lungs and long-term maintenance. Through World War II the provision of care was the NFIP's greatest success, and research remained somewhat haphazard, distracted by the differing approaches of scientists. After the war, O'Connor determined to give the research effort more focus. The disease affirmed his decision by striking ever more children: 25,000 in 1946 rising to 58,000 in 1952. It was the fastest growing infectious disease, but the chances of dying or even being crippled remained quite small. The real impact was psychological and driven by Foundation public relations. From 1951 to 1955, the NFIP raised the then-enormous sum of $250 million, much of which flowed into research.

The search for a vaccine followed two paths: live **virus** and killed virus. Advocates for the former, led by **Albert Sabin** of the University of Cincinnati, argued that dependable, long-term immunity could best be established by exposure to a weakened but living strain of the virus. Unfortunately, a weakened virus might regain strength as it passed through the human system, and it would take some years to perfect. Development of a killed virus vaccine was less creative scientifically but quicker. **Jonas E. Salk** at the University of Pittsburgh spearheaded this work. Less well known than Sabin, Salk started with the tedious task of identifying the types of the virus—there turned out to be three—and then got funding from the NFIP for vaccine research. By 1951 Salk was ready to test his vaccine, though the Foundation's Immunization Committee favored the live virus version. The tests were conducted privately with only a few of Foundation's leaders involved. Although the trials of Salk's vaccine were positive, Sabin and the Immunization Committee remained dubious about long-term acquired resistance. Nonetheless, O'Connor reported to the NFIP trustees that a breakthrough had occurred. O'Connor was determined to move ahead rapidly with the Salk vaccine. A new committee was created to get around bickering in the Immunization Committee, and large-scale field tests were planned for 1954. Some committee resignations resulted from the decision, as did much debate over test protocols. Should all possible children receive the vaccine, with their results compared to the unvaccinated? Or should some be given a placebo to allow for comparison within a particular group? The former meant that more children would get the possible protection, whereas the latter was more scientifically sound. In the end they followed popular opinion and used a combination of the two methods. Opinion was polarized because Sabin openly attacked the Salk virus, and influential gossip columnist Walter Winchell (1897–1972) called it deadly. Test results turned out quite positive, though the vaccine did not produce immunity in all recipients.

Not surprisingly, the nation was ecstatic. Popular demand clamored for **vaccination**, but the federal government headed by President Dwight Eisenhower (1890–1969) stuck to its conservative philosophy. It had made no preparations, preferring to allow **capitalism's** market supply and demand to control availability. Eventually, the President decided that wealth should not determine health. Manufacturers rushed to produce the vaccine, and in one case ignored industry standards: some children actually contracted polio from the vaccine made by Cutter Laboratories in California. Although properly manufactured vaccine was safe, the tragedy shook public confidence. Public reluctance to get vaccinated resulted in unnecessary outbreaks in 1955, but thereafter incidence dropped virtually to zero in the United States. By comparison, meticulous government planning, control, and vaccination in Canada resulted in elimination of the disease without a hitch. By 1961 Albert Sabin had completed his live oral virus vaccine. Eliminating the need for booster shots, which the Salk vaccine required, the Sabin version replaced Salk's, despite its very slight risk of inducing polio.

Buoyed by the progress of the global effort to eradicate smallpox (the last reported case was in 1979), in 1974 the World Health Assembly (WHA) decided to diversify the program and created the Expanded Program on Immunization (EPI). This sought to provide basic childhood disease immunizations worldwide. This was reinforced in 1985, when the **World Health Organization** and UNICEF established the Universal Childhood

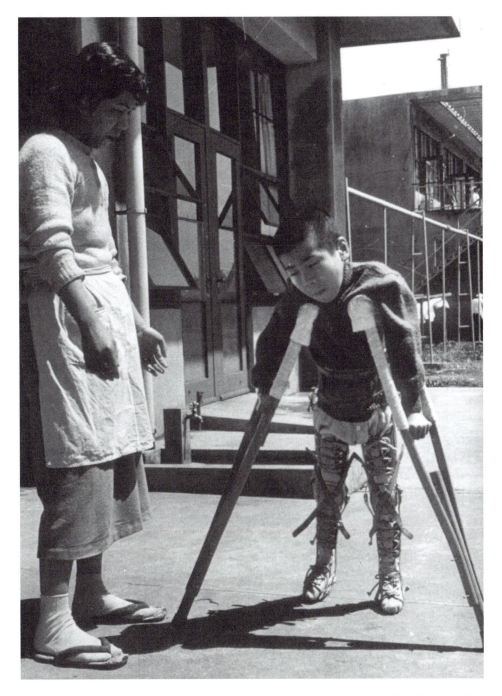

A nurse is ready to offer assistance to a young boy struggling to walk with the aid of crutches and leg braces in Tokyo, Japan. Courtesy of the National Library of Medicine.

Immunization Initiative, and the Pan American Health Organization declared its initiative to eliminate polio from the Americas by 1990 (certified accomplished in 1994). Launching the Global Polio Eradication Initiative in 1988, the WHA announced its goal of worldwide polio eradication by 2000. National Immunization Days in countries such as India and China began in the mid-1990s, and in 1996 the Organization of African Unity initiated the campaign to "Kick Polio out of Africa." In addition to providing four doses of the oral vaccine to infants with later supplementals, the global eradication campaign includes close surveillance for naturally occurring cases, and, when these are found, "mopping up" by targeted immunizations. By 2006 over $5 billion, including $247 million from Rotary International, had been spent worldwide immunizing over 2 billion children. In 1988 some 350,000 children in 125 countries suffered from endemic polio; less than two decades later, it was endemic in only Afghanistan, India, Nigeria, and Pakistan, with a worldwide count of fewer than 2,000 reported cases. In November 2007 the Bill and Melinda Gates Foundation joined Rotary International in committing an additional $200 million to supplement dwindling funds. The target date for eradication has been extended to 2015. *See also* Measles, Efforts to Eradicate; Pharmaceutical Industry; Poliomyelitis and American Culture; Smallpox Eradication.

Further Reading

Finger, Anne. *Elegy for a Disease: A Personal and Cultural History of Polio.* New York: St. Martin's, 2006.

Kluger, Jeffrey. *Splendid Solution.* New York: Berkley Books, 2004.

Oshinsky, David M. *Polio: An American Story.* New York: Oxford University Press, 2005.

Shell, Marc. *Polio and Its Aftermath.* Cambridge, MA: Harvard University Press, 2005.

Fred R. van Hartesveldt

POPULAR MEDIA AND EPIDEMIC DISEASE: RECENT TRENDS. Plagues, **viruses**, and **epidemic** disease feature regularly in popular media and provide audiences with dramatic and gripping plots. Epidemic disease frequently functions as a catalyst to the overall narrative shedding light not only on motivations and struggles of the individual to survive but also on wider societal reactions to infection and containment. In popular media, the epidemiological specificities of the plague, epidemics, or diseases are often less important than the aftermath of epidemic disease and the social disruption that they cause.

Thus filmmakers are able to address wider questions about society, "normal" life, and powerful institutions. Fictional portrayals raise important questions including the search for appropriate solutions. In so doing, our "normal" codes of behavior can be interrogated: What is permissible or appropriate? What does it mean to be human? In addition, epidemic disease operates as a metaphorical device that allows critiques of contemporary society that reflect upon existing cultural, social, and political institutions in ways that would not otherwise be possible in factual media. The origins of disease and measures to contain such outbreaks frequently reveal a deeply pessimistic view of institutions (scientific, medical, political), social divisions, and the individual will for survival. By contrast, in popular fictional television, particularly soap operas, the focus concerns individual experience of disease. Thus, medical **diagnosis** can facilitate discussion of issues that would typically be taboo and transgressive in entertainment media.

Race for the Vaccine.   Epidemic disease forms the basis of a number of popular **cinema** films. Frequently, the main protagonists are engaged in a desperate search for infected victims (often the first victim "patient zero"), and potentially lethal contact with the infected is required if a cure is to be developed. Narrative pace stems from the constraints of "time" where infection must be contained before it spreads to the wider population. Such themes can be identified in films as early as docudrama style thriller *Panic in the Streets* (1950), in which medical and police officers have just 48 hours to locate all those who came into contact with a man infected with **pneumonic plague** before an epidemic is unleashed. This theme of "race against time" is prevalent in cinematic representations of plague and disease, with many such films alluding to the **Ebola fever** and evoking global public fears and anxieties about the epidemic. Thus, in the film *Outbreak* (1995), a married couple who work for a federal disease laboratory must search for an infected monkey and a vaccine before the town is bombed by the military, which considers this to be the only solution.

Showing Not Telling: Destruction of the Body.   Themes of epidemic disease can be identified across other cinematic genres, particularly within the contemporary horror film in which the theme of destruction of the body plays less on the broad fear of death than on the fear of one's own body, of how one controls and relates to it. Showing rather than telling is directly related to the destruction of the body. The movies of the film trilogy by George Romero—*Night of the Living Dead* (1968), *Dawn of the Dead* (1978), and *Day of the Dead* (1985)—are cult horror classics dealing with an unknown infection that turns people into zombies. These films are highly regarded for their gory and explicit visual references to "body horror" mixed with dark humor and social satire. Others such as horror science-fiction film *28 Days Later . . .* (2002) and the sequel *28 Weeks Later* (2007) build on Romero's mix of gore and social commentary offering a nightmare vision of a post-apocalyptic society caused by the release of diseased chimps infected with a "Rage" virus from a laboratory by environmental terrorists. As most of the population becomes infected, survivors must evade not only those infected but also the frequently draconian military efforts to contain the epidemic. The sequel *28 Weeks Later* deals with the repopulation of urban areas and depicts England under surveillance by American-led NATO forces. These films raise pessimistic questions of human nature, as social order breaks down bringing increased lawlessness, sexual violence, and looting, thus playing on our fears about human nature in crisis.

Lack of Trust in Military and Science.   Plague and disease are commonly used as metaphors to address war and political issues, including political disappearances in Argentina, as in *The Plague* (1993). Sometimes the origins of plague are unknown, but a number of popular films involve human-engineered infections. In *The Crazies* (1973), a biological weapon is accidentally transferred to the drinking water of a small town. Dramatic tension stems from conflict between survivors and the military, and the subsequent breakdown in social order reveals scientists, military personnel, and survivors as unable to cooperate. Negative repercussions of biological warfare form the basis of *Omega Man* (1971), in which a military scientist survives and must evade flesh-eating zombies and find a cure. The use of viruses in **bioterrorism** features in *Twelve Monkeys* (1995) with a deliberately released lethal virus wiping out most of the population and forcing survivors to live underground. In *I am Legend* (2008) a human-made virus designed to cure cancer results in transmitting an infectious disease that turns recipients into mutants. The theme of fear of technological advances is similarly exploited in *The Andromeda Strain* (1971), in which a team of scientists struggle to contain an extraterrestrial molecular virus. This film is based on medically trained Michael Crichton's novel and has been praised for its attention to scientific detail.

The AIDS Body and HIV Infection.   During the early 1990s, a number films emerged that focused on the **HIV** and AIDS epidemic. Some, such as *Longtime Companion* (1990) and *Philadelphia* (1993), deal with the discrimination, stigma, and prejudice experienced by those affected. Such portrayals of people living with AIDS aimed to highlight the human dimensions of the problem and sought to counteract the very negative media reporting which could be identified in the news media in which gay men (and injecting drug users) were positioned as "deserving victims." The representing of AIDS traverses difficult territory, in that it is sexually transmitted, and popular media struggled to depict gay relationships in any detail. More overtly political messages in *And the Band Played On* (1993) reflect on the first five years of AIDS in the United States. The conservative political climate is held responsible for the delayed reaction to the epidemic and the reluctance to direct resources to medical research.

Telling in Popular Television.   Popular television miniseries have dealt with epidemic disease in terms of conspiracy and corruption; for example, in *Virus* (1995), a doctor tries to uncover why a strain of **Ebola** is spreading among the urban population of the United States and in so doing uncovers corruption and conspiracy within the medical profession and senior hospital administrators. Television drama provides important opportunities for long-term discussion of health issues through characters with whom audiences can identify. The medical drama *ER* (NBC) featured Dr. Jeanie Boulet, who contracts HIV from her sexually promiscuous husband. Heterosexual risk was similarly highlighted in soap operas *The Young and the Restless*, *All My Children*, and *Another World*, all of which featured women with HIV/AIDS. In the British soap opera *EastEnders* (BBC1) Mark Fowler was forced to challenge his own prejudices against gay people and intravenous drug users when he contracted HIV heterosexually. These socially realistic storylines represent an important commitment to social realism and were developed to counter public misconceptions of the disease as a "gay plague."

Accuracy, Sensationalism, and Impact on Audiences.   The representation of infectious disease in popular film and television is frequently criticized by members of the medical and scientific profession for perpetuating scientific inaccuracies and for playing on public anxieties that may fuel panic in the event of an actual outbreak of epidemic disease. Yet popular representations of epidemics in popular media cannot be assessed on the grounds of accuracy and bias. Such representations are not perceived by audiences in the same way as factual reporting in news and documentary. As noted above, these fictional stories allow us to tackle other deep-rooted issues in society. This is not to argue that such portrayals have no impact on public understandings. Indeed, audience research studies have found that stories involving health and illness topics can have a positive and lasting impact, particularly in terms of understanding the psycho-social repercussions of infectious disease and in challenging sociocultural attitudes toward those affected. *See also* AIDS, Literature, and the Arts in the United States; Cinema and Epidemic Disease; Disease, Social Construction of; Literature, Disease in Modern; Poliomyelitis and American Popular Culture.

Further Reading

Brophy, Philip. "Horrality: The Textuality of Contemporary Horror Films." *Screen* 27 (1986): 2–13; reprinted in *The Horror Reader*, edited by Ken Gelder, pp. 276–284. New York: Routledge, 2000.

Cook, Pam. *The Cinema Book*, 3rd edition. London: British Film Institute, 2007.

Henderson, Lesley. *Social Issues in Television Fiction*. Edinburgh: Edinburgh University Press, 2007.

Miller, David. *The Circuit of Mass Communication: Media Strategies, Representation and Audience Reception in the AIDS Crisis*. New York: Sage Publications, 1998.

Pappas, G. "Infectious Diseases in Cinema: Virus Hunters and Killer Microbes." *Clinical Infectious Diseases* 37 (2003): 939–942.

Seale, Clive. *Media and Health*. New York: Sage Publications, 2002.

Tulloch, John, and Deborah Lupton. *Television, AIDS and Risk*. Chicago: Allen and Unwin, 1997.

LESLEY HENDERSON

POVERTY, WEALTH, AND EPIDEMIC DISEASE.   Death comes to all, but the poor often die younger and from different illnesses than the non-poor. Since ancient Greece, **physicians** have noted that social conditions shape the **epidemiology** and outcome of disease. **Hippocrates**, writing in 400 BCE, noted that any proper medical investigation must "explore the mode in which the inhabitants live, and what are their pursuits." The yawning gap between health outcomes for the indigent and the wealthy has become more pronounced as public health and medical knowledge have advanced, enabling those with financial resources to protect themselves from acquiring disease and preventing themselves from succumbing to disease. Indeed, as Paul Farmer, a professor of social medicine at Harvard University, observes "the spectacular successes of biomedicine have in many instances further entrenched medical inequalities."

Poverty, Wealth, and Health.   The positive correlation between health and wealth is shown in the accompanying box. This graph plots average life expectancy, a commonly used measure of a population's health, versus income per capita, a common indicator of national wealth. The figure demonstrates that residents of high-income countries enjoy better health, on average, than residents of lower-income countries.

According to the World Bank statistics for 2004, low-income countries (defined as countries with an average income per capita less than $875 annually and encompassing more than 2 billion people) have an average life expectancy of 58.8 years, whereas high-income countries (defined as countries with an income per capita greater than $10,726) have an average life expectancy of 78.7 years.

There are many possible factors driving the relationship shown in the graph. Perhaps it is mere coincidence. This seems unlikely given the robustness and reproducibility of the correlation over time. Traditionally, economists have interpreted the association as evidence that higher incomes lead to improved population health. The intuitiveness of this perspective is attractive. Wealth could reduce the risk of sickness, injury, and death through myriad pathways. Financial resources may be used to purchase clean water and sanitation, a comfortable home in a crime-free neighborhood, an adequate and nutritious **diet**, a health club membership, insurance, and high-quality medical care. Wealthier individuals often have more access to health information through media outlets or their social networks. The wealthy also tend to have more political clout—allowing them to advocate for better schools, a cleaner **environment**, and health benefits. A disproportionate share of medical research funds is allocated toward health concerns of the wealthy. In 1990 the Commission on Health Research for Development estimated that less than 10 percent of global health research resources were being applied to the health problems of developing countries, which accounted for over 90 percent of the world's health problems. This observation became known as the 10-90 gap. More current estimates suggest that over U.S. $105 billion is being spent on research and development for neglected diseases, yet the imbalance between disease burden and research funding persists.

However, the relationship between wealth and health may be more complex than originally thought. More recent economic and epidemiologic data support the view that the relationship between socioeconomic status and health is bidirectional. Health may induce wealth, but illness could also lead to indigence. A robust, fit individual is more capable of becoming an educated, productive, and higher-earning member of society than is one who is debilitated or diseased. Moreover, disease can impoverish households via medical and funeral expenses, lost wages, and the erosion of social networks. At the societal level, disease can interrupt supply networks, increase worker turnover, deter foreign investment, and hinder national savings. The shift in perspective, from viewing health as merely a byproduct of economic growth to an engine of development, was reflected in the 2001 **World Health Organization** (WHO) Report chaired by economist Jeffrey Sachs and entitled *Macroeconomics and Health: Investing in Health for Development*. Since 2000 a consensus has emerged that health and wealth, sickness and poverty, can lead to either a virtuous cycle of development and longevity or a vicious cycle of destitution and premature mortality. The eight Millennium Development Goals (MDGs), agreed to by all member states of the United Nations, as well as the leading international financial institutions form a blueprint for extending prosperity to the world's poor. Half of the MDGs are directly concerned with health issues—further evidence of the central role health has assumed in development circles.

However, it is not only absolute poverty that places individuals at greater risk for premature morbidity and mortality—relative position in society also appears to be important. Sir Michael Marmot (b. 1945) has been at the forefront of health inequalities research since the 1970s. Marmot was the principal investigator for a famous study involving thousands of British civil servants, known as the Whitehead study. The study demonstrated an inverse relationship between social class (proxied by employment grade) and the prevalence of multiple medical conditions. Marmot believes there is a connection between the adverse health outcomes for the disadvantaged in developing and developed worlds: "both low-grade civil servant and slum dweller lack control over their lives; they do not have the opportunity to lead lives they have reason to value." Philosophically, Marmot's conception of poverty and development is aligned with that of Amartya Sen (b. 1933), the Nobel Prize-winning (1998) economist. Sen argues that the enduring deprivations caused by poverty, hunger, and the violation of basic liberties are common in rich and poor countries. It follows that freedom from such deprivations is necessary to achieve human development.

Poverty and Epidemics: AIDS and Obesity.   Over 40 percent of the world's population, or 2.5 billion people, live on less than $2 a day. The depredations of destitution lead to increased severity and vulnerability to epidemic disease. **Rudolf Virchow**, a renowned nineteenth-century German **physician**, is often cited as one of the first individuals to identify the social origins of epidemic disease. In today's world, the spread of the **human immunodeficiency virus** (HIV) is a conspicuous example of how socioeconomic status affects susceptibility to infectious disease. According to 2006 figures from the Joint United Nations Program on HIV/AIDS (UNAIDS), 39.5 million people were living with HIV. In 2006 over 4 million individuals were newly infected with the virus, and 3 million individuals died from AIDS and its related complications. Sub-Saharan Africa is the epicenter of the global AIDS **pandemic**. In 2006 two-thirds of all HIV-infected individuals

LIFE EXPECTANCY VERSUS INCOME, 2004

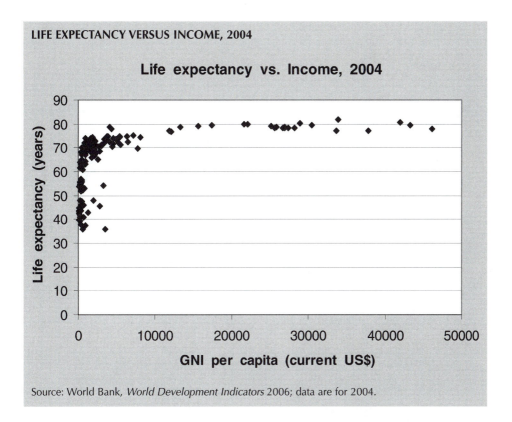

Source: World Bank, *World Development Indicators* 2006; data are for 2004.

(about 25 million people) and the majority of HIV-related deaths occurred in Sub-Saharan Africa. Not surprisingly, Sub-Saharan Africa is also the poorest place in the world: over half of continent's 650 million people live on less than U.S. $1 a day (the definition of extreme poverty). Of the 48 poorest countries in the world, 32 are located in this region. Poverty can increase vulnerability to HIV through many different mechanisms. Poverty prevents people from accessing regular medical and prenatal care. Without treatment for sexually transmitted infections (STIs), the indigent develop ulcerated and denuded genital mucosa, thus facilitating transmission of the AIDS virus. Expectant women may not be able to afford the medicines necessary to prevent viral transmission to their children during pregnancy or parturition. Preventing viral transmission through breast milk is only achievable if the mother has access to safe water for preparing infant formula, a luxury many cannot afford.

The global AIDS pandemic exemplifies the bidirectional relationship between disease and poverty. Winford Masanjala, an economist from Malawi, has summarized the effects of HIV at the household level: "AIDS undermines livelihoods by eroding affected households' resource base, thereby raising vulnerability to future collapse of livelihoods." Masanjala explains how AIDS erodes the four basic components of livelihood: human capital (via death of individuals), financial capital (via income depletion from death of breadwinners and diversion of resources toward health-care and funeral costs), agricultural resources (via the loss of livestock and labor), and social capital (via the loss of relatives and via disease-related stigma). At the macroeconomic level, AIDS strikes those in

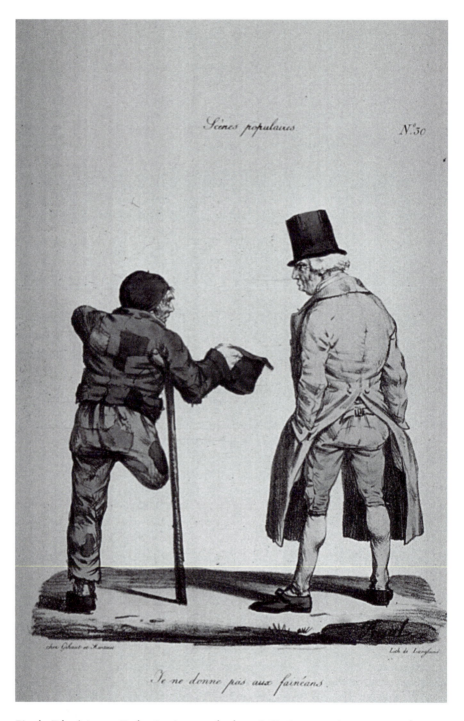

Pigal, Edmé Jean, "I don't give to slackers." Caricature: An amputee beggar holds out his hat to a well-dressed man. Courtesy of the National Library of Medicine.

the prime of their productive life—killing farmers, teachers, political leaders, and doctors. A population of orphans and elderly is left behind. Such a radical demographic shift stymies income growth and could lead to economic collapse.

Yet it is not only infectious disease that stalks those living in poverty—obesity is becoming more prevalent among the relatively poor. According to Dr. Benjamin Caballero, director of the Center for Human Nutrition at Johns Hopkins Bloomberg School of Public Health, "The relationship between obesity and poverty is complex: being poor in one of the world's poorest countries (i.e., in countries with a per capita gross national product [GNP] of less than $800 per year) is associated with underweight and malnutrition, whereas being poor in a middle-income country (with a per capita GNP of about $3,000 per year) is associated with an increased risk of obesity. Some developing countries face the paradox of families in which the children are underweight and the adults are overweight. This combination has been attributed by some people to intrauterine growth retardation and resulting low birth weight, which apparently confer a predisposition to obesity later in life through the acquisition of a "thrifty" phenotype that, when accompanied by rapid childhood weight gain, is conducive to the development of insulin resistance and the metabolic syndrome." The Whitehead study showed that those on the lower rung of the socioeconomic ladder living in developed countries were more susceptible to chronic lung disease, cancer, and bronchitis and were more likely to engage in high-risk behaviors such as smoking, a high-fat **diet**, and a sedentary lifestyle.

Thus, the relationship between poverty and epidemic disease is bidirectional and observed across countries at every level of development. Using the expanded definition of poverty as lack of autonomy, empowerment, and freedom, we observe that premature morbidity and mortality plague the poor wherever they live. Recognizing that epidemic disease is shaped by socioeconomic realities allows effective interventions aimed at correcting both medical and social inequities to be envisioned. Acknowledging the role epidemic disease plays in economic development may provide the impetus for such interventions to be funded and enacted. *See also* AIDS in Africa; Capitalism and Epidemic Disease; Colonialism and Epidemic Disease; Environment, Ecology, and Epidemic Disease; Human Papilloma Virus and Cervical Cancer; Industrialization and Epidemic Disease; International Health Agencies and Conventions; Irish Potato Famine and Epidemic Disease, 1845–1850; Medical Ethics and Epidemic Disease; Pest Houses and Lazarettos; Race, Ethnicity, and Epidemic Disease; Scapegoats and Epidemic Disease; Sexuality, Gender, and Epidemic Disease; Urbanization and Epidemic Disease; War, the Military, and Epidemic Disease; Water and Epidemic Diseases.

Further Reading

Alsan, M., D. Bloom, D. Canning, and D. Jamison. "Health and Economic Performance." In *Health, Economic Development and Household Poverty: From Understanding to Action*, edited by Sarah Bennett, Lisa Gilson, and Anne Mills. (London: Routledge, forthcoming).

Anderson, Gerard, and Edward Chu. "Expanding Priorties: Confronting Chronic Diseases in Countries with Low-income." *New England Journal of Medicine* 356 (2007): 209–211.

Bloom, David E., and David Canning. "Epidemics and Economics," online at http://www.hsph.harvard.edu/pgda/BLOOM_CANNING%20Epidemics%20and%20Economics%2024%20may%2006.pdf

Caballero, Benjamin. "A Nutrition Paradox: Underweight and Obesity in Developing Countries." *New England Journal of Medicine* 352, 15 (2005): 1514–1515.

Farmer, Paul. *Infections and Inequalities: The Modern Plagues.* Berkeley: University of California Press, 1999.

Hossain, Parvez, Bisher Kawar, and Meguid El Nahas. "Obesity and Diabetes in the Developing World—A Growing Challenge." *New England Journal of Medicine* 356 (2007): 213–215.

Marmot, Michael. "Health in an Unequal World." *Lancet* 368 (2006): 2081–2094.

Masanjala, Winford. "The Poverty-HIV/AIDS Nexus in Africa: A livelihood approach." *Social Science and Medicine* 64 (2007): 1032–1041.

Sen, Amartya. *Development as Freedom.* New York: Alfred A. Knopf, 1999.

UNAIDS Joint United Nations Programme on HIV/AIDS. *AIDS Epidemic Update.* 2006. http://data.unaids.org/pub/EpiReport/2006/2006_EpiUpdate_en.pdf

MARCELLA ALSAN

PRESS. *See* News Media and Epidemic Disease.

PROTOZOON, –ZOA. Protozoa are unicellular organisms with a nucleus. There are over 200,000 species, of which about 10,000 are parasitic, and some infect all species of vertebrates and many invertebrates. However, the majority of significant human infections are caused by only a dozen or so species. There are three pathways into the human body: oral, sexual, or by a blood-sucking vector, usually an insect. Some of the intestinal protozoa can form cysts and live for years outside of their host.

There are four groups of protozoa, organized according to their means of motion. Sarcodina—amoeba or rhizopods—use pseudopods to move and are the most primitive protozoa. Mastigophora (flagellates) use whip-like flagella for motion, and Ciliophora (ciliates) use hair-like cilia. Sporozoa is the smallest of protozoa and is not motile in its adult stage.

The most widely dispersed severe disease from amoeba, amebiasis, is caused by *Entamoeba histolytica.* It affects about 10 percent of the world's population, causes a bloody diarrhea, and results in about 40,000 to 110,000 deaths per year. African Trypanosomiasis **(sleeping sickness)** is caused by two species of flagellates, *Trypanosoma brucei gambiense* and *T. brucei rhodesiense,* found in central Africa, transmitted by the tsetse fly, and causing 100,000 new cases per year. American Trypanosomiasis (Chagas' disease), found in Mexico and Central and South America, is caused by *Trypanosoma cruzi* and transmitted by the triatomid **insect.** About 24 million people are infected, and there are 60,000 new cases per year.

Leishmaniasis, also called Kala-azar (black fever) or Assam fever, is caused by *Leishmania donovani,* is transmitted by sand flies, and is located in Asia, Europe, Africa, and Latin America. About 12 million people are infected, and it causes a skin disease or a disseminated disease. *Toxoplasma gondi,* a sporozoa, can infect and reproduce in any mammalian cell. That makes it the most widely distributed parasite in the world. It infects about one-third of the world's human population and may cause death or congenital defects of fetuses or newborns. Most mammals and many birds can be infected, and a common reservoir is the intestinal tract of the domestic cat. Thus, cat feces play a large role in the transmission; however, some infections are transmitted by ingestion of undercooked meat.

Malaria is caused by four *Plasmodium* species (sporozoa) that are transmitted by the female *Anopheles* mosquito. About 500 million people are infected, and between 1 and 3 million people (mostly children) die each year from this protozoon. Malaria was described as far back as 2700 BCE and by **Hippocrates** in the fifth century BCE. It remains the leading parasitic cause of death in the world and is endemic in Africa, Asia, and Latin America.

Further Reading

Despommier, Dickson D., et al. *Parasitic Disease*, 5th edition. New York: Apple Trees Productions, 2005.

McPherson, Richard A., and Matthew R. Pincus. *Henry's Clinical Diagnosis and Management by Laboratory Methods*, 21st edition. Philadelphia: Saunders Elsevier, 2007.

Ryan, Kenneth J., and C. George Ray. *Sherris Medical Microbiology: An Introduction to Infectious Disease*, 4th edition. New York: McGraw-Hill, 2004.

MARK A. BEST

PUBLIC HEALTH AGENCIES IN BRITAIN SINCE 1800.   The history of public health agencies in Britain reflects wider shifts in attitudes toward state intervention in the lives of individuals and the centralization of political and economic power. The idea of public health as one of the responsibilities of a modern state emerged in France in the early nineteenth century, under the social reforms of Napoleon Bonaparte (1769–1821). European intellectuals and reformers were quick to adopt this idea: the German physiologist **Rudolf Virchow's** claim that "medicine is politics" reflected a growing sense that European citizens could expect their governments to get involved in maintaining and promoting the health of the nation.

But in Britain the notion of state intervention in the lives of individuals was widely seen as an infringement of **personal liberty**, running against the spirit of *laissez-faire* **capitalism**. Before the 1840s, British governments took little interest in centrally organized public health measures. Rapid **industrialization** and **urbanization** in the early nineteenth century, and terrible **poverty** in new industrial cities, generated some support for government action on this subject, as did a series of **cholera epidemics** in the 1830s and 1840s. The 1848 Public Health Act, passed against great opposition in Parliament, established a General Board of Health under the civil servant and sanitary reformer **Edwin Chadwick**, with the London **physician** John Simon (1816–1904) appointed Medical Officer for the City of London.

Simon's program of reforms became a model for subsequent British public health agencies. Though he was a physician, his work was based on public sanitation and statistical analyses of demographic data rather than on developments in medical theory and practice. Like Chadwick, Simon sought to improve the urban **environment** by removing sewage and providing clean water. The 1848 Act established the principle of central governmental intervention in public health. In 1872, following the success of this approach, a further Public Health Act required local councils throughout the country to appoint Medical Officers of Health (MOsH).

For the next 50 years, MOsH were the cornerstone of British public health. Their role was initially preventative—to identify, trace, and prevent local outbreaks of epidemic diseases such as cholera. Their work was supported by two central agencies. The General Register Office collected and published demographic data on health and disease, and the Local Government Board coordinated public health at a national level. The "bacteriological revolution" of the late nineteenth century, associated with the work of the French chemist **Louis Pasteur** and the German biologist **Robert Koch**, had little immediate impact on British public health. MOsH were, in general, more influenced by local social and economic factors than by developments in scientific theory. Despite the growing acceptance of state intervention in public health, it remained a controversial subject.

Fierce debates over the Contagious Diseases Acts in the 1860s and 1870s reflected continuing concern for individual freedom.

In the closing decades of the nineteenth century, Simon's "environmental" approach to public health was augmented by a new focus on poverty. Journalists, novelists, and social reformers drew attention to the health problems associated with poverty and to the plight of poor children in particular. Successive governments made many attempts to improve the health of children: compulsory primary education in the 1870s and 1880s, the central provision of milk for infants in the 1890s, free school meals in 1906, and the Schools Medical Service 1907. These measures culminated in the 1911 National Insurance Act, introduced by the first Liberal government in Britain, which provided old age pensions, medical care, and unemployment benefit for all—the Welfare State.

A new Ministry of Health, established at the end of the First World War (1914–1918), provided a fresh governmental focus for a multi-agency approach to public health in Britain. MOsH continued to support improvements in sanitation and housing and to monitor infectious diseases. The Schools Medical Service monitored the health, development, and nutrition of local children and coordinated health education. More widely, the apparatus of the Welfare State—pensions, unemployment benefits and health insurance— aimed to lift the working classes out of poverty by improving the environment in which they were born, grew up, and worked. But this apparent cooperation masked a growing tension between local and central agencies. The 1929 Local Government Act, an attempt to centralize power and financial authority, actually reduced the funds available to the poorest areas.

Despite these tensions, by the mid-twentieth century, the environmentalist approach to public health was widely seen as being successful. Epidemic diseases had largely been eradicated, and, despite the economic depression of the 1930s, the worst Victorian urban poverty had been eradicated. New ideas of citizenship emphasized the responsibility of individual citizens to look after their own health. Public health was increasingly redefined as "community medicine," with a new focus on the chronic disorders of old age and "diseases of affluence." This new approach was embodied in the National Health Service, established in 1948. Much authority and financial control over public health was transferred from local councils and MOsH to the Ministry of Health. The Ministry used general practitioners, now working under the National Health Service, and the increasingly influential mass media to encourage the public to take responsibility for their own health through healthy eating, exercise, and participation on state health programs such as **vaccination** and maternity care.

Since its foundation, the National Health Service has undergone an almost continuous process of reform. The balance has shifted back and forth between local and central control of public health, but the Service has remained under the supervision of the Ministry of Health and its satellite agencies. Current enthusiasm for local control of funds and medical policy means that public health is more than ever in the hands of individual British citizens. *See also* Cholera: First through Third Pandemics, 1816–1861; Cholera: Fourth through Sixth Pandemics, 1862–1947; Demographic Data Collection and Analysis, History of; Germ Theory of Disease; Hospitals since 1900; Irish Potato Famine and Epidemic Disease, 1845–1850; Literature, Disease in Modern; Personal Hygiene and Epidemic Disease; Pharmaceutical Industry; Sanitation Movement of the Nineteenth Century.

Further Reading

Berridge, Virginia. *Health and Society in Britain since 1939*. New York: Cambridge University Press, 1999.

Harris, Bernard. *The Origins of the British Welfare State: Social Welfare in England and Wales, 1800–1945*. Basingstoke, England: Palgrave Macmillan, 2003.

Wohl, Anthony. *Endangered Lives: Public Health in Victorian Britain*. Cambridge, MA: Harvard University Press, 1983.

RICHARD BARNETT

PUBLIC HEALTH AGENCIES, U.S. FEDERAL.   The origins of the United States Public Health Service may be traced back to the passage of an act "for the relief of sick and disabled seamen," signed into law by President John Adams (1735–1826) on July 16, 1798. This original legislation was not actually concerned with public health, which was not a concern of the federal government at the end of the eighteenth century, but was motivated by a recognition on the part of the leaders of the young American nation that a healthy merchant marine was necessary to protect the economic prosperity and national defense of the country. There was no mechanism at the time for providing health care to sick American merchant seamen when their ships docked in American ports. The 1798 law, based on a British model, created a fund to be used by the federal government to provide medical services to merchant seamen in American ports. The Marine Hospital Fund was administered by the Treasury Department and originally financed through a monthly deduction from the wages of the seamen (although later the federal government provided the full funding for the program). Medical care was provided through contracts with existing hospitals and, increasingly as time went on, through the construction of new hospitals for this purpose.

The earliest marine hospitals were located along the East Coast, with Boston being the site of the first such facility. Hospitals were soon also established in a number of other cities on the eastern seaboard, such as Newport, Rhode Island, and Norfolk, Virginia. In time, hospitals were also established along inland waterways, on the Great Lakes, on the Gulf Coast, and finally on the Pacific Coast. The marine hospitals hardly constituted a system in the pre-Civil War period. Funds for the hospitals were inadequate, political rather than medical reasons often influenced the choice of sites for hospitals and the selection of **physicians**, and the Treasury Department had little supervisory authority over the hospitals. During the Civil War (1861–1865), the Union and Confederate forces occupied the hospitals for their own use, and in 1864 only 8 of the 27 hospitals listed before the war were operational. In 1869 the Secretary of the Treasury commissioned an extensive study of the marine hospitals, and the resulting critical report led to the passage of reform legislation in the following year.

The 1870 reorganization converted the loose network of locally controlled hospitals into a centrally controlled Marine Hospital Service, with its headquarters in Washington, D.C. The position of Supervising Surgeon (later Surgeon-General) was created to administer the Service. John Maynard Woodworth (1837–1879) was appointed as the first Supervising Surgeon in 1871, and he moved quickly to reform the system. He adopted a military model for his medical staff, instituting examinations for applicants and putting his physicians in uniforms. Woodworth created a cadre of mobile, career service physicians who could be assigned and moved as needed to the various marine hospitals. The uniformed services component of the Marine Hospital Service was formalized as the Commissioned Corps by legislation enacted in 1889.

The scope of activities of the Marine Hospital Service also began to expand well beyond the care of merchant seamen in the closing decades of the nineteenth century, beginning with the control of infectious disease. Responsibility for **quarantine** was originally a function of the states rather than the federal government, but an 1877 **yellow fever epidemic** that spread quickly from New Orleans up the Mississippi River served as a reminder that infectious diseases do not respect state borders. The epidemic resulted in the passage of the National Quarantine Act of 1878, which conferred quarantine authority on the Marine Hospital Service. Because the Service already had hospitals and physicians located in many port cities, it was a logical choice to administer quarantine at the federal level. Over the course of the next half a century, the Marine Hospital Service increasingly took over quarantine functions from state authorities.

As immigration increased dramatically in the late nineteenth century, the federal government also took over the processing of immigrants from the states, beginning in 1891. The Marine Hospital Service was assigned the responsibility for the medical inspection of arriving immigrants. Immigration legislation prohibited the admission of persons suffering from "loathsome" or dangerous contagious diseases, those who were insane or had serious mental deficiencies, and those who were likely to become public charges (e.g., because of a medical disability). Officers of the Marine Hospital Service were assigned to immigration depots to examine immigrants for medical fitness. The largest center of immigration was Ellis Island in New York, where Service physicians would examine 5,000 or more immigrants on a busy day. The Service also operated hospital facilities on Ellis Island to provide care for those arriving immigrants who needed to be hospitalized.

The newly emerging science of bacteriology was just beginning to make its impact felt on medicine in the late nineteenth century (e.g., by aiding in the **diagnosis** of infectious diseases). In 1887 the Service established a bacteriological laboratory at the marine hospital at Staten Island, New York. Originally concerned mainly with practical problems related to the diagnosis of disease, the Hygienic Laboratory, as it was called, was moved to Washington, D.C., in 1891 and became a center for biomedical research, eventually known as the National Institutes of Health.

Because of the broadening responsibilities of the Service, its name was changed in 1902 to the Public Health and Marine Hospital Service. The Service continued to expand its public health activities as the nation entered the twentieth century. For example, Service physicians cooperated with local health departments in campaigns against **bubonic plague** and yellow fever in cities such as San Francisco and New Orleans in the early part of the century. The increasing involvement of the Service in public health activities led to its name being changed again in 1912 to the Public Health Service (PHS). At the same time, the PHS was given clear legislative authority to "investigate the diseases of man and conditions influencing the propagation and spread thereof, including sanitation and sewage and the pollution either directly or indirectly of the navigable streams and lakes of the United States." Thus, any kind of illness, whatever the cause (including environmental pollution), now came within the purview of the PHS.

During World War I (1914–1918), some PHS-commissioned officers were detailed to the Army and the Navy, but most PHS staff were involved in **war**-related efforts on the home front. The Service was given the responsibility of working with local health departments to keep the areas around military training camps free from disease. Venereal disease was a particular concern to the military, and a PHS Division of Venereal Disease was established in 1918 to control the spread of "social disease." The wartime concern with potential industrial hazards for workers served to stimulate PHS activities in the field of industrial hygiene. Following the war, the PHS was given the responsibility for the care of all returning veterans for a brief time, until the Veteran's Bureau was created in 1921.

In the two decades between the two world wars, the PHS expanded the population to which it provided health care beyond the traditional categories of merchant seamen and the Coast Guard. In 1921 the PHS assumed responsibility for individuals suffering from Hansen's disease when it converted the state **leprosy** facility in Carville, Louisiana, to a national leprosy hospital. Under the PHS, the hospital at Carville carried out pioneering research on the nature and treatment of leprosy. In 1928 the Service detailed a commissioned officer to serve as Director of Health of the Bureau of Indian Affairs of the Department of Interior, as well assigning a number of other officers to the Bureau to provide medical assistance in the field. The law creating the Federal Bureau of Prisons in 1930 included provisions for the assignment of PHS officers to supervise and provide medical and psychiatric services in Federal prisons, thus adding another category of beneficiaries to the roster of those served by the PHS.

The Public Health Service also increased its involvement in this period with issues of drug abuse and mental health. A Division of Narcotics was created in 1929, and the following year it was given the broader name of Division of Mental Hygiene (although drug abuse remained its major focus for some years). The 1929 law that established the Division also authorized the creation of two hospitals for the treatment of narcotics addicts, and these facilities were opened in Lexington, Kentucky, and Fort Worth, Texas, in the 1930s.

Under the New Deal, the PHS became more involved in the broader health concerns of the nation. The Social Security Act of 1935 provided the PHS with the funds and the authority to build a system of state and local health departments, an activity that it had already been doing to some extent on an informal basis. Under this legislation, the Service provided grants to states to stimulate the development of health services, train public health workers, and undertake research on health problems. These new authorities were embraced by Thomas Parran (1892–1968), who was appointed as PHS Surgeon-General in 1936. Venereal disease was an area of particular concern to Parran, who sought to focus the battle against **syphilis** and **gonorrhea** on scientific and medical grounds. He played a major role in breaking down the taboo against the discussion of the subject in the **popular media**, and his efforts were instrumental in leading to the passage of the National Venereal Disease Control Act in 1938.

After being housed in the Treasury Department ever since its establishment, the PHS suddenly found itself in a new administrative home as the result of a government reorganization in 1939. President Franklin D. Roosevelt (1882–1945) aligned the PHS along with a number of social service agencies, such as the Social Security Board, in a newly created Federal Security Agency. The reorganization had little effect, however, on the functions and operation of the Service.

With the entry of the country into World War II (1939–1945), some PHS officers were detailed to the military services. The Coast Guard was militarized in November 1941, and 663 PHS officers served with the Guard during the war, four of them losing their lives. A concern about a wartime shortage of **nurses** led to the passage of the Nurse Training Act of 1943, creating a program known as the Cadet Nurse Corps, administered by the PHS. The program provided participants with a tuition scholarship and a small monthly stipend while attending a qualified nursing school. In return for this support, the Cadets agreed to

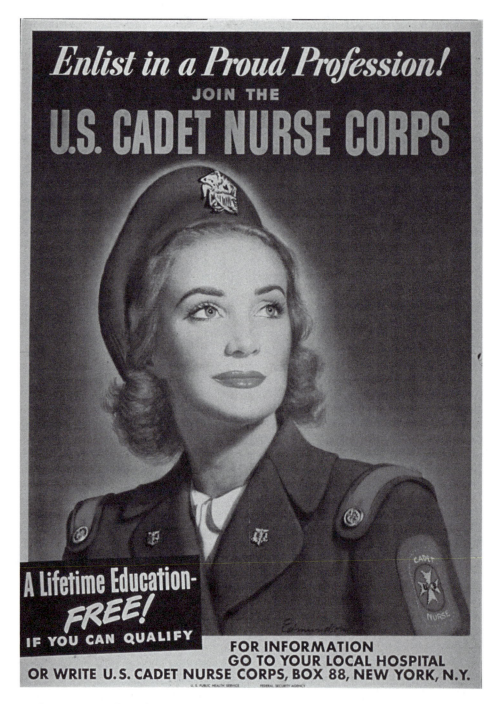

"Enlist in a Proud Profession!" An advertisement for the U.S. Cadet Nurse Corps. Courtesy of the National Library of Medicine.

work after graduation in essential nursing services for the duration of the war, whether in the military or in civilian life. By the time that the program was terminated in 1948, over 124,000 nurses (including some 3,000 African Americans) had graduated.

The war contributed to expansion in the Service's programs and personnel and also increased the involvement of the Service in international health activities. The 1944 Public Health Service Act codified on an integrated basis all of the authorities of the Service and strengthened the administrative authority of the Surgeon-General. This act also provided the authority under which the PHS developed a major postwar program of grants for medical research through the National Institutes of Health, building upon the earlier example of the extramural grants for cancer research given by the Service's National Cancer Institute since its creation in 1937.

Another legacy of World War II grew out of a wartime program of the PHS to control **malaria** in areas around military camps and in maneuver areas in the United States, most of which were established in the South. Over the course of the war, the Malaria Control in War Areas program, based in Atlanta, expanded its responsibilities to include the control of other communicable diseases such as yellow fever, **Dengue**, and **typhus**. The program was converted in 1946 to the Communicable Disease Center (CDC). The mission of the CDC continued to expand over the next half-century, going beyond the bounds of infectious disease to include areas such as nutrition, chronic disease, and occupational and environmental health. To reflect this broader scope of the institution, its name was changed to the Center for Disease Control in 1970. It received its current designation, Centers for Disease Control and Prevention (retaining the acronym CDC), in 1992.

In 1946 two major legislative acts had a significant impact on the PHS. The National Mental Health Act greatly increased PHS involvement in the area of mental health. The Act supported research on mental illness, provided fellowships and grants for the training of mental health personnel, and made available grants to states to assist in the establishment of clinics and treatment centers and to fund demonstration projects. It also called for the establishment within the PHS of a National Institute for Mental Health, which was created in 1949. The Hospital Survey and Construction Act, more commonly referred to as the Hill-Burton Act, authorized the PHS to make grants to the states for surveying their hospitals and public health centers, for planning construction of additional facilities, and to assist in this construction.

The Federal Security Agency was elevated to cabinet status as the Department of Health, Education, and Welfare (DHEW) in 1953, but this change in status of the Service's parent organization had little direct impact on the PHS at the time. The Service did assume several new tasks, however, in the 1950s and 1960s. For example, it became responsible for the health of American Indians in 1955, when all Indian health programs of the Bureau of Indian Affairs were transferred to the PHS. A new Division of Indian Health (now the Indian Health Service) was established to administer these programs. The Food and Drug Administration was made a part of the PHS in 1968, thus involving the PHS much more heavily and visibly in the area of regulation.

While expanding its responsibilities in a number of areas, the PHS also saw its activities circumscribed in one field in this period, namely environmental health. In the 1960s, water pollution control was moved from the PHS to the Department level, and eventually transferred to the Department of Interior. The creation of the Environmental Protection Agency (EPA) in 1970 led to the loss of PHS programs in areas such as air pollution and solid waste to the new agency. Although some PHS-commissioned officers were detailed to the EPA to assist it in its work, the Service had lost its role as the leader of the federal environmental movement.

A major reorganization in 1968, prompted by the concerns of some that the PHS needed to be more responsive to the policies of elected public officials and more of a modern political bureaucracy, dramatically changed the leadership structure of the Service. From the reorganization of 1870 through the middle of the 1960s, the PHS had been led entirely by career commissioned officers (who represented less than 20 percent of PHS employees by the 1960s), with no member of the civil service having ever run a bureau. The Surgeon-General, although appointed by the president, had always been a career member of the Commissioned Corps. The 1968 reorganization transferred the responsibility for directing the PHS from the Surgeon-General to the Assistant Secretary for Health (a political appointee position). For the first time, a non-career official became the top official in the PHS. Although the Assistant Secretary for Health could come from the ranks of the PHS Commissioned Corps, this has not typically been the case. The Surgeon-General was no longer responsible for the management of the PHS but became largely an advisor and spokesperson on public health matters. Candidates for the position of Surgeon-General no longer necessarily came from the ranks of the Corps but were often appointed from outside the PHS and commissioned upon their appointment.

A series of further reorganizations over the next three decades continued to reshape the structure, but not the major functions, of the PHS. The PHS did assume responsibility for the first time for the health of certain members of the general public (as opposed to specific groups such as seamen or prisoners or Indians) with the creation of the National Health Services Corps (NHSC) in 1970. Under this program, the PHS sent physicians and other health professionals into clinical practice in areas where there were critical health humanpower shortages. Beginning in 1972, the PHS could offer health professional students scholarships in exchange for a commitment to serve in the NHSC. A decade later, however, the PHS lost another group of patients when the health care entitlement for merchant seamen was terminated. By that time, the provision of health care to merchant seamen played only a small part in the work of the PHS, but nevertheless the closing of the remaining 8 marine hospitals and 27 clinics in 1981 represented the end of the activity for which the Service was originally created.

There has been no lack of challenges for the PHS since that time, with the **HIV/AIDS** epidemic being just one example of the health-care issues confronting the Service. The Service today, with some 50,000 employees, remains a component of the Department of Health and Human Services (DHHS), as the DHEW was renamed upon the creation of a separate Department of Education in 1980. A major reorganization in 1995 once again changed the leadership structure of the PHS. The PHS agencies, by this time numbering eight, no longer reported to the Assistant Secretary for Health, but directly to the Secretary of the DHHS. The eight agencies, or operating divisions, together with the Office of Public Health and Science (headed by the Assistant Secretary for Health and including the Surgeon General), compose today's Public Health Service. *See also* Hospitals in the West to 1900; Hospitals since 1900; Influenza Pandemic, 1889–1890; Influenza Pandemic, 1918–1919; Leprosy in the United States; Poliomyelitis, Campaign Against; Public Health Agencies in Britain since 1800; Public Health Boards in the West before 1900; Trade, Travel, and Epidemic Disease; Venereal Disease and Social Reform in Progressive-Era America; Yellow Fever in the American South, 1810–1905.

Further Reading

Furman, Bess. *A Profile of the United States Public Health Service 1798–1948*. Washington, DC: U.S. Department of Health, Education, and Welfare, 1973.

Mullan, Fitzhugh. *Plagues and Politics: The Story of the United States Public Health Service*. New York: Basic Books, 1989.

Parascandola, John. "Public Health Service." In *A Historical Guide to the U.S. Government*, edited by George T. Kurian, pp. 487–493. New York: Oxford University Press, 1998.

Ward, John W., and Christian Warren, eds. *Silent Victories: The History and Practice of Public Health in Twentieth-Century America*. New York: Oxford University Press, 2007.

Williams, Ralph C. *The United States Public Health Service 1798–1950*. Washington, DC: Commissioned Officers Association of the United States Public Health Service, 1951.

JOHN PARASCANDOLA

PUBLIC HEALTH BOARDS IN THE WEST BEFORE 1900. The ancient Greeks and Romans rightly associated the preservation of health with clean living **environments**, healthy **diets**, and fresh **water**. Roman *aediles* were public officials charged with maintaining public sanitation, baths, drinking water supplies, and reasonably fresh food, and Rome's first emperor, Augustus Caesar (r. 31 BCE–14 CE) organized their efforts in the Eternal City and provincial capitals. Rome's Byzantine and Islamic successors retained some of this structure, adding hospices, **hospitals**, and **bimaristan** to care for the ill. In the Latin West the revival of Roman law and the development of cities needful of sanitary legislation and oversight were delayed until the twelfth and thirteenth centuries. Beginning in Italy, city councils and their officers oversaw rudimentary attempts to keep streets clean, drainage and sewage flowing, and food sold in markets healthy. Occupational guilds oversaw the practices of **physicians, surgeons**, and **apothecaries**, but there was little in the way of organized public health. Guilds and philanthropists supported poor relief, **leprosaria**, and hospitals, largely as means of maintaining social order.

The **Black Death** in the late 1340s ushered in a new age of concern and public health organization. Many Italian city-states appointed temporary, ad hoc committees of non-medical expert laymen to oversee intensified sanitation and charity efforts, and to protect the property of those who had fled or died. The Venetian Republic's temporary board closed its port, and, after a few bouts of plague, began **quarantine** practices. The Milanese dukes acted decisively in closing the city gates, isolating early plague cases in their houses, establishing a **pest house** outside the city and forcibly relocating the sick, and maintaining a **cordon sanitaire** at the edge of their duchy. Elsewhere in Continental Europe, city governments adopted the ad hoc committee approach, though very slowly, appointing the politically significant who relied on physicians for framing temporary policies and laws. Permanent health boards, still dominated by non-medical experts, began to appear in Italy from the later fifteenth century. Ducal Milan and newly ducal Florence (1527) led the way, with subject towns and cities following their leads. These early magistracies sent investigators around the territories and collected reports on sanitary and health conditions, and when plague or another **epidemic** hit, they appointed the necessary officials to affected locales and enacted appropriate legislation to prevent the spread of disease. By the seventeenth century, their authority trumped that of local church officials, who often wanted to hold religious gatherings the boards felt dangerous to public health. It was no coincidence that small monarchical states pioneered these coercive means and measures. In England the Tudor monarchs' Privy Councils handed down "orders" during plague times. These applied foremost to London, but even there compliance was relegated to the parish level of municipal organization.

From the sixteenth through the eighteenth centuries, maintenance of public health and reaction to epidemic disease remained largely local concerns, despite the flourishing of new and reemerging infectious diseases (the **English sweat, typhus, syphilis, bubonic plague, smallpox**, scarlet fever). Though little changed administratively, a number of individuals made important contributions to public health thinking during the period, sometimes referred to as the **Scientific Revolution**. Many of these ideas resonated with the leaders of states that considered their populations to be economic and political resources to be protected and fostered. **Girolamo Fracastoro** developed an unprecedentedly coherent theory of **contagion**. Englishmen William Petty (1623–1687) and John Graunt (1620–1674) respectively constructed the bases for accurate population data collection and its analysis. In the wake of the **Great Plague of London** in 1665, Petty proposed the establishment of a permanent Health Council for the capital, as well as the construction of public plague isolation hospitals. Wealthy Quaker John Bellers (1654–1725) in his *Essay toward the Improvement of Physick* promoted a comprehensive national health service that would provide well-trained physicians, hospitals, and medical research into diseases. On the continent, the absolutist states took a paternalistic approach to the welfare of their people, but theory rarely translated into action. Germans Veit Ludwig von Seckendorff (1626–1692) and Gottfried von Leibniz (1646–1716) developed early statistical methods and advocated a state health council to oversee public health. Conrad Behrens of Hildesheim (1660–1726) wrote that a state had the obligation to provide for the good health of its people as a mater of natural law, and this meant preventing illness where possible, and treating the suffering to the extent possible.

Humanitarian and Lockean (classical liberal) strains of the eighteenth-century Enlightenment shifted the focus to the individual's right to protection by the state. Enlightened absolutists in Germany set up "medical police," and prison reformer John Howard (1726–1790) inspected prisons and pest houses from Ireland to the Black Sea and reported his findings on the human misery he witnessed. Public-spirited Quakers supported hospitals and trustworthy water supplies for the cities that were growing in number and size. In Germany, Johann Peter Frank (1748–1821) composed a meticulously detailed, nine-volume work outlining a system of state-controlled public welfare that relied on professionals and their emerging sciences. The French Revolution (1789–1796) established France's first national Health Committee, but it took Napoleon (1769–1821) to organize the ad hoc *bureaux de santé* (bureaus of health), commissioned in times of epidemics, under a central council—though only in Paris. A few other French cities followed suit in the 1820s and 1830s. Following the Revolution of 1848, the French government created a system of provincial health councils consisting of health professionals in each *département*. It also created a permanent advisory committee on public health that reported to the Minister of Agriculture and Commerce. The same revolution sparked a public health reform movement in Germany, one of whose leaders was Prussian **Rudolf Virchow**. Though crushed by the royal reaction, a quarter century later, Virchow in Berlin and **Max von Pettenkoffer** in Munich were cleaning up their respective capitals under the authority of new German Empire's Reich Health Office, a creation of the liberal Chancellor Otto von Bismarck (1815–1898).

Both the French and German advances were inspired by changes in England that began in the 1830s and constituted part of the so-called **Sanitation Movement**. **Edwin**

Chadwick shared the popular notion that physical and social environments determined good or bad health, and that poverty and filth contributed directly to disease. This included the dreaded **cholera** that struck London in 1831 and 1832. The capital had undergone intense **urbanization**, and the whole country **industrialization**, and these processes aggravated living conditions across the isle. Chadwick was key actor in drafting the reformative Poor Law Act of 1834, and he served on the Poor Law Commission that oversaw reform activity. A second commission, the Health of Towns Commission, followed in 1843, and, finally, a General Board of Health was established by the Public Health Act in 1848 (not coincidently a year of epidemic cholera). Though it lasted only five years (at which point its initial mandate ran out), it established and directed local boards of health that were responsible for water, sewage, cemeteries, and other sanitary matters. Health matters reverted to the Privy Council until a royal commission report on sanitary administration led to the creation of the Local Government Board in 1871. Four years later, the Public Health Act created a full framework that directed all local boards of health, thus creating a meaningful national health oversight system.

Colonial America had relied on ad hoc committees to see the colonists through epidemic seasons, and by 1830 only five cities had boards of health. New York City began with a City Inspector of Health in 1804, but immigration, growth, industrialization, and the health and social problems and dangers that accompanied these outpaced a single official. By the 1840s the New York slums and recurring outbreaks of **yellow fever**, typhus, **typhoid**, smallpox, and cholera caused deep concern, as chronicled in physician and health inspector John Griscom's (1809–1874) *Sanitary Conditions of the Laboring Population of New York* (1848). As did other Sanitationists of the era, Griscom believed that most disease was preventable, and he outlined the steps to a cleaner and healthier city. Citizen committees picked up much of the slack until the New York Metropolitan Board of Health was established in 1866. It had a geographically wide mandate that was narrowed in 1870. The new New York City Health Department was presided over by a political appointee and consisted of four doctors who served as health commissioners, four police commissioners, and the health officer of the Port of New York. The post-Civil War years also saw the development of state health departments. Between 1869, when Massachusetts began the trend by following the recommendations of Boston's Lemuel Shattuck (1793–1859), and 1877, eight states and the District of Columbia established boards of health. This was followed in 1879 by the creation of the U.S. National Board of Health. *See also* Cholera: First through Third Pandemics, 1816–1861; Demographic Data Collection and Analysis, History of; Epidemiology, History of; Industrial Revolution; International Health Agencies and Conventions; Personal Liberties and Epidemic Disease; Plague and Developments in Public Health, 1348–1600; Plague in Britain, 1500–1647; Plague in Europe, 1500–1770s; Plague in Medieval Europe, 1360–1500; Public Health Agencies in Britain since 1800; Public Health Agencies, U.S. Federal; Public Health in the Islamic World, 1000–1600; Syphilis in Sixteenth-Century Europe; Yellow Fever in the American South, 1810–1905.

Further Reading

Cipolla, Carlo M. *Fighting the Plague in Seventeenth-Century Italy.* Madison: University of Wisconsin Press, 1981.

Duffy, John. A *History of Public Health in New York City, 1625–1866.* New York: Russell Sage Foundation, 1968.

————. *The Sanitarians: A History of American Public Health*. Chicago: University of Illinois Press, 1990.

Hamlin, Christopher. *Public Health and Social Justice in the Age of Chadwick*. New York: Cambridge University Press, 1997.

Porter, Dorothy. *Health, Civilization and the State*. New York: Routledge, 1999.

————, ed. *The History of Public Health and the Modern State*. Atlanta: Editions Rodopi, 1994.

Rosen, George. *A History of Public Health*. Expanded Edition. Baltimore: Johns Hopkins University Press, 1993.

JOSEPH P. BYRNE

PUBLIC HEALTH IN THE ISLAMIC WORLD, 1000–1600. Although structured and extensive **public health** organizations are products of modern states, there was a continuous concern for preserving the health of communities in the Islamic world, as there was in Europe, before the modern era. A variety of cultural and religious practices, such as circumcision or prohibition of eating pork, either attempted to or in effect served to preserve **personal hygiene** and communal health in medieval Islamic society.

Islamic disease theory and medicine, which was largely based on **Galen**ic teachings of **humoral theory**, stressed the importance of preserving health and restoring the balances of the body's humors. Eating a well-balanced diet; bathing and purging regularly; and observing moderation in physical exercise, sexual intercourse, sleep, and emotions were recommended for maintaining good health.

The earliest Islamic hospitals—**bimaristan**—date to the tenth century. Early hospitals were founded in several major cities of the Islamic world including Baghdad, Damascus, and Cairo, and later in several Anatolian cities. Although these foundations grew in number and quality of organization, it is debatable to what extend medieval Islamic hospitals served as public health institutions.

As in neighboring Europe, epidemic disease appears to have been the most important factor that prompted the formation of public health measures in the Islamic world. The **Black Death (1347–1352)** and its recurrent waves affected the Islamic world immensely, as it did the rest of the Old World, and it pressed hard the various governing bodies to adopt measures to monitor, control, and fight the disease. As such, historical analyses of the chain of events in the medieval and early modern Islamic world allow one to document the extent to which the **plague and developments in public health** have been intertwined in the Old World. Practices such as **quarantine**, records of death tolls, control of burying of the dead, and maintenance of urban hygiene were some of the common measures adopted during epidemics.

Quarantine, which required that people and goods be detained and isolated for a number of days before they would be allowed to enter a town, was commonly practiced in the Mediterranean world. This ancient custom had been well known in the Islamic world since antiquity. Although there are occasional references to this custom in the sources, it is hard to determine to what extend regulations were being systematically enforced.

During outbreaks of plague, it was also a common practice for governments to monitor the death toll. Daily death tolls were meticulously kept in many cities of the Islamic world in an effort to observe the progress of the plague infestations. For instance, during the plague in Mamluk Cairo, the death toll was recorded for tax registers. Similarly, in sixteenth-century Istanbul, the number of dead bodies that were taken outside of city walls was recorded on a daily basis.

Because of the supposed connection between **corpses and epidemic disease**, quick and effective burying of the dead was one of the primary concerns during outbreaks. At times, meeting the increased need for labor to carry out burying duties presented a serious challenge to governments. In early fifteenth-century Cairo, for example, the Mamluk Sultan hired the city's poor and beggars and paid them high wages to bury the dead and perform Muslim burial rituals. In another case, during a violent outbreak of plague in late fifteenth-century Istanbul, the city appears to have been nearly deserted as a result of communal **flight**, and chronicles describe the struggle of the government to find the necessary labor force to bury the dead.

As cities grew, maintaining urban hygiene became a major task for governments. For instance, the early modern Ottoman government began to give greater care to public sanitation: it sought to dry up marshy lands, keep water resources clean, and regulate garbage disposal practices in the Empire's cities. From the sixteenth century onward, local judges were made responsible for monitoring and controlling urban hygiene in Ottoman cities. They were also responsible for resolving legal disputes among individuals, which could also entail issues of health. For instance, local judges were consulted for obtaining a report confirming the health status of an individual or his/her illness.

Although the link between **personal hygiene and epidemic disease** was not accurately established in the early modern period, we do see an emphasis on domestic hygiene in most extant Islamic plague treatises. It was recommended, for example, to clean houses by sprinkling vinegar, sandalwood, and rosewater.

The rise of hospitals also helped the emergence and development of institutional **medical education** in the Islamic world. The first medical school opened in Damascus in the early thirteenth century, and new medical schools were established in various cities of the Islamic world. Islamic medical education reached its apogee in the sixteenth century with the establishment of Süleymaniye hospital and medical school in Ottoman Istanbul. Through establishing medical schools and patronizing medical works, the early modern Ottoman state was able to exert control over the production of medical knowledge. From the late fifteenth century onward, for instance, Ottoman plague treatises legally authorized the need to exit a plague-infested city, in contrast to the earlier treatises written in the Islamic world, which strictly forbade this practice.

From the last years of the fifteenth century, the early modern Ottoman state established the post of the Chief **Physician**, who was responsible for administering all health affairs of the empire. The Chief Physician was also responsible for appointing physicians to hospitals in the empire. These health measures paved the way for a gradual institutionalization of medicine and the public health in the Islamic world. *See also* Apothecary/Pharmacist; Black Death, Economic and Demographic Effects of; Hospitals in the West to 1900; Plague in the Islamic World, 1360–1500; Plague in the Islamic World, 1500–1850; Public Health Boards in the West before 1900.

Further Reading

Conrad, Lawrence I. "The Arab-Islamic Medical Tradition." In *The Western Medical Tradition: 800 BC to AD 1800*, edited by Lawrence et al., pp. 93–138. New York: Cambridge University Press, 1994.

Dols, Michael W. *The Black Death in the Middle East*. Princeton, NJ: Princeton University Press, 1977.

Leiser, G. "Medical Education in Islamic Lands from the Seventh to the Fourteenth Century." *Journal of the History of Medicine and Allied Sciences* 38 (1983): 48–75.

Pormann, Peter E., and Emilie Savage-Smith. *Medieval Islamic Medicine.* Washington, DC: Georgetown University Press, 2007.

NÜKHET VARLIK

PUBLIC HEALTH POSTERS.   Publicly displayed health warnings go back at least to Roman times. But public health posters as we know them today, especially following their extensive use in campaigns against **AIDS**, are scarcely a century old. A variant of posters in general (essentially large announcements, usually with a pictorial element, and usually mass-produced on paper for display on walls or billboards to a general audience), they made their debut in the first decade of the twentieth century when health campaigners began to adopt the techniques of mass commercial advertising. During the First World War (1914–1918), they came to be more widely relied upon, particularly in France where a tradition of poster art was exploited for an anti-**tuberculosis** campaign financed by the

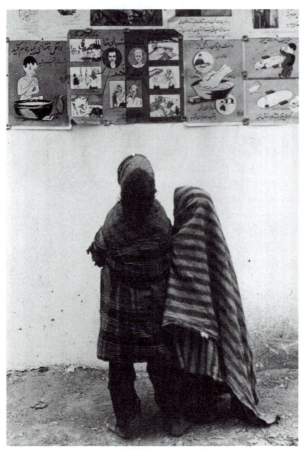

Two Iranian children look at educational posters depicting healthy practices. Photo by Marc Riboud. Courtesy of the National Library of Medicine.

Rockefeller foundation. They were also extensively deployed during the Russian Civil War (1918–1921) and in the new Soviet Union, above all in the battle against the rickettsial **typhus** louse. Unlike wartime propaganda posters, public health posters did not suffer the backlash of informational distrust, in part because in most liberal democracies during the interwar period they continued to be mainly produced and distributed by voluntary organizations such as the **Red Cross** and were perceived as educational tools in a humanitarian interest. By the Second World War (1939–1945) they were increasingly under the aegis of state health authorities, military and civilian, and were as frequently used in campaigns against rats and vermin, as in soliciting blood donation or informing on the dangers of sexually transmitted disease. Whereas in Africa and impoverished countries they continued to be important in campaigns against **smallpox**, **malaria**, and various other infectious diseases, in the West, where infectious diseases were thought to be all but conquered by the 1960s, they were often directed to the dangers of smoking. Ironically, with the advent of AIDS, in the context of the retreat of many Western nations from public health and welfare programs, state initiatives in health poster production were dramatically increased (albeit usually in multimedia campaigns franchised to major advertising companies who could utilize the latest production technologies and marketing strategies). Subsequently, their production in the West tended to revert to voluntary organizations whose audiences are no longer the homogeneous "public" of mid-century, but targeted groups perceived to be at risk. Thus, public health posters have been transformed into health posters for different "publics."

Public health posters might be said to operate by evoking a controlled form of fear and anxiety for the purpose of the rational governance of personal and/or national life. It remains an open question, however, how far this or any other emotional response to them can be generalized, either in terms of the intent to instill it by the producers of posters, or in terms of viewers' reactions. Quintessentially ephemeral objects—disposable, defaceable, and over-paste-able—intended to make an impression and then disappear (as, indeed, many of them have), it is almost impossible historically to measure their behavioral impact. Indeed, just how "public" their circulation was before the time of AIDS (and which posters, when and where) is not readily established. Historically, their greatest power may have been not with regard to public and preventive health, but rather, in destigmatising certain corporeal discussions and in consolidating discourses and authority structures around the body in health and illness. *See also* Disease, Social Construction of; Non-Governmental Organizations (NGOs) and Epidemic Disease; Personal Hygiene and Epidemic Disease; Poliomyelitis, Campaign Against.

Further Reading

Helfand, William H. "Art in the Service of Public Health: The Illustrated Poster." *Caduceus* 6 (1990): 1–37.

Jarcho, Saul. *Italian Broadsides Concerning Public Health*. New York: Blackwell, 1986. (Texts in Italian.)

Porter, Dorothy. *Health, Civilization and the State: A History of Public Health from Ancient to Modern Times*. New York: Routledge, 1999.

ROGER COOTER

PUBLIC HEALTH SERVICE, U.S.   *See* Public Health Agencies, U.S. Federal.

Q

QUACKS, CHARLATANS, AND THEIR REMEDIES. Quackery or charlatanism can be defined in simple terms as a pretense to medical skill, usually by those lacking a formal or credible **medical education**. Although both are pejorative terms, charlatan is more often associated with itinerant healers who exhibited a flair for the theatrical. Historically, accusations of quackery or charlatanism often formed part of larger social and cultural interactions among medical professionals. Any number of practitioners accused their contemporaries of quackery and were themselves accused in turn by their rivals, as part of wider professional conflicts and turf wars or as retribution for perceived slights. In fact, though pretenders to medical skill and knowledge have existed throughout the history of medical practice, it is largely within the context of these professional interactions and rivalries that quackery has assumed particular importance. Accusations of charlatanism became a way for some medical practitioners to establish and defend their professional prerogatives by excluding other, rival, practitioners as "medical pretenders."

The writings of ancient Greek **physicians** indicate that concerns about medical charlatanism date back to the very roots of Western medicine, but it is important to note that charlatanism was by no means unique to the West. For example, when Arabic physicians in the medieval Islamic world discussed quackery, they framed it in terms of fraud and ignorance—for them, the charlatan was someone who deliberately deceived his patients with a pretense to medical skill. It could also, however, be someone whose medical ideas were not based in what was understood to be the legitimate canon of medical literature, derived in large part from classical authors such as **Galen**. Those who were viewed by the predominantly male, Muslim professional class as "others" were also attacked as medical pretenders, particularly women, Christians, and Jews. Some Arabic authors viewed attempts by women to practice medicine as a dangerous form of deception and quackery; their gender was in itself sufficient to brand them as incompetent and illegitimate. By the same token, cultural attitudes toward Jews, in particular, and toward Christians as well, colored the ways Muslim physicians discussed and portrayed Jewish and Christian practitioners.

That Arabic physicians discussed and debated the problem of medical charlatanism for centuries tells us that, in spite of their best efforts, they never entirely succeeded in eliminating rival practitioners. The same can be said for practitioners in Europe, who struggled with similar problems. In the European context, it became increasingly common from the Middle Ages for physicians to identify the self-taught and untraditional practitioners known as **empirics** as quacks and charlatans; the faults ascribed to empirics were almost universally applied to quacks, and vice versa. In seventeenth-century France, a small but powerful coterie of professional physicians railed against a long list of illegitimate practitioners, including foreigners, priests, and women, as well as empirics, alchemists, and **Paracelsians**. They published dozens of pamphlets attacking these practitioners and even appealed to the king in their efforts to eradicate them, but like their Arabic predecessors, they met with little success.

It could be argued that quacks were, in fact, the entrepreneurs of the medical marketplace, which explains why they were so numerous in both Western and non-Western contexts. Because their advertising was cheap and widely circulated, and their services and remedies were affordable, they were more widely consulted by the popular classes than were the more expensive physicians, and as a result, they were often an important part of the medical response to widespread medical crises such as plague and pestilence.

In fact, historians have noted that quacks and charlatans often abounded in times of plague, no doubt seeing a ready market for their cures in an increasingly panicked and fearful populace. During the great **London plague** of 1665–1666, for example, contemporaries recorded numerous instances of quacks and mountebanks advertising both prophylactic measures to ward off the plague and cures for those who had already contracted it. Some of these remedies included powdered unicorn horn and stones extracted from the intestines of camels, both of which would have carried an appealing veneer of exoticism for Londoners. Based on ancient notions of sympathy, the flesh of poisonous animals like vipers and toads was thought to attract the pestilential poison from the air and thereby protect those carrying or consuming it, which explains why quacks and mountebanks sold numerous amulets that contained traces of toad poison or arsenic. Significantly, many professional physicians and **apothecaries** advocated the same types of prophylaxis and treatment.

Undoubtedly, some charlatans preyed on popular fears of plague in order to turn a tidy profit. Accounts from the London plague of 1665–1666 report that some were selling an ounce of the miraculous (but useless) *aurum potabile*, or potable gold, for 5 pounds—a huge sum of money in an age when most household servants earned no more than 10 pounds a year. These abuses led a number of prominent intellectuals to test claims of miracle cures, subjecting them to the new fashion for experimentation that was becoming popular in the latter half of the seventeenth century as part of the **Scientific Revolution**. Unsurprisingly, they discovered that unicorn horn, camel stones, and the rest had no discernible therapeutic properties, a conclusion that nonetheless did little to deter the throngs of paying customers.

As with empirics, however, quacks and charlatans could become useful in times of **epidemic** disease. Towns and cities sometimes turned to alternative practitioners for help when disease threatened to overwhelm the capabilities of legitimate physicians, and this

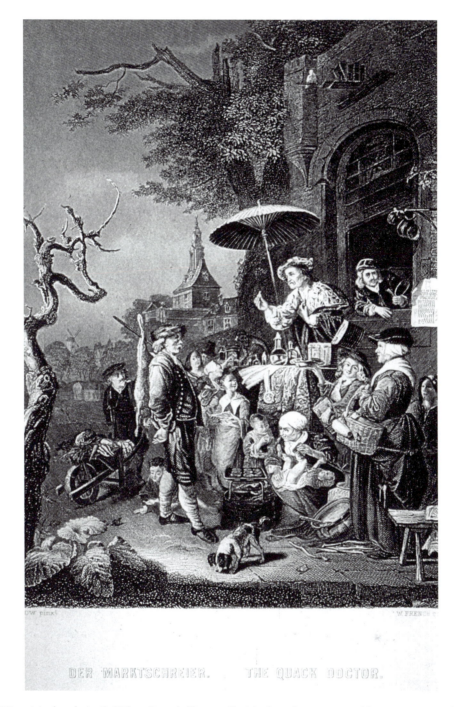

"Der Marktschrier" ("The Quack Doctor"). Market-day scene with a seventeenth-century quack doctor behind his stand. Engraving by W. French after a seventeenth-century painting by Gérard Dou. Courtesy of the National Library of Medicine.

in turn helped at least some of these alternative practitioners to secure footholds in the medical profession. In Italy, physicians attempted to regulate charlatans and quacks by actually issuing them with licenses to practice specific kinds of medicine, such as operations on the eye or the removal of diseased teeth. This seemed to reflect a widespread attitude among physicians that controlling and supervising alternative practitioners was a more practical measure than a futile effort to eradicate them altogether. This attitude, combined with the perceived utility of quacks during periods of epidemic disease, permitted an important degree of professional inclusion for alternative practitioners, which increased during the eighteenth and nineteenth centuries.

As the medical marketplace has become increasingly professionalized in the modern era, the policing of medical practice has assumed greater importance, a task taken up today by organizations such as the state licensing boards in the United States or the General Medical Council in Britain. In other countries, however, medical charlatanism remains a serious problem. For example, some of those with **HIV** or AIDS in parts of Africa have been encouraged by a wide range of charlatans to abandon Western medicines and to turn instead to a host of alternative remedies, often including homemade concoctions that patients are induced to buy but which have no demonstrated therapeutic benefit. Similarly, in parts of India and Southeast Asia where **dysentery** remains a serious health problem, charlatans masquerading as traditional healers have duped thousands of suffering patients into paying for ineffective remedies. Without a centralized and effective means of countering such practices, many physicians worry that this brand of modern-day quackery will only worsen the spread of epidemic disease. *See also* Folk Medicine; Magic and Healing; Medical Ethics and Epidemic Disease.

Further Reading

Gambaccini, Piero. *Mountebanks and Medicasters: A History of Charlatans from the Middle Ages to the Present.* Jefferson, NC: McFarland and Co., 2004.

Gentilcore, David. *Medical Charlatanism in Early Modern Italy.* New York: Oxford University Press, 2006.

Lingo, Allison Klairmont. "Empirics and Charlatans in Early Modern France: The Genesis of the Classification of the 'Other' in Medical Practice." *Journal of Social History* 19 (1986): 583–603.

Pormann, Peter. "The Physician and the Other: Images of the Charlatan in Medieval Islam." *Bulletin of the History of Medicine* 79 (2005): 189–227.

Porter, Roy. *Quacks: Fakers and Charlatans in Medicine.* Stroud, UK: Tempus, 2000.

MARK WADDELL

QUARANTINE.   Quarantine is the enforced temporary isolation of humans (and animals) suspected of carrying a disease because of public health concerns. Quarantine is not the same as enforced isolation of those who are already sick in **leprosaria, pest houses, hospitals, sanatoria,** or their own homes. The practice of isolating and avoiding the ill, or those suspected of being ill, has a long history. The first recorded testimonies come from the Hebrew Bible (Old Testament) and there are examples of quarantining in the writings of **Hippocrates**, Thucydides (460–400 BCE), and **Galen**. In 549 the Byzantine Emperor Justinian (c. 482–565) produced the first effective quarantine laws. Such legislation established that travelers coming from territories struck by the plague should be isolated and avoided. As in Byzantium, China and other countries in Asia and Europe practiced some form of quarantine during the **first plague pandemic**, seven centuries before the **Black Death** visited Europe.

Most scholars agree that source of the term was the city-state of Venice. In 1377 Venetian officials established a waiting period of 40 days for ships seeking entry to the port of Ragusa controlled by Venice. This prohibition included all goods, animals, crews, and passengers, and it was called *quarantine* or *quaranta giorni* (40 days). More controversial is the explanation behind the 40 day length that the isolation lasted. Some scholars maintain that the duration of the quarantine relates to the prevalent medical theory of the time, Hippocratic theory. Hippocrates set at 45 days the limit distinguishing between chronic and acute diseases, a distinction discussed in Europe from the later sixteenth century. Others relate it to the symbolic 40 days of Jewish ritual purification, of Jesus's time in the desert, and the 40 days of the Lenten season.

Of all the measures put in place to contain the spread of the plague that repeatedly struck Europe from 1347 on, quarantine appeared to be the most effective. As in the example of Venice, quarantine aimed to satisfy two main purposes. The first was to allow time for medical inspectors to examine the crew, passengers, and animal cargo of the vessel; the second (and most important) was to permit the development of any incubating disease the ship's passengers and crew might have brought with them.

A modified type of procedure was put in practice in the new world to protect the human cargo that European slave-traders forcefully transported from Africa to the Americas. After major **smallpox** and **typhus** epidemics in the seventeenth century hit the major slave trade ports of the new world, such as Havana, Cartagena, Rio de Janeiro, and Portobelo, all vessels, and more specifically all slave ships, were subjected to a quarantine period and to a careful inspection by physicians of the colonial medical corps. The main task for the medical inspectors was to ensure that the human cargo was free of any signs of epidemic disease. The slightest suspicion could result in the vessel's lying at anchor offshore for weeks. Naturally, quarantines, which by the mid-seventeenth century had become common all over the Caribbean, stimulated the smuggling of slaves and all sort of goods in the Americas, as well as the practice of bribery as a way of doing business in the region.

During European colonial rule, quarantine became standard in the cities and plantations of the Western Hemisphere, as a way of dealing with the threats of **yellow fever, cholera**, smallpox, and typhus. Quarantine was also widely used in France, Britain, Austria, Germany, Russia, and many other European and Asian nations from the fourteenth century on. Even though the microbiological revolution that linked germs with disease would not come until late in the nineteenth century, quarantine was enacted as an effective sanitary measure, and it became mandatory especially during epidemic times, such as during the cholera pandemics of the 1800s.

In the United States, quarantine facilities were first established in port cities from the early eighteenth century. They proved especially important as immigration increased and after the first cholera epidemics struck New York City in the mid-nineteenth century. Quarantining in the United States, even after Pasteur's bacteriological revolution, became a form of social stigmatization. "Undesirable immigrants," such as Russians, Italians, Austrians, Hungarians, and Irish, came to be regarded not only as symbols of disease, but as a menace to American social structure. They were picked out for quarantine in the ships coming from Europe, whereas passengers on the upper decks were allowed to disembark. Also, they were singled out in American cities and quarantined in secluded locations outside the city limits.

From the 1870s, quarantining of animals became a standard practice to prevent the spread of **animal diseases**, ranging from rabies to mad cow disease. It also has been consistently applied to astronauts after returning from space.

More recently, in an age when quarantine was thought to be a primitive tool for the control of disease, only necessary before the rise of modern medicine, humans were faced with the apparently unavoidable fate of quarantining. The late-twentieth-century epidemics of **AIDS, Ebola** virus, and especially **SARS**, prompted governments, of both developed and underdeveloped countries (though not the United States), to enact stringent quarantines. Quarantine, regardless of scientific and medical advances, will long remain the only effective defense against the spread of some diseases, particularly those associated with epidemic spread and high mortality. *See also* Cordon Sanitaire; Hospitals in the West to 1900; Leprosy, Societal Reactions to; Personal Liberties and Epidemic Disease; Plague and Developments in Public Health, 1348–1600; Plague: End of the Second Pandemic; Poverty, Wealth, and Epidemic Disease; Public Health Boards in the West before 1900; Slavery and Disease; Trade, Travel, and Epidemic Disease.

Further Reading

Alchón, Suzanne A. *A Pest in the Land: New World Epidemics in a Global Perspective*. Albuquerque: University of New Mexico Press, 2003.

Alexander, John T. *Bubonic Plague in Early Modern Russia: Public Health and Urban Disaster*. Baltimore: Johns Hopkins University Press, 1980.

Borodi N. K. "The Quarantine Service and Anti-epidemic Measures in the Ukraine in the Eighteenth Century." *Soviet Studies in History* 25 (1987): 24–32.

Fee, Elizabeth, and Daniel Fox. *AIDS: The Burdens of History*. Berkeley: University of California Press, 1988.

Gehlbach, Stephen H. *American Plagues: Lessons from Our Battles with Disease*. New York: McGraw-Hill, 2005.

Markel, Howard. *Quarantine: East European Jewish Immigrants and the New York City Epidemics of 1892*. Baltimore: Johns Hopkins University Press, 1997.

Rosenberg, Charles. *The Cholera Years: The United States in 1832, 1849 and 1866*. Chicago: University of Chicago Press, 1987.

Rothenberg, Gunther. "The Austrian Sanitary Cordon and the Control of Bubonic Plague: 1710–1871." *Journal of the History of Medicine and Allied Sciences* 28 (1973): 15–23.

Sehdev, P. S. "The Origin of Quarantine." *Clinical Infectious Diseases* 35 (2002): 1071–1072.

Watts, Sheldon J. *Epidemics and History: Disease, Power, and Imperialism*. New Haven, CT: Yale University Press, 1997.

PABLO F. GOMEZ

R

RACE, ETHNICITY, AND EPIDEMIC DISEASE. Race is among the most controversial factors used for understanding and tracking diseases in human populations. The classification of human groups under racial labels is largely a cultural creation and does not strictly correspond with biology. **Epidemic** disease factors previously thought to be related to race are now known to be caused by cultural behaviors, socioeconomic conditions, and environmental factors. Nonetheless, race has been, and continues to be, used for scientific, political, religious, social, and cultural classification of human populations.

Hippocrates used the Greek term for "race" in the first classical medical texts, and **Galen** perpetuated its use in the Western medical tradition from 170 CE on. The definition of "race" is, however, highly unstable and can change even within a single generation: for example, not long ago "Jewish" and "Irish" were considered racial categories. Also, because of such variability, race has worked as an effective tool in creating **scapegoats** for the appearance of epidemics. History is full of such examples and even today the subtle force of racial categorization assigns a racial determinant to diseases such as **HIV/AIDS**.

Differences in socioeconomic conditions and geographical patterns of longstanding human settlements—traditionally ascribed to race—have influenced patterns of epidemics' distribution. The interaction between humans and the **environment**, which is studied through economic and sociocultural modeling, slowly shapes immune system characteristics, and these changes make certain human populations more susceptible to disease than others. Thus, diseases that are endemic in certain territories became epidemic when introduced to immunologically "naïve" populations. Most notable among these examples is the sixteenth-century collapse of Native American populations caused by epidemics of **smallpox, measles, tuberculosis**, and other "Old World diseases."

By the time Europeans began their colonization of the Americas, they had lived in settled communities for centuries. This close-range association of humans and animals, fostered by European economic and social models, permitted the biological interchange of **bacteria, viruses,** and parasites among multiple animal species and humans. Diseases such as tuberculosis, the common cold, and smallpox originated in animals and, over centuries of close contact, became endemic in European human communities, where children acquired them at an early age.

The behavior of most infectious illnesses, and the immune reaction to them, varies considerably depending on the age at which the person is first infected. Infections that are mild if first encountered in infancy can be deadly when humans encounter them in adulthood. This is particularly true for smallpox.

With the European colonization of the New World, Native American groups encountered for the first time diseases that had become endemic in the Old World after centuries of close cohabitation between animals and humans, and they suffered dearly from it. The 1507 smallpox epidemic on the island of Hispaniola—today's Haiti and Dominican Republic—marked the beginning of a demographic catastrophe in which almost 80 percent (in some cases, such as the Brazilian smallpox epidemic of 1660, as much as 90 percent) of the original inhabitants of the Americas perished. Thus, differences in immune characteristics, as defined by human groups' particular interaction with the environment, were behind the demise of Native Americans and the consequent rise of African **slavery** in the Americas.

It was precisely in the slave ships that **yellow fever** came to America. Until the sixteenth century, yellow fever affected mostly Europeans visiting the West coast of Africa, and the first recorded epidemic in the Americas struck the island of Barbados in 1647. Like smallpox, yellow fever is a milder disease when acquired during childhood, but it is vicious when acquired later in life. Most Africans, and later in the eighteenth-century European and Native Americans, living in the New World became immune to the disease by acquiring it during infancy and developing a lifelong immunity. Thus, "the disease of the strangers," as contemporary inhabitants of the West Indies called yellow fever, became a disease of new European colonists and invaders. This lesson was relearned the hard way by the British and French armies in their multiple, failed assaults on Caribbean cities and in later militarized colonization of western Africa, when they were defeated mainly by the endemic yellow fever virus.

In other historical cases, the assignment of particular diseases to particular human groups, as defined by their "race," does not correlate with any biological explanation. For instance, when the **Black Death** struck Europe in the fourteenth century, terrified Christians used ethnicity and religion to explain the origin of the disease. Though defended by royal and religious authorities, Jews in many parts of Europe were accused of "poisoning" "Christian" water supplies to initiate the waves of pestilence over European cities. Because of these claims, mobs murdered hundreds of Jews, while local magistrates imprisoned and exiled others during the plague epidemics of the fourteenth centuries. In Spain the concept of "purity of blood" (*limpieza de sangre*) reinforced the intolerance for Jews that led to their expulsion in the late fifteenth century.

European racial and ethnic prejudices accompanied the settlement of America. The inhabitants of nineteenth-century American cities affected by the **cholera** pandemics associated cholera with moral degeneracy, impiety, filth, and race and ethnicity. After striking New York in 1832, cholera became a symbol of the moral degeneracy of the city and its inhabitants. Throughout the nineteenth century, the Irish in particular were blamed as the spreaders of cholera's scourge. Stereotyped Irish characteristics, such as alcoholism, moral degeneracy, and filthiness, were linked to the disease. Similarly, toward the end of the nineteenth century, immigrant Jews, Italians, and Asians came to be seen as carriers of disease, including **typhus**, cholera, and plague. Hundreds were quarantined, either after being evicted from their houses or upon their arrival at American ports.

As had cholera, AIDS has also been associated with race. AIDS had its origins in Africa, and because of specific sociocultural and economic circumstances, people of African descent have been disproportionably affected by the AIDS pandemic. But there is no definitive evidence linking African descent with increased propensity toward infection by the virus. The mechanisms behind this link are probably similar to the ones through which every major pestilence has been ascribed to particular ethnic groups, including particular socioeconomic conditions and cultural behaviors.

The association of race with epidemics has a long history. However, it was not until the nineteenth century, with the work of the German naturalist J. F. Blumenbach (1752–1840), that race achieved its current status in the categorization of human groups. Nonetheless, a nuanced analysis of the history of epidemic diseases shows that rather than being definitive, race is a temporal and fluid category, one that is not objective and does not relate to biological characteristics that determine susceptibility to disease. Although it is undeniable that differences in immune responses have been responsible for the behavior of epidemic diseases around the globe, such differences are the result of cultural patterns or geographical location and not racial characteristics. *See also* AIDS in America; Black Death, Flagellants, and Jews; Colonialism and Epidemic Disease; Disease, Social Construction of; Human Immunity and Resistance to Disease; Human Subjects Research; Irish Potato Famine and Epidemic Disease, 1845–1850; Latin America, Colonial: Demographic Effects of Imported Diseases; Mallon, Mary; Medical Ethics and Epidemic Disease; Poverty, Wealth, and Epidemic Disease; Yellow Fever in Colonial Latin America and the Caribbean.

Further Reading

Alchón, Suzanne A. *A Pest in the Land: New World Epidemics in a Global Perspective.* Albuquerque: University of New Mexico Press, 2003.

Aly, Götz, et al. *Cleansing the Fatherland: Nazi Medicine and Racial Hygiene.* Baltimore: Johns Hopkins University Press, 1994.

Briggs, Charles, and Clara Mantini-Briggs. *Stories in the Time of Cholera: Racial Profiling during a Medical Nightmare.* Berkeley: University of California Press, 2002.

Gehlbach, Stephen H. *American Plagues: Lessons from Our Battles with Disease.* New York: McGraw-Hill, 2005.

Hogan, Katie. *Women Take Care: Gender, Race, and the Culture of AIDS.* Ithaca: Cornell University Press, 2001.

Humphreys, Margaret. *Intensely Human: The Health of the Black Soldier in the American Civil War.* Baltimore: Johns Hopkins University Press, 2007.

———. *Malaria: Poverty, Race, and Public Health in the United States.* Baltimore: Johns Hopkins University Press, 2001.

LaVeist, Thomas A., ed. *Race, Ethnicity, and Health: A Public Health Reader.* Hoboken, NJ: Jossey-Bass, 2002.

Levine, Philippa. *Prostitution, Race and Politics: Policing Venereal Disease in the British Empire.* New York: Routledge, 2003.

McBride, David. *From TB to AIDS: Epidemics among Urban Blacks since 1900.* New York: State University of New York Press, 1991.

Molina, Natalia. *Fit to Be Citizens?: Public Health and Race in Los Angeles, 1879–1939*. Berkeley: University of California Press, 2006.

Rosenberg, Charles. *The Cholera Years: The United States in 1832, 1849 and 1866*. Chicago: University of Chicago Press. 1987.

Shah, Nayan. *Contagious Divides: Epidemics and Race in San Francisco's Chinatown*. Berkeley: University of California Press, 2001.

Troesken, Werner. *Water, Race, and Disease*. Cambridge, MA: MIT Press, 2004.

Washington, Harriet A. *Medical Apartheid: The Dark History of Medical Experimentation on Black Americans from Colonial Times to the Present*. New York: Doubleday, 2006.

Watts, Sheldon J. *Epidemics and History: Disease, Power, and Imperialism*. New Haven, CT: Yale University Press, 1997.

PABLO F. GOMEZ

RED CRESCENT.   *See* Non-Governmental Organizations (NGOs) and Epidemic Disease.

RED CROSS.   *See* Non-Governmental Organizations (NGOs) and Epidemic Disease.

REED COMMISSION.   *See* Yellow Fever Commission.

REED, WALTER (1851–1902).   After being imported into the Western Hemisphere from Africa via the slave trade, **yellow fever**, with a mortality rate of 20 percent, went unchecked for about 400 years. Recognition of the mosquito vector and its breeding ground, and the disproving of the fomite (infectious object or substance) or **contagion theory**, proved invaluable to eliminating this disease. Though others played key roles, the **physician** and medical researcher Walter Reed gets the most credit for this advance in public health, as well as for greater understanding of **typhoid fever**.

Walter Reed was born in Belroi, Virginia. He obtained a two-year medical degree in only one year at age 18, from the University of Virginia, and is the youngest person ever granted a M.D. from that university. Wanting more clinical experience, he obtained a second M.D. degree from Bellevue Medical College in 1870, because it had an associated hospital. He then went on to serve an internship at Kings County Hospital and Brooklyn City Hospital. He was noted for his conversational skills, optimism, and enthusiasm. After joining the Army, he practiced medicine at various frontier Army posts. His later years were spent conducting medical research activities in **epidemiology** and infectious disease. In 1890–1891, Reed studied pathology and bacteriology at the Johns Hopkins University Pathology Laboratory. In the last decade of his life, the targets of his investigations included **yellow fever**, typhoid, **cholera**, erysipelas, **malaria**, and **smallpox**.

Reed is most noted for his contributions to our understanding of the etiology (cause) and spread of typhoid and yellow fever (yellow jack) as a key member on both the Typhoid Board (1898) and the **Yellow Fever (Reed) Commission** (1900). Between 1596 and 1900, 90 waves of yellow fever hit what is now the United States, resulting in an estimated 100,000 deaths. During the American military preparation and campaigns in Cuba in 1898, diseases such as yellow fever and typhoid killed more America soldiers than did the enemy. The generally accepted theory at that time was that fomites (clothing or bedding) transmitted the disease from one person to another. From his research, however, Reed disproved the fomite theory and identified the causative agent as being in the blood, with the *Aedes aegypti* mosquito as the vector of yellow fever (a discovery pioneered in 1881 by Cuban physician Carlos Finlay [1833–1915]) and the housefly as one means of passing typhoid fever. Reed's research on yellow fever, based in Cuba, resulted in a campaign to eliminate bodies of standing **water** that were **insect** breeding places, thus decreasing the disease incidence. Years later, this approach was introduced to Panama during the construction of the Panama Canal. A vaccine for yellow fever was first produced in 1937.

Reed died in 1902 from a ruptured appendix at age 51 and was buried in Arlington National Cemetery. The epitaph on his monument states: "He gave to man control over that dreadful scourge, yellow fever." The Walter Reed Army Medical Center is named in tribute to this remarkable man, soldier, physician, pathologist, and medical researcher. *See also* Colonialism and Epidemic Disease; Environment, Ecology, and Epidemic Disease; Germ Theory of Disease; Sanitation Movement of the Nineteenth Century; War, the Military, and Epidemic Disease; Yellow Fever in Latin America and the Caribbean, 1830–1940; Yellow Fever in the American South, 1810–1905.

Further Reading

Bean, William B. *Walter Reed: A Biography*. Charlottesville: University of Virginia Press, 1982.

Pierce, John R., and James V. Writer. *Yellow Jack: How Yellow Fever Ravaged America and Walter Reed Discovered Its Deadly Secrets*. Hoboken, NJ: John Wiley & Sons, 2005.

Walter Reed Army Medical Center. http://www.wramc.amedd.army.mil/visitors/visitcenter/history/pages/biography.aspx

Mark A. Best

RELAPSING FEVER.   The most distinctive feature of relapsing fever can be discerned in its name. The disease, which is caused by the spirochete *Borrelia* **bacterium**, has a cycle of recurrent bouts of fever. Between each relapse is a period of a few days during which the victim appears to have returned to normal good health. The deceptive lull is then followed by another round of the fever's symptoms, with each recurrence becoming increasingly less virulent as the patient slowly becomes immune to the disease.

Relapsing fever takes on two forms based on the type of carrier that is present. One form is carried by ticks and the other by body lice. They both have the bacteria in their bodies and can infect humans by injecting the *Borrelia* into the bloodstream. The two types of relapsing fever can best be symbolized by the settings in which each thrives. The tick-borne variety is found in remote mountainous or desert regions, especially in North America. Victims are typically people who utilize isolated cabins or explore caves where rodent hosts have nested leaving behind the *Borrelia*-carrying ticks. This type tends to be endemic in nature. The **epidemic** form is the louse-borne relapsing fever, the outbreaks of which are far more deadly and fearsome. The louse-borne fever is a disease of poverty, overcrowding, poor **personal hygiene**, and poor health standards. It is often associated with **typhus**, another louse-borne disease that has some symptoms that are similar to relapsing fever. The two diseases sometimes travel together and can be clearly distinguished by the latter's recurrent cycles and by the presence of jaundice not found with typhus. Louse-borne relapsing fever is perhaps most prevalent during **war**time, with refugees and returning soldiers helping to spread the fever. Arguably, the worst outbreaks have occurred in Africa following World War I (1914–1918) and, especially, World War II (1939–1945). In North America, where it is rare, it can be linked to the **Irish potato famine** immigration in the mid-nineteenth century.

The symptoms of relapsing fever begin with the sudden onset of a fever, one that can range as high as 102.5°F or more. This is followed by headaches, stiff neck, nausea, and vomiting, as well as sore, aching muscles and joints. It can escalate to unsteadiness, seizures, facial droop, and even coma. The first bout of fever takes place about two weeks after infection, and it can last three to five days. In both types of relapsing fever, the initial febrile attack can end in a "crisis" phase that lasts approximately 30 minutes and can include severe shaking and chills followed by sweating accompanied by falling temperature and blood pressure. It is this stage that causes death in 10 percent of cases. This cycle of symptoms reoccurs within seven to ten days following the seeming disappearance of the disease. The number of such relapses can range from one, typical of the louse-borne type, to up to ten for the tick-borne variety. The entire series of relapses can continue for as long as 50 or more days, but the average is 18 to 20 days. This relapse cycle is caused by the ability of the *Borrelia* bacteria to create clones that evolve to ward off antibodies. Once the first round of bacteria has been dealt with by the body's immune defense system, variations of the original are created. Thus, as one type is cleaned out, other, initially less prominent, clones take over and multiply, triggering another round of relapsing fever.

The long-term effects can include problems of the central nervous system that could result in seizures or stupor. *Borrelia* can also invade heart and liver tissue and produce inflammation. Relapsing fever is particularly dangerous for **children** and pregnant women. In the latter it can cause a spontaneous abortion or lead to stillbirth. The bacteria can also be passed on to the fetus, who would then have the disease at birth.

The average mortality rates for relapsing fever range around 5 percent and, with treatment, are as low as 1 percent. However, particularly with the louse-borne type, the death toll can be much higher especially among infants, the very old, and those who are malnourished and debilitated. It would not be unusual for such victims to die even before the first relapse, a fact that, on occasion, made it difficult to identify the disease. During the epidemic in Africa in the 1940s, the mortality rates went as high as 10 to 15 percent.

The **transmission** of the fever bacteria requires a reservoir host for the tick-borne type, usually some variety of rodent, including mice, squirrels, or chipmunks that carry the infected ticks. The louse-borne fever requires no such host animal because it feeds on the human body and is transported by it. This is what makes louse-borne relapsing fever so prone to erupt into an epidemic. The lice pick up the disease from humans who are already infected and feverish and then transport it to other humans, especially in areas that are unhygienic or severely overcrowded. The infection enters the human body when the lice are crushed into a bite-wound or into an area made raw from scratching. From there, it goes into the bloodstream eventually to start the relapsing cycle.

Whereas lice infestation of the body is very obvious, the bite of a tick carrying the fever often is not. The tick bites are painless and occur at night when the **insect** feeds. Thus, the victim may not even know that the infection has begun. The ticks acquire the disease from rodent hosts and pass it on to humans through saliva during feeding. The transmission can take place within minutes. When rodents leave a cabin or other vacant building, the humans who may move in become the ticks' only available host.

A diagnosis of the disease involves a combination of a patient's recent history and travel locations for the tick-borne fever and a visual discovery of body lice for the louse-borne fever. Clinically, relapsing fever can be confirmed through staining blood smears that will detect the spiral form of the *Borrelia* bacteria type. The blood work has to be performed during one of the victim's febrile periods. Modern treatment includes the use of **antibiotics** such as doxycycline or tetracycline. Such treatment is generally very successful, and there is rarely any antibiotic resistance. What has been learned, however, is that tetracycline can set off a Jarisch-Herxheimer Reaction, which triggers an increase in the symptoms of relapsing fever. This can occur within two hours of administering the antibiotic, and it can sometimes be fatal.

Prevention of relapsing fever differs depending on the type. With the tick-borne variety, it involves a common sense approach to utilizing wilderness areas, particularly if using remote cabins. Avoidance of rodents, the use of insect repellent such as DEET, and the wearing of proper clothes that cover the skin can help. This is particularly true while sleeping because of the nighttime feeding habits of ticks. Buildings or crawlspaces that may harbor rodents should be sprayed with a 0.5 percent solution of malathion insecticide. The louse-borne type thrives in more horrific environments where prevention demands a good deal of vigorous social and political activity. The disease must be combated by relieving overcrowded living conditions, by improving levels of personal hygiene in often-difficult conditions, and by the systematic disinfecting of camps and dwelling places. Once an epidemic starts, it also becomes necessary to use thorough de-lousing procedures of the clothes and bodies of the general population.

Further Reading

Burgdorfer, Willy. "The Epidemiology of Relapsing Fever." In *The Biology of Parasitic Spirochetes*, edited by Russell C. Johnson. Orlando: Academic Press, 1976.

Humphries, Margaret. "A Stranger to Our Camps: Typhus in American History." *Bulletin of the History of Medicine* 80 (2006): 269–290.

Kirksville College of Osteopathic Medicine. *Relapsing Fever.* http://www.kcom.edu/faculty/chamberlain/website/lectures/lecture/relapfev.htm

Merck Pharmaceuticals. *Relapsing Fever.* http://www.merck.com/mmpe/sec14/ch174/ch174f.html

National Library of Medicine. *Medline Plus.* http://www.nlm.nih.gov/medlineplus/encyc/article/001350.htm

ERIC JARVIS

RELIGION AND EPIDEMIC DISEASE.   Religious beliefs have always been a primary lens through which people have viewed and understood the experience of **epidemic** disease. Religion entails the cultural practices and beliefs that have as their goal relationship and communication between human beings and those (usually) unseen spiritual entities or forces that are believed to affect their lives. As anthropologists have noted, the dominant motif of a religion—its fundamental characteristics—is often most clearly revealed in the ways in which it explains misfortune and sickness and by the steps recommended to avert them. Classifying such beliefs as "primitive" or "civilized" according to the degree to which they approach or diverge from some external, imposed ideal (whether monotheism or modern scientific medicine) is less useful than recognizing the extent to which all religions have offered a way of making sense of common human experiences of danger, suffering, and disease.

In the case of epidemics, religious beliefs are forged in the furnace of catastrophic mass disease and high mortality, affecting not just one or two unfortunates but large numbers of sufferers at the same time. For many societies, this represents a qualitatively different situation from individual experience of sickness and health, generating different explanations and responses. Because epidemics affect entire communities at a time, prescribed actions are most often public and collective rather than private and individual, because the goal is to end the epidemic and restore health for the entire group.

Religion may offer more than one possible reading of events and could be integrated within or coexist alongside other, more empirically inflected, ideas of epidemic disease causation and cure. Ancient Assyria, for example, is known for its extensive medical corpus of naturalistic therapies, but Assyrian scholarly healers were also exorcists and priests who performed propitiatory rituals to soothe the angered gods and made no distinction between natural and supernatural causes of disease. Similarly, religious and naturalistic interpretations and practices have coexisted in Indian **Ayurvedic** medicine, Confucian China, medieval Islam and Christendom, early modern Europe, and in many societies today. Religion is thus not necessarily monolithic as an explanatory model, nor is it automatically exclusive of other models. Most often, people will find explanations that work for their particular set of imperatives. Being conscious of such diversity and pluralism of understandings allows us to recognize the robust creativity and resilience of human responses to epidemic disease across time and space.

Understanding Causes: A Twofold Model.   The most important role that religion played in relation to epidemics was in explaining what was happening in terms that made sense to that particular culture. Usually, such explanations were two-pronged, looking upward to the supernatural realm and outward (or perhaps better, inward) to contemporary society. Epidemics were usually understood as having been let loose upon the world by supernatural forces: one or many gods, demons, or spirits of the dead. In most cases, these heavenly beings were not seen as acting randomly, but as responding to particular human actions that offended them. A society's identification of the behaviors that would prompt the infliction of mass suffering and death upon an entire people reveals a great deal about the values and worldview of that culture. These vary considerably among cultures, but usually revolve around definitions of the sacred—which could be polluted, profaned, or neglected by deliberate or inadvertent actions—and of acceptable standards of moral behavior within the community.

For all cultures, explaining epidemic disease is less focused on addressing the disease symptoms of individual sufferers, and much more about the cosmic disorder that such diseased bodies manifest. Epidemic disease represents the world out of joint, a disastrous upset of the expected cosmic harmony. Religion aims to identify the causes, redress the problem, and restore good relations between heaven and earth. To do this, adherents draw on specially designated human intermediaries. These men and women—priests, chanters, oracles, diviners, seers, prophets, soothsayers, exorcists, and other specialists—are attributed with special skills and status that enable them to clarify the wishes of the supernatural powers and identify the human failings responsible. From these individuals, too, would often come specific recommendations for remedial devotional and ritual action.

Divine Agency and Divine Cure.   When epidemics are viewed as divine punishments for human error, the gods that send the disaster are also those who will lift it, if correctly approached. In both heavenly pantheons and monotheism, the gods are inherently dualistic, both benevolent and punitive, the source of the scourge and the means of deliverance. In ancient Mesopotamia (modern Iraq), the underworld god Nergal was a benefactor of humanity and protector of kings, as well as a "destroying flame" and "mighty storm," a fearsome warrior god who looses war, pestilence, and devastation upon the land. His destructive powers are enthusiastically celebrated in a hymn in his honor from the second millennium BCE:

Lord of the underworld, who acts swiftly in everything, whose terrifying anger smites the wicked, Nergal, single-handed crusher, who tortures the disobedient, fearsome terror of the Land, respected lord and hero, Nergal, you pour their blood down the wadis [gullies] like rain. You afflict all the wicked peoples with woe, and deprive all of them of their lives.

Such hymns were part of placatory rituals designed to mollify the angry gods and restore their good humor by heaping up their praises.

This dualism is not unique to ancient Mesopotamia. Greco-Roman Apollo was god of learning and the arts, as well as the death-dealing archer raining plague arrows on those who offended him, as he did upon the Greeks at Troy. Yoruba divinities supervise all aspects of human existence, but punish with misfortune, disease, and epidemics. The most feared is Shopona, powerful as a whirlwind, who attacks by sending **smallpox**, insanity, and other crippling diseases. Judaism, Christianity, Islam, and monotheistic African religions like those of the Neer and the Masaai, have all recognized the supreme creator God as both author of their devastation and source of their liberation. In India, Sitala has been venerated since the sixteenth century as the goddess of smallpox. The heat of her anger causes the disease when she possesses the body, but if she is appeased and cooled by human propitiation, she will leave, and the sufferer will recover. Today, she is the major village deity in Bengal and elsewhere, annually celebrated as "the mother" of the village, who takes away the fear of smallpox.

Arguing One's Case before an Angry God: The Plague Prayers of King Mursilis. Some of the earliest and most vivid examples of prayers composed to request divine aid against an epidemic come from ancient Anatolia (the Asian part of modern Turkey), from the reign of the Hittite king Mursilis II (r. c. 1321–1295 BCE) (see sidebar). Faced with a devastating 20-year pestilence, the king appeals to

---

THE PLAGUE PRAYERS OF HITTITE KING MURSILIS, FOURTEENTH CENTURY BCE

O, Stormgod of Hatti, my Lord, and gods of Hatti, my Lords, Mursilis your servant has sent me, (saying) go and speak to the Stormgod of Hatti and to the gods, my Lords, as follows: What is this that you have done? You have let loose the plague in the interior of the land of Hatti. And the land of Hatti has been sorely, greatly oppressed by the plague. Under my father (and) under my brother there was constant dying. And since I became priest of the gods, there is now constant dying under me. Behold, it is twenty years since people have been continually dying in the interior of Hatti. Will the plague never be eliminated from the land of Hatti? I cannot overcome the worry from my heart; I cannot overcome the anguish from my soul.

Translated at http://www.utexas.edu/cola/centers/lrc/eieol/hitol-8-X.html

. . . See! I lay the matter of the plague before the Stormgod of Hatti, my Lord. Hearken to me, Stormgod of Hatti, and save my life! This is what I (have to remind) you: The bird takes refuge in (its) nest, and the nest saves its life. Again: if anything becomes too much for a servant, he appeals to his lord. His lord hears him and takes pity on him. Whatever had become too much for him, he sets right for him. Again: if the servant incurred a guilt, but confesses his guilt to his lord, his lord may do with him whatever he pleases. But, because (the servant) has confessed his guilt to his lord, his lord's soul is pacified, and his lord will not punish that servant. I have now confessed my father's sin. It is only too true. I have done it . . . Stormgod of Hatti, my Lord, save my life! Let this plague abate again in the land of Hatti.

Translated by Albrecht Goetze in *Ancient Near Eastern Texts Relating to the Old Testament*, 3rd revised edition, edited by James B. Pritchard (Princeton: Princeton University Press, 1969) pp. 395–96.

the gods through the intermediary of a priest reciting the prayer aloud. He begins with a dramatic evocation of unending death, reproaching the gods for their harshness—even, one might say, for their irresponsibility—in allowing the plague to last so long. He comes to the gods as an urgent petitioner, seeking answers to a terrible situation.

Like a defendant in a law case, Mursilis uses every means he can to present his case favorably to the gods ranged in judgment. He stresses his piety and devotion to the temples of all the gods, and his many attempts, so far unsuccessful, to convince them to lift the plague. He points out that the epidemic is against the gods' own self-interest, since so many have died that there is no one left alive to honor them. In the divine court, the accused must admit guilt. Consultation of oracles has revealed that Mursilis's father angered the storm god by breaking a treaty oath (sworn on the gods) and failing to maintain certain rites. Though himself blameless, Mursilis accepts that punishment of his father's sin has fallen on him. Moreover, because the king is the priestly representative of his people before the gods, royal offenses implicate the whole society in their punishment.

Confession disarms the angry judges, who are further appeased with the offering of gifts, in the form of sacrifices and libations. The identified offenses are rectified—the king repairs the broken oath and promises to restore the neglected rites. Finally, Mursilis reminds the gods to be merciful, like a good patron with an erring dependent. Gods and humans exist in a hierarchical but reciprocal relationship, which imposes responsibilities on each party: the king to admit faults and rectify offenses, the gods to be compassionate and receptive to pleas for help. The king has fulfilled his side of the bargain, and it is now time for the gods to do their part.

Heavenly Bookkeeping.   Heavenly pantheons are envisaged in terms that make sense to a particular society. In China, from the twelfth century CE, the influence of Confucian ideals led to belief in a hierarchically organized celestial bureaucracy, with a Ministry of Epidemics presided over by five powerful deities, the Commissioners of Epidemics. These divine bureaucrats drew up heavenly balance sheets of good and evil deeds for every person on earth, rewarding meritorious acts with health and sending disease when the balance tipped too far toward the negative. Epidemics occurred when the score sheets of an entire community were so unfavorable as to be judged beyond saving. Like bureaucrats everywhere, the Commissioners themselves stayed in their offices and sent their assistants to earth to carry out their commands. A host of plague gods (*wenshen*) acted as their emissaries, carrying out annual inspections of morals and inflicting epidemics on those deserving of punishment.

As the active causative agents, it is the *wenshen* who receive cultic veneration. Images of the plague gods were set up to receive homage and worship, and festivals in their honor were held around the time when they were believed to be making their annual tours of inspection, to persuade them to return to heaven without marking the community down in their black books. Similar festivals were also held when an epidemic broke out. Prayers and ceremonies of cleansing and purification culminated in a procession to drive out demons (who could be enlisted by the plague gods) and see the gods on their way. The gods' departure was visibly enacted by placing images of the *wenshen* on boats made of paper or grass that were then floated away or burnt.

What Makes the Gods Angry?   Crimes that stir up the gods vary according to cultural priorities. In the plays of the Greek poet Sophocles (496–406 BCE), Oedipus's murder of his father, the king, and his marriage with his mother, though unwitting, polluted the land in the sight of the gods and cried out for vengeance. Only the suicide of the queen and

Oedipus's own blood offering (he blinds himself) and banishment could begin to wipe the stain clean. Disrespect or profanation of a divinity's cult was equally fatal. In the *Iliad*, Apollo inflicts an epidemic on the Greek army at Troy after their king, Agamemnon, captures the daughter of the priest of Apollo and refuses to ransom her back to her father. Yoruba deities were angered not by moral shortcomings but by failure to maintain their cult properly, including neglect, disrespect, and breaking taboos. Hindu and Buddhist ideas of reincarnation and inherited karma raised the possibility that epidemics could be heaven-sent punishments for unrighteousness or misdeeds in a previous life.

Judaic understanding of the causes of epidemics was determined by Israel's sense of mission as God's chosen people. Directed against Israel's enemies, pestilence was an aspect of God's unique sovereignty, his unlimited power over all creation, and his ability to trump the gods of any other peoples. Yet Yahweh could also turn this fearful weapon upon his own people. This was the burden as well as the promise of the covenant between nation and God, a mutual agreement that promised divine favor and protection on condition that Israel faithfully obeyed the divine commandments. The polarities of judgment and deliverance, destruction and sustenance, are thus central to the relationship between God and his people: "I will kill and I will make to live, I will strike, and I will heal, and there is none that can deliver out of my hand" (Deuteronomy 32:39–41). The only hope is repentance of sin and cleaving once more to God, for he has promised compassion after judgment, rewards after suffering, the renewal of divine favor, and blessing upon a chastised and penitent nation.

This concept of a God at once merciful and severe, who punishes his people for their own good, is also a central feature of Christian and Islamic understandings of epidemic disease. When plague broke out in the mid-third century CE, Christianity was a minority religion in a hostile Roman world. According to bishops Cyprian of Carthage (d. 258) and Eusebius of Caesarea (c. 260–340), although the epidemic appeared to strike down pagan and Christian indiscriminately, the purposes and end results for each were very different. For the enemies of Christ, the plague was a justly deserved punishment that led straight to eternal torment. But for Christians, the plague was to be welcomed as a way of testing one's faith and making sure the believer followed Christ's injunctions to care for the poor and the sick. Christians who died were called to paradise and eternal rest, and those who died caring for others were equal to the martyrs in the way they testified to the faith at the cost of their own lives. Thus, a paradoxical interpretation of hope and mercy was wrested from a seemingly calamitous situation. Early Islamic teachers similarly viewed epidemic disease as differentially freighted according to belief: for infidels, plague was a punishment and a disaster, but for faithful Muslims, it was a mercy and a reward, a martyrdom sent by God that led directly to paradise.

When Christianity became the state religion of the Roman Empire, this kind of dialectic explanatory model was less appropriate. Instead, like the Israelites, Christians recognized God was punishing them for their sins, chastising them into better behavior. Thus, Pope St. Gregory the Great (c. 540–604), in a sermon preached in Rome during an episode of the **Plague of Justinian** in 590, stated, "May our sorrows open to us the way of conversion: may this punishment which we endure soften the hardness of our hearts." Interior repentance and conversion of morals had to be proven by collective rituals performed under the divine gaze by a united and reformed community, "so that when he seeth how we chastise ourselves for our sins, the stern Judge may himself acquit us from the sentence of damnation prepared for us." Some later Islamic authorities also interpreted plague as divine castigation of sins, such as adultery, prostitution, usury, or drinking alcohol, with a consequently greater emphasis on reformation of morals, as well as individual prayer and collective processions.

Spirits of the Dead: Community beyond the Grave.   As agents of epidemic disease, the ancestor spirits of certain African religions share many characteristics with the gods: they watch over the living and expect to be honored with correct cultic veneration. Like the gods, they are both agents of affliction and sources of healing. They are angered by neglect of their rites, breaches of taboo, and flouting of acceptable behavior. Like the relatives they once were, they can be difficult, exacting, and demanding, holding grudges until they are properly propitiated. Kongo *nikisi* spirits, the oldest and most powerful of a hierarchically ranked series of ancestor spirits, are each associated with a particular disease. Epidemics are caused by Mayimbi spirits, particularly potent *nikisi* who belong to a family of "smashers." Severe epidemics are the work of male Mayimbi, whereas less serious outbreaks are attributed to female Mayimbi spirits. To appease their anger and give them the honor and respect they require, these spirits must be invoked and propitiated by sacrifices.

Ancestor spirits may also be more constrained than gods by close-knit ties of kinship joining the living and the dead in community, with their sphere of abilities limited to their own living relatives. In societies with strong traditions of sacred kingship, even if disrupted or abolished by colonial rule, such as the Sukuma and the Kongo, only the spirits of deceased chiefs can cause an epidemic afflicting many families at once. During their lifetimes, chiefs were religious representatives of the entire territory, responsible for the correct performance of rituals maintaining the health of the community, and this power continues after death.

Elsewhere, relations between the living and the dead could be more fraught, as in the Chinese belief in hostile or hungry ghosts, vengeful spirits of the unquiet dead, who had suffered premature or violent deaths. Their bodies unclaimed, their rites neglected, they cannot return home, but instead roam the countryside, searching for victims. Alone, they inflict disease on individuals, but joined together in packs, they are even more dangerous, capable of causing epidemics. These spirits are the polar opposites of African ancestor spirits, unconstrained by family ties, representing an uncontrollable, potentially lethal supernatural force, defining these particular dead as more demonic than human.

Hostile Demons and How to Get Rid of Them.   As supernatural agents of epidemic disease, gods and ancestors share the essential quality of moral duality: they might punish, but they will also heal. Humans enter into cultic relations with them as a way of keeping the lines of communication open, so that disagreements can be resolved and harmony restored. But demons are another matter, fundamentally malevolent and chaotic. Different strategies are therefore required. Where gods and ancestors are praised and petitioned, demons are exorcised, battled, and even tricked. In Vedic India (c. 1700–800 BCE) and in China from at least the sixteenth century BCE, all diseases, including epidemics, were thought to be caused by demons, who attacked the body from outside and possessed it. A Chinese dictionary from the second century CE defined epidemics as corvée, or harsh servitude from which there is no escape, clarifying that "it refers to the corvée exacted by demons." With incantations and prayers, Vedic and Chinese healers engaged in a ritual battle to expel demons from the body. Subsequently, in China, belief in demonic origins of epidemics existed alongside or was combined with the heavenly bureaucracy discussed above. Demons might act on their own, but more often they were thought to be under the control of the *wenshen*, or plague gods.

Demons sometimes appear in Christian art as secondary supernatural agents of the plague. However, if demons are allowed to harry humanity with epidemic disease, it is only because God has given permission for them to do. The demons act not in their own right but as part of the divine plan. Sometimes they cooperate with angels in imposing punishment on sinful humanity. Nevertheless, such a withdrawal of active divine agency from the task of chastising sinners does leave open the possibility for others, such as saints and holy people, to wrest control from the demons and provide protection from the plague.

Heavenly Helpers. In addition to the supernatural beings who cause the plague, many religions provide for lower-level heavenly helpers. Bhaiajyaguru, the medicine Buddha, dispenses a range of healing benefits, including protection against epidemics. Until the decline of smallpox as a serious threat in the modern era, several Shinto deities in Japan were petitioned for protection against smallpox and other epidemics. Both the Christian belief in a triune godhead and the cult of the saints offered many possibilities for playing one heavenly power against another. Before an angry God the Father, Christians could appeal for relief to Christ the merciful son. If Christ is enraged, then one might invoke his mother, the Virgin Mary, known to be especially forgiving of sinners and enjoying a mother's privilege in overriding or deflecting her son's destructive impulses. As the special friends of God, the saints were also well placed to intercede with the deity, acting as impassioned advocates before the throne of the divine judge. Whether name saints, local patrons, or specialist healing and plague saints, they could be relied upon to respond to their worshippers' appeals.

Religion as Help and Hindrance. By providing an explanation of events that was judged meaningful and satisfactory by a particular society, and by offering concrete solutions that were believed to avert or change events, religion has offered believers a way of making sense of the world and thereby, perhaps, gaining some measure of control over it. In times of epidemics, religion often functions as a significant coping strategy. Such positive psychological effects have sometimes been paid insufficient attention when historians have considered the psychological effects of epidemics upon any given society.

Many religions emphasize care of the sick as part of their work in the world and have contributed significantly to the creation of institutions and personnel providing much-needed nursing and medical care of victims of epidemic disease. In some instances, such as the practice of variolation as a part of the worship of the smallpox goddess Sitala in India, or the emphasis of cleansing and ritual purity, religious beliefs can have demonstrable positive therapeutic effects.

Conversely, religious rituals involving the coming together of many worshippers at a time, such as processions and **pilgrimages**, often facilitate the spread of epidemic disease. Along with conquering armies, missionaries can be the cause of spreading epidemic diseases to previously unexposed populations they are attempting to convert (though modern Christian missionaries usually shared the miracles of modern medicine along with those of the Gospel). All too often, conquering Europeans interpreted the resulting catastrophic mortality of indigenous peoples in waves of epidemic diseases as divine judgment on the savage heathens. This use of religious beliefs to justify stigmatization and persecution of minorities and outsiders—Jews, women, the poor, the lower classes, foreigners, racial minorities, homosexuals, practitioners of other religions—of whom the dominant group does not approve is the most troubling element of the encounter of religion and epidemics, and as the recent history of the **AIDS** epidemic has demonstrated, it remains very much with us today. In sum, religion cannot be ignored in any attempt to understand past, present, and future encounters with epidemic disease. *See also* AIDS in America; Astrology and Medicine; Biblical Plagues; Black Death (1347–1352); Black Death and Late Medieval Christianity; Black Death, Flagellants, and Jews; Black Death: Literature and Art; Chinese Disease Theory and Medicine; Colonialism and Epidemic Disease; Contagion Theory of Disease, Premodern; Disease, Social Construction of; Hospitals in the West to 1900; Islamic Disease Theory and Medicine; Leprosarium; Leprosy, Societal Reactions to; London, Great Plague of (1665–1666); Non-Governmental Organizations (NGOs) and Epidemic Disease; Plague Literature and Art, Early Modern European; Plague Memorials; Public Health in the Islamic World, 1000–1600; Race, Ethnicity, and Epidemic Disease; Scapegoats and Epidemic Disease; Syphilis in Sixteenth-Century Europe.

Further Reading

Amundsen, Darrel. *Medicine, Society and Faith in the Ancient and Medieval Worlds.* Baltimore: Johns Hopkins University Press, 1996.

Arnold, David. *Colonising the Body: State Medicine and Epidemic Disease in Nineteenth-century India.* Berkeley: University of California Press, 1993.

Benedict, Carol. *Bubonic Plague in Nineteenth-Century China.* Stanford: Stanford University Press, 1996.

Brown, Peter. *The Cult of the Saints: Its Rise and Function in Latin Christianity.* Chicago: University of Chicago Press, 1981.

Conrad, Lawrence, and Dominik Wujastyk, eds. *Contagion: Perspectives from Pre-modern Societies.* Aldershot: Ashgate, 2000.

Dols, Michael. *The Black Death in the Middle East.* Princeton: Princeton University Press, 1977.

Hanson, Kenneth. "When the King Crosses the Line: Royal Deviance and Restitution in Levantine Ideologies." *Biblical Theology Bulletin* 26 (1996): 11–25.

Kee, Howard. *Medicine, Miracle and Magic in New Testament Times.* New York: Cambridge University Press, 1986.

Marshall, Louise. "Manipulating the Sacred: Image and Plague in Renaissance Italy." *Renaissance Quarterly* 47 (1994): 485–532.

Nicholas, Ralph. "The Goddess Sitala and Epidemic Smallpox in Bengal." *The Journal of Asian Studies* 14 (1981): 21–44.

Selin, Helaine, and Hugh Shapiro, eds. *Medicine across Cultures: History and Practice of Medicine in Non-Western Cultures.* Dordrecht: Kluwer, 2003.

Westerlund, David. *African Indigenous Religions and Disease Causation: From Spiritual Beings to Living Humans.* Leiden: Brill, 2006.

Zysk, Kenneth. *Asceticism and Healing in Ancient India: Medicine in the Buddhist Monastery.* New York: Oxford University Press, 1991.

LOUISE MARSHALL

RHAZES (ABU BAKR MUHAMMAD IBN AKRIYYA AL-RAZI; 865–925). The Persian Al-Razi, known in the West as Rhazes, studied medicine in Baghdad and became one of the greatest **physicians** of the medieval period, writing over 200 works. Half of them were on medicine, but others covered topics including philosophy, mathematics, and astronomy. He was named after the place where he was born and died, Rayy, near Tehran in modern Iran.

The largest and most important of his medical works, *Kitab al-Hawi fi al-tibb* (The Comprehensive Book of Medicine), is a collection of notes he made from everything he

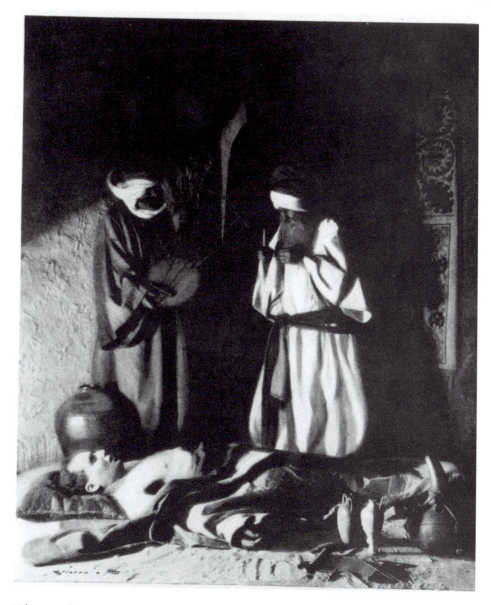

"Rhazes of Baghdad Used Harp Strings for Sutures." Courtesy of the National Library of Medicine.

had read, as well as observations from his own medical experience. Alone among his contemporaries, Rhazes names every author he quotes, and when the statement is his own, he prefixes it with the word "mine". Translated into Latin in the thirteenth century, *Kitab al-Hawi* was repeatedly copied and had a major influence on medical practice in Europe. In the famous first chapter of Volume XVII of this work, "On **Smallpox, Measles** and Plagues," which circulated separately, Rhazes described the symptoms of smallpox and measles as constant fever, inflammation, itchy nose, severe backache, and disturbed sleep. He added that a sure sign of an impending smallpox **epidemic** is an exceptionally hot autumn followed by a dry winter. When a rash erupted, he advised patients to keep warm and not to breathe cold air; for scars, he recommended peanut-oil paste. To prevent spreading of the rash into sensitive parts of the face, he recommended a special kohl for the eyes, sucking pomegranates for the mouth and throat, and an ointment containing horned poppy for the nostrils. Rhazes adopted the theory that pestilence is caused by corrupt **air** (miasma) and, contrary to Muslim opinion at the time, he strongly advocated **flight** to avoid epidemic disease.

Rhazes states that pestilence occurs at the end of summer and autumn when the wind is southerly and the air heavy. To avoid hot, contaminated air, he wrote, houses should be built on high ground, facing north; infection with **leprosy**, scabies, **tuberculosis**, and plague occurs in confined places. To lessen the effect of putrid air, he recommended fumigation with sandalwood and camphor, and sprinkling the place with rosewater. The patient should drink chilled water and take a mixture of aloes, saffron, and myrrh daily; from **Galen**, Rhazes also recommended a potion of Armenian clay with vinegar, or snake theriac.

Toward the end of his life, Rhazes went blind from cataracts; he must have died frustrated and unhappy, for he refused treatment, saying he had seen enough of the world. *See also* Diet, Nutrition, and Epidemic Disease; Humoral Theory; Islamic Disease Theory and Medicine.

Further Reading

Iskandar, A. Z. "Al-Razi–Biography and Religious Views." In *The Cambridge History of Arabic Literature*, edited by M. J. L. Young, J. D. Latham, and R. B. Serjeant, pp. 370–377. New York: Cambridge University Press, 1990.

Pormann, Peter E., and Emilie Savage-Smith. *Medieval Islamic Medicine*. Edinburgh: Edinburgh University Press, 2007.

Richter-Bernburg, L. "Abu Bakr Muhammad Al Razi's (Rhazes) Medical Works." *Medicina nei secoli* 6 (1994): 377–392.

SELMA TIBI-HARB

ROCKEFELLER FOUNDATION.   *See* Non-Governmental Organizations (NGOs) and Epidemic Disease.

ROMANTICISM.   *See* Tuberculosis and Romanticism.

ROSS, RONALD (1857–1932).   A **Physician** and malariologist of Scottish origin, Ross was the son of General Sir Campbell Claye Grant Ross (b. 1824), an officer of the British Army stationed in India. Encouraged to study medicine, Ross duly entered London's

St. Bartholomew's Hospital medical school in 1874. He began his career in the Indian Medical Service in 1881. After four months at the Army Medical College at Netley, he was commissioned to Madras. Over the next seven years, he served in Vizianagram, Moulmein, Burma, and Port Blair. On a leave of absence in 1888, Ross studied bacteriology at his former medical school. Upon returning to India, he was appointed Acting Garrison Surgeon in Bangalore, which he considered "the best station" in southern India, and where he developed an interest in the breeding habits of mosquitoes.

Ross published his first medical paper in 1893 on the subject of **malaria**. This led him to correspond with **Patrick Manson**, a London-based authority on tropical medicine. During a visit to London in 1894, Ross met Manson, who disclosed his view that malaria was transmitted by mosquitoes. In 1895 Ross returned to India where he continued his malaria research under Manson's guidance; their correspondence generated 173 letters over the next four years. Initially using *Culex* mosquitoes, the carriers of **bird** malaria, Ross's research became productive in 1897 when he was posted to Ootacamund, a malarial region. In Secunderabad, Ross first began to experiment with the "dapple-winged," or *Anopheles*, mosquito. Dissections of the **insect's** gastrointestinal tract eventually

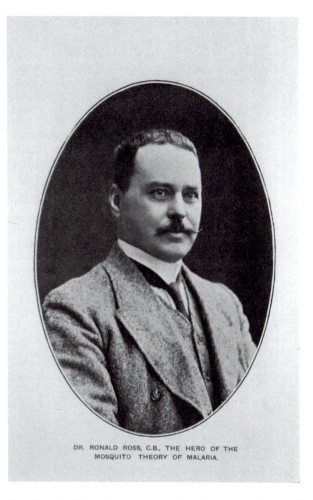

DR. RONALD ROSS, C.B., THE HERO OF THE MOSQUITO THEORY OF MALARIA.

Dr. Ronald Ross. Courtesy of the National Library of Medicine.

revealed the malaria parasite. Ross continued his work throughout 1898 in Calcutta, where he used birds to research the parasite's life cycle. Working in a disused laboratory, he traced the parasite to the *Anopheles*' salivary glands. By July 1898, he could prove that avian malaria was transmitted from infected birds to healthy ones through the vector's bite. Ross communicated a full account of his work to Manson, who presented his findings before the new tropical diseases section at the British Medical Association's annual meeting. The research was subsequently published in leading British medical periodicals.

In February 1899, Ross retired from the Indian Medical Service and was appointed to a lectureship at the newly founded Liverpool School of Tropical Medicine. Subsequent publications, including *The Prevention of Malaria* (1910), laid the foundations for combating malaria. In 1901 Ross was elected a Fellow of both the Royal College of Surgeons and the Royal Society; he was Vice-President of the latter between 1911 and 1913. In 1902 Ross became the first Briton to be awarded the Nobel Prize in Physiology and

Medicine. The same year, he was appointed to the Order of Bath and was knighted in 1911. In 1912 he was made an honorary chair at the University of Liverpool, where he taught until 1916. Four years earlier, he had relocated to London, when he was appointed as a consultant physician to King's College Hospital. During World War I (1914–1918) he was appointed as a malaria consultant to Indian troops. A final memorial to his achievements came in 1926 when the Ross Institute opened in Putney; it moved to Bloomsbury in 1934. Soon after the institute's inauguration, Ross suffered a stroke and was confined to a wheelchair. Eager to secure his role in the discovery of malaria's transmission, Ross published his memoirs in 1930, minimizing both Manson's and Italian entomologist Giovanni Batista Grassi's (1854–1925) contributions to tropical medicine. He died two years later on September 16 at the Ross Institute. *See also* Colonialism and Epidemic Disease; Malaria and Modern Military History.

Further Reading

Bynum, W. F., and Caroline Overy. *The Beast in the Mosquito: The Correspondence of Ronald Ross and Patrick Manson*. Amsterdam: Rodopi, 1998.

Chernin, E. "Sir Ronald Ross, Malaria, and the Rewards of Research." *Medical History* 32 (1988): 119–141.

Nye, Edwin R., and Mary E. Gibson. *Ronald Ross: Malariologist and Polymath, a Biography*. New York: St. Martin's Press, 1997.

Ross, Ronald. *Memoir: With a Full Account of the Great Malaria Problem and its Solution*. London: John Murray, 1923.

JONATHAN REINARZ

RUSH, BENJAMIN (1746–1813). Both a political leader and **physician**, the Philadelphian Benjamin Rush promoted clinical research despite the fact that his advocacy of **humoral theory**–based "depletion" therapies (such as bloodletting) were ultimately harmful. Educated at the College of New Jersey (Princeton) and taking a medical degree at the University of Edinburgh, Scotland, Rush returned to practice medicine in Philadelphia while teaching chemistry and writing extensively on medical topics. His fame spread as a result of his scores of publications, and he eventually taught several thousand students over the course of his career. Both civic-minded and a champion of **inoculation**, in 1774 he was one of the founding physicians of Philadelphia's Society for Inoculating the Poor.

Rush was also a member of the Continental Congress and a signer of the Declaration of Independence. In the first years of the Revolutionary War, he served as surgeon general and physician general for the army, but resigned in 1778 in protest over what he saw as the mismanagement of army hospitals then under the supervision of an officer appointed by George Washington (1732–1799). Nonetheless, he remained a consultant to the Congress on military medicine, and his important *Result of Observations* outlines the means by which American troops could best be protected form the ravages of disease.

The careful observations Rush made during the Philadelphia **measles** epidemic of 1789 reflect the high medical standards developed during the Scottish Enlightenment. These were included in his *Medical Observations and Inquiries*, which he later expanded and republished. During the great Philadelphia **yellow fever epidemic** in 1793, Rush proposed that treatment had to be calibrated to the severity of fever: the higher the fever, the stronger the therapy, which in Rush's view, meant purgatives and bloodletting (which he even applied to himself). However benighted these treatments seem to modern readers, Rush was nonetheless tireless in his care for victims of the epidemic and recorded meticulous notes on its progress. His publication of the account written for a general lay audience, *An Account of the Bilious Remitting Yellow Fever, as It Appeared in the City of Philadelphia, in the Year 1793* (1794), made him famous internationally. The book provides a narrative of the epidemic's appearance and progress, attributes its cause to "exhalations" from rotting produce and swamps (akin to the "bad air" or *malaria* that provided the name of that other tropical disease in which mosquitoes are the vector of transmission), observes quite accurately the two stages of the disease in patients, and carefully charts the daily death rates of the epidemic. Although the book reflects the Enlightenment's penchant for meticulous (and sometimes irrelevant) recording of data, it is also a defense of Rush's views on the origins and effective treatment of the epidemic.

At the time of the epidemic, Philadelphia was the capital of the new republic, its largest city, and its busiest **trade** port, intensifying the notoriety of and anxiety about the mosquito-borne tropical disease, probably carried there by refugees from political turmoil in Haiti. Eventually many citizens, including members of Congress and President Washington, fled the city. To his credit, Rush remained treating the sick, putting himself at risk since nearly a tenth of the population died.

Later in his life, Rush became an ardent abolitionist and enlisted the help of African Americans during the yellow fever epidemic. *See also* Demographic Data Collection and Analysis, History of; Measles in the Colonial Americas; Medical Education in the West, 1500–1900; Scientific Revolution and Epidemic Disease; Yellow Fever in North America to 1810.

Further Reading

Brodsky, Alyn. *Benjamin Rush: Patriot and Physician.* New York: Truman Talley, 2004.

Gehlbach, Stephen H. *American Plagues: Lessons from Our Battles with Disease.* New York: McGraw Hill, 2005.

Haakonssen, Lisbeth. *Medicine and Morals in the Enlightenment: John Gregory, Thomas Percival and Benjamin Rush.* Amsterdam: Editions Rodopi, 1997.

Kopperman, Paul E. "'Venerate the Lancet': Benjamin Rush's Yellow Fever Therapy in Context." *Bulletin of the History of Medicine* 78, 3 (Fall 2004): 539–574.

Powell, John Harvey. *Bring Out Your Dead: The Great Plague of Yellow Fever in Philadelphia in 1793.* Philadelphia: University of Pennsylvania Press, 1993.

THOMAS LAWRENCE LONG

S

SABIN, ALBERT (1906–1993). Albert Sabin is best known for the development of an oral, attenuated-live-**virus** vaccine against **poliomyelitis**. An outstanding contributor to virology and **epidemiology**, he championed the vaccine for mass **vaccination** programs to achieve eradication of the disease in the United States and around the world. He vehemently opposed the use of the killed-virus vaccine developed by **Jonas Salk** and never acknowledged that his own vaccine can mutate back to virulence and cause paralysis. Nevertheless, the Sabin vaccine remains the preferred vaccine worldwide.

Sabin was born in Bialystok, Poland, where his parents were silk weavers. After immigrating to the United States in 1921, he earned his medical degree from New York University in 1931. Fresh out of medical school, in a decision that changed the course of his life, he postponed his residency and began working with polio during a major **epidemic** in New York City. He continued his research starting in 1935 at the Rockefeller Institute for Medical Research in New York. Four years later, eager to combine laboratory research with patient care, he moved to the University of Cincinnati College of Medicine and the associated Children's Hospital. During World War II (1939–1945) Sabin spent time in North Africa with the U.S. military studying polio and documenting his confirmation of **Wade Frost's** model of the virus as an intestinal pathogen spread through tainted water supplies. His research continued in Cincinnati, where he developed the polio vaccine. This he accomplished in 1956, just as the world hailed the first successful vaccine by Salk.

After field testing his oral vaccine in the Soviet Union, Sabin oversaw successful mass immunization campaigns in Europe, South and Central America, Asia, and the Soviet Union. In 1960 the U.S. Public Health Service approved the use of the vaccine in the United States. It became the essential tool for the defeat of polio in the Western Hemisphere and in Europe. Sabin urged vehemently that his vaccine was more effective, cheaper, and easier to administer than the Salk vaccine. But the overriding advantage was the vaccine's ability to induce immunity in the gut, which is where poliovirus multiplies.

As it disseminates in the feces, it might, he believed, naturally immunize nonvaccinated persons. This, he concluded, was essential to preventing the spread of wild poliovirus in communities. To facilitate its universal use, in 1972 he donated the rights to the vaccine to the **World Health Organization** (WHO). In 1988 the WHO—following the model of the eradication of smallpox—set the goal for polio's worldwide eradication for the year 2000. The goal was not realized, and its feasibility remains in question.

Although Sabin understood the potential for large-scale vaccination programs, he remained narrow-minded when it came to the merits of his own vaccine. Though it is cheap and easy to administer, in very rare cases it can revert to virulence—an outcome that is prompting research into new vaccines. Sabin disputed the evidence for reversion and continued to research this problem until his death. Though he had a difficult personality, his exceptional contribution to the epidemiology and eradication of poliomyelitis is undisputed. *See also* Children and Childhood Epidemic Diseases; Human Immunity and Resistance to Disease; Immunology; Personal Hygiene and Epidemic Disease; Poliomyelitis and American Popular Culture; Poliomyelitis, Campaign Against; Salk, Jonas E.; Smallpox Eradication.

Further Reading

Allen, Arthur. *Vaccine: The Controversial Story of Medicine's Greatest Lifesaver.* New York: W. W. Norton, 2007.

Oshinsky, David. *Polio: An American Story.* New York: Oxford University Press, 2005.

Shell, Marc. *Polio and Its Aftermath: The Paralysis of Culture.* Cambridge, MA: Harvard University Press, 2005.

ANGELA MATYSIAK

ST. VITUS' DANCE.   St. Vitus' Dance refers to an historical condition that included the uncontrollable compulsion to dance, hop, and leap, which could last for days and sometimes caused the sufferer's death from exhaustion. The term is today synonymous with "**Sydenham's** chorea," but it derived from a series of dancing **epidemics** that struck Europe during the medieval and early modern periods. In 1021, chroniclers tell us, several people began dancing outside a church in the town of Kölbigk in Saxony. An angry priest cursed them to dance for a year, which they did. Some argue that this is the first case, albeit distorted into allegory, of a dancing epidemic. In Maastricht, Netherlands, in 1278, 200 are said to have drowned after the collapse of a bridge on which they had been dancing emphatically and perhaps uncontrollably. The largest epidemic began in 1374 and ended in 1378, extending from Aachen in the north of Germany to Strassburg (Strasbourg) in the southwest. Chroniclers talk of thousands of dancers, screeching with pain, begging bystanders to tie sheets tightly around their waists while they called on the mercy of saints. Most assumed that they were possessed by demons, and the chronicles speak of many deaths. A small outbreak occurred around 1463 when several people danced compulsively near Trier, Germany. Better documented is a Strasbourg epidemic that began in mid-July 1518. As many as 400 people danced uncontrollably for days or even weeks. Isolated cases, affecting one or a few people, have also been recorded in fifteenth-century Switzerland and twentieth-century Turkey. No more epidemics of dancing occurred in Europe after 1518, but reports of "Tigretier" in Abyssinia, Africa, in the nineteenth century sound very much like St. Vitus' Dance, as does a major outbreak of dancing in

Madagascar in 1863. Chronicles and medical reports are unequivocal in stating that the victims of these outbreaks danced. They may have twitched and convulsed as well, but their movements were quite recognizable as dancing. Indeed, the Dutch artist Pieter Brueghel drew victims of what he called victims "St. John's Dance" during the 1540s. He shows them performing the semblance of a dance, although they are clearly distracted and in pain.

There is little consensus as to the cause of these outbreaks. It has been claimed that the dancers suffered from ergot poisoning. Yet **ergotism** is not compatible with sustained dancing. Equally unsatisfactory is the claim that the dancers were members of a religious cult. The dancers did not dance voluntarily, and the church did not consider them heretical or blessed. Many have opted for the category of hysteria or conversion disorder, seeing the dance as a response to intolerable stress, a physical manifestation of despair. This is plausible: it seems that during the 1500s some expected to develop St. Vitus' Dance every year after feeling mounting anxiety lasting weeks. This is strongly reminiscent of the Italian tradition of the tarantella dance, for which preexisting psychological stress was an important element. Indeed, like those who performed the traditional tarantella, the St. Vitus dancers may have been in a state of trance, a conclusion also supported by chroniclers' reports and the otherwise astonishing endurance of the dancers. Those in a state of trance usually behave in ways consistent with their own and their culture's expectations. It may therefore be significant that there was a well-established belief, especially in the Rhine region, in the danger of a compulsive dance being inflicted by St. Vitus, St. John, or the Devil. Those whose resistance to such beliefs had been lessened by hunger, poverty, and religious crisis, may have succumbed to a trance state in which they behaved according to such deeply laid fears. This would also explain why exorcism rituals and visits to St. Vitus shrines so often cured the afflicted. Importantly, similar beliefs in the possibility of unwanted possession leading to dance seem to have existed in the popular cultures of Abyssinia and Madagascar. If this interpretation is correct, St. Vitus' Dance is an example of a reprobate trance, and its disappearance is explained by the fading away of the mystical or demonological beliefs that made it possible. *See also* Social Psychological Epidemics.

Further Reading

Hecker, J. F. C. *The Dancing Mania of the Middle Ages.* Translated by B. G. Babington. Honolulu: University Press of the Pacific, 2004. (German original 1832.)

Midelfort, H. C. Erik. *A History of Madness in Sixteenth-Century Germany.* Palo Alto, CA: Stanford University Press, 1999.

JOHN WALLER

SALK, JONAS E. (1914–1995).   Dr. Jonas Salk developed the first safe and effective vaccine against **poliomyelitis**. The introduction of the inactivated polio vaccine in 1955 was one of the most important medical advances of the twentieth century.

Jonas Salk was born in 1914 in New York City to Russian immigrant parents. He was a young child during the beginnings of **epidemic** polio, which mostly affected the children of the United States. Jonas Salk attended New York University School of Medicine and became a **physician**, but he was drawn to research rather than to direct patient care. Salk's interest in virology (the study of viruses) was piqued by a lecture in medical school. The

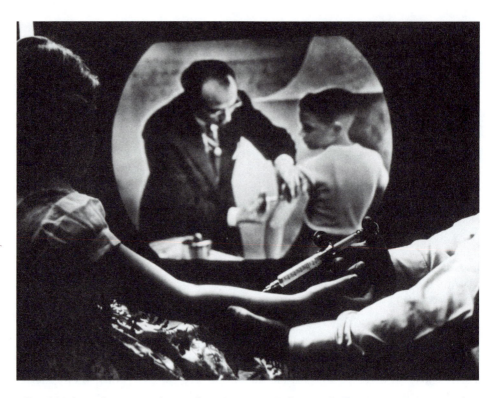

Cheryl Halpin (foreground) watches Dr. Jonas Salk on television in 1955, inoculating a child with polio vaccine, as part of a closed-circuit television show from the University of Michigan. Courtesy of the National Library of Medicine.

lecturer stated that the only way for a person to become immune to a viral disease was to suffer the disease, because a killed vaccine would not work on **viruses**. In addition, he said that it was possible to make a person immune to the bacterial disease **diphtheria** by **inoculation** with a vaccine made from killed **bacteria**. Salk felt that both statements could not be true. After completing his medical training, he entered the University of Michigan and assisted in research to develop a successful killed influenza virus.

Salk was then recruited to the University of Pittsburgh in 1947. He received a research grant to participate in a poliovirus-typing project commissioned by the National Foundation for Infantile Paralysis (NFIP). A new technique was adopted in Salk's lab that allowed the growth of the virus on monkey kidney tissue. Polio virus could suddenly be grown in large amounts, reducing time and costing less money, and reducing the sacrifice of monkeys. After the development of this technique, he killed the virus with formalin and ensured that no live virus remained in the vaccine preparation. After testing successfully in rhesus monkeys, a small trial was conducted using previously infected children. Salk vaccinated the children with the same type of polio that they had previously been exposed to and measured the increase in immunity. This ingenious approach ensured that the children were exposed to no risk. The pivotal placebo-controlled trial of the vaccine involved 1.8 million American children in 1954. **Vaccination** provided a greater than 80 percent protection rate against infection from epidemic polio. In 1956 **Albert Sabin** completed a live-virus oral vaccine in an effort to create mass immunizations. Controversy thus ensued over which kind of vaccine was better, and today Salk's original vaccine is still used, though Sabin's is preferred. Five years after introduction of the Salk vaccine, the incidence of poliomyelitis cases dropped 90 percent, and the vaccine proved to be safe, potent, and effective.

In 1960 Jonas Salk established the Salk Institute in California, a nonprofit research institution devoted to biological research related to health. After his work on the polio virus, Salk began research on the AIDS virus and contributed his remaining career in search of a cure. *See also* Animal Research; Children and Childhood Epidemic Diseases; Human Immunity and Resistance to Disease; Human Subjects Research; Poliomyelitis and American Popular Culture; Poliomyelitis, Campaign Against; Sabin, Albert.

Further Reading

Bredeson, Carmen. *People to Know: Jonas Salk Discoverer of the Polio Vaccine*. Berkeley Heights, NJ: Enslow Publishers Inc., 1993.

Kluger, Jeffrey. *Splendid Solution: Jonas Salk and the Conquest of Polio*. New York: G. P. Putnam's Sons, 2004.

Martin, Wayne. *Medical Heroes and Heretics*. Old Greenwich, CT: The Devin-Adair Company, 1977.

LARA J. KUNSCHNER

SANATORIUM.   A sanatorium (pl. –toria) is a place to which sick people go to recuperate or recover from disease. Nineteenth-century Germans who pioneered the use of the term, derived from the Latin *sanare* (to heal), distinguished sanatorium from sanitarium—derived from *sanitas* (health)—though Americans have often blurred the distinction. A sanatorium utilizes a regimen of rest, diet, exercise, and other forms of therapy in aiding recovery. These facilities may be dedicated to any physical problem, from venereal disease to broken limbs, but sanatoria were most often built to aid early-stage pulmonary **tuberculosis** (TB) patients.

Before the discovery of the tubercle bacillus by **Robert Koch** in 1882, Western medicine understood the disease in traditional, Galenic terms and emphasized rest, clean **air**, and special **diets** as treatment. Seventeenth-century English **physician Thomas Sydenham** and his friend, physician and philosopher John Locke (1632–1704), recommended horseback riding as a suitable passive exercise. In 1791 Quaker physician and founder of the Medical Society of London John Coakley Lettsom (1744–1815) opened the Royal Sea Bathing Infirmary at Margate in Kent, England, for patients with scrofula, a form of TB. Sea air had long been recommended to wealthy English patients, but Lettsom designed Margate for London's poorer denizens. Residents bathed in the sea and slept in the open on covered verandas, and by 1800 the number of beds had risen from 36 to 86. Sir James Clark's (1788–1870) *Sanative Influence of Climate* (1841) opened a new chapter in residential treatment of TB. The same year saw the opening of the Brompton Hospital for Consumption near London, and of the first Swiss sanatorium in Davos, later made famous by German novelist Thomas Mann (1875–1955) in *Magic Mountain* (1924). German physician Hermann Brehmer (1826–1889) devoted his 1853 dissertation to the advantages of high altitude treatment for pulmonary TB. He noted that autopsied TB victims had small hearts and concluded that the thinner air would reduce pressure on the organ and help cure patients. Brehmer opened the first sanatorium for pulmonary TB at Görbersdorf in the mountains of Bavaria in 1854. Linking atmosphere with diet and advocating walking for exercise, he invented for the weary the park bench placed alongside the path.

Tuberculosis grew increasingly common in later nineteenth-century Europe and America, becoming the leading cause of death among adults. The Romantic Movement in the arts clasped the wan consumptive to its breast and provided a model of the "recuperative power of nature" for treatment. *Abandon the filth and stress of the urban cesspool and embrace the clean, health-restoring nature of flashing sea or majestic mountaintop; and do so under the strict regimen of a sanatorium,* it seemed to advise. Of course, who but the well-off could afford to travel, let alone pay for such treatment? The tubercular poor remained all but invisible.

In the United States, tuberculosis patients, such as the gambler, gunslinger, and dentist "Doc" Holliday (1851–1887), sought the dry desert air of the frontier Southwest or Colorado. New Yorker Edward Livingston Trudeau (1848–1915) contracted TB while tending his consumptive brother in the 1860s. Gaining nothing by a stay in the South, he decided to live out his days in the Adirondack Mountains, where he had vacationed as a child. He was soon showing signs of improvement, regaining weight and strength. In 1882 he read about both Brehmer's theories and his sanatorium, as well as about Koch's discovery of the **bacterium** causing tuberculosis. Collecting funds from friends, Trudeau purchased property on Saranac Lake and in 1884 opened the Adirondack Cottage Sanatorium. Fascinated by Koch's findings, he furnished his establishment with a research laboratory, putting his medical experience—and **microscope**—to good use. By 1900 Saranac had 12 buildings and served as a model for other nearby sanatoria as well as for facilities in Pennsylvania and other neighboring states. Across the United States in 1900 there were 34 sanatoria with 4,485 beds, most in the Northeast with a few in arid western states. In 1904 there were about a hundred American sanatoria, and by 1910 another 300. America was participating in the so-called Sanatorium Movement that followed Koch's discovery. Sanatoria now not only served the patient with a restful, healthful environment, but it also isolated him or her from wider society, a growing concern as microbiologists uncovered the mysteries of the disease and its transmission.

The 1890s witnessed a worldwide concern for both consumptives and lepers, and the decade saw a parallel flourishing of **leprosaria** and sanatoria. In 1901 the editor of *The Sanitarian* magazine reported on European and American progress in establishing sanatoria. England had about 2,000 beds (this number would double over the next decade), whereas France had well over 3,000 and was building or had finished 10 new facilities. Czarist Russia had five facilities, with more "under way," and Italy had eight new sanatoria under construction. The Netherlands, Norway, Denmark, Sweden, Spain, Portugal, and the Habsburg Empire each had one or more sanatoria for consumptives being built, most with royal funding. The French tended toward smaller facilities, with contemporary medical opinion favoring 12 to 20 patients, whereas the German Heidehaus near Hanover, founded in 1907, had four physicians and ten nurses tending 200 patients in 1914. Canada's first antituberculosis society appeared in 1895 and created the Cottage Sanitarium on Muskoka Lake, Ontario, two years later. By 1901 Canada had two facilities with a total of 75 beds, whereas New York State alone had ten private sanatoria with 600 beds and a new state institution "projected." The first state facility in the United States was the Sharon Sanatorium, founded in 1898 some 18 miles from Boston.

By the early twentieth century, Romanticism had run its course, **germ theory** had established itself, and the **Sanitation Movement** had established links among disease, **poverty**, and filth. Tuberculosis slowly morphed from a fashionable disease of aesthetes to a pestilence of the urban poor. The Sanatorium Movement became linked to social philanthropy and public health, and newer sanatoria were increasingly urban and institutional rather than rural and idyllic. By 1910, 61 of Britain's 90 TB sanatoria were public. When physician Hermann M. Biggs (1859–1923), Public Health Officer for New York City, established a rural sanatorium at Otisville, he instituted a "work cure" instead of the typical "rest cure" for the city's lower class consumptives. Shortly after, he had Riverside set up as a virtual prison for nonvoluntary committals who presented a public health risk to New York. Although charitable, religious, and for-profit sanatoria continued to thrive, the percentage of beds in public facilities continued to climb even faster. Between 1907 and 1916, Pennsylvania had the largest state system of sanatoria; between 1904 and 1919, its number of beds increased from 660 to 3,972. Pennsylvania's public sector controlled 32 percent of beds in 1904, 50 percent in 1908, and 73 percent in 1919. Camp Mont Alto grew from 28 to 730 patients between 1907 and 1910, and housed

---

HOW TO REST IN AN AMERICAN SANATORIUM (1909)

Rest out of doors is the medicine that cures consumption. Absolute rest for mind and body brings speedy improvement. It stops the cough and promotes the appetite. The lungs heal more quickly when the body is at rest. Lie with the chest low, so the blood flow in the lungs will aid to the uttermost the work of healing. The rest habit is soon acquired. Each day of rest makes the next day of rest easier, and shortens the time necessary to regain health. The more time spent in bed out of doors the better. Do not dress if the temperature is above 99 degrees, or if there is blood in the sputum. It is life in the open air, not exercise, that brings health and strength. Just a few minutes daily exercise during the active stage of the disease may delay recovery weeks or months. Rest favors digestion, exercise frequently disturbs digestion. When possible have meals served in bed. Never think the rest treatment can be taken in a rocking-chair. If tired of the cot, shift to the reclining chair, but sit with head low and feet elevated. Do not write letters. Dictate to a friend. Do not read much and do not hold heavy books. While reading, remain in the recumbent posture.

Once having learned the simple facts that must be noted and the simple laws that must be followed, once having placed oneself in a position to secure the rest, the fresh air, and the health diet, no better next steps can be taken than to observe the closing injunction in the rules for rest:

> There are few medicines better than clouds, and you have not to swallow them or wear them as plasters,—only to watch them. Keeping your eyes aloft, your thoughts will shortly clamber after them, or, if they don't do that, the sun gets into them, and the bad ones go a-dozing like bats and owls.

From William H. Allen, *Civics and Health* (Boston: Ginn and Co., 1909) online at http://chestofbooks.com/health/

1,150 in 1916, making it the largest sanatorium in the country. Still, in 1916 there was but one bed for every three Pennsylvanians who died of TB that year. Those sanatoria that admitted African Americans generally segregated blacks and whites, and the first public sanatorium specifically for black Americans was established near Burkeville, Virginia, in 1917. By 1925 there were 536 sanatoria in the United States with a total of 73,338 beds, or an average of 137 per institution.

The 1920s saw a slowdown in the creation of new sanatoria in Europe as the incidence of the disease fell. The movement had its impact on architectural style, however, as

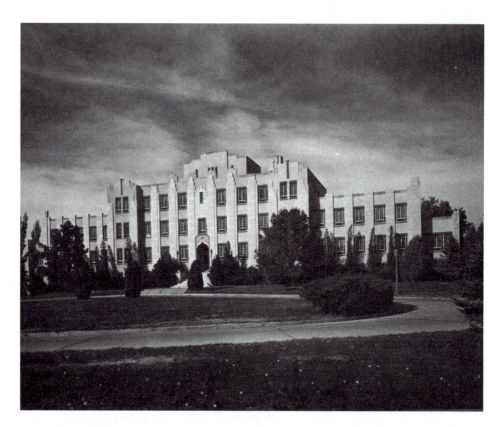

Sanatorium, Albuquerque, New Mexico, built in 1934. Courtesy of the National Library of Medicine.

architects adopted the clean, smooth, include-nothing-on-which-dust-might-accumulate imperative in Bauhaus and other modernist styles. For example, pioneer Finnish architect Alvar Aalto (1898–1976) designed Paimio Sanatorium (1929–1932) 20 miles from Helsinki.

The introduction of streptomycin as a relatively effective treatment against TB in 1943, and its even more effective combination with para-aminosalicytic acid (PAS) in 1948, brought the age of the sanatorium to a close. An experiment in Madras, India, in 1959 showed that outpatient treatment with the new medications could be as effective as hospitalization. Mountain health resorts were transformed into playgrounds for winter sports—a role Davos plays just as well as it ever served as a health resort. Although sanatoria disappeared from or changed functions in most national landscapes, only the Soviet Union and post-Soviet states retained the facilities and regimens for TB into the twenty-first century. *See also* Disease, Social Construction of; Environment, Ecology, and Epidemic Disease; Industrialization and Epidemic Disease; Industrial Revolution; Leprosy in the United States; Leprosy, Societal Reaction to; Tuberculosis and Romanticism; Tuberculosis in England since 1500; Tuberculosis in North America since 1800; Urbanization and Epidemic Disease.

Further Reading

Bates, Barbara. *Bargaining for Life: A Social History of Tuberculosis, 1876–1938.* Philadelphia: University of Pennsylvania Press, 1992.

National Tuberculosis Association. *A Directory of Sanatoria, Hospitals and Day Camps for the Treatment of Tuberculosis in the United States.* New York: For the Association, 1919. Google Book: http://books.google.com/

Rothman, Sheila. *Living in the Shadow of Death: Tuberculosis and the Social Experience of Illness in America.* New York: Basic Books, 1994.

Taylor, Robert. *Saranac: America's Magic Mountain.* Boston: Houghton-Mifflin, 1985.

Warren, P. "The Evolution of the Sanatorium: The First Half-Century, 1854–1904." *Canadian Bulletin of Medical History* 23 (2006): 457–476.

Worboys, Michael. "The Sanatorium Treatment for Consumption in Britain, 1890–1914." In *Medical Innovations in Historical Perspective*, edited by John V. Pickstone, pp. 47–73. London: Macmillan, 1992.

JOSEPH P. BYRNE

SANITATION MOVEMENT OF THE NINETEENTH CENTURY. The sanitation movement of the mid-nineteenth century in Europe and the United States had at its heart a profound tension between the classic nineteenth-century principle of **personal liberty** and the growing importance of collective health and citizenship. The sociopolitical ramifications of this tension played a major part in determining the course of the movement. From it emerged a highly influential view of the proper relationship between medicine and the state, one mediated in Europe and the United States by the creation and expansion of new **public health agencies**.

But this movement did not exist in isolation. It was part of a broader aspiration among the newly affluent middle classes—initially in Britain, the first Western country to industrialize, and later in Europe and the United States—to place their own standards of morality, civility, and hygiene at the heart of life in industrial societies. Sanitation reform became, in the words of the contemporary historian Anthony Wohl, "a kind of *fundamental* reform," one necessary to improve not only health but also wealth, welfare, and morality.

Industrialization and Urban Poverty.   In 1800 80 percent of the British population lived in rural villages. By 1900, 80 percent lived in towns and cities. This startling statistic reflects the dizzying social and economic transformations of the Industrial Revolution in the nineteenth century. **Industrialization** and continued **urbanization** brought great wealth for the middle and upper classes, but also levels of urban **poverty**, squalor, and disease never before experienced in Europe. **Epidemic** diseases such as **cholera**, first seen in Britain in 1831, swept through overcrowded slums. Industrialization made the country as a whole rich, but its poor—the workforce on which industry depended—were sick and getting poorer.

A key question for nineteenth-century intellectuals was how to respond to this new industrial poverty. In the early decades of the century, *laissez-faire* **capitalism**—the principle that trade and industry should be subject to as few regulations as possible—dominated British public life. This idea was embodied in the work of the British economists Adam Smith (1723–1790) and Thomas Malthus (1766–1834), who argued that free trade was the basis of Britain's industrial success. According to **Malthusianism**, poverty indicated a moral failure on the part of the poor to learn the lessons of the free market.

One expression of *laissez-faire* capitalism was in the provision of fresh **water** and the disposal of sewage in the new industrial cities. Water was provided by private companies or from communal street pumps, and sewage was collected in cesspools or emptied into rivers—often the only source of drinking water. Through the lens of modern bacteriology, it seems obvious that this cycle of contamination was implicated in the transmission of epidemic diseases. But to the inhabitants of these cities, sewage disposal was only one aspect of urban life, all of which seemed dirty and diseased. Overcrowded slum housing, slaughterhouses, and heavy industries, the pigs and chickens kept by the poor, the three million tons of dung deposited by horses on British streets every year—early sanitation reformers saw all aspects of the urban **environment** as causes of disease.

Sanitation Reform and Social Reform.   Many social reform movements in this period were based on the new Christian evangelical movements of the 1830s and 1840s. The sanitation movement possessed this element of **morality**: epidemics were seen not as God's punishment of sin, but rather as the failure of humans to look after His creation and His poor. This reflects a gradual movement away from *laissez-faire* ideology, as the middle classes began to take a paternalistic—some said patronizing—interest in the health and welfare of the industrial poor.

Two strands, one public, one private, characterized the sanitation movement. The public strand, led by members of the urban middle classes such as physicians, politicians, and journalists, emphasized the material, collective aspects of sanitation—sewers, clean water, and so on. The private strand, associated with groups of middle-class women such as the Ladies Sanitary Association, took an interest in individual behavior and circumstances. These groups entered and inspected the homes of the poor and offered education in cleaning and cooking. These strands were not separate but rather complementary, and their interests coalesced on many subjects. In the 1830s, for example, both were involved in a campaign to provide public washhouses in which the poor could wash themselves and their clothes.

A leading figure in the public strand of the British sanitation movement was the lawyer and civil servant **Edwin Chadwick**. Chadwick had been a student of the English Utilitarian philosopher Jeremy Bentham (1748–1832), and he adopted the Utilitarian principle of using government to produce "the greatest happiness of the greatest number." From 1834 Chadwick worked for the Poor Law Commission, a government organization investigating poverty in Britain. From 1837 the British government introduced official registration of births and deaths. Early returns from this scheme revealed a very high infant death rate in poor urban areas—153 infant deaths per 1,000 live births, compared with fewer than 16 per 1,000 in the West today. This, and Chadwick's work for the Commission, convinced him that disease was associated with poverty.

Chadwick's Report.   In 1839 Chadwick was asked to investigate the health of the British working class, and in 1842 he published a *Report on the Sanitary Condition of the Labouring Population of Great Britain*. His main conclusion was that rotting organic matter such as sewage and food waste released a smelly and poisonous "**miasma**," and that this form of air pollution was responsible for transmitting infectious epidemic diseases such as cholera. In his view, slums were not only a danger to those who inhabited them: the miasma they generated could spread disease to a whole town. This "miasmatic" model of disease provided a rationale for Chadwick's proposed program of "environmental" sanitation reform—improving water supplies, building sewers and drains, regulating refuse disposal, and controlling industrial pollution.

Though widely seen as a challenge to personal liberty, Chadwick's program of reform received governmental approval with the 1848 Public Health Act. The Act established a General Board of Health to oversee public health and sanitation reform, with Chadwick as chairman and the London physician John Simon (1816–1904) as medical officer. But many local authorities resented Chadwick's autocratic chairmanship, and in 1855 he was forced to resign. Despite his pioneering work in this field, the most radical sanitation reforms took place under Simon's supervision after Chadwick had left the Board. Simon favored a neo-**contagionist** model of epidemic disease, in which disease was spread from case to case by waterborne particles, and this model provided an equally strong rationale for sanitation reform.

In 1858 the engineer Joseph Bazalgette (1819–1891) was commissioned to build a massive integrated sewer system for London. In the hot summer of that year, the level of the River Thames fell, and the smell of rotting sewage on its banks caused Parliament to be suspended for several weeks. Several years of these "great stinks" and a major cholera epidemic in 1866, brought home the need for further sanitation reform and the urgent completion of Bazalgette's scheme. The swift change in public attitudes toward sanitation reform in this period is illustrated by the fact that the 1866 Sanitary Act, though far more interventionist than Chadwick's 1848 Public Health Act, faced little opposition in parliament and the press.

The Sanitation Movement in Europe and the United States.   Both Europe and the United States experienced cholera epidemics in the first half of the nineteenth century, but it was not until the 1870s that the condition of their industrial cities began to reach crisis point. And political instability—particularly the European revolutions of 1848 and the American Civil War—complicated sanitation reform. The emergence of bacteriology and new theories of disease transmission in France and Germany in the late nineteenth century added a scientific dimension to the activities of the sanitation movement in these countries. In Germany sanitation reform became part of Otto von Bismarck's (1815–1898) program of political unification, industrial modernization, and social welfare. In France, meanwhile, two "great stinks" in Paris in the 1880s triggered a nationwide program of sewer construction and slum clearance. But this aggravated underlying class tensions in French society. Could working-class neighborhoods—seen by many as the principal source of smell and disease—be cleaned up without alienating and radicalizing their inhabitants?

Though Chadwick's work had inspired some sanitation reformers in the United States in the 1840s and 1850s, the social and political turmoil of the Civil War hampered their efforts to establish a federal agency for sanitation reform. In the aftermath of the war, many cities and states established health boards, which oversaw food quality, water supplies, and the containment of epidemic disease. The National Board of Health, established in 1879, took responsibility for coordinating scientific research into contagious diseases and sanitation engineering at a national level. As the influence of the sanitation movement spread across Europe and the United States, the incidence of epidemic diseases declined sharply. Public health reformers began to shift their emphasis away from sanitation reform, embracing a wider concern for the social and medical problems associated with urban poverty.

Interpreting the Sanitation Movement.   Historians have traditionally seen the sanitation movement as a straightforward battle between "miasmatists" and "contagionists." But its impact remains controversial. Recent research suggests that the story is more complex, reflecting the success of social, economic, and administrative reform rather than the triumph of science and medicine over disease. The sanitation movement reflected the cultural, social, religious, and political concerns of those involved. Its success owed as much to new techniques of data analysis and the skill of sanitation engineers as to any developments in medical practice or scientific theory. *See also* Capitalism and Epidemic Disease; Cholera: First through Third Pandemics, 1816–1861; Cholera: Fourth through Sixth Pandemics, 1863–1947; Demographic Data Collection and Analysis, History of; Disinfection and Fumigation; Environment, Ecology, and Epidemic Disease; Industrial Revolution; Personal Hygiene and Epidemic Disease; Public Health Agencies in Britain since 1800; Public Health Boards in the West before 1900; Religion and Epidemic Disease.

Further Reading

Barnes, David. *The Great Stink of Paris and the Nineteenth-Century Struggle Against Filth and Germs.* Baltimore: Johns Hopkins University Press, 2006.

Chadwick, Edwin. *Report on the Sanitary Condition of the Labouring Population of Great Britain, 1842.* Edited by Michael Flinn. Edinburgh, UK: Edinburgh University Press, 1965.

Duffy, John. *The Sanitarians: A History of American Public Health.* Urbana: University of Illinois Press, 1990.

Fee, Elizabeth, and Dorothy Porter. "Public Health, Preventive Medicine and Professionalization: England and America in the Nineteenth Century." In *Medicine in Society: Historical Essays*, edited by Andrew Wear, pp. 249–75. New York: Cambridge University Press, 1992.

Hardy, Anne. *The Epidemic Streets: Infectious Disease and the Rise of Preventive Medicine, 1856–1900.* Oxford: Clarendon Press, 1993.

LaBerge, Ann Elizabeth Fowler. *Mission and Method: The Early Nineteenth-Century French Public Health Movement.* New York: Cambridge University Press, 2002.

Worboys, Michael. *Spreading Germs: Disease Theories and Medical Practice in Britain, 1865–1900.* New York: Cambridge University Press, 2000.

RICHARD BARNETT

SARS.   *See* Severe Acute Respiratory Syndrome.

SCAPEGOATS AND EPIDEMIC DISEASE.   Epidemics generate profound social disorder. In response, the individuals who risk infection during **epidemic** episodes seek explanations for the fundamental causes of disease outbreaks. Throughout history, societies have created scapegoats by blaming otherwise innocent people in order to rationalize and explain the origins and course of disease outbreaks. These patterns of scapegoating often mirror existing social prejudices, as the socially disempowered become objects of blame. The designation of certain groups or individuals as scapegoats may be based partially in fact. Poor living conditions, for example, put some at greater risk for infection and mortality; these demographic realities thus made it appear logical that such individuals were particularly dangerous. In other cases, persecution stems from existing cultural biases with perceptions of danger bearing little relation to actual disease risk. Religious, ethnic, political, economic, and sexual prejudices all factor into the process of scapegoating, and these affiliations are not mutually exclusive. Though not intended to be exhaustive, the following representative cases of epidemic scapegoating demonstrate its long history across time and place.

People often turn to religion to explain disease outbreaks. By extension, religious persecution has been a frequent response to epidemics. During the **Black Death**, Christian majorities accused Jews of poisoning wells and spreading plague in Strasbourg, Basle, Mainz, and other sites. Likewise, when **cholera** struck the United States in the 1830s, many Americans believed the epidemic was a divine punishment for immorality. Protestants blamed cholera on individuals who disobeyed God's law, including the population of Irish Catholics in the nation. In the 1980s and 1990s, fundamentalists such as Pat Robertson and Jerry Falwell defined **AIDS** as divine retribution against homosexuals.

As the above examples illustrate, religious scapegoating overlaps with other discrimination. Ethnic scapegoating targeted Jewish and Irish Catholic immigrants to the United States as inherently diseased. The perceived links between disease and ethnicity have changed over time, as cultural and biological understandings of difference give new meanings to prejudices. In sixteenth- and seventeenth-century Geneva and Milan, Spaniards and other foreigners found themselves accused of conspiracy to spread plague among locals. By the nineteenth century, new biological understandings of **race** and **heredity** linked certain ethnic groups to specific diseases. Eastern European Jews were blamed for spreading **typhus** and cholera in 1890s New York, whereas whites targeted residents of San Francisco's Chinatown for spreading and concealing plague in the early 1900s. In the 1980s, attempts in the United States to explain the source of **HIV** focused on Haitians, although it would later be clear that the disease probably spread *from* the United States to the Caribbean instead. The perceived connection between disease and foreigners persists.

Epidemic scapegoating also stems from political and socioeconomic conflicts. Many infectious diseases disproportionately affect people who lack decent housing, nutrition, or sanitation. Furthermore, many people blame **poverty** on individual moral failings, and thus hold poor people responsible for their disease-ridden living conditions. As diseases spread to other parts of the community, the more affluent classes are prompted to see the poor as harboring disease. **Mary Mallon**, or "**Typhoid** Mary," has come to typify the links between working classes and infectious disease. Mallon, a typhoid carrier, worked as a cook for wealthy New Yorkers and unknowingly contaminated dozens. Public health authorities blamed her refusal to stop cooking on ignorance and disregard for others' lives, while ignoring the economic constraints that obliged Mallon to make a living through cooking. Likewise, disease outbreaks such as **cholera**, **tuberculosis**, and hookworm, transmitted more easily in overcrowded living conditions, are often blamed on lower economic classes.

Socioeconomic and political scapegoating does not always target lower classes. Disempowered people have also blamed dominant groups for introducing disease. Disease here is understood as a conspiracy to exterminate certain peoples. Citizens of many Allied nations accused Germany of creating **influenza** as a biological weapon during World War I, and the British were blamed for importing cholera and **malaria** to Egypt after World War II (1939–1945). Leonard Horowitz and others have argued that the U.S. Government created HIV as a tool to commit genocide against African Americans and Hispanics. In many cases, distrust stems from historically hostile relations between groups; indeed, some conspiracy theories have a basis in past or present intimidation and threats. Whatever the reality, political and class distrust creates miscommunications that hamper effective public health initiatives.

Like politics and economics, gender profoundly affects assumptions about contamination. During the second plague pandemic, women blamed for spreading plague were accused of witchcraft and executed. In the late fifteenth century, **syphilis** became a major problem in Europe, and many female prostitutes were condemned as sources of venereal infection. Likewise, in the 1860s, the British Parliament passed a series of Contagious Disease Acts for both Britain and its colonies. This legislation held female prostitutes (rather than their male patrons) responsible for infecting soldiers and civilians. Women have not been the only sexual scapegoats. In the early 1980s, scientists and civilians considered homosexual men as the prime casualties of HIV (initially termed Gay-Related Immunodeficiency). When heterosexual individuals began to acquire the disease, members of the gay community became scapegoats. Gender and sexuality continue to create the basis for scapegoating in epidemic diseases.

As the above examples illustrate, many different factors combine to construct the epidemic scapegoat. Mary Mallon, for example, was a poor, Irish Catholic immigrant woman and a threat to middle class, Anglo-Saxon Protestant norms on many levels. Similarly with HIV, religious, political, and gendered beliefs weave together to shape perceptions of risk.

In epidemic scapegoating, individuals attempt to impose order during a period that is fundamentally disordered and to assign blame for a seemingly random disease to a definable target group of individuals. Yet infectious diseases are always more complex sociological phenomena, the causes of which are never so simply defined. *See also* AIDS in Africa; AIDS in America; Biblical Plagues; Black Death, Flagellants, and Jews; Leprosy, Social Reactions to; Mallon, Mary; Personal Liberties and Epidemic Disease; Poison Libels and Epidemic Disease; Religion and Epidemic Disease; Sanitation Movement of the Nineteenth Century; Sexual Revolution.

Further Reading

Douglas, Tom. *Scapegoats: Transferring Blame.* London: Routledge, 1995.

Hays, J. N. *The Burdens of Disease: Epidemics and Human Response in Western History.* New Brunswick: Rutgers University Press, 1998.

Kraut, Alan. *Silent Travelers: Germs, Genes, and the Immigrant Menace.* Baltimore: The Johns Hopkins University Press, 1995.

JULIA F. IRWIN

SCHAUDINN, FRITZ RICHARD (1871–1906). Fritz Richard Schaudinn's brief career focused on protozoology (the study of **protozoa**) and parasitology. His research culminated with the identification of the bacterial cause of venereal **syphilis**. Schaudinn was born in the village of Roesiningken in East Prussia. In 1890 he matriculated into Berlin University with the intention of studying philology, but he was soon drawn to zoology and studied protozoa with his mentor, Franz Eilhard Schulze (1840–1921). He received his doctorate in 1894 and in 1901 he was appointed director of the German-Austrian zoological station in the town of Rovigno near Venice, Italy. Here he conducted research on the etiology of **malaria** and proved that an amoeba is the cause of tropical **dysentery**. Schaudinn was recalled to Berlin in 1904 to head the newly created parasitology laboratory at the Imperial Health Office, and it was here that he started his investigations into the cause of syphilis. In the following year, he was appointed director of the Research Institute for Naval and Tropical Diseases in Hamburg, but he died from sepsis following a pararectal abscess before he could assume this post.

In early 1905, John Siegel (1861–1941), a parasitologist under the direction of Franz Schulze at Berlin, published a series of papers in which he pointed to *Cytorrhyctes luis* as the cause of syphilis. As part of his duties with the Imperial Health Office, Schaudinn was called upon to confirm Siegel's findings. He started by investigating biopsy materials from syphilitic patients, provided by Erich Hoffmann (1868–1959), a clinical dermatologist and syphilologist. Rather than confirming Siegel's claims, however, he discovered a different microorganism in his syphilitic samples, which he initially named *Spirochaeta pallida*. In March 1905 Schaudinn and Hoffmann presented their results and noted that they had repeatedly found *Spirochaeta pallida* in their syphilitic materials, but they cautiously chose not to declare it the cause of the disease. Over the next few months, Schaudinn continued to study this microorganism and determined that based on its structure it was actually a new genus of protozoa, so he renamed it *Treponema pallidum*. Then, on May 17, 1905, Schaudinn publicly presented his discovery to the Berlin Medical Society and revealed research that more clearly identified *Treponema pallidum* as the causative agent of syphilis. Despite his initial caution, Schaudinn met with sharp criticism from Siegel and his supporters, including their shared mentor, Franz Schulze, who continued to advocate for the causal role of *Cytorrhyctes luis* in syphilis. Over the next few months, however, researchers from around the world confirmed Schaudinn's observations. Tragically, because of his untimely death, Schaudinn did not witness **Paul Ehrlich's** development of a cure for syphilis that depended on his identification of the microorganism that caused the disease.

Further Reading

Lindenmann, Jean. "Siegel, Schaudinn, Fleck and the Etiology of Syphilis." *Studies in the History and Philosophy of Biology and Biomedical Science* 23 (2001): 435–455.

Quétel, Claude. *History of Syphilis.* Baltimore: Johns Hopkins University Press, 1990.

Stokes, John H. "Schaudinn: A Biographical Appreciation." *Science* 74 (1931): 502–506.

Thorburn, A. Lennox. "Fritz Richard Schaudinn, 1871–1906." *British Journal of Venereal Disease* 47 (1971): 459–461.

WILLIAM H. YORK

SCHISTOSOMIASIS.   Schistosomiasis is a parasitic disease afflicting over 200 million people throughout the world, principally in areas of **poverty** and inadequate public health facilities. The causative agents are species of trematodes, or flukes, in the genus *Schistosoma*. *Schistosoma mansoni, S. hematobium,* and *S. japonicum* cause the vast majority of infections, with *S. mekongi* and *S intercalatum* accounting for the rest. *S. japonicum* also infects a variety of domestic animals and therefore has epidemiologic significance. *S. mansoni* is the only species found in the western hemisphere and is seen in Brazil, Venezuela, Surinam, and parts of the Caribbean. *S. mansoni* and *S. hematobium* are both encountered in most African countries and on the Arabian peninsula, with *S. hematobium* found alone in parts of the Middle East. *S. japonicum* is found in China, the Philippines, and parts of Indonesia. *S. mekongi* is found in Laos and Cambodia, and *S. intercalatum* in Sub-Saharan Africa. Many other species infect birds, sheep, cattle, dogs, cats, and other mammals, but not humans. Most trematodes are bisexual, but *Schistosoma* are unisexual and reproduce by mating.

History.   Schistosomiasis is an ancient disease. Eggs have been found in Egyptian mummies of the twelfth century BCE, and ancient Egyptian papyri describe hematuria. The first description of the adult worm (*S. hematobium*) was made in 1851 by Theodor

Bilharz (1825–1862), a German physician working in Cairo, who also described its terminal (end)–spined eggs. Other than the additional finding of lateral (side)–spined eggs (perhaps another species) no further progress was made until the turn of the century. In 1904 S. japonicum was described by John Catto; the circle was closed in 1913 when Japanese biologist Keinosuka Miyairi (d. 1946) found the intermediate host of S. japonicum to be a freshwater snail. This work was confirmed by British biologist Robert Leiper (1881–1969), and differentiation of S. mansoni and S. hematobium into two distinct species was confirmed by noting specific intermediate host snails for each. By the close of World War I (1914–1918), the three major species and their life cycles were known, and efforts could be directed at prevention and treatment.

However, progress was slow because of lack of effective therapeutic drugs and difficulties with snail control. Not until the 1970s, when drugs such as niridazole, metrifonate, and oxamniquine appeared, were greater strides made. These were effective, were less toxic than previous pharmaceuticals, and could be orally administered. Praziquantel, developed in the 1970s and in use by the 1980s, proved to be superior because it covered all three species and was low in cost and toxicity. It is the mainstay of most control programs today.

Life Cycle.   Like other trematodes, Schistosoma have a life cycle involving two separate hosts. On exposure to freshwater, free-swimming larvae, called cerceriae, penetrate the skin within three to five minutes of contact. The larvae, now called schistosomulae, make their way into the circulation system through the heart and lungs and terminate in the portal circulation in about five to ten days. Here the larvae grow to adults and mate. The females migrate upstream to venules (small veins) around the intestinal or bladder walls. There, about four to six weeks after initial skin penetration, eggs are laid, about half of which pass upstream to lodge in the portal venules of the liver (in S. mansoni and japonicum). The other half penetrates the venules and the bladder or intestinal wall to be passed to the outside world. S. haematobium are passed in urine, whereas the other species are passed in the stool. Adult worms live an average of 3 to 7 years, though exceptional life spans of up to 30 years have been reported.

If the eggs reach freshwater, they hatch, releasing another larva, the miracidium. The miracidia penetrate the soft parts of certain species of snails and develop into sporocysts. These give rise to numerous daughter sporocysts, which grow and migrate out of the snail to become the cerceriae that reinitiate the cycle. In the case of S. japonicum, a similar life cycle exists in domestic animals, including cattle, water buffalo, pigs, dogs, and cats, whose eggs contribute to the disease burden.

Human Pathology and Disease.   The life cycle of the Schistosoma parasite determines the clinical and pathologic findings. Penetration of the cerceriae for the first time often elicits little reaction. Repeated exposure results in an allergic reaction, cercarial dermatitis, an inflammatory papular rash limited to the exposed area of skin. It may also result from repeated exposure to nonhuman cerceriae, most commonly from birds, and it is often referred to as "swimmer's itch."

Passage of the larvae through the lungs is usually silent, but heavy infections cause symptoms and signs of inflammation (pneumonitis). Cough, wheeze, and scattered X-ray changes may be noted.

The onset of egg laying, in a heavy infection, is associated with an allergic reaction known as acute schistosomiasis or the "Katayama syndrome." It is most commonly seen with S. japonicum but occurs with the other varieties as well. Symptoms and signs are fever, pneumonitis with cough and X-ray changes, abdominal pain, diarrhea, and enlargement of the liver, spleen, and lymph nodes. In light infections this stage may pass unnoticed, and it is less often seen in endemic areas.

Subsequent stages, referred to as chronic schistosomiasis, take months to years to manifest. The pathology is almost entirely the result of inflammatory changes from the eggs, which secrete enzymes and other antigens that provoke a granuloma-forming inflammatory reaction. The most common early symptom of urinary tract involvement is hematuria, whereas prolonged infections may result in bladder cancer and urinary tract obstruction at various points along the tract. The intestinal forms are characterized by intermittent diarrhea, abdominal discomfort, and intermittent blood loss. In these, about 50 percent of eggs laid pass upstream to the liver where they elicit a similar inflammatory reaction around the portal venules. Less commonly, eggs may be found in "ectopic" foci, such as the spinal cord, brain, lungs, and genitalia, with symptoms dependent on the location.

In general, the symptoms of schistosomiasis are mild and chronic, and the economic impact of the disease is hard to estimate. Studies have shown evidence of growth retardation and decline in cognitive function in heavily infected children. There is some dispute about how much disability on a global scale is attributable to schistosomiasis, partly because of the nonspecific nature of the symptoms and the frequent coexistence of other diseases.

There is an immune response to this infection, but it is incomplete and complex. Research in this area is ongoing in hopes of developing a vaccine. Initial infections in childhood trigger an antibody response that facilitates removal of new invading schistosomulae, but this seems to have little effect on adult worms, which are thought to be resistant to immune mechanisms. A portion of acquired immunity may be related to age alone.

Diagnosis and Treatment.   The diagnosis of schistosomiasis is best made by finding the eggs in stool or urine samples. Light infections may require more sensitive procedures such as rectal (or colon) biopsy. Blood serum tests are helpful, especially as screening tests or for epidemiological studies. Antibody tests generally take two to three months to become positive (thus, they are of limited help in acute cases), and they are subject to some error. Antibodies remain measurable for up to two years after successful treatment. Measurement of the antigen in the bloodstream is possible and quite specific, but it may miss light infections. Ultrasound studies of the liver are helpful as screening tests, but they are not precise in finding the parasite.

Great progress has been made in recent decades in the treatment of schistosomiasis. The drug of choice today is praziquantel, which is administered orally in one or two daily doses and is effective against all three major species. Side effects are mild enough for the drug to be used in mass treatment campaigns, and it is considered safe in pregnancy. Praziquantel is not effective, however, against the schistosomula stage.

Assessing cure requires follow-up stool or urine samples at three or more months after treatment and an assessment of the viability of any eggs found. There is generally good reversal of bowel and urinary tract pathology after treatment, and improvement is seen in liver inflammation, if it is not too far advanced.

Epidemiology and Control.   The geographic distribution of schistosomiasis is dependent on the distribution of the intermediate host snails. Human contact with water that is contaminated with human, and in some cases (particularly in the Orient) animal excreta,

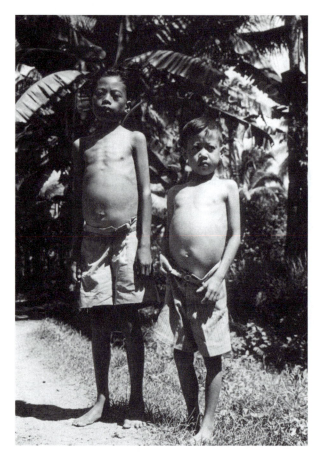

Two young children suffering from schistosomiasis, a debilitating water-borne disease. WHO photo. Courtesy of the National Library of Medicine.

perpetuates the infection. This combination occurs commonly in poor environments, where sewage disposal is primitive, and farming practices, swimming, and bathing enhance water contact. It is generally an endemic disease, though outbreaks have occurred, such as the outbreak in troops in the Philippine Islands during World War II and an occurrence that spread upstream in the 1990s after the damming of the Senegal River. The highest prevalence and intensity of infection is generally in 8- to 12-year-olds. The prevalence and intensity tend to decline later in life, perhaps as a result of reduced exposure to freshwater (because of new occupations, etc.) and of a partial immunity that develops over time. Endemic populations often have prevalence rates (of egg excretion) in the range of 30 percent to 50 percent, but lifetime infection rates of over 90 percent.

Strategies to control this disease require interruption of the life cycle at one or more points. Such strategies generally include the following approaches: sewage management to avoid contaminating water, provision of clean water for washing and bathing, drug therapy, and education programs. Work with mollusk poisons to control the snails is in less favor today because of cost and environmental concerns. The efficacy, relative cheapness, and safety of praziquantel have made drug therapy with this agent, combined with education measures and provision of clean water, the most cost-effective approach today. A serious concern in all programs employing praziquantel is the emergence of **drug-resistant** parasites. These have been reported, and failures of treatment are seen, but thus far, resistance does not seem to be increasing. Caution and surveillance are, however, in order.

Great progress has been made in recent years in controlling schistosomiasis in the Orient, South America, Caribbean, and North Africa, utilizing the aforementioned control measures. Less successful has been control in Sub-Saharan Africa, where little progress has been made. The **World Health Organization** estimates that of the 200 million cases in the world, 150 million occur in Sub-Saharan Africa; there, 70 million have had hematuria, 10 million have had hydronephrosis, and 130,000 have hematemesis yearly. In response, the recently constituted Schistosomiasis Control Initiative, a mix of public and private consortiums funded primarily by the Melinda and Bill Gates Foundation, is addressing this deficiency. The goal is to select high-risk groups as primary targets for control programs and help local governments to implement these programs. The initiative includes research, surveillance, chemotherapy, education, and other measures.

Research on a vaccine against schistosomiasis is being actively pursued, but thus far there is nothing available. Some candidate vaccines are in early stages of trial. *See also* Children and Childhood Epidemic Diseases; Diagnosis and Diagnostic Tools; Ectoparasites; Environment, Ecology, and Epidemic Disease; Human Body; Human Immunity and Resistance to Disease; Personal Hygiene and Epidemic Disease; Pilgrimage and Epidemic Disease; Vaccination and Inoculation; Water and Epidemic Diseases.

Further Reading

Centers for Disease Control and Prevention. *Schistosomiasis.* http://www.cdc.gov/ncidod/dpd/parasites/schistosomiasis/default.htm

Fenwick, A., and J. P. Webster. "Schistosomiasis: Challenges for Control, Treatment, and Drug Resistance." *Current Opinion in Infectious Disease* 19 (2006): 577–582.

Gryseels, B., et al. "Human Schistosomiasis." *Lancet* 368 (2006): 1106–1118.

World Health Organization. *Schistosomiasis.* http://www.who.int/topics/schistosomiasis/en/

J. GORDON FRIERSON

SCIENTIFIC REVOLUTION AND EPIDEMIC DISEASE. Historians use the term Scientific Revolution to describe a radical shift in human understanding of nature and natural processes during the later European Renaissance and Early Modern periods. Lasting from the mid-sixteenth through the seventeenth centuries, this revolution was the work of scientists, physicians, and other researchers who moved away from the medieval and Renaissance natural philosophy, based on classical knowledge, religion, and folklore, toward a discipline of science based on principles of empiricism, experimentalism, and the communication of one's findings, often summarized by the term scientific method. This overthrow of tradition resulted in the emergence of new systems of knowledge. These were proposed by a range of innovative thinkers who challenged both the utility of ancient philosophy and the accumulated authority on which that philosophy rested. Some of the foremost exponents of these "new philosophies" included the French mechanical philosophers Pierre Gassendi (1592–1655) and René Descartes (1596–1650), the astronomers Nicolaus Copernicus (1473–1543) and Johannes Kepler (1571–1630), the Italian mathematician and astronomer Galileo Galilei (1564–1642), and the English virtuosi Robert Boyle (1627–1691) and Isaac Newton (1642–1727).

In the field of medicine, prominent reformers included the Flemish anatomist Andreas Vesalius (1514–1564), whose *Workings of the Human Body* (1543) revolutionized the study of anatomy, and the English physician William Harvey (1578–1657), who first described the circulation of the blood. Other prominent medical reforms were linked to the rise of **Paracelsianism** and its novel theory of disease. Originally proposed by German **empiric Paracelsus** and taken up by followers such as Jan Baptista van Helmont (1577–1644), this new theory rejected the dominant **humoral theory** of **Galen** and sought to explain illness as the disruption of an internal vital principle called the *archaeus*, which could be negatively affected by "seeds" of disease entering the body from the external environment. Paracelsians rejected traditional organic remedies for inorganic metals and salts in tiny doses.

Atomism, Mechanism, and Fermentation.   Paracelsus and his followers were not the only thinkers to propose the idea of disease "seeds." In the early sixteenth century, for example, the Veronese physician **Girolamo Fracastoro** applied the ancient philosophy of atomism to the problem of disease and proposed that **syphilis** and other **epidemic** diseases could be explained by the presence of *seminaria*, or "tiny seeds," which were responsible for sickening otherwise healthy individuals. As part of the **miasma theory** of disease, he suggested that these seeds or particles were part of the "bad air" generated by certain **environments** and pollutants, but Fracastoro combined this idea with **contagion theory** by observing that these *seminaria* could be passed from one individual to another, particularly with diseases like syphilis. Fracastoro's notion of a material cause for disease transmission is viewed by some as a direct ancestor of modern **germ theory**.

More than a century after Fracastoro, atomism came more prominently into vogue. Arguably the most significant of the "new sciences" that emerged during the Scientific Revolution was the materialistic mechanical philosophy, which sought to explain all natural phenomena in terms of matter and motion. Pierre Gassendi, a French Catholic priest, revived the atomism of the ancient Greek philosopher Epicurus (341–270 BCE), in which phenomena were explained by the movement of atoms through a void; differing in their size, shape, and weight, these atoms could combine and disperse to an almost infinite degree. At the same time, the French philosopher René Descartes proposed a system in which phenomena as disparate as light, magnetism, and sound were explained by the movement and contact of corpuscles, or tiny pieces of matter.

These ideas had a profound effect on thinkers in the seventeenth century, and so it is unsurprising that, like Fracastoro, some philosophers would seek to apply atomistic or mechanical explanations to the problem of epidemic diseases. For example, Robert Boyle, often considered the father of modern chemistry, considered that **bubonic plague** might be transmitted by discrete corpuscles. To Boyle, these "plague corpuscles" seemed the most likely explanation for the manner in which the plague appeared to move between individuals and places. Atomism in particular became strongly linked with miasmatic theories of transmission, in which it was generally assumed that tiny particles of disease could attach themselves to persons exposed to miasmas, or pockets of "bad air." These particles could remain attached to a person's clothing or hair for some time, affecting them and others around them even once clear of the miasma, making travel through congested urban areas such as London a potentially hazardous exercise.

Not all notions of epidemic disease were linked with corpuscularian or atomistic theories, however. The English physiologist Thomas Willis (1621–1675) was, like Boyle, a member of the Royal Society of London (founded in 1660) and an avid experimentalist, placing him squarely at the epicenter of the Scientific Revolution. He was also a vocal disciple of Paracelsus and sought to explain vital processes such as respiration and digestion by means of a chemistry of fermentation. Observing that fevers often accompanied diseases like plague, Willis suggested that the active fermentation of the blood, producing a high fever, was the body's attempt to expel the "pestilential poison" of the disease. The innovative theories advanced by Boyle, Willis, and their contemporaries would reshape general understanding of physiology and of the body's response to disease.

New Technologies.   The Scientific Revolution spawned not only radical changes in ideas about the world, but the advent of new technologies as well. Prominent among these was the telescope, used by Galileo around 1609 to discover the four largest moons of Jupiter, and the **microscope**, which was to play an important role in the study of living things and, importantly, diseases such as plague.

The advent of the microscope in particular was closely linked to prevailing ideas concerning the particulate or corpuscularian nature of disease in the seventeenth century. The English journalist Marchamont Nedham (1620–1678) took his cue from Girolamo Fracastoro's notion of *seminaria* and looked for visual evidence of what he described as "certain Atoms, Corpuscles, or Particles, sometimes animated into little invisible worms as in the case of Pestilential infection." In his *Medela Medicinae: A Plea for the free Profession, and a Renovation of the Art of Physic Tending to the Rescue of Mankind from the Tyranny of Diseases* (1665), Nedham noted that these "little worms" had also been observed by the eminent German Jesuit philosopher and polymath Athanasius Kircher (1602–1680), who had examined human blood under the microscope and reported, according to Nedham, that "upon the opening of buboes and tumors, they have been found full of innumerable vermicules [little worms] indiscernible by the eye." Dutch scientist **Antony van Leeuwenhoek**, famed today for his close observation of spermatozoa under the microscope, also reportedly observed what he described as "animacules"—tiny animals—when examining the blood of an infected individual. The increasing use and sophistication of these technologies would eventually have a profound effect on **epidemiology** and the subsequent treatment of epidemic disease.

Organization, Communication, and the State.   Because most scientists were not connected with the academic life of universities, they needed to create new methods of communicating their findings and discoveries. Scientific societies like the privately organized Royal Society in London, the state-directed French Academy of Science (1666), and several independent Italian academies were organized to facilitate discussion and the sharing of information and to promote scientific endeavors. Beginning in 1453, books by researchers and practitioners began to be printed in large numbers, and they increasingly appeared in vernacular languages for wide national audiences. Within these audiences were leaders and bureaucrats in the rapidly evolving European states. Information was power, and states began collecting data on, for example, epidemic death tolls, in attempts to rationalize and centralize state responses to disease. In the seventeenth century, mathematics—from Descartes's coordinate geometry to Newton's calculus—became a tool for scientists and a language for communicating information. Both probability theory and statistical method emerged around mid-century and helped lay the groundwork for epidemiology. One of the earliest examples of statistical analysis was English haberdasher *cum* demographer John Graunt's 1662 study of the London Bills of Mortality, which had been started under King Henry VIII (1491–1547) and listed the weekly numbers of dead by cause of death. Governments also gave greater weight to medical expertise, and in the sixteenth century, physicians began appearing on health boards and health magistracies, and their developing theories on contagion helped spur the widespread use of such measures as **quarantines** and isolation, and the institution of **pest houses** and *cordons sanitaires*. *See also* Colonialism and Epidemic Disease; Demographic Data Collection and Analysis, History of; Greco-Roman Medical Theory and Practice; Medical Education in the West, 1500–1900; Plague in Europe, 1500–1770s; Public Health Boards in the West before 1900.

Further Reading

Applebaum, Wilbur. *The Scientific Revolution and the Foundations of Modern Science.* Westport, CT: Greenwood, 2005.

French, R. K., and Andrew Wear, eds. *The Medical Revolution of the Seventeenth Century.* New York: Cambridge University Press, 1989.

Jardine, Lisa. *Ingenious Pursuits: Building the Scientific Revolution.* New York: Anchor, 2000.

Shapin, Steven. *The Scientific Revolution.* Chicago: University of Chicago Press, 1998.

Temkin, Owsei. *Galenism: The Rise and Decline of a Medical Philosophy.* Ithaca: Cornell University Press, 1973.

Wear, Andrew, et al., eds. *The Medical Renaissance of the Sixteenth Century.* New York: Cambridge University Press, 1985.

MARK A. WADDELL

SCROFULA.   *See* Tuberculosis.

SECOND PLAGUE PANDEMIC.   *See* Black Death (and related articles); Plague: End of the Second Pandemic; Plague in Britain, 1500–1666; Plague in China; Plague in Europe, 1500–1770s; Plague in Medieval Europe, 1360–1500; Plague in the Islamic World, 1360–1500; Plague in the Islamic World, 1500–1850.

SEMMELWEIS, IGNAZ (1818–1865).   Ignaz Semmelweis is most famous for advocating sanitary techniques, but his true innovation was redefining a disease in terms of a single cause, which, by definition, made the cause universal and necessary. This opened the way to systematic prophylaxis (prevention) and treatment and to coherent explanations of disease phenomena.

Semmelweis was born in Budapest, Hungary. After completing an M.D. degree at the University of Vienna, he was appointed an assistant in the Viennese maternity hospital. There he confronted the horrible reality of childbed fever. Childbed fever, now called puerperal sepsis, ravaged European maternity clinics. In some years, some facilities had mortality rates above 70 percent, but the Viennese clinic maintained a relatively favorable rate of about 8 percent. The situation in Vienna, however, was unusual: its maternity facility had two divisions. In the first, staffed by obstetricians, mortality averaged about 10 percent, whereas in the second division, which utilized midwives, mortality averaged about 2 percent. Semmelweis tried desperately to understand the higher mortality rate in his division. He required that all procedures be the same in both divisions—even to the extent that all patients received the same food and were delivered from the same position. Nothing helped.

When Semmelweis's colleague Jakob Kolletschka (1803–1847) died after being accidentally cut while performing an autopsy, his corpse revealed morbid remains similar to those found in deceased maternity patients. Semmelweis speculated that, if the remains were similar, perhaps the cause was the same. In Kolletschka's case, the cause was contamination by decaying matter from a cadaver. Semmelweis realized that his first division maternity patients were also exposed to decaying organic matter conveyed on the hands of medical personnel. This did not happen in the second division because the midwives did not conduct autopsies. In May 1847, Semmelweis began requiring everyone to wash regularly in a chlorine solution. Within days, the morality rate dropped to the same level as in the midwives' division.

The chlorine washings, which Semmelweis probably adopted from the British, were tried here and there throughout Europe. However, in presenting his results, Semmelweis insisted that every case of childbed fever had the same one cause—decaying organic matter. This claim was inconsistent with the traditional view that every disease could have various causes, and initially both those who accepted chlorine washings and those who did not rejected it. Beginning in the mid-1860s and continuing through the century, however, Semmelweis's views were repeatedly discussed in German and French medical literature. Gradually, his way of thinking prevailed.

Frustrated at what he saw as reluctance to accept new ideas, Semmelweis's writings became strident. By 1865 he may have become deranged (although the evidence is inconclusive). In August he was committed to an asylum in Vienna where he was forcibly restrained. Two weeks later he died, probably from wounds inflicted in the asylum. *See also* Children and Childhood Epidemic Diseases; Contagion and Transmission; Disinfection and Fumigation; Germ Theory of Disease; Hospitals in the West to 1900.

Further Readings

Carter, K. Codell, and Barbara R. Carter. *Childbed Fever: A Scientific Biography of Ignaz Semmelweis.* New Brunswick, NJ: Transaction Publishers, 2005.

Loudon, Irvine. *The Tragedy of Childbed Fever.* New York: Oxford University Press, 2000.

Semmelweis, Ignaz. *The Etiology, Concept and Prophylaxis of Childbed Fever.* Translated by K. Codell Carter. Madison, WI: University of Wisconsin Press, 1983.

K. Codell Carter

SEPTICEMIC PLAGUE.   *See* Pneumonic and Septicemic Plague.

SEVERE ACUTE RESPIRATORY SYNDROME (SARS).   Severe Acute Respiratory Syndrome (SARS) originated in southern China in November 2002 and rapidly swept the globe to appear on five continents. From February to July 2003, it affected over 8,000 people worldwide, leaving at least 774 dead (including 349 in China, 299 in Hong Kong, 44 in Canada, 39 in Vietnam, 37 in Taiwan, and 33 in Singapore). A few sporadic cases continued to appear in China and Taiwan until April 2004.

A highly contagious lung infection, the illness was characterized by fever, cough, and difficulty breathing. It could result in hindrance to breathing such that death resulted in 10 percent or more of cases, even when good medical care was available. With a predilection for infants and the elderly, SARS also affected many health-care workers including **physicians, nurses**, and their family members.

After a few false leads, laboratories working independently on three continents identified the causative agent in late March 2003. It was new a strain of coronavirus, called SARS CoV. Such RNA **viruses** are named for their "crown-like" (corona) appearance on electron microscopy.

However, a pathogen is only one cause of any infectious disease; it is necessary for infection and spread, but it is not always sufficient to trigger an outbreak. **Environmental** and social factors also contribute to the appearance and spread of disease. In the wake of the September 11, 2001, attacks on the United States, some people wondered if this new disease was a deliberate act of **bioterrorism**. Their suspicions were soon dispelled.

Global air **travel** was another important factor in the spread of SARS. Initially unrecognized as a distinct new disease, SARS began in the southern Chinese province of Guangdong. An ailing doctor from Guangdong went to Hong Kong where he stayed on the ninth floor of the Metropole hotel. Sixteen hotel guests and visitors to that floor acquired the infection, probably while waiting for the elevator. Some carried the disease home to Vietnam, Singapore, or Canada. Many other cases arising in those countries would eventually be traced back to links with the Metropole hotel.

Disease can also be spread by technology and health workers. It was possible to transmit infection by care-giving and through special instruments for investigating and treating breathing disorders. Furthermore, health successes may backfire. The concept of pathocenosis, elaborated by medical historian Mirko Grmek (1924–2000), suggests that in any given time and place, prevailing diseases exist in a kind of harmony. When one condition disappears, another can come along to take its place. As a result, we can ask if SARS exploited a window of opportunity in the developed world created by the systematic use of **vaccinations** against **influenza** and childhood illnesses.

There is no specific treatment for SARS. In every center, the outbreak was contained by traditional methods: isolation of sufferers, **quarantine** of contacts, and use of protective clothing and sterile techniques by caregivers. Sick people were supported by oxygen and artificial respiration. Hospital security was increased; visiting was prohibited. Upon arrival each day, workers were required to have their temperatures taken and to **disinfect** their hands. All schools were closed in Singapore, Beijing, and Hong Kong, whereas isolated school closures were implemented in other centers. Consideration was given to closing airports, but health screening was preferred. Air passengers were monitored for fever and questioned about symptoms. Research on a vaccine continues.

SARS taxed the chronically underfunded public health services of several countries, and in its wake it left many other sequelae: medical, social, economic, political, and legislative. Medically, the outbreak made heavy demands of public health workers and infectious disease specialists. In Canada, cases appeared in Vancouver and Toronto, but the impact was much wider. For example, hospitals across the entire province of Ontario were quarantined for many weeks resulting in emotional turmoil. New rituals of handwashing and temperature control were implemented. Some patients with SARS had access to specialized technologies for respiratory support, but it became clear that a larger outbreak would soon exhaust existing resources. Too often neglected, disease prevention grew in importance.

Socially and culturally, SARS unleashed personal fears and irrational xenophobia. Travelers from Asia and people of Asian origin experienced outright discrimination, as they were wrongly thought to be carriers of the pathogen. Questions were raised about normally harmless customs. Who should attend funerals for those dead of SARS? Should common communion cups be dispensed with in Christian services? Should collective prayer be banned?

Economically, SARS resulted in massive disruption, directly because its costs and indirectly through its effects. Concerts, plays, and conferences were cancelled, and normally busy hotels, theatres, and restaurants stood empty. This situation was thought to have been aggravated by **World Health Organization** travel advisories against Hong Kong, Beijing, and Toronto. Some of the direct expenditures were later found to have been unnecessary. For example, sales of costly N95 face masks escalated, and supplies were depleted, although those masks were later shown to offer no advantage over others. The perceived need to stimulate travel to Toronto prompted a mega-concert by the Rolling Stones on July 20, 2003 Nevertheless, some evidence suggests that the financial hardship resulting from SARS was shorter lived and less severe than had been predicted.

Politically and legislatively, SARS revealed flaws in the existing safety nets for infection control. The disease occurred only in a few cities, but its legislative and policy impact was felt on a global scale. In its wake, more funding was directed to public health agencies, "**pandemic** planning" became standard practice, and restructuring of government ministries occurred.

Finally, SARS highlighted the continued vulnerability of the human organism to natural pathogens. When in the following year avian flu emerged as a health concern, the serious attention it received from media and governments, despite a paucity of human cases, was prompted by the recent passage of SARS. Looking back, many experts believe that a devastating pandemic was avoided more by good luck than by good management. Even as they deal with the nature and control of the disease, publications about SARS also emphasize the "lessons learned" from its brief but sharp debut in 2003.

Further Reading

Abraham, Thomas. *Twenty-First Century Plague: The Story of SARS*. Baltimore: Johns Hopkins University Press, 2005.

Brookes, Tim, and Omar Khan. *Behind the Mask: How the World Survived SARS, the First Epidemic of the 21st Century*. Washington, DC: American Public Health Association, 2004.

Duffin, Jacalyn, and Arthur Sweetman, eds. *SARS in Context: Memory, History, Policy*. Montreal: McGill Queen's University Press and Queen's School of Policy Studies, 2006.

Fidler, David P. *SARS, Governance and the Globalization of Disease*. New York: Palgrave Macmillan, 2004.

Greenfield, Karl Taro. *China Syndrome: The True Story of the 21st Century's First Great Epidemic*. San Francisco: HarperCollins, 2006.

History Now—SARS and The New Plagues [film]. History Channel, 2006.

MacDougall, Heather. "Toronto's Health Department in Action: Influenza in 1918 and SARS in 2003." *Journal of the History of Medicine & Allied Sciences*. 62 (2007): 56–89.

McClean, Angela, et al., eds. *SARS: A Case Study in Emerging Infections*. New York: Oxford University Press, 2005.

Serradell, Joaquima. *SARS*. Philadelphia: Chelsea House, 2005.

JACALYN DUFFIN

SEXUALITY, GENDER, AND EPIDEMIC DISEASE. The association of sexuality or gender with epidemic disease has an ancient pedigree in the Western world. Two themes seem to dominate: transgressions of sexual taboos or moral prohibitions are seen as causing disease, and stigmatized categories of people are viewed as particularly dangerous vectors of **transmission** or reservoirs of disease. Of course, issues of taboo and stigma aside, a large number of potentially fatal diseases are simply transmitted through the sex act, ironically making the act of procreation a potentially deadly one.

The Linguistic Production of "Plague" and "Pestilence". The neutral medical term "epidemic" (*epi* + *dēmos* meaning "around or close to the people") appears in English in the early seventeenth century. Its coinage at the dawn of modern science suggests a turn away from the prevailing notion of widespread disease as a divine punishment that is contained in the far older medieval term "plague," which appears in French and English in the fourteenth century. The term "pestilence" (the condition of plague, particularly **bubonic plague**) has a similar linguistic history to that of "plague," appearing in English in the early fourteenth century, at which point it already appears to have had a figurative sense of "that which is morally pestilent or pernicious; moral plague or mischief, evil conduct, wickedness; that which is fatal to the public peace or well-being" (Oxford English Dictionary). By the use of such terms for phenomena that were mysterious, unpredictable, and uncontrollable, premodern societies were able to attribute meanings to widespread diseases, often at the expense of socially marginalized people (such as women) or socially stigmatized behaviors (such as sexual relations).

The Ancient World.   The Hebrew Scriptures provide numerous instances of plague as the visitation of divine punishment, often associated with gender and sex. Genesis 12, for example, narrates Abraham's removing to Egypt during a famine, where his wife Sarah poses as his sister only to be brought into the pharaoh's house, ostensibly to become a concubine, for which God sends a plague upon Pharaoh. In Numbers 25:1–2 the association of plague with sexual transgressions and gender is explicit: "And Israel abode in Shittim, and the people began to commit whoredom with the daughters of Moab. And they called the people unto the sacrifices of their gods: and the people did eat, and bowed down to their gods"(King James Version). In this instance and in the vast Hebrew prophetic literature, intermarriage with non-Hebrew tribes is metaphorically configured as religious apostasy, and religious apostasy is metaphorically configured as consorting with prostitutes.

If Classical Greco-Roman cultures failed to associate epidemic disease with moral error or sin, they nonetheless understood plagues as divine punishments for displeasing the impetuous gods by acts often involving sexual elements. In Homer's (c. 8th century BCE) *Iliad,* for example, the god Apollo hurls a plague upon the Greeks camped outside of Troy because of the trophy abduction of a virgin daughter of a priest of Apollo. Similarly, the incestuous patricide Oedipus at the beginning of Sophocles' (c. 495–406 BCE) *Oedipus Rex* confronts a plague sent to punish his kingdom for its having harbored the murderer of his predecessor on the throne.

Although the Christian scriptures seem to make little of disease as a divine punishment, the last book of the Christian scriptures, the apocalyptic Book of Revelation, includes nearly a dozen verses describing end-times plagues. Not surprisingly, these are associated with the allegorical figure of the Whore of Babylon, who rides upon a symbolic Beast and who carries a defiling cup of iniquity. Thus, the most mythological of Christian scriptures associates plague with both divine judgment for sin and perverse female sexuality.

The Medieval and Early-Modern Worlds.   In medieval Western Europe, which was dominated by Roman Catholic Christianity, epidemic disease was often understood as the product of immorality as well as an occasion for repentance. The association of sin and sickness provided more than an **epidemiology** in the medieval mind. Sin itself was viewed as a soul sickness, and in medieval Christian theology the most pervasive epidemic disease was Original Sin, the result of Adam and Eve's fall, infecting all humans. Both the seven deadly sins and a multitude of physical illnesses were understood as symptomatic of the epidemic Original Sin, which is transmitted to the next generation of humans through the sexual intercourse of their parents. God's displeasure with moral transgressions including prostitution and adultery led to plague, and plague led in many late medieval and early modern cities to the closing of brothels and to intense sermons against sexual sin.

At the end of the fifteenth century, the emergence of a new venereal pox epidemic, **syphilis**, coincided with new historical and social forces, including the rise of imperial ventures (expanding international travel) and the birth of Protestantism. **Syphilis in sixteenth-century Europe** was frequently attributed to infection by foreigners. Moreover, women were viewed as dangerous reservoirs of the disease. Protestant moralism, which particularly took aim at what it considered the sexual license and corruption of Roman Catholicism, militated against prostitutes and brothels. Medical authorities even argued whether or not remedies should be attempted, not because of questions about medical efficacy but because they viewed the disease as a divine judgment for lust in which the physician should not intervene.

Modern Medicine, Primitive Metaphors.   Moralizing epidemiology did not end with the eighteenth-century Enlightenment and the development of modern medical science, including **germ theory**, which attributes a microbial cause to epidemic disease. Perhaps the most iconic epidemic disease of the nineteenth century, **tuberculosis** (known more commonly at the time as "consumption"), was associated with women (particularly high-strung or high-living women) and with effeminate men (who lacked the manly virtues of self-control and restraint and who were prone to hysteria). A product of a bacterial infection that was assisted by the explosive growth of urban dwellers during the **Industrial Revolution**, tuberculosis figured prominently in the era's Romantic novels, melodramas, and operas as the affliction of ruined women and weak men.

Across the twentieth-century Western world, sexual taboos tended to dissolve, especially during the 1920s and from the early 1960s on (the Sexual Revolution). In both cases, increased social options for women (and in the latter the birth control pill) led to freer and often riskier sexual activity. Though increasingly controllable, **sexually transmitted disease** case rates grew, often dramatically, and new forms of venereal disease emerged.

AIDS: Postmodern Plague.   Since its emergence in the early 1980s, **acquired immune deficiency syndrome** (AIDS) has also absorbed numerous metaphorical meanings because of its association with stigmatized behavior (for example, intravenous drug use, anal sex, or sex with multiple partners) and stigmatized or marginalized social groups or populations (gay men, urban African Americans, Caribbean immigrants, and Africans). Few epidemics have become as deeply entangled in attitudes toward sexuality and gender roles as has AIDS, in discussions of both its epidemiology and its prevention. The fact that some body fluids (like semen, vaginal secretions, and blood) are vectors of transmission for the human immunosuppressive virus (HIV) has meant that public health education required a frank discussion of the containment of these fluids to prevent HIV infection. *See also* Biblical Plagues; Disease, Social Construction of; Gonorrhea and Chlamydia; Religion and Epidemic Disease; Scapegoats and Epidemic Disease; Sexual Revolution; Venereal Disease and Social Reform in Progressive-Era America; Tuberculosis.

Further Reading

Allen, Peter Lewis. *The Wages of Sin: Sex and Disease, Past and Present.* Chicago: University of Chicago Press, 2000.

Gilman, Sander L. *Disease and Representation: Images of Illness from Madness to AIDS.* Ithaca: Cornell University Press, 1988.

Leavy, Barbara Fass. *To Blight with Plague: Studies in a Literary Theme*. New York: New York University Press, 1992.

Long, Thomas L. *AIDS and American Apocalypticism: The Cultural Semiotics of an Epidemic*. Albany: State University of New York Press, 2005.

Mack, Arien, ed. *In Time of Plague: The History and Social Consequences of Lethal Epidemic Disease*. New York: New York University Press, 1991.

Sontag, Susan. *Illness as Metaphor* and *AIDS and Its Metaphors*, double edition. New York: Picador, 2001.

THOMAS LAWRENCE LONG

SEXUAL REVOLUTION.   The sexual revolution is the global shift in attitudes, behaviors, and legal regulations that occurred with respect to sexuality in the 1960s and 1970s. Born out of the broader "rights" movements of the era (i.e., the civil rights, feminist, gay rights, peace, and counterculture movements), the sexual revolution has had a major impact on **epidemiology**, as well as on the **diagnosis** and treatment of venereal and nonvenereal diseases and **epidemics**.

A Brief History of the Sexual Revolution.   Most historians define 1960 as the start of the sexual revolution because it marks the year in which the **pharmaceutical** company Searle released the birth control pill. The pill had an immediate social impact: it was the most effective form of contraception (up to 99 percent when used properly) in history, and gave women extraordinary control over their bodies. For the first time, women could engage in sex without the fear of becoming pregnant, while the development of **antibiotics** in the 1940s made the most dreaded venereal diseases, such as syphilis curable. The fear of **AIDS** would not become a major concern for another two decades. This led to an explosion in sexual experimentation and the number of professional women who could now enter the workforce without worrying about motherhood.

Through his magazine *Playboy*, Hugh Hefner (1926–) promoted the findings of Alfred Kinsey (1894–1956; *Sexual Behavior in the Human Male*, 1948; *Sexual Behavior in the Human Female*, 1953) and Masters and Johnson (*Human Sexual Response*, 1966) as evidence that a sexual revolution was well under way. *Sex and the Single Girl* (1962), written by Helen Gurley Brown (1922–), the editor of *Cosmopolitan* magazine, echoed the message that was being conveyed by her male counterpart Hefner. Seen by conservative segments of society as promoting promiscuity and adultery, most young, single, sexually liberated urban women used the book as a "how to" manual to guide them through professional and romantic relationships.

With the threats of pregnancy, disease, and social stigmatization gone, many of the traditional restrictions on sexuality seemed no longer justifiable. With the birth control pill came the legitimization of feminism and reproductive rights (especially abortion). As women became more concerned with reclaiming power over their lives and bodies, they began questioning sexual expression and the social construction of medicalized sexuality. They began seeking advice about sexual health from laywomen and exploring alternative treatments to gynecological diseases; the Boston Women's Health Book Collective's *Our Bodies Ourselves*, first published in 1970, addressed both of these concerns. Feminists also began promoting the exploration of sexuality—especially through mainstream texts such as *The Female Eunuch* (1970) by Australian scholar Germaine Greer (1939–) and Alex Comfort's (1920–2000) *The Joy of Sex* (1972).

More radical men and women explored their sexuality through the "free love" movement. Free love and other sexual movements, such as "swinging" in Britain, became prominent strains of the counterculture movement especially after the "Summer of Love" (1967), when peace activists and hippies merged to chant the famous 1960s slogan "make love not war." In between anti-Vietnam protests (in the United States) and anti-nuclear demonstrations (in the United Kingdom), the men and women of this branch of the counterculture movement began exploring their sexuality without the constraints of marriage and monogamy. Popular modes of sexual expression included interracial, homosexual, and bisexual relationships; open cohabitation of unmarried couples; communal living; casual sexual encounters; and political "love-ins." These were popularized by celebrities such as John Lennon (1940–1980) and Yoko Ono (1933–), who held a "Bed-in for Peace" in their honeymoon suite at the Amsterdam Hilton Hotel in March 1969. Another component of the hippie/free love lifestyle was illegal drug use. Drugs of choice included marijuana and harder psychedelics such as LSD and mescaline; in the 1980s, cocaine, crack, and heroine became the drugs of choice for individuals still practicing this lifestyle. The sexual revolution thus contributed to the transformation of illicit drug use into a national, and global, **epidemic**, especially as the hippie movement spread to Canada, Denmark, the Netherlands, Australia, New Zealand, Brazil, Mexico, and Japan.

The sexual revolution also had a profound impact on same-sex relationships. Sensing a window of opportunity, gays, lesbians, bisexual, and transgendered individuals began to seek equal civil and political rights. After the New York City Stonewall Riots of 1969, activists formed the Gay Liberation Front (GLF), which spearheaded the burgeoning gay rights movement. The GLF's activism was quickly inherited by a number of other consciousness-raising groups, a technique that gay activists borrowed from feminists. Both feminists and gay activists used the sexual revolution to bring down social and legal barriers that had been restricting their activities for centuries: homosexuality was finally demedicalized in the 1970s (up until late 1974, the American Psychiatric Association considered it a psychiatric disorder), and American women were given the unfettered right to have an abortion through the 1973 U.S. Supreme Court decision in *Roe v. Wade*.

The open discussion of pornography and the legitimization of some aspects of the sex trade were also outcomes of the sexual revolution. Magazines such as *Playboy* had succeeded in making sexual expression and the display of nude bodies commonplace. No longer a taboo subject, pornography went from being a sin to being a "tasteful" form of adult entertainment. Even though their freedom of speech was protected by the First Amendment of the U.S. Constitution, Hefner, and his more controversial competitor Larry Flynt (1942–), publisher of *Hustler* magazine, faced scrutiny from feminists, such as Gloria Steinem (1934–), who described pornography—even soft-core pornography—as a form of violence against women.

As sex on the silver screen became a prerequisite for a box-office hit, Westerners became more and more comfortable with the commercial sex trade. Prostitution was decriminalized in a number of countries, including regions of Australia, as well as Germany, Switzerland, and the Netherlands. In the last nation, prostitutes even became unionized, tax-paying workers. The sex trade, like pornography, also attracted the attention of activists, such as Andrea Dworkin (1946–2005), who maintained that the selling of female bodies only increased the exploitation and violence that women were already facing in society.

The Impact of the Sexual Revolution on Epidemic Disease.   Although some scholars continue to debate whether or not there actually *was* a sexual revolution, one fact is
undeniable: the changes in sexual attitudes and activities revolutionized the way societies
think about epidemics, plagues, and diseases. The sexual revolution profoundly impacted
the way in which men, and especially women, perceive their bodies. Before the 1960s,
modern society permitted only physicians to examine, diagnose, and treat ailments of the
female body. The women's health movement, which was an offshoot of the second wave
feminist movement of the 1960s and 1970s, gave women the power, and the permission,
to bypass doctors and heal themselves.

One radical branch of the women's health movement, self-help gynecology, which was
promoted by Carol Downer (1933–) and Lorraine Rothman (1932–), even taught women
how to perform self-breast and cervical examinations. Although the former has now
become part of standard medical practice, at the time, touching one's breast, or looking at
one's cervix in order to detect possible abnormalities (such as cysts and tumors) was
unheard of. These self-help groups made women more aware of their health and more
knowledgeable about epidemic diseases, such as breast and cervical cancer, and their
causes (i.e., **HPV, heredity**, the **environment**). Women are now active participants in
their own health care and routinely seek medical attention for these epidemics by request-
ing testing such as pap smears and mammograms.

The consciousness-raising that was promoted by feminist groups eventually served as
the foundation of the men's health movement, which rose to prominence in the early
1980s. During the 1960s and 1970s, very few individuals thought about sexually transmitted diseases while experimenting with their sexuality. Antibiotics had, after all,
eliminated the consequences of venereal diseases such as **syphilis, gonorrhea**, and
chlamydia; antiviral medicines would tame herpes and **hepatitis** B. Even so, the increase
in sexual activity meant significant increases in cases of sexually transmitted diseases.
Everything changed when AIDS entered the scene in the early 1980s. Initially branded a
homosexual disease because of its incidence in the promiscuous gay population, AIDS
actually helped create an organized men's health movement. Although its main focus was
originally the AIDS **pandemic**, the men's health movement has, over the past decade,
begun to branch out into other areas such as prostate cancer and heart disease prevention.
Leading the way are groups such as the Gay Men's Health Crisis (established in New York
in 1982), the Men's Health Forum (established in the United Kingdom in 1994), and the
Men's Health Network (established in Toronto in 2000).

Free love and the liberalization of sexual relations also transformed the ways in which
epidemic diseases are diagnosed and treated. Because individuals are, in the post–sexual
revolution era, far more likely to have multiple sex partners, epidemiologists usually treat
the identification of sexually transmitted diseases as they would any other outbreak. In
other words, they routinely identify the common (or point) source (i.e., the diagnosed
patient), and then try to determine how the disease might have propagated (i.e., they
determine with whom the diagnosed individual had sexual relations). This approach,
especially if it concerns a patient diagnosed with HIV/AIDS, usually involves contacting
and testing other potentially infected individuals, as well educating the local community.
It is here, more than with any other disease, that personal privacy rights conflict with
public safety mandates.

Liberalized prostitution, one of the outcomes of the sexual revolution, has long been
demonized as a major contributor to the spread of epidemic diseases. However, it is

unclear whether or not this is true because it is difficult to study prostitutes and disease transmission. Nevertheless, in an effort to reduce the spread of epidemic disease through prostitution, nations have taken one of three approaches to the sex trade: outlawing it completely; instituting regulations to monitor the health of sex workers; and/or educating sex workers about treatment and prevention. Prohibiting prostitution is probably the least effective approach because it only drives the practice underground, where epidemic diseases, such as HIV and hepatitis, can spread even more rapidly. This is especially true when unprotected sex is combined with intravenous drug use. The rationale behind regulation is that because the sex trade is impossible to eliminate, the best way to deal with it is to reduce its negative ramifications. The Netherlands, for example, requires routine health check-ups from prostitutes. If they fail an examination, or do not submit to state requirements, they could lose their licenses. The U.S. state of Nevada and the nation of Australia, where prostitution is legal, have been particularly successful in educating prostitutes about safe sex. *See also* AIDS, Literature, and the Arts in the United States; Cinema and Epidemic Disease; Human Papilloma Virus and Cervical Cancer; Medical Ethics and Epidemic Disease; Pharmaceutical Industry; Personal Liberties and Epidemic Disease; Public Health Agencies, U.S. Federal; Sexuality, Gender, and Epidemic Disease.

Further Reading

Allyn, David. *Make Love Not War: The Sexual Revolution, an Unfettered History*. New York: Routledge, 2001.

Brandt, Allan M. *No Magic Bullet: A Social History of Venereal Disease in the United States since 1880*. New York: Oxford University Press, 1985.

D'Emilio, John, and Estelle B. Freedman. *Intimate Matters: A History of Sexuality in America*. Chicago: University of Chicago Press, 1998.

Kimball, Roger. *The Long March: How the Cultural Revolution of the 1960s Changed America*. New York: Encounter Books, 2001

Petersen, James. *The Century of Sex: Playboy's History of the Sexual Revolution, 1900–1999*. New York: Grove Press, 1999.

Rosen, Ruth. *The World Split Open: How the Modern Women's Movement Changed America*. New York: Viking Press, 2000.

Tone, Andrea. *Devices and Desires: A History of Contraceptives in America*. New York: Hill and Wang, 2002.

Watkins, Elizabeth Siegel. *On the Pill: A Social History of Oral Contraceptives, 1950–1970*. Baltimore: Johns Hopkins University Press, 1998.

TANFER EMIN TUNC

SIMOND, PAUL-LOUIS (1858–1947). Paul-Louis Simond was a French **physician** who discovered that the rodent flea transmitted the plague **bacterium** and was thus responsible for human cases of **bubonic plague**. Born to a French Protestant clergyman in Beaufort-sur-Gervanne, Simond graduated as a **physician** from the French Naval Medical School at Bordeaux in 1887. His medical thesis on **leprosy** in French Guyana won a prize, and he was posted to Indochina and the South China coast. His career changed dramatically after he took the course in bacteriology in 1895–1896 at the Pasteur Institute of Paris, where he was assigned to the laboratory of Elie Metchnikoff

(1845–1916). In 1897 the Pasteur Institute sent him to India to relieve **Alexandre Yersin** and to continue the latter's program of administering the Pasteur antiplague serum to Indian patients. In 1898 Simond developed his flea transmission theory after he noticed that a small blister-like lesion was usually found on the foot or leg of Indian plague patients. In his makeshift laboratory, he discovered organisms resembling the plague bacillus in the stomach of fleas that had fed on infected rats. The *Annales de l'Institut Pasteur* published his article in 1898. It stated boldly, on the basis of a limited number of experiments, that the bite of rat fleas constituted the mode of infection for both rats and humans. Elated at his discovery, Simond could not resist remarking that he "had uncovered a secret that had tortured man since the appearance of plague in the world."

Such luminaries as **Robert Koch** and **Patrick Manson** were partial to Simond's theory but wanted more evidence. They formed a small minority. Experts on the German and Indian Plague Commissions disregarded the flea and held that although rats were important during initial outbreaks, thereafter human agency played the greater role in spreading bubonic plague. It was not until the second Indian Plague Commission of 1905 conducted its own field and laboratory experiments that Simond began to receive scientific credit. It took a further three years before the conservative Indian Medical Service finally accepted the flea's role in plague transmission.

From India, Simond went to Indochina (Vietnam) where he was named Director of the Pasteur Institute's branch in Saigon (1898–1900). His next Pasteurian assignment took him to Brazil from 1901 to 1905 where, together with Emile Marchoux (1862–1943) and Alexandre Salimbeni (1867–1942), he formed a three-man team assigned to study the **yellow fever** control methods of Oswaldo Cruz (1872–1917) in Rio de Janeiro. Simond was able to apply these methods in the French colony of Martinique in the Caribbean in 1908–1909.

His final posting was as Director of Health Services for the French Colonial Army in Indochina during the First World War. In 1917, a falling-out with military authorities led him to resign his military commission. Too often neglected in general medical histories, Simond deserves a place beside his fellow Pastorian Alexandre Yersin in the history of bubonic plague.

Further Reading

Crawford, Edward A., "Paul-Louis Simond and his work on Plague." *Perspectives in Biology and Medicine* 39 (1996): 446–458.

Marriott, Edward. *Plague: A Story of Science, Rivalry, and the Scourge that Won't Go Away.* New York: Metropolitan Books, 2002.

MYRON ECHENBERG

SIMPSON, WILLIAM JOHN RITCHIE (1855–1931). An expert on hygiene and control of **epidemic** diseases (in particular **bubonic plague**) in the tropics, William Simpson was a professor of public health and an advisor to British colonial governments. Born in Scotland, he graduated from the University of Aberdeen and in 1880 was awarded his M.D. degree along with a diploma in public health from Cambridge University. He served as a Medical Officer of Health, first in Aberdeen from 1881 to 1886 and then in Calcutta in 1886–1897. He moved to London in 1897 and joined **Patrick Manson** to establish the

London School of Tropical Medicine in 1899. Simpson also held the Chair in Hygiene at King's College, London. From 1900 to 1929 he took brief trips to advise colonial governments on the control of plague or sanitation more generally, including to Cape Town (1901), Hong Kong (1902), Singapore (1906), the Gold Coast, Sierra Leone, and Southern Nigeria (1908), Uganda and Zanzibar (1913), the Gold Coast (1924), and Northern Rhodesia (1929).

As Medical Officer of Health in Aberdeen, Simpson developed an interest in epidemics through his study of outbreaks of diseases characterized as zymotic (including **smallpox, measles,** scarlet fever, **diphtheria, typhoid fever, typhus,** and **whooping cough**). These were believed to result from chemical reactions acting as catalysts for a chain of disease processes. He also began to study **germ theories** of disease that developed from laboratory research, although he was at first skeptical about the value of such research for public health practice. By the time he helped found the London School, he had become a lifelong advocate of laboratory research. He related many of his findings in *A Treatise on Plague Dealing with the Historical, Epidemiological, Clinical, Therapeutic and Preventive Aspects of the Disease* and in *The Maintenance of Health in the Tropics,* both published in 1905.

On his trips abroad, Simpson put into practice ideas about plague control from research at the London School. For example, in Cape Town he drew on the newest laboratory research to institute a plague **vaccine** campaign. His medical colleagues and other citizens, however, found the campaign suspect, and it died away. In contrast, his colleagues and colonial authorities wanted to rely on a much older method of plague control: the separation of those they deemed dangerous, in this case all black Africans, whether they were healthy or not. Although he considered it inadequate, Simpson sanctioned the segregation. At issue was the local belief that black Africans were to blame for the epidemic's severity and Simpson's belief that segregation or isolation was only one of several means to control plague.

As do contemporary international health experts who travel from one epidemic to another, Simpson tried to reconcile practices to control plague that were new—such as plague vaccines—with older, established practices, such as segregation and isolation. *See also* Colonialism and Epidemic Disease; Disease, Social Construction of; Pest Houses and Lazarettos; Plague in Africa: Third Pandemic; Race, Ethnicity, and Epidemic Disease; Scapegoats and Epidemic Disease.

Further Reading

Baker R. A., and R. A. Bayliss. "William John Ritchie Simpson (1855–1931): Pubic Health and Tropical Medicine." *Medical History* 31 (1987): 450–465.

MARY SUTPHEN

SLAVERY AND EPIDEMIC DISEASE.   Slavery is an ancient practice. Even two centuries after the abolition of slavery in Europe and the Western hemisphere, numerous societies still have state-sponsored slavery or sustain slave-like working conditions. Though defined by the slave's status as chattel property, the physical circumstances of slavery have often included overcrowding, forced labor, poor nutrition and sanitary conditions, and forced travel through or to vastly different ecological **environments**. These provide the perfect environment for the emergence and proliferation of **epidemic** diseases.

Slavery was common in antiquity and the Middle Ages, and Arab slavers notoriously removed millions of Central and East Africans to North Africa, Arabia, and the Indian Ocean. In Western Europe the practice of slavery waned with the practice of serf labor but was revived to address the huge labor shortages caused by the **Black Death** and the late medieval colonial developments in the eastern Mediterranean and Atlantic isles. It was not until the mid-sixteenth century, however, that massive epidemics occurred in association with the slave trade. The surge is related to Europeans' transformation of slavery into a transatlantic enterprise. This followed their discovery that the natives of the Western Hemisphere made very poor slaves; in no small part this was because of the natives' susceptibility to European diseases. And so the Europeans turned to Africa for labor. The process of capture, enslavement, and forced **migration** of approximately 12 million West Africans to the Americas over three centuries defined the "New World" culturally and socially and was responsible for an unprecedented intercontinental biological interchange.

Bacteria, viruses, and parasites were transported in the ships linking Africa, the Americas, and Europe. These biological entities, regardless of their alleged origin, had been confined to geographic and human reservoirs for millennia, and human populations living with these microorganisms evolved to develop specific immune characteristics that kept germs at bay. Like the common cold today, their presence was endemic, and the usual presentation of the diseases they caused mild, when compared to the crippling symptoms of an epidemic. The transatlantic biological interchange set in motion by the colonization of the Western Hemisphere and by the slave trade put human populations and the germs associated with them into contact—populations that had been separately evolving, culturally, socially and biologically, for millennia. This set the perfect stage for an explosion of epidemics for which the only precedent in mortality and in geopolitical and social impact was the Black Death.

The introduction of African slavery to the New World was intimately related to the interchange of pathogens that caused native Central and South Americans' demographic collapse. Disease did not spare any group. Africans died by the thousands of **smallpox**, the same Old World disease that obliterated Incan, Mayan, and Aztec civilizations. However, Africans brought with them their own share of pestilences such as **malaria, yellow fever**, and filariasis, among others. But if there were one pestilence that was central in the shaping of the South American continent, it was yellow fever.

Yellow Fever is a mild affliction in its endemic state, but it became vicious when it traveled. It first emerged as a source of epidemics in the port cities of West Africa where enslaved Africans were appraised, sold to merchants, and shipped to the New World. Thousands of sailors died during the middle passage (the journey from Africa to the slave trade ports in the Caribbean and in South and North America), and many others once ashore. Slave ships, with their crew of susceptible European hosts and half-empty **water** casks, provided with the perfect transcontinental transport system for the yellow fever virus and its fastidious vector, the mosquito *Aedes*. The disease needed to survive in the body of susceptible hosts, jumping from one European to another after either killing them or immunizing them, for the 12 weeks that the middle passage usually lasted.

In 1647 yellow fever arrived at Barbados. Its pronounced symptoms and high mortality (approximately 10 percent) terrorized Native Americans, Europeans, and Creoles all the same, whereas immune Africans could ignore it. Yellow fever spread throughout the ports of the Americas as far north as Boston and New York in the English Colonies. It even reached Europe and struck Lisbon, Barcelona, St. Nazaire in France, and Swansea in

Wales. Although this very African epidemic did not seem to affect Africans, the story of malaria was different.

Even though Africans had been living with malaria for millennia, the parasitic characteristics of the *plasmodium* (the parasite causing malaria) did not allow African bodies to acquire immunity. Thus, malaria's scourge came within slaves' bodies and became endemic on the American continents. Though not immune, Africans had undergone a process of natural selection that made them able to survive the quartan fevers of the *falciparum* variant of the disease, but with one drawback. The special malaria-resistant red blood cells Africans developed were less effective at withstanding low blood oxygen concentration, hypoxemia, or body stress's hormone's surge and acidic conditions. These sickle-shaped cells are responsible for the condition known as sickle cell anemia, a disease specific to those of African descent.

In the New World, slavery also provided the perfect infrastructure for disease dissemination. Most African slaves were brought to the Americas to labor in two particular working spaces, the plantation and the mine. European colonists created or controlled both of these ecologically disruptive spaces, which proved to be perfect breeding grounds for the native *Anopheles* mosquito. These mosquitoes proliferated in close proximity to humans in the warm residual waters re-collected in the ubiquitous white clay receptacles used on the sugar plantations and in the rainwater-filled ponds left by silver and gold mining. From here, scores of *Anopheles* emerged and feasted on humans, while transmitting the deadly *falciparum*.

Four out of ten Africans died between the time they embarked from African shores and the end of their first year in the New World. Although there are no reliable statistics, it is not a stretch to say that most of these men, women, and children—predominantly men because of the nature of the demand for field hands—died of disease. Two epidemic diseases share responsibility for this humanitarian catastrophe: smallpox and **typhus**.

Sailors and captains; British, Portuguese, French, and Spanish governmental officers; **physicians** of European royal medical corps such as the Spanish *protomedicato*; and clergymen such as the Jesuit priests Alonso Sandoval (1577–1652) and Pedro Claver (1581–1654), all testify to the common occurrence of smallpox among African American slave populations. The conditions in which Africans were shipped from Africa made of the middle passage a truly Darwinian selective rite of passage in which only the strongest survived. African slaves were confined in overcrowded quarters for three or more months. In the poorly ventilated stowage decks of the slave ships, they shared everything from blankets to eating utensils. These are, of course, the perfect conditions for the dissemination of smallpox and epidemic typhus, among other diseases.

Sailors and captains of vessels under all flags left testimony about the terrifying experience of smallpox epidemics on board the slave ships and the economic catastrophe that it represented, in their desperate diary entries. After major smallpox epidemics struck cities such as Havana, Portobello, Rio de Janeiro, and Cartagena, authorities prohibited infected slave ships from unloading their cargoes in any American ports until after a strict **quarantine** period and careful inspections by medical officers. Unwilling to undergo this hardship, captains took no risks, and thousands of slaves were thrown overboard in the middle of the Atlantic at the slightest symptom of disease.

The arrival of new African slaves brought virgin material for the smallpox virus. Epidemics shook all the major cities of the New World until late in the nineteenth century, after decades of vaccination and, most importantly, the abolition of slavery. Slave owners considered epidemics in slaves' quarters catastrophic, more often because of their economic impact than because of humanitarian concerns. Compulsory inoculation of the susceptible population became standard in North America after 1816 and in the rest of the Americas somewhat later. But there was no procedure that could protect slaves from the "ship's disease," a pestilence that roamed between the decks where they were confined in their passage from Africa to the Americas.

Epidemic typhus, the violent version of the milder endemic typhus is caused by *Rickettsia prowazekii*. The conditions predominating in the slave ships were perfect for the transmission of this affliction, one that prefers filthy environments and bodies. The unhygienic conditions in the lower decks of the *negreros* (Black slave) ships were perfect for the blistering spread of the *Rickettsia* through its vector, the human louse *Pediculus humanus corporis*. Scores of slaves perished because of the ship's disease, many of them even before reaching the shores of the New World. The terrifying symptoms brought on by the louse-borne typhus, the high fevers and unmistakable rash, signaled the fate of scores of slaves who were thrown overboard in a desperate measure to save the cargo.

Cholera also deeply concerned slave traders and owners in the Americas. The unsanitary conditions in both rural and urban slave quarters in North and South America facilitated the spread of cholera's *Vibrio* bacteria. As in the rest of the world, the **pandemics** that raged in the New World during the nineteenth century were not ameliorated until 1853, when **John Snow** associated cholera dissemination with contaminated water sources. The bacterium would remain undiscovered until late in the century. Thus, during the first half of the century, measures that had proven to be at least partially effective against diseases such as smallpox or yellow fever were fruitlessly implemented when cholera struck. Contemporary conceptions of the disease's etiology and racial associations tinged the reports of the cholera epidemics in the Americas. As cholera was thought to be associated with filth, moral degeneracy, and degraded conditions, Euro-Americans and Europeans categorized it as a "black" disease. Though African slaves and even freed slaves, because of their diminished living conditions, were more prone to come in contact with *Vibrio cholerae*, the disease was very democratic, sparing no segment of society. Nineteenth-century reports attributed higher cholera rates among African Americans to slaves' dietary preferences and to inferior moral conditions. However, it was slaves' living conditions that really put them in harm's way. On the plantations of the Americas, most slaves lived in crowed quarters with minimal sanitary facilities, and when living in urban settlements, slaves and freed blacks were confined to the most impoverished neighborhoods. This, added to slaves' chronic malnourishment and strenuous working conditions, made them an easy prey for the cholera germs.

The **"pest houses"** that had been created for pox quarantine were now used to isolate slaves who were stricken by the disease. Cholera prompted town councils to establish public health boards and appropriate money for the treatment of the destitute, including slaves. Owners of slaves closed factories and plantations and urged "their" blacks to stay in quarters while paying especially good attention to cleanliness and Christian moral standards of living. In the end, society's preoccupation with the unfathomable characteristics of cholera's contagion, the puzzlement it caused by affecting black and white, moral and immoral, all the same, helped to elevate the standards of living of slaves in British and Spanish colonies. *See also* Cholera: First through Third Pandemics, 1816–1861; Colonialism and Epidemic Disease; Insects, Other Arthropods, and Epidemic Disease; Latin America, Colonial: Demographic Effects of Imported Diseases; Malaria in the Americas; Poverty, Wealth, and Epidemic

Disease; Race, Ethnicity, and Epidemic Disease; Smallpox in Canada and the United States since 1783; Smallpox in Colonial Latin America; Smallpox in Colonial North America; Yellow Fever in Colonial Latin America and Caribbean; Yellow Fever in North America to 1810; Yellow Fever in the American South, 1810–1905.

Further Reading

Alchón, Suzanne A. *A Pest in the Land: New World Epidemics in a Global Perspective*. Albuquerque: University of New Mexico Press, 2003.

Bewell, Alan. *Medicine and the West Indian Slave Trade*. London: Pickering & Chatto, 1999.

Cook, David Noble. *Born to Die: Disease and New World Conquest 1492–1650*. New York: Cambridge University Press, 1998.

Curtin, Philip D. "Epidemiology and the Slave Trade." *Political Science Quarterly* 83 (1968): 190–216.

———. *Migration and Mortality in Africa and the Atlantic World, 1700–1900*. Burlington, VT: Ashgate/Variorum, 2001.

Fett, Sharla M. *Working Cures: Healing, Health, and Power on Southern Slave Plantations*. Chapel Hill: University of North Carolina Press, 2002.

Gehlbach, Stephen H. *American Plagues: Lessons from Our Battles with Disease*. New York: McGraw-Hill, 2005.

Kiple, Kenneth F., and Stephen V. Beck. *Biological Consequences of the European Expansion, 1450–1800*. Brookfield, VT: Ashgate/Variorum, 1997.

Watts, Sheldon J. *Epidemics and History: Disease, Power, and Imperialism*. New Haven: Yale University Press, 1997.

PABLO F. GOMEZ

SLAVES.   *See* Slavery and Epidemic Disease.

SLEEPING SICKNESS.   The term African sleeping sickness comprises two fairly distinct clinical and epidemiologic disorders caused by **protozoa** of the genus *Trypanosoma* and spread by the tsetse fly. The two causative organisms, *T. brucei gambiense* and *T. brucei rhodesiense*, are considered subspecies of the *T. brucei* complex. A third member of the complex, *T. brucei brucei*, only infects **animals**. *Gambiense* disease occurs in central and West Africa, whereas *rhodesiense* disease is found in eastern and southern Africa, all within about 15 degrees north and south of the Equator.

History.   African sleeping sickness is an old disease. The first written notation is by the fourteenth-century Arab writer Al-Qualquashaudi, who commented on "a sleeping sickness" common around the kingdom of Mali, but it was not until the eighteenth century that Europeans took notice. In 1742 John Atkins, a British naval **surgeon**, first described its presence on the coast of Guinea. In 1803 Thomas Winterbottom (1765–1854), working in the newly organized colony for freed slaves in Sierra Leone, described the same disorder and noted the presence of enlarged cervical (neck) lymph nodes, later called "Winterbottom's sign." In the last quarter of the nineteenth century, when the European rush to colonize vast areas of Africa prompted large population shifts and severe economic disruption, infected Africans and colonists introduced many new cases of sleeping sickness into virgin tsetse fly areas, creating epidemic conditions. Mortality estimates in central Africa in the years 1895–1905 run as high as 500,000. In 1901 a huge epidemic of sleeping sickness, possibly of the *rhodesiense* type, broke out on the north shore of Lake Victoria and eventually took about 200,000 lives. During this outbreak, Aldo Castellani (1874–1971), a bacteriologist and member of a team sent by the London School of Tropical Medicine to investigate, first found trypanosomes in the spinal fluid of victims. Further work, encouraged by the arrival in Uganda of David Bruce (1855–1931), a British doctor who had discovered trypanosomes as the cause of an African cattle disease called "nagana," clarified their importance. Trypanosomes were also found in cases in West and Central Africa.

By 1909 the full cycle of the parasite in Glossina flies was elucidated. In subsequent decades the disease distribution was more clearly mapped, and its two forms established. Control measures were instituted, and the epidemics subsided, though later relaxation of surveillance resulted in subsequent outbreaks. Early treatment with atoxyl, an arsenic derivative important also in the history of syphilis treatment, was moderately effective but could cause blindness. Bayer 205 (Germanin) and tryparsamide followed, and Melarsoprol, currently in use today, was developed in the 1940s. Eflornithine, originally developed as a possible anti-cancer drug, became available in the 1980s for late stage *gambiense* disease.

Organism and Vector.   Glossina (tsetse) flies live in vegetation around rivers and lakes and do not venture far away, which accounts for the localized nature of disease distribution. The protozoa enter the digestive tract of the fly when the fly bites and sucks the blood of an infected victim. The protozoa multiply in the fly's midgut and migrate to the salivary glands where they develop to an infective stage 18 to 35 days after initial feeding. New bites introduce the organisms into new hosts, where they circulate as motile forms characterized by a flagellum and undulating membrane, which propel them. They also migrate to lymph nodes and eventually to the central nervous system (CNS).

Parasites often cause harm over a period of time because they have mechanisms to survive for a long time in their "host." For survival in the host's body, the trypanosome's outer membrane is coated with a layer of "variant surface protein" (VSP) that protects it from the host's immune system. The human host manufactures antibodies to attack the protein, only to find that the parasite can produce new variants of this protein.

Pathology and Clinical Disease.   Two different human organ systems are particularly affected by in sleeping sickness. Early in the disease, the victim's lymph nodes and spleen enlarge as a result of inflammation induced by the parasite. All three layers of the heart suffer an inflammatory reaction, including the conduction system that governs the heart's contractions. Inflammatory changes in the central nervous system involve the covering layers of the brain and around blood vessels, leading to clots, small hemorrhages, and localized areas of inflammation.

Different strains of the organism lead to different disease patterns. *T. b. gambiense* infection follows a chronic course. For months to years victims have no symptoms, even though trypanosomes may be found in blood or lymph nodes. At some point nonspecific symptoms appear, consisting of mild fever, headaches, and fatigue, which come and go. During this phase the lymph nodes begin to enlarge, especially in the neck (referred to as Winterbottom's sign). Only years after onset, the symptoms of **encephalitis**—decreased thinking ability, sleepiness, tremor, and sometimes psychosis—gradually appear. Eventually severe somnolence prevails, the victim becomes wasted from poor nutrition, and he or she often succumbs to pneumonia.

T. b. rhodesiense infection, however, is a more acute disease, lasting weeks to months. Initially a dark red, painful swelling (chancre) around the tsetse fly bite can appear and

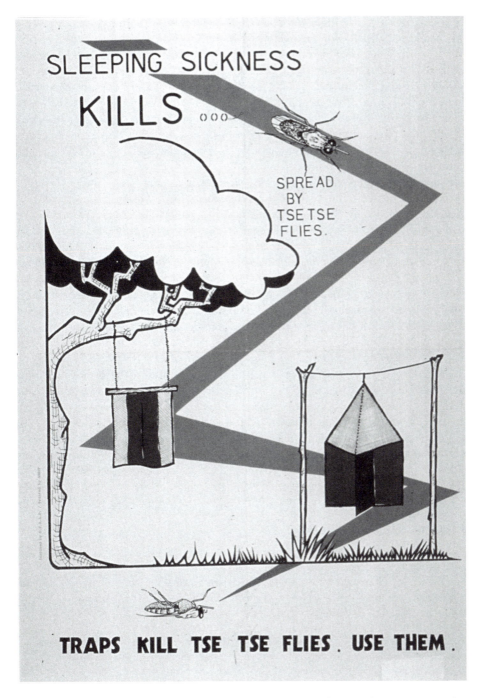

Poster distributed by the African Medical and Research Foundation in Nairobi, Kenya displaying that the use of traps kills tsetse flies that spread sleeping sickness. Courtesy of the National Library of Medicine.

last two to three weeks. With or without a chancre, fever begins within one to three weeks of the bite. Lymph nodes may enlarge. Invasion of the CNS follows fairly shortly, characterized by headache, then signs of encephalitis (as noted above) which progress more rapidly to death. An irregular, faintly pink rash may be seen in lighter skinned persons.

Diagnosis and Treatment.   Today the diagnosis of sleeping sickness is made with a combination of clinical and laboratory findings. Some factors—geographic location, the chancre and rash (if visible), and enlarged lymph nodes—remain important features in suspecting sleeping sickness, but specific diagnosis rests on demonstrating the presence of the parasite. Treatment of trypanosomiasis is still difficult because we do not have simple, nontoxic medicines that kill the parasites.

Epidemiology and Control.   Sleeping sickness is acquired only where tsetse flies live and is therefore what epidemiologists term a "focal disease." Larger outbreaks occur when parasite-infested individuals move into uninfected tsetse fly areas and/or when control efforts are neglected. The two types of sleeping sickness do not overlap, and Uganda is the only country where both are found (in different foci). Animals constitute the major reservoir of *rhodesiense*, whereas humans (and to some extent pigs) are reservoirs of *gambiense*. Control efforts have utilized a combination of finding and treating cases, fly trapping, clearing of fly breeding areas, and animal destruction. Today most programs emphasize case finding and treatment, coupled with varying degrees of fly control. Because this disease is linked to specific vectors, controlling the flies during outbreaks helped to eliminate the disease from the Gambia, Senegal, Ghana, Sierra Leone, and Guinea-Bissau. Because of political unrest and lapse of control programs there was resurgence in central African states in the 1990s, peaking at over 37,000 reported cases in 1998 (estimated to be a fraction of the total). More recently, as a result of better control measures, the outbreaks have been subsiding rapidly. Vaccine development is unlikely because of the parasite's ability to alter its VSP. Development of cheaper, safer drugs should put even more emphasis on case finding and treatment. *See also* Colonialism and Epidemic Disease; Environment, Ecology, and Epidemic Disease; Insects, Other Arthropods, and Epidemic Disease; Pesticides; Urbanization and Epidemic Disease.

Further Reading

Centers of Disease Control and Prevention. *African Trypanosomiasis.* http://www.cdc.gov/ncidod/dpd/parasites/trypanosomiasis/default.htm

Fèvre, E. M., et al. "Reanalyzing the 1900–1920 Sleeping Sickness Epidemic in Uganda." *Emerging Infectious Disease* 10 (2004): http:www.cdc.gov/ncidod/EID/vol10no4/02-0626.htm.

Ford, John. *The Role of Trypanosomiasis in African Ecology: A Study of the Tsetse Fly Problem.* New York: Oxford University Press, 1971.

Ford, Lea Berrang. "Civil Conflict and Sleeping Sickness in Africa in General and Uganda in Particular." *Conflict and Health* (2007): http://www.conflictandhealth.com/content/1/1/6

Hide G. "History of Sleeping Sickness in East Africa." *Clinical Microbiology Reviews* 12 (1999): 112–125.

Lyons, Maryinez. *The Colonial Disease: A Social History of Sleeping Sickness in Northern Zaire, 1900–1940.* New York: Cambridge University Press, 1992.

McKelvey, John J. *Man against Tsetse: Struggle for Africa.* Ithaca: Cornell University Press, 1973.

Musere, Jonathan. *African Sleeping Sickness: Political Ecology, Colonialism and Control in Uganda.* New York: Edwin Mellen, 1990.

Perleth, Matthias. *Historical Aspects of American Trypanosomiasis (Chagas' Disease)*. Frankfurt-am-Main: Peter Lang, 1997.

World Health Organization. *African Trypanosomiasis (Sleeping Sickness)*. http://www.who.int/mediacentre/factsheets/fs259/en/

J. Gordon Frierson

SMALLPOX.   Smallpox is the only infectious disease that has been eradicated as a human infection by medical intervention. Smallpox was a disease characterized by fever and eruptive rash caused by infection with the *variola* **virus**, principally by *Variola major*, its most virulent form. *Variola* is a member of the poxvirus family and is a relatively large, brick-shaped, envelope-coated DNA virus. *Variola* has no other host than human beings, the characteristic that made smallpox a candidate disease to be eliminated from the human population. It was primarily transmitted to a new host via inhalation of droplets from an infected person at close range, although it was also possible to transmit the disease through contact with infected clothing or bedding.

After an incubation period of about 12 days, the onset of smallpox was abrupt and debilitating, marked by a high fever, headache, muscle and back pains, and occasionally vomiting and convulsions. Two to five days after onset, the characteristic rash erupted, and in a few more days, pustules formed. In uncomplicated cases, just over a week after the first eruptions, the pustules began drying and forming scabs. By the third or fourth week after onset of the disease, the scabs fell off, and the victim was well again with lifetime **immunity** to the virus.

Smallpox caused by *Variola major* had a mortality rate of 25 to 30 percent. Fatal cases progressed more rapidly and dramatically. Blood poisoning could lead to massive hemorrhaging into the skin and internal organs followed by rapid death. In other cases, the pustules, which appeared more densely on the face, the palms of the hands, and the soles of the feet than on the trunk, became confluent and signaled a lethal infection. The pustules often left a scarred or "pocked" face that marked the victim for the rest of his or her life. Smallpox could also cause blindness and male infertility.

In the late nineteenth century, a milder form of smallpox first appeared in southern Africa, later spreading to Brazil, North America, and parts of Europe. Caused by a less virulent strain of *Variola* known as *Variola minor*, its mortality rate was 1 percent or lower.

History.   There are accounts of many ancient **epidemics** that might have been caused by smallpox, but none described the symptoms sufficiently to permit accurate diagnosis in hindsight. The first medical account comes from **Rhazes**, a ninth-century physician in Baghdad, who differentiated between smallpox and **measles** and described smallpox as a common, nonlethal disease of **children** in southwest Asia. Not until the sixteenth and seventeenth centuries in Europe did it emerge as a feared epidemic disease. There is debate among scholars as to whether *Variola major* mutated into a more virulent form at that time or whether previous diagnoses of smallpox were wrong.

Beginning in the sixteenth century, however, smallpox played a deadly role in the efforts of European nations to colonize other areas of the world. Native American tribes with no immunity were decimated as Spanish, Portuguese, French, and English explorers marched across North, Central, and South America. In 1630 native Siberians were decimated when Russian colonists triggered the first smallpox epidemic in that region. In 1713 the Dutch brought the disease to South Africa and decimated the native Khoikhoi, and in 1789 Australian aborigines were felled by smallpox after English settlers landed at Sydney.

Smallpox was also known in Asian cultures. By the thirteenth century, the Chinese practiced *variolation*—the **inoculation** of a healthy person with smallpox from a diseased person with the desire to cause a mild form of the disease, induce immunity, and prevent a possibly lethal case. Smallpox remained endemic in the cities of China and, like the Great Wall itself, served as a barrier against Mongols and others who might try to invade. Indeed, after conquering the western Mongols, the Chinese excused them from making obeisance to the Emperor in Beijing, accepting their tributes at sites north of the Great Wall in order to protect them from the disease.

It is not known exactly when or where variolation was developed, but by the early eighteenth century, it was being practiced by wealthy Europeans such as Lady Mary Wortley Montagu (1689–1762) and in colonial North America by the Massachusetts minister **Cotton Mather**. The practice was not embraced widely because there always remained the danger that an inoculated person could infect others and set off an epidemic.

Near the end of the eighteenth century, physician **Edward Jenner** noticed that variolation failed to produce symptoms in people who had previously contracted cowpox, and that milkmaids and others who contracted cowpox did not contract smallpox during epidemic outbreaks. Jenner conducted a trial of a procedure he termed "**vaccination**," from the Latin word *vacca*, "cow." He inoculated individuals with cowpox matter and later conducted traditional variolation. The variolation failed to produce any signs of illness in those vaccinated.

In 1798 Jenner published his results, and by 1801 more than 100,000 people in England had been vaccinated. Millions across Europe were vaccinated by 1815. In 1840 an act of Parliament made variolation illegal in England and empowered local officials to vaccinate the poor from public funds. Between 1853 and 1873, vaccination in England became compulsory, with civil fines levied for failure to comply. Prussia likewise pursued compulsory vaccination, and the result for both England and Prussia was the near **eradication** of the disease by 1900.

Resistance to compulsory vaccination grew in the last quarter of the nineteenth century. Anti-vaccinationists argued that healthy children should not be forcibly injected with an agent that caused cowpox. The smallpox vaccine, known officially as "calf lymph" and produced commercially by scraping infected matter from cowpox pustules from infected calves, was subject to contamination at many points in production. By 1895, the governments of France, Germany, Italy, and Russia had enacted laws requiring vaccines and antitoxins, known collectively as *biologics* or *biologic products* because they were injected into the human body, to be licensed by government laboratories. In the United States, however, no oversight was enforced until 1902, following the deaths of 13 children in one city who received **diphtheria** antitoxin contaminated with tetanus spores. Initially, the law required proof that the vaccine was not contaminated during production. In 1934 a further regulation was issued in the United States requiring proof that commercially produced vaccines were effective.

Edward Jenner realized that his cowpox vaccine had the potential to annihilate smallpox, even if it did not happen quickly. Smallpox vaccination eliminated the disease from Britain by 1940, from the United States by 1950, and from China by 1965. In 1972 the United States ended the routine use of smallpox vaccine. Ten years later, the vaccine was no longer even available to civilians in the United States, and in 1990 the U.S. Department of Defense discontinued vaccinating military recruits.

Since 1979 samples of *Variola major* have been maintained in freezers at the U.S. Centers for Disease Control in Atlanta, Georgia, and in the Moscow Research Institute for

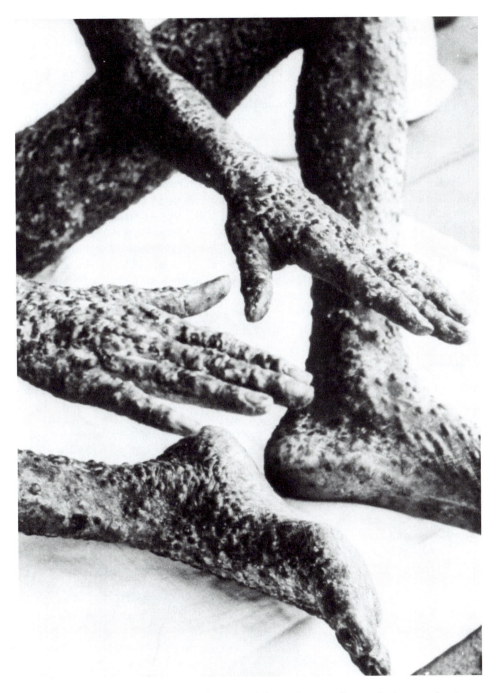

The heavily pockmarked hands, legs, and feet of a smallpox victim on the Ivory Coast. WHO photo. Courtesy of the National Library of Medicine.

Viral Preparation's High Containment Laboratories. The genome of the virus has been sequenced, and numerous discussions have occurred about whether the frozen samples should be destroyed, lest they accidentally be released into a nonimmune population. After the terrorist attacks in the United States of September 11, 2001, and the anthrax attacks shortly thereafter, there was considerable fear that smallpox virus had been obtained and stored illegally and thus might be used as a **bioterror** agent. The Public Health Security and Bioterrorism Preparedness and Response Act of 2002 included provisions for supporting smallpox vaccine development. Vaccinations for first responders began in January 2003, but within months, concerns arose about vaccine safety after reports that some recipients had suffered fatal heart attacks. Congress enacted a vaccine compensation plan for those injured, but by June 2003, a Federal Advisory Committee on Immunization Practices recommended that the program be ended. Since that time, the United States and the **World Health Organization** have moved to establish stockpiles of smallpox vaccine in the event that *Variola major* is released as a bioterror agent. *See also* Animal Diseases (Zoonoses) and Epidemic Disease; Biological Warfare; Colonialism and Epidemic Disease; Diagnosis of Historical Diseases; Public Health Agencies, U.S. Federal; Smallpox Eradication; Smallpox in Canada and the United States since 1783; Smallpox in Colonial Latin America; Smallpox in Colonial North America; Smallpox in European Non-American Colonies; Smallpox in Premodern Europe; Smallpox in the Ancient World.

Further Reading

Baciu, Alina, Andrea Pernack Anason, Kathleen Stratton, and Brian Strom, eds. *The Smallpox Vaccination Program: Public Health in an Age of Terrorism*. Washington, DC: National Academies Press, 2005.

Centers for Disease Control and Prevention. *Smallpox*. http://emergency.cdc.gov/agent/smallpox/

Crosby, Alfred W. *Ecological Imperialism: The Biological Expansion of Europe, 900–1900*. New York: Cambridge University Press, 1986.

History's Mysteries—Smallpox [film]. History Channel, 2006.

Hopkins, Donald R. *The Greatest Killer: Smallpox in History*. Chicago: University of Chicago Press, 2002.

Mayo Clinic. *Smallpox*. http://www.mayoclinic.com/health/smallpox/DS00424

National Museum of Health and Medicine. http://nmhm.washingtondc.museum/ collections/archives/ agalleries/smallpox/smallpox.html

World Health Organization. *Smallpox*. http://www.who.int/csr/disease/smallpox/en/

VICTORIA A. HARDEN

SMALLPOX AND THE AMERICAN REVOLUTION. By 1775 **smallpox** had long been endemic in England, but colonials were rarely immunized against it by natural exposure as children. Adults could be inoculated and suffer a weak but **immunity**-conferring case, but this required a four-week **quarantine** while the patient was contagious. Many of Continental Army General George Washington's (1732–1799) rural recruits had been isolated from the colonial urban outbreaks, and natural infection by the **virus** would send these men reeling, exacting a mortality rate of around 14 percent.

In the summer of 1775, at the outset of the **war**, Washington acted very cautiously as smallpox ravaged Boston, the British-held city around which his army was positioned. Knowing firsthand what damage smallpox could inflict, Washington did all he could to isolate his army from the disease that wracked the civilian population. "Camp followers" who cooked and did laundry underwent close medical scrutiny and surveillance. Access to American camps was restricted, and refugees from Boston were checked closely for signs of disease: he knew that the British might use infected citizens as a type of biological weapon. Above all, he refused to assault the city, a decision that prolonged the siege to nine months and allowed the redeployment of the British Army rather than its defeat or surrender. British troops had often been exposed to smallpox as children, and the besieged commanders had no issue with inoculating those who had not.

When British Commander General William Howe (1729–1814) finally evacuated Boston on March 17, 1776, Washington remained convinced that he had left the city poisoned with smallpox. Only troops who had been immunized were allowed to take the heights directly overlooking the city, and as late as July, only immunized or immune troops could enter liberated Boston. At first reticent to hobble his army with recuperating inoculation patients, Washington rapidly embraced the practice, and only 1 in 500 American troops died of the virus.

While Washington was settled in around Boston, the American Northern Army led by General Richard Montgomery (1736–1775) headed north to seize Montreal and Quebec and bring Canada into the war on America's side. Had this ploy succeeded, Canadian provinces might have emerged as U.S. states. As with Boston, Quebec was suffering an outbreak of smallpox, and American leaders suspected spies of spreading the disease to the vulnerable American siege lines around the city. When the American assault took place on the night of December 30–31, 1775, 300 of the 1,100 colonials were laid up sick. The attack failed, and Montgomery was killed. American General Benedict Arnold (1741–1801) continued the siege, but smallpox and other diseases ravaged his shrinking army. Men succeeded in

---

GEORGE WASHINGTON'S ORDER TO INOCULATE RECRUITS FOR SMALLPOX (1777)

To Doctor William Shippen, Junior.

Head Quarters, Morristown, January 6, 1777.

Dear Sir: Finding the small pox to be spreading much and fearing that no precaution can prevent it from running thro' the whole of our Army, I have determined that the Troops shall be inoculated. This Expedient may be attended with some inconveniences and some disadvantages, but yet I trust, in its consequences will have the most happy effects.

Necessity not only authorizes but seems to require the measure, for should the disorder infect the Army, in the natural way, and rage with its usual Virulence, we should have more to dread from it, than the Sword of the Enemy. Under these Circumstances, I have directed Doctr. Bond [Dr. Nathaniel Bond], to prepare immediately for inoculating this Quarter, keeping the matter as secret as possible, and request, that you will without delay inoculate all the Continental Troops that are in Philadelphia and those that shall come in, as fast as they arrive. You will spare no pains to carry them thro' the disorder with the utmost expedition, and to have them cleansed from the infection when recovered, that they may proceed to Camp, with as little injury as possible, to the Country thro' which they pass. If the business is immediately begun and favored with common success, I would fain hope they will soon be fit for duty, and that in a short space of time we shall have an Army not subject to this, the greatest of all calamities that can befall it, when taken in the natural way.

[Signed by Washington.]

From *The Writings of George Washington*, edited by John C. Fitzpatrick (Washington: U.S. Government Printing Office, 1931–1944) 6: 473–74.

inoculating themselves but failed to isolate themselves while infectious, spreading the disease to their comrades. Bostonian rebel John Adams (1735–1826) was prompted to write, "This pestilence completed our destruction." American General John Thomas (1724–1776) took command in early May with some 1,900 men, about half of whom were sick at any given time; he, too, took ill and died after a month. Fully 30 percent of the American Northern Army died of disease, and the Americans were in full retreat from Canada by late June 1776.

In July 1781, British General Alexander Leslie in Portsmouth, Virginia, wrote to his colleague General Charles Cornwallis (1738–1805) in Yorktown: "Above 700 Negroes are come down the River in the Small Pox—it will ruin our market, which was bad enough before. I shall distribute them about the Rebell Plantations." From the time of Benjamin Franklin (1706–1790) to the present colonial historians have believed this to mean that Leslie was going to use infected slaves to spread the pox. Recently, however, historian Philip Ranlet viewed this in a different light, interpreting Leslie to mean that escaped slaves who had caught the pox in Portsmouth would be returned to their owners, who presumably would have them isolated for recuperation. The harried British had no interest in weakened laborers and few supplies to spare for their care. When Leslie's troops relocated to Yorktown, they left the ailing African Americans behind. Even so, some who accompanied Leslie were carriers and spread the disease further. Cornwallis expelled hundreds of sickened blacks as his own troops suffered from diseases other than smallpox, for which they had been inoculated. *See also* Colonialism and Epidemic Disease; Slavery and Epidemic Disease; Smallpox in Colonial North America; War, the Military, and Epidemic Disease.

Further Reading

Becker, Ann M. "Smallpox in Washington's Army: Strategic Implications of the Disease during the American Revolutionary War." *The Journal of Military History* 68 (2004): 381–430.

Cash, P. "The Canadian Military Campaign of 1775–76: Medical Problems and Effects of Disease." *Journal of the American Medical Association* 236 (1976): 52–56.

Elizabeth A. Fenn. *Pox Americana: The Great Smallpox Epidemic of 1775–82.* New York: Hill & Wang, 2003.

Ranlet, Philip. "The British, Slaves, and Smallpox in Revolutionary Virginia." *The Journal of Negro History* 84 (1999): 217–226.

JOSEPH P. BYRNE

SMALLPOX ERADICATION.   **Smallpox** is thus far the only infectious disease to have been eliminated by human activity from nature. Following an exhaustive study of documentation gathered from several countries where smallpox had been endemic, a Global Commission composed of international experts certified the disease eradicated in December 1979, after they felt confident enough to announce that there had been no cases in the world for two years. This momentous announcement, which many observers had considered impossible, was ratified by the 33rd World Health Assembly gathered in the **World Health Organization's** headquarters in Geneva, Switzerland, in 1980.

It is generally accepted that the successful **eradication** of smallpox across the world was a result of an unprecedented level of international cooperation—apart from the World Health Organization (WHO), assistance was also provided by other United Nations' agencies like UNICEF; in addition, countries like the United States and the former Soviet Union provided financial and infrastructural aid on a global scale. Although the WHO played an important role as a manager of resources, directing personnel, vaccine, and money to national and local contexts where this assistance was required, a range of national public health and funding agencies made significant contributions as well. Although workers associated with a range of organizations were regularly posted to the WHO's headquarters or regional offices, several personnel continued to represent formally—and serve—the governments of the countries where systematic smallpox eradication efforts were initiated. All these efforts led to the creation of a series of carefully planned national smallpox eradication programs involving teams composed of international staff and local workers; the dedicated efforts of all these personnel, who came from a range of educational and social backgrounds, over the course of a period of more than a decade made the dream of smallpox eradication a reality.

The calls for the global eradication of smallpox were made relatively early within the WHO. During World Health Assembly meetings held as early as the late 1950s, officials representing the USSR started arguing that such a world-

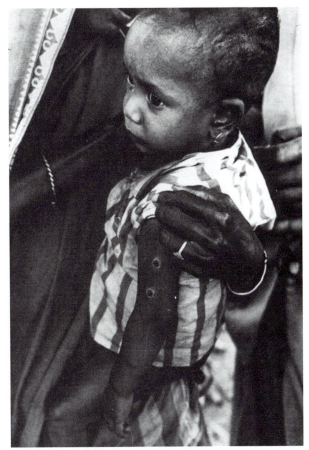

Positive reactions from two vaccinations leave visible scars on the arm of a little boy in Bangladesh. WHO photo. Courtesy of the National Library of Medicine.

wide campaign was feasible. These calls were not ignored, and some senior officials in the WHO headquarters embarked on a relatively small feasibility study, involving discussions with officials associated with the regional offices and specific national governments. These engagements carried on right through the first half of the 1960s and revealed deep rifts in viewpoint, both within and outside WHO structures, about important elements of the proposed project. These included the shape and the timing of the planned smallpox eradication program, its funding modalities, and, not least, questions of management and leadership. This resulted in weak initial efforts in countries such as India. Although the country's federal authorities agreed to a series of proposals made by the WHO, the implementation of policies was whimsical. As a result, the goal of mass immunization against smallpox, which was generally seen in the early 1960s as the means of achieving eradication, was not met.

These trends resulted in a reexamination of the goals and the structures of the planned global smallpox eradication program. Relevant administrative structures within the

WHO were revamped from the mid-1960s onward, leading to a series of personnel changes that would turn out to be crucial to the successful completion of the campaign. **Donald A. Henderson**, who was at that time associated with the U.S. **Centers for Disease Control** (CDC), was posted to the WHO offices in Geneva and asked to set up a Unit to plan and manage a world program for the smallpox eradication. This went hand in hand with the reform of administrative structures in the WHO regional offices, whose personnel were encouraged to collaborate closely with Henderson and his team. These initiatives were accompanied by negotiations with funding agencies, vaccine donors, and national governments; efforts were consistently maintained to raise money and stocks of reliable smallpox vaccine, which were then promised by the WHO to different national governments in return for their cooperation. National governments and local donor agencies did, of course, also make crucial donations, in the form of vaccine and finance, at important junctures of the campaign. The result was the creation of a reenergized global smallpox eradication program from 1966 onward, straddling Latin America, Africa, and Asia.

Numerous technological and strategic adaptations helped move the eradication program forward. The availability of large stocks of heat-stable, freeze-dried smallpox vaccine proved an enormous boon. These prophylactics were donated in huge quantities by the USSR (to the WHO or to individual countries) and were also purchased from private companies like Connaught (Canada) and Wyeth (United States) for use across the globe; it is, of course, important to note that many of the countries with endemic smallpox also developed the capacity of produce freeze-dried vaccines, with assistance from countries like Denmark, the USSR, the United States, and the United Kingdom, and these stocks were also used to good effect in the program. Another major technological adaptation was the bifurcated needle, which allowed for two extremely important developments: the introduction of less painful immunization methods and the ability to make available stocks of vaccine last much longer. Yet another adaptation, which is generally considered to be crucial to the achievement of smallpox eradication, is the strategy of "surveillance-containment." Accepting the principle that mass immunization was unnecessary after about 70 to 80 percent vaccinal coverage had been achieved, the strategy was based on the understanding that the main objectives were to find smallpox cases, isolate them, and then vaccinate all contacts. When this was achieved, it was argued and later proven, the chain of smallpox transmission could be broken and the disease eradicated. This strategy was utilized and refined in several contexts by CDC teams working in western Africa, and also by WHO-funded teams of national and international workers in the Indian state of Madras in the 1960s. In practice, surveillance-containment was adapted to the needs of myriad localities by teams of workers, after significant debates with the supporters of mass immunization (who were never completely silenced), in response to the needs and feelings of local collaborators and the civilian populations being targeted. Indeed, it was not unknown for teams of international workers to carry out mass vaccinations in the villages of South Asia in the 1970s; this was often in response to concerted civilian demand for immunization against smallpox, but there were also instances in which entire villages were surrounded and forcibly vaccinated.

These multifaceted efforts paid rich dividends. In countries like Brazil, Pakistan, India, Bangladesh, Ethiopia, and Somalia, smallpox had been endemic, had caused loss of life, and had also been the source of exportations of the disease to the Americas and Europe. Now, one after the other at different points in the 1970s, each was declared free of the errant *variola* virus. *See also* Measles, Efforts to Eradicate.

Further Reading

Bazin, Hervé. *The Eradication of Small Pox: Edward Jenner and the First and Only Eradication of a Human Infectious Disease.* New York: Academic Press, 2000.

Bhattacharya, Sanjoy. *Expunging Variola: The Control and Eradication of Smallpox in India, 1947–77.* New Delhi: Orient Longman, 2006.

Fenner F., D. A. Henderson, I. A. Arita, Z. Jezek, and I. D. Ladnyi. *Smallpox and Its Eradication.* Geneva: WHO, 1988.

Greenough P. "Intimidation, Coercion and Resistance in the Final Stages of the South Asian Smallpox Eradication Campaign, 1973–75." *Social Science and Medicine* 41 (1995): 633–645.

Koplow, David A. *Smallpox: The Fight to Eradicate a Global Scourge.* Berkeley: University of California Press, 2004.

Naraindas, H. "Crisis, Charisma and Triage: Extirpating the Pox." *Indian Economic and Social History Review* 40 (2003): 425–458.

SANJOY BHATTACHARYA

SMALLPOX IN CANADA AND THE UNITED STATES SINCE 1783. By 1783 **smallpox** already had a long history in British North America, but within the next two decades there would evolve a significant medical discovery that could successfully combat the disease. As a result of the work of **Edward Jenner** in England, a far safer and more reliable preventative was developed, one that injected harmless cowpox **virus** into a patient that would provide immunity from smallpox. Because of its source it became known as "vaccine," and the process "**vaccination**." After Jenner published his findings, in 1798 the treatment came to North America.

Jenner sent a copy of his report and some of the vaccine to a **physician** friend, the Rev. John Clinch (1749–1819) in Trinity, Newfoundland. He became the first person in North America to attempt vaccination, eventually performing the procedure on several hundred people, including his own child. The technique was lost in Trinity for a few years, but it was picked up in Massachusetts, where another of Jenner's correspondents, a respected doctor named Benjamin Waterhouse (1754–1846), received both Jenner's findings and a vaccine sample. In 1800 Waterhouse performed the first vaccination in the United States on his six-year-old son. He also wrote about and promoted Jenner's system in the United States, and one of his contacts was President Thomas Jefferson (1743–1826), who subsequently began a personal correspondence with Jenner. Jefferson was completely won over to vaccination and became one of its strongest advocates.

Urban Epidemics of the Nineteenth Century. A number of American and Canadian cities experienced smallpox epidemics in the first half of the nineteenth century, including Philadelphia, Quebec City, Boston, and Baltimore. New York City suffered through nine outbreaks, the worst occurring in 1853–1854, that killed nearly a thousand people. Native Americans continued to die in large numbers from the disease, especially those in the Great Plains and on the west coast. There were two major pandemics among the native populations, the first in 1801 and the second in 1836–1840. The areas hit also included Mexican California, Russian Alaska, and British Columbia. Overall, an estimated 300,000 native people died.

Smallpox was a problem during the American Civil **War**, particularly in the South, which recruited unvaccinated soldiers and which possessed unreliable vaccine stocks. It did not help that new supplies of vaccine were stopped from entering the Confederacy because of the Union blockade of its coastline. By the end of the war, the situation had become so desperate that variolation—purposeful infection with the variola virus—rather than vaccination had to be used, with very poor results. Smallpox spread to the North carried by freed slaves and by Confederate prisoners of war who were kept in transit camps and prisons in a number of northern states. One of the victims in the North was Abraham Lincoln (1809–1865) who fell ill while returning to Washington after having delivered the Gettysburg Address in November of 1863. Although it proved to be a mild case of the disease, he did develop a characteristic rash within two days and was unable to perform his duties for four weeks. Lincoln, of course, survived, but his black valet caught the disease and died. After the war, smallpox was carried all over the nation with returning soldiers and by a substantial movement of people, both black and white, that occurred in the war's wake.

In the latter nineteenth century, smallpox outbreaks increased in many areas of North America with the growing number of immigrants, particularly those from Europe. The disease could also be spread more expeditiously by the growing network of railroads that crisscrossed the continent. These factors played a role in the epidemics of the early 1870s that seemed to originate from the turmoil of the Franco-Prussian War of 1870–1871 and subsequent population movements spawned by it. Nearly 2,000 died of smallpox in Philadelphia in 1871, and 1,500 in Baltimore in 1872 and 1873. Other urban areas that suffered heavy losses included New Orleans (1872–1875) with 1,400 victims and New York City (1874–1875) with 1,700. Another wave of the disease occurred in 1881–1883 centering on the Midwest, the South, and New England, causing some health officials, especially in the last region, to enforce moribund vaccination regulations.

One reason for the relative failure of vaccination to stem smallpox outbreaks completely during the late nineteenth and early twentieth century was the continuing controversy surrounding the procedure. The growth and influence of anti-vaccination organizations, often led by medical men, had a negative impact on its universal use. There was a fear that vaccination could cause infections from other diseases, a phenomenon that occurred in a small number of cases. Linked to that was the age-old debate involving mandatory vaccination and its violation of **personal liberty** that could result in violent resistance. The problem tended to intensify with the swelling tide of immigrants coming into pre–World War I America and Canada. Many had not been vaccinated before and simply did not trust government encroachment into their lives.

Two famous smallpox outbreaks in the late nineteenth century brought this debate clearly and vividly into focus. Both Milwaukee in 1894–1895 and Montreal in 1885–1886 had to live through not only severe epidemics but also vigorous reaction to public health authorities who tried to combat the disease. In most American and Canadian cities, health officials had established a program of activities to deal with such a situation. They moved to stop the spread of smallpox by the use of mass vaccinations, the removal of victims to isolation hospitals, and the **quarantine** of infected families or businesses. Resistance to these policies first arose over whether the vaccinations were to be enforced by law. The isolation hospitals were unwanted in most neighborhoods, and victims saw them simply as horrible places where no one survived. Quarantines meant the limitation of freedom of movement, and for businesses, a loss of revenue. All these actions could lead to emotional resentment against the boards of health and police.

During the Montreal epidemic of 1885–1886 it was the French Canadian portion of the city's population that harbored doubts about vaccinations. The attempt by public health administrators to enforce necessary vaccinations to prevent the spread of disease was met in the French wards with rioting and armed violence against police. There was well-publicized resistance to the forced removal of victims to the isolation hospital, especially the separation of infected **children** from their parents. Eventually troops had to be called out to restore order and to enforce the vaccination of over 80,000 people. In the end, within a city of 168,000 residents, over 10,000 had been infected with smallpox, and 3,164 had died. It proved to be Montreal's (and Canada's) last major smallpox epidemic.

A similar dislike of vaccination and isolation hospitals caused a reaction during the smallpox epidemic in Milwaukee in 1894–1895. Again, ethnic divisions motivated events as immigrants from Germany and Poland were vociferous in opposing the health board's policies. Riots broke out, health officers were attacked, and a political battle ensued in city council, where representatives of the ethnic wards successfully challenged the city's health commissioner. In the end, the powers of the health board were cut back, and a victory of sorts for the anti-vaccinationists was won. It was an example of how ethnicity and politics could dominate a smallpox epidemic.

A New Strain of Smallpox.   Not all events involving smallpox at the end of the nineteenth century were so demoralizing. A genuine success story occurred in Puerto Rico soon after its capture and annexation by the United States at the conclusion of the Spanish-American War in 1898. A systematic vaccination drive was undertaken, and nearly 80 percent of the population was vaccinated. It meant that the island was one of the first areas of North America to eradicate smallpox from its society. Also, two years earlier, with little initial publicity, a major change emerged in the nature of the disease itself. A weaker strain of the virus, soon to be called *Variola minor*, found its way into mainland North America and would soon be far more prevalent than its virulent relative, *Variola major*. The increasing ubiquity and the uniform mildness of the new strain set the context for how smallpox epidemics would be dealt with into the twentieth century.

Variola minor was first reported in Pensacola, Florida, in 1896. Although it caused many of the signs of smallpox, it often did not cause serious illness. As a result, a person with *Variola minor* often continued to move around, not even knowing at first that he or she was carrying smallpox. Because of this, the strain spread very quickly across the United States and Canada. *Minor* could leave scars, but it was not nearly as disfiguring as *Variola major*. The new strain's mortality rate was approximately 1 percent, as opposed to the old strain's 15 to 30 percent. By the 1920s, *Variola minor* had become the most prevalent form of smallpox on the continent. From 1900 to 1939, the number of reported cases of *Variola minor* grew to 20 times that of *major*. Because of this, the numbers dying of smallpox declined sharply, from 20 percent in 1896 to 4 percent in 1900 to just 0.6 percent in 1906. These figures were reassuring, but they did not mean that the danger from smallpox was over.

The Twentieth Century.   Epidemics of *Variola major* did continue to break out. The worst occurred from 1901 to 1903 in a number of large cities including Philadelphia, Boston, and New York. In the last city, a significant number of victims lived in various ethnic wards, and in Boston the outbreak resulted in an important pathological study of those who had died of the disease. Overall, there were 16,000 cases of *Variola major* across America and Canada, with over 3,500 deaths. It was a shocking throwback to the outbreaks of the nineteenth century. In addition, *Variola major* was still active in Mexico, and from its base there, the strain was imported to the United States. From 1915 to 1929, there were 23 occurrences of *Variola major* in the United States, 14 of which had originated in Mexico. Also, it became clear that the two strains could appear at the same time in different regions of the continent.

The last great wave of epidemic smallpox in the United States and Canada took place during the 1920s. Hundreds of thousands of cases of *Variola minor* were reported, and in 1924–1925, 7,400 cases of *Variola major*, especially in cities such as Cleveland, Pittsburgh, and Detroit. The latter epidemic also spilled over the border into Windsor, Canada. During the twenties, a clear pattern for vaccinations became evident. In the face of a *V. Major* attack, the number of vaccinations increased dramatically; with a *Variola minor* outbreak, they increased very little.

In 1926 there were two well-publicized outbreaks of smallpox in the United States with an epidemic of *Variola minor* in Florida and one of *Variola major* in California. In that year, Florida was experiencing a significant decline from the land-boom era of the early twenties. One of the last things that promoters of the state wanted to hear was that a possible smallpox epidemic was afoot. Nonetheless, Florida eventually recorded 2,525 cases, more than any other state in the union during 1926. Still, the Florida epidemic was at least *Variola minor*; California was not so lucky. That state had the second largest number of smallpox cases with 2,432, and unfortunately it was the *Variola major* variety. Only six people had died in the Florida epidemic, but 231 died in California. Therefore, *Variola major* could still strike and still kill, but during and after the 1920s, *Variola minor* continued to dominate, and the number of outbreaks of both strains continued to decline.

In the post–World War II era, smallpox became much less of a threat. There were still outbreaks in Mexico, and on occasion even *Variola major* could be brought into the United States from there. For instance, this happened in 1947 when a businessman arriving from Mexico arrived in New York City carrying *Variola major*. In response, over 6 million residents of the city were vaccinated, and 12 people died. The last reported outbreaks of either strain in the United States or Canada was in 1949. In 1950 the Pan American Sanitary Organization moved to eliminate smallpox from all of the Americas. By the end of 1958, the disease had been eliminated in North America.

In 1980 the **World Health Organization** announced that following a long eradication process the world was now free of smallpox. Previously, in 1972, the United States and Canada had already ended the policy of smallpox vaccination, arguing that it was simply no longer necessary. Thus, after that year, for the first time since Jenner, North Americans would no longer need to procure their own immunity. However, if smallpox ever reappeared, the U.S. and Canadian populations would be nearly as vulnerable to the disease as the native people had been prior to the arrival of Europeans. It was this sobering fact, coupled with the fear of the use of bioweapons by terrorists, that raised concerns during the 1990s. Outside of the two official repositories of smallpox virus in the United States and Russia, were there any other samples that could have gotten into the wrong hands? After 9/11 these fears heightened considerably, beginning a move back to reactivating programs of ring, and even mass, vaccinations.

By 2006 the United States had produced and stockpiled enough smallpox vaccine to vaccinate every person in the country. Also instituted was a policy of vaccinating frontline personnel who would have to deal with an outbreak in an emergency situation. Incredibly, because of the difficult and dangerous milieu of the twenty-first century, the ancient, dreaded disease of smallpox has been placed back into the spotlight once again. *See also* Biological Warfare; Bioterrorism; Colonialism and Epidemic Disease; Public Health Agencies, U.S. Federal; Race, Ethnicity, and Epidemic Disease; Smallpox Eradication; Smallpox in Colonial North America; Trade, Travel, and Epidemic Disease.

Further Reading

Bliss, Michael. *Plague: A Story of Smallpox in Montreal*. New York: HarperCollins, 1991.

Fenn, Elizabeth Anne. *Pox Americana: The Great Smallpox Epidemic of 1775–82*. New York: Hill and Wang, 2002.

Glynn, Ian, and Jennifer Glynn. *The Life and Death of Smallpox*. New York: Cambridge University Press, 2004.

Grob, Gerald N. *The Deadly Truth: A History of Disease in America*. New York: Cambridge University Press, 2002.

Hopkins, Donald R. *The Greatest Killer: Smallpox in History*. Chicago: University of Chicago Press, 2002.

Leavitt, Judith W. "Politics and Public Health: Smallpox in Milwaukee, 1894–1895." In *Health Care in America*, edited by Susan Reverby and David Rosner. Philadelphia: Temple University Press, 1979.

Robertson, R. G. *Rotting Face: Smallpox and the American Indian*. Caldwell, ID: Caxton Press, 2001.

ERIC JARVIS

SMALLPOX IN COLONIAL LATIN AMERICA.   **Smallpox**, commonly known as *viruelas* in Spanish America and *huitzahuatl*, translated awkwardly by the Spanish as "great **leprosy**," (*lepra*; measles was "little leprosy") among the Aztecs of Mexico, first appeared on the island of Hispaniola in 1518. From there, the disease spread throughout the Caribbean and onto the Mexican mainland by 1520. During the sixteenth, seventeenth, and eighteenth centuries, major **epidemics** of smallpox occurred every 10 to 20 years throughout the Spanish and Portuguese colonies. The most severe outbreaks often claimed 25 to 50 percent of those infected, leading to long-term demographic decline among native populations in many areas. The introduction of smallpox and other previously unknown diseases, in conjunction with the violence of European conquest and colonization, ultimately led to drastic cultural, economic, political, and social changes in indigenous societies throughout Latin America.

Historical Record.   The nature and scope of the evidence available on epidemics of smallpox in colonial Latin America varies widely by region. In general, the most numerous and detailed accounts, especially for the sixteenth and seventeenth centuries, come from central Mexico and the Andean highlands, areas with the largest indigenous and European populations. Jesuit missionaries in Brazil also recorded detailed descriptions of a number of outbreaks during the second half of the sixteenth century.

The historical record also varies over time, as the number of descriptions and the amount of detail included tended to increase throughout the colonial period. Although a few illustrations by indigenous and European artists survive, almost all of what we know about the history of smallpox in colonial Latin America comes from documents written by Europeans. Some of these documents include eyewitness accounts, whereas others are based on secondhand reports. In some areas such as the Andean highlands of the Inca Empire, the historical record includes transcriptions of oral traditions describing possible epidemics of smallpox that occurred shortly before the arrival of Spaniards in the early 1530s. European explorers, conquerors, settlers, and priests wrote many of the earliest accounts, and, especially in colonial Spanish America, government officials often included information on outbreaks of smallpox and other diseases in their reports.

Some of the earliest accounts are brief and include only vague descriptions of the symptoms of the disease. As a result, confusion often exists as to the exact disease responsible for some of these epidemics. Similarly, many descriptions contain only vague references to rates of mortality and morbidity, whereas others do not include any references to death rates at all.

The introduction of the smallpox virus to the Americas triggered a series of virgin-soil epidemics that resulted in extremely high rates of morbidity and mortality. Sixteenth-century accounts described skin eruptions that covered the bodies and faces of the sick, and several illustrations also depict the pustules characteristic of the disease. Other symptoms included fever and body pain, and in some areas severe nosebleeds were also common. Most victims died within days of manifesting symptoms. Records indicate that the disease spread rapidly and widely and that the majority of individuals in infected, indigenous communities became ill, with mortality rates averaging between 25 and 50 percent.

Origins and Spread.   The first documented appearance of smallpox in the Americas occurred in 1518 when the disease was introduced from Europe onto the island of Hispaniola. According to several witnesses, the disease spread quickly, claiming one-third of the native population. Some Spaniards also became ill, but according to all accounts, none died. The fact that smallpox had not arrived earlier in the New World is not surprising since the **virus** requires three weeks to complete its cycle—a ten- to twelve-day incubation period, followed by the onset of illness, including the appearance of a rash or pustules, that often lasted two weeks. Lengthy transatlantic voyages and childhood immunities already acquired by most Europeans delayed the transfer of the disease to the New World for over two decades. On Hispaniola, this first epidemic of smallpox coincided with the forced resettlement of natives into communities closer to Spanish towns, and the violence and disruption resulting from this policy significantly exacerbated mortality rates once the epidemic had begun.

From Hispaniola, the disease spread to the neighboring islands of Puerto Rico, Jamaica, and Cuba, where it left a similar path of devastation. In 1520 smallpox arrived in Mexico with the expedition of Panfilo de Narvaez (1470–1528), dispatched by the governor of Cuba to arrest Hernán Cortés (1485–1547), the soon-to-be conqueror of the Aztecs. Although some accounts blame the introduction of smallpox in Mexico on an African slave, others argue that the infection arrived with natives from Hispaniola who accompanied the Narvaez expedition. The epidemic, which claimed between 25 to 50 percent of the population according to several accounts, broke out during the Spanish siege of the Aztec capital, Tenochtitlán, claiming the life of the Aztec emperor, Cuitlahuac (r. 1520), and many Indian nobles. The power vacuum that resulted from the deaths of Aztec leaders during the epidemic led to a collapse of political authority and organization, and as a result, many enemies of the Aztecs allied themselves with the Spanish. In addition to the catastrophic loss of life that resulted from both warfare and disease, the collapse of Aztec imperial authority played an important role in Spain's defeat and subjugation of the Aztecs.

From central Mexico, the epidemic spread out, moving south into Central America, where an epidemic, possibly of smallpox, claimed the lives of many Guatemalans in 1520–1521. Whether or not smallpox continued south through Central America at this time is not clear, but one historical account states that the disease was responsible for an epidemic that occurred in Panama in 1527.

The arrival of smallpox in South America is less clearly documented. Some scholars have argued that in the decade following its introduction to the Caribbean, smallpox became **pandemic**, spreading throughout large sections of the Americas, eventually reaching as far south as the Andes. Both Spanish and Inca chroniclers recorded the impact of an epidemic that occurred several years before the arrival of Europeans. According to these accounts, the disease arrived in the Inca Empire sometime between 1524 and 1530, claiming a significant portion of the population, including members of the Inca royal family. This set off a civil **war** that ultimately weakened the political structure of the empire and contributed to its conquest by the Spanish several years later. In this case, smallpox could have arrived along the coast of Peru on ships coming from Central America; or the infection could have arrived overland from Panama.

Permanent Portuguese settlement of the Brazilian coast began in the 1550s, and the first recorded epidemic of smallpox in Brazil occurred in 1562, although it is possible that the disease may have arrived earlier. Indigenous residents of the missions and those enslaved on Bahia's sugar plantations succumbed in large numbers, leading to severe labor shortages. Labor shortages led to dwindling food supplies, starvation, and further increases in mortality. According to eyewitness accounts, between 25 and 50 percent of the native population died as a result of this initial epidemic.

Because virgin-soil epidemics of smallpox appeared in conjunction with Spanish and Portuguese campaigns of conquest and colonization, the stresses on indigenous populations were extreme. In many cases, basic social services such as the provision of food and **water** broke down completely, increasing morbidity and mortality rates. Throughout the colonial period, major epidemics of smallpox broke out every 10 to 20 years, providing sufficient time between episodes to allow partial recovery of native populations. When the next wave of the disease struck, individuals born since the previous epidemic proved especially susceptible. Although Europeans and Africans also succumbed to the smallpox **virus**, many possessed at least partial immunity to the disease, owing to its presence among Old World populations for many generations. As a result, the infection was often less severe, with correspondingly lower rates of morbidity and mortality.

Individual and Societal Reactions.   Both Native Americans and Europeans interpreted epidemics of smallpox and other infectious diseases as divine punishment. But whereas Europeans believed that their Christian god was responsible for sending epidemics of smallpox among nonbelievers, for indigenous peoples the situation was more complicated. Following their conquest by Europeans, two sets of gods, Christian and indigenous, had the power to inflict punishment, and thus both had to be propitiated. Terror, confusion, and despair, all common human reactions to catastrophic events, were frequently noted among Native American populations, especially during the sixteenth and seventeenth centuries. And in several areas, messianic movements appeared in response to the turmoil created by war and disease. When smallpox first appeared in Brazil in 1562, for example, a messianic movement, the *Santidade*, attracted many Indians and slaves with promises of turning masters into slaves and slaves into masters. During this same period, a similar movement appeared in the southern highlands of Peru, posing a serious challenge to Spanish authority in the region. European observers often commented on the tendency of natives to flee in an attempt to avoid infection. This strategy had the consequence, however, of spreading the disease more widely and quickly.

For their part, Europeans responded to epidemics of smallpox in a variety of ways: priests organized religious processions and ministered to the sick and dying, whereas government officials and wealthy citizens often collected donations for charity hospitals. In response to a particularly severe outbreak in 1589, the viceroy of Peru issued a series of specific medical instructions intended to help regional governments mitigate the impact of the epidemic. On the advice of several Lima **physicians**, the viceroy ordered local officials throughout the Andes to **quarantine** all native communities in the hope of preventing the spread of the disease. He also recommended specific medical measures including bleeding and a **diet** of meat as preventative measures, and he urged families to limit contact in order to avoid spreading infection among themselves. Quarantines proved largely unenforceable, however, and as a result, Spanish and Portuguese officials seldom attempted to implement them.

Historical Effects. The introduction of smallpox and other diseases of Old World origin transformed the complex disease environment of the Americas to one of extreme virulence by the middle of the sixteenth century. The devastation wrought by the introduction of smallpox and other diseases from the Old World, in conjunction with the depredations of European **colonialism**, ultimately reduced most Native American populations by 75 percent or more during the course of the colonial period. This demographic catastrophe triggered many wide-ranging alterations in the social, political, and economic order of indigenous life. Waves of native migration throughout Latin America transformed both communities and families. Because adult males often chose to abandon home and family in response to the crushing fiscal and labor demands of colonial settlers, female heads-of-household became more common, and birth rates dropped in many areas. In the wake of major epidemics, labor shortages often materialized, leading to dwindling food supplies and rising prices. In addition, the crisis precipitated by European colonialism also transformed indigenous political structures, as colonial officials replaced traditional native leaders with individuals willing to collaborate with colonial administrators. The long-term impact of the introduction of smallpox and other diseases from the Old World was drastic population decline and traumatic social change within indigenous societies throughout colonial Latin America. *See also* Contagion Theory of Disease, Premodern; Diagnosis of Historical Diseases; Disease in the Pre-Columbian Americas; Flight; Historical Epidemiology; Latin America, Colonial: Demographic Effects of Imported Diseases; Malaria in the Americas; Measles in the Colonial Americas; Religion and Epidemic Disease; Slavery and Epidemic Disease; Smallpox in Colonial North America.

Further Reading

Alchón, Suzanne Austin. *A Pest in the Land: New World Epidemics in a Global Perspective*. Albuquerque: University of New Mexico Press, 2003.

———. *Native Society and Disease in Colonial Ecuador*. New York: Cambridge University Press, 1991.

Cook, Noble David. *Born To Die: Disease and New World Conquest, 1492–1650*. New York: Cambridge University Press, 1998.

McCaa, Robert. "Spanish and Nahuatl Views on Smallpox and Demographic Catastrophe Mexico." *Journal of Interdisciplinary History* 25 (1995): 397–431.

Verano, John W., and Douglas H. Ubelaker. *Disease and Demography in the Americas*. Washington, DC: Smithsonian Institution Press, 1992.

SUZANNE AUSTIN

SMALLPOX IN COLONIAL NORTH AMERICA.

Before 1492, North America was free from **smallpox**. Because the *variola* **virus** had to be transmitted from an actively ill patient to a fellow human via breath, touch, or material contaminated with the virus, the Atlantic and Pacific Oceans had served as effective barriers to the spread of smallpox from the Old World.

Beginning with Christopher Columbus (1451–1506), however, each shipload of European colonizers and their African slaves to arrive in the Western Hemisphere became a potential vector of the disease. Very soon, the Americans learned to recognize the symptoms so well-known in Europe, Africa, and Asia: an intense fever and headache, pain in the midsection, a thoroughly justified sense of dread, and the characteristic rash of pustules (the pox) that especially attacked the face, palms, soles, back, and the mucous membranes of mouth and nose.

Lacking the genetic resistance common among groups in which smallpox had been endemic for centuries, American native populations constituted "virgin soil" for the virus. They often suffered the disease in its worst forms, and they died in terrible numbers. Although the American-born children of Europeans and Africans were somewhat more likely than Amerindians to survive smallpox (often with disfigurement and blindness), each new generation to grow up without exposure to smallpox represented a large pool of possible victims for the next outbreak.

Smallpox in Fifteenth-, Sixteenth-, and Seventeenth-Century North America. Within 15 years of Columbus's first voyage, the first recorded American outbreak of *viruela* (the Spanish term) in 1507 proved deadly to the Arawak people of the Caribbean. The 1519–1520 epidemic, carried from Cuba to Mexico by a slave in Hernán Cortés's (1485–1547) army, enabled Cortés to conquer Mexico City. Two decades later, the Spanish chronicler, Fray Toribio Motolinía (d. 1568) wrote that "in most provinces more than half the population [had] died," and still more had perished from starvation "because, as they were all taken sick at once, they could not care for each other." That pattern was repeated in native American communities for centuries to come.

Hernando de Soto's (1496–1542) 1539 expedition carried smallpox inland to native populations from Florida to the Carolinas, and westward to the Mississippi and Texas. The Spanish slave trade, soon joined by the Dutch, French, and English, was a continuing source of new smallpox infections in the New World.

England's first attempts at American settlement in the 1580s may have brought smallpox to North Carolina and the Chesapeake Bay: both the English settlers and the Algonquins observed that Indian villages near the Roanoke colony were struck by fatal fevers a few days after visits from the English. Although Jamestown seems to have escaped smallpox until the late seventeenth century, smallpox is often blamed for the death of the most famous figure in Jamestown history, Pocahontas (1595–1617), who was struck down just as she was about to return from London to her native Virginia. John Lawson (1674–1711), the surveyor-general of North Carolina, declared in his *Account of the Indians of North-Carolina* (London 1709), "The Small-Pox and Rum have made such a Destruction . . . that, on good grounds, I do believe, there is not the sixth Savage living within two hundred Miles of all our Settlements, as there were fifty Years ago" (Lawson, 140).

Shortly before English colonists arrived in New England in 1620, an **epidemic** of "sores"—quite possibly smallpox brought by English fishermen—killed thousands of Narragansetts. In 1634, the Narragansetts were further devastated by confluent smallpox, the worst form. Although both the Pilgrims and the Puritans suffered from deadly smallpox

WILLIAM BRADFORD DESCRIBES SMALLPOX AMONG THE NATIVES IN MASSACHUSETTS (1633)

This spring, also, those Indians that lived aboute their trading house there fell sick of the small poxe, and dyed most miserably; for a sorer disease cannot befall them; they fear it more then the plague; for usualy they that have this disease have them [pocks] in abundance, and for wante of bedding and linning and other helps, they fall into a lamentable condition, as they lye on their hard matts, the poxe breaking and mattering [suppurating], and runing one into another, their skin cleaving (by reason therof) to the matts they lye on; when they turne them[selves], a whole side will flea of at once, (as it were,) and they will be all of a gore blood, most fearfull to behold; and then being very sore, what with could and other distempers, they dye like rotten sheep. The condition of this people was so lamentable, and they fell downe so generally of this diseas, as they were (in the end) not able to help on another; no, not to make a fire, nor to fetch a litle water to drinke, nor any to burie the dead; but would strivie as long as they could, and when they could procure no other means to make fire, they would burne the woden trayes and dishes they ate their meate in, and their very bowes and arrowes; and some would crawle out on all foure to gett a litle water, and some times dye by the way, and not be able to gett in againe.

From *Bradford's History of Plymouth Plantation, 1606–1646, Vol. 6, Original Narratives of Early American History*, edited by W. T. Davis (Charles Scribner's Sons: New York, 1908), pp. 312–13.

outbreaks (on shipboard and in five major episodes in Boston between 1630 and 1702), they regarded smallpox's continuing mortality among the native inhabitants as a sign of God's blessing on their own colonial enterprise.

In the Mid-Atlantic colonies, settled by the Dutch, Swedes, French Huguenots, Germans, and English Quakers during the seventeenth century, a 1633 smallpox epidemic proved disastrous to the Pequots and Lenape. Pehr Kalm (1716–1779), a Swedish naturalist who visited the Delaware Valley in 1748–1751, ascribed the disappearance of Indians from the region chiefly to smallpox, unknown before the Europeans came. He added the grim detail that wolves devoured the corpses and attacked the survivors.

In New France, smallpox came with French settlers as early as 1616 and quickly spread to the Maritimes, along the St. Lawrence River, and to the Great Lakes. The Hurons associated smallpox with the French Jesuit missionaries and with the nuns who provided care in Québec's first hospital. The French government's plan to improve relations with the Labrador "Esquimaux" by educating some of their children ended when all the children died from smallpox.

Smallpox in Eighteenth-Century North America. Although figures are uncertain, it appears that the rapid rise in immigration, settlement, trade, and warfare in eighteenth-century North America was accompanied by an increase in the number and geographic spread of smallpox outbreaks. Outbreaks typically began in crowded ports with arrival of a ship carrying someone infected with smallpox. The 10- to 14-day incubation period gave people who unwittingly harbored the virus time to travel many miles by water, road, or trail before the first symptoms struck. For the next two to three weeks of sickness, they, the air they breathed, and everything their bodies touched was a danger to others.

Boston's colonial records show that, out of every 1,000 inhabitants, 37 died from smallpox in an ordinary year. In 1721, the city's worst eighteenth-century epidemic, that rate nearly tripled. Among the approximately 10,000 residents who stayed in the city (1,000 had fled), more than half fell ill, and more than one in seven died: 844 deaths among 5,900 cases of smallpox over the course of a year. Presumably most of those who did not fall ill had survived earlier exposure to the disease.

The 1721 epidemic is notable for the first use of **inoculation** (also called variolation) in North America to prevent smallpox. Of the 244 Bostonians who tried the controversial new method advocated by the minister-scientist **Cotton Mather** and carried out by Dr. Zabdiel Boylston (c. 1677–1766), only six died (anti-inoculation **physicians** disputed Boylston's figures).

The troop movements and battles on the fronts of the French and Indian Wars (1754–1760) brought smallpox inland in the mid-eighteenth century. The British commander-in-chief, Lord Jeffrey Amherst (1717–1797), is notorious for urging the deliberate spread of smallpox among Indians. Both the English and the French used the **biological warfare** technique of introducing infected prisoners or blankets among the enemy at least once.

Despite the increasing use of inoculation as a private and public health measure, smallpox continued to spread through North America. Documenting the 1775–1782 outbreaks that reached much of the North American continent (Mexico to Northern Canada, the Eastern seaboard, the Great Lakes, the Great Plains, and the Northwest coast) in 1775–1782, the historian Elizabeth A. Fenn argued that smallpox was so rampant that the pestilence should be regarded as a pandemic. Moreover, coinciding with the Revolutionary War and propelled by it, the pandemic had an impact on history that was as far-reaching as the war and American independence. Smallpox unquestionably affected the conduct of the American Revolution. British soldiers in the war were either immune or inoculated in England, but thousands of American Indians and slaves recruited to the Loyalist side died miserably from smallpox. General Charles Cornwallis's (1738–1805) inability to draw on these troops was a major factor in his surrender at Yorktown in 1782.

At the outset, the Continental Army had been far more vulnerable than the British to smallpox. The future President John Adams (1735–1826) blamed the failure of the 1776 siege of Québec on the "Cruel small Pox" that had killed an American general and forced the Americans into "precipitate Retreat." Nonetheless, General George Washington (1732–1799), who had survived the disease as a young man, resisted inoculating his soldiers for fear that the English would descend on the weakened army. Facing a smallpox outbreak in January 1777, Washington declared he had "more to dread from it, than from the Sword of the Enemy." Even then he did not order his recruits to be isolated for the month required to go through inoculation until harsh winter conditions prevented the British from taking advantage of the situation.

Treatment and Prevention. Neither the Native American healer nor the physician trained in European medicine could offer any effective treatment to smallpox victims. Traditional Indian methods of relieving fever by sweat-baths and cold plunges seemed to increase their mortality from smallpox, European observers felt. In the first medical work published in British North America, *A Brief Rule to Guide the Common-People of New-England How to Order Themselves and Theirs in the Small-Pocks, or Measles* (Boston, 1677), the pastor-physician Thomas Thacher (1620–1687) advised fellow Bostonians during an epidemic to keep patients in cool rooms and give them a simple **diet** of cool drinks, corn-meal gruel, and boiled apples. Adapting the advice of his English contemporary Dr. **Thomas Sydenham** (who in turn had followed the medieval Muslim physician, **Rhazes**), Thacher warned against bloodletting, purges, vomits, and other common European treatments of fevers.

To protect their communities, colonial authorities tried to impose quarantines on incoming travelers and sometimes set guards on households where the disease had struck.

A self-imposed isolation stopped young men from going to European universities where they would be almost certain to encounter smallpox. Colonial Americans understood that smallpox survivors could not catch the disease again or spread it. Consequently, slave-owners paid a premium for African slaves whose pockmarks testified to immunity. (Pockmarks also served to identify runaway servants, slaves, and criminals.)

Early in the eighteenth century, Cotton Mather learned from two very different sources about the **folk** practice of inoculation—the deliberate insertion of a bit of smallpox scab or pus under the skin to induce a mild case of the disease. His slave Onesimus described his own inoculation in Africa, and Mather read reports of successful inoculations in Turkey and Greece, published in the scientific journal *Philosophical Transactions of the Royal Society* in 1714 and 1716. Throughout the eighteenth century, American families, officials, and physicians argued over the risks of inoculation. The hoped-for mild case could turn deadly. The artificially induced case was as contagious as smallpox contracted "in the natural way" and just as dangerous to the susceptible bystander. Inoculation was expensive in doctor's fees and time lost from work. (Rhode Island's delegate to the Continental Congress in Philadelphia felt he could not spare the time—and died during Philadelphia's 1774–1776 outbreak.) To many, inoculation seemed an unnatural, impious challenge to God's will. Massachusetts, Virginia, and the cities of Charleston and New York severely restricted or banned inoculation. Elsewhere, inoculators set up makeshift isolation hospitals where their patients could "go through" the illness.

These arguments lost force with Dr. **Edward Jenner's** breakthrough discovery of **vaccination**. North Americans quickly recognized that vaccination was far simpler, safer, and surer than inoculation. Six months after Jenner's first experiment in 1796, his former schoolmate Dr. John Clinch (1749–1819) received samples of the vaccine and began vaccinating patients in Newfoundland—well before Dr. Benjamin Waterhouse (1754–1846) of Boston read Jenner's *Inquiry into the Causes and Effects of the Variolae Vaccinae* (1800) and actively promoted vaccination in the United States. As early as 1803, a humanitarian medical mission brought the vaccine to Abenaqui communities in Upper Canada, and the Balmis Expedition supplied it to the Caribbean and Mexico. Although smallpox continued to be a major threat to health into the twentieth century, the first step in **smallpox eradication** in the American colonies and former colonies had been taken. *See also* Colonialism and Epidemic Disease; Contagion and Transmission; Latin America, Colonial: Demographic Effects of Imported Diseases; Race, Ethnicity, and Epidemic Disease; Slavery and Epidemic Disease; Smallpox and the American Revolution; Smallpox in Canada and the United States since 1783; Smallpox in Colonial Latin America; Smallpox in Premodern Europe; Trade, Travel and Epidemic Disease; War, the Military, and Epidemic Disease.

Further Reading

Fenn, Elizabeth A. *Pox Americana: The Great Smallpox Epidemic of 1775–82.* New York: Hill and Wang, 2001.

Harvard University Library. *Contagion.* http://ocp.hul.harvard.edu/contagion/smallpox.html

Hopkins, Donald R. *The Greatest Killer: Smallpox in History.* Chicago: University of Chicago Press, 2002.

Lawson, John. *Account of the Indians of North-Carolina.* London: 1709.

McIntyre, John W. R., and C. Stuart Houston, "Smallpox and Its Control in Canada," *Canadian Medical Association Journal* 161, 12 (December 14, 1999): 1543–1547.

Smallpox in Colonial America [collection of pamphlets by Thacher, Boylston, and three others]. New York: Arno Press, 1977.

Winslow, Ola Elizabeth. *A Destroying Angel: the Conquest of Smallpox in Colonial Boston*. Boston: Houghton-Mifflin, 1974.

KAREN MEIER REEDS

SMALLPOX IN EUROPEAN NON-AMERICAN COLONIES.   The age of European discovery and expansion began in the late fifteenth century, at a time when the dreaded disease **smallpox** was common if not endemic in Europe. Spanish, Portuguese, French, and English explorers and colonists, and infected African slaves, brought smallpox to the New World of the Western Hemisphere with devastating results for the native Americans—north and south—who had no resistance to the virus. **Smallpox in the colonial Americas** defaced, blinded, and killed millions, and it long remained a threat to colonists raised in isolation from the disease. European contact with Africans, South Asians, Australians, and Pacific Islanders also often resulted in the importation of the disease, but the range of effects was much wider and more complex. Some of these regions presented, like the Americas, "virgin soil" for smallpox, whereas others had had long histories with the disease. From at least 1800, colonial authorities attempted to prevent and, to a lesser extent, treat smallpox. These efforts had mixed results in the short run, but they laid the groundwork for the **eradication of smallpox** in the 1970s.

Europe.   Europe clearly suffered from smallpox in late antiquity and in the early Middle Ages, but for several centuries before the era of the Crusades, little was reported of the disease. A Danish ship brought smallpox to Iceland for the first time in the mid- or late 1200s—sources disagree on the date—with a (probably exaggerated) death toll of 20,000. The island suffered recorded outbreaks in 1430–1432, 1462–1463 (with 1,600 deaths), and 1472. Iceland's worst **epidemic**, the "Great Pox," occurred in 1707–1709, when nearly all of its 50,000 inhabitants (its first census was in 1703) were affected, and between 16,000 and 18,000 died. It took a century to recover. Shortly after 1430, many believe, smallpox struck Greenland from Iceland and essentially wiped out the colonial population. Having been restocked with Danes, the island underwent another epidemic in 1733 when a Greenlander returned from Denmark (probably via Iceland) with the disease. Three-quarters of the white population suffered, and between 2,000 and 3,000 died. Isolation and low population density on both islands generally meant long periods—decades instead of years—between major outbreaks, and thus grew large segments of the population that had not been immunized by previous exposure to the disease. When smallpox hit, the mature as well as the young were susceptible.

Seventeenth-century Russian exploration of and expansion into Asian Siberia brought the **virus** into "virgin soil," paralleling the American experience. Beginning around 1630, thousands of Ostyak, Tungus, Yakut, and Samoyed natives fell ill, with a mortality rate reported at nearly 50 percent. Further expansion meant further devastation, and in an early example of international public health cooperation, in 1724 the Chinese sent **physicians** to inoculate Siberians during one of the epidemics that recurred every two or three decades. In 1768–1769 Kamchatka lost two-thirds to three-quarters of its native population to *ospa*, and in the later nineteenth century, the Yukaghirs, who had controlled a huge region east of the Lena River basin were reduced to a mere 1,500 souls. Such depopulation allowed for Russia's rather easy absorption of nearly half a continent.

An epidemic in 1856 killed an estimated 100,000 Russians despite enlightened Imperial laws mandating smallpox **vaccination** from as early as 1812.

India and the Indian Ocean Region.   India had had long experience with smallpox when the Portuguese established their colony at Goa in 1510. In many parts of the subcontinent, smallpox was endemic and directly related to the goddess Sitala, who was believed by Hindus to possess the body of the victim. **Inoculation** with smallpox material was thus a ritual, and religious action related more to the goddess cult than to medical prophylaxis. A class of professional inoculators made a good living performing the procedures. Of course, those inoculated could very easily die, and while getting over the infection, they were themselves contagious and needed to be isolated. Inoculation was never systematic, and young children tended to be spared inoculation, which is why most of the 8,000 who died in Portuguese-controlled Goa over three months in 1545 were children.

After the British ran the French out of India and established the ascendancy of the British East India Company in 1764, observers in Bengal noted that smallpox recurred roughly every seven years, in the spring, prompting the colonials to take **flight** to the countryside. In 1769–1770 an epidemic struck the Bengali capital and claimed 63,000 lives, while more widely an estimated third of the Bengali population, or 3 million, died. Bengal was said to have had among the highest regional levels of inoculation: it may well have been that the practice itself helped spread the disease. In 1802 the first **Jenner**-type vaccine arrived in Bombay via Vienna and Baghdad (being transferred arm-to-arm in vaccinated people), and variolation was banned by law in 1804. Though the British saw this as the height of rationality and generosity, native Indians, especially the inoculators and devotees of Sitala, saw the attempt to replace a religious ritual with a rather disgusting secular therapy as demeaning and impious. The fact that the vaccine was a cow product did not help matters. The law was ignored by Indian and colonist alike.

Though vaccination made some inroads, by 1855 a total of about 1.5 percent of the native Indian population had undergone the procedure. Calcutta suffered through smallpox epidemics that killed 11,000 in a population of 350,000 between 1837 and 1850. 1850 saw a pan-Indian epidemic of smallpox and a revival of the previously ignored anti-variolation law. A widespread epidemic around Bombay inspired the regional 1877 Vaccination Act that required all infants to be vaccinated before the age of six months. Bengal followed with the broader 1880 Bengal Vaccination Act, which required the vaccination of all residents and all newcomers. The gradual replacement across colonial India of variolation with vaccination resulted in a drop in smallpox deaths of 75 percent between 1870 and 1930. The colonial Indian Medical Service (established 1887) continued the vaccination program to the end of British rule, vaccinating about 10 percent (4.3 million) of the population annually between 1936 and 1945, and in its last year—1947—a total of 21.3 million. Still, epidemics recurred every five to eight years, and until 1975 India remained the world's main reservoir for the disease. A major reason for this was the unwillingness of either British or Indian authorities to impose strict, compulsory isolation of patients until the 1960s. Though never popular, this measure inhibited the circulation of the disease among the nonimmunized.

The people of Borneo suffered from smallpox for so long that their mythology connected the disease with creation itself. Every 40 years, they believed, the demon was unleashed on the island and took away half of the population. They refused to touch pox-scarred **corpses** and utilized a primitive form of *cordon sanitaire*. Low population densities probably prevented smallpox from becoming endemic, whereas the "40-year cycle" had to have been marked by sea-borne importations. This cycle was accelerated with colonization, and despite a decades-long program of vaccination, East Java in 1913 suffered an estimated 18,000 cases and 5,000 deaths. A better vaccine, which could be dried and vacuum packed, arrived in Borneo in the late 1920s, and Dutch authorities all but eliminated smallpox from the island by the later 1930s.

As in India, on the largely Muslim island of Ceylon (Sri Lanka) smallpox had long been endemic—and inoculation practiced—when the Portuguese arrived around 1500. A key part of a wide trading network, and factionalized into warring native and colonial social and political groups, the Ceylonese were subjected to regular epidemic outbreaks under both the Portuguese and the Dutch (1658–1800). When British colonial officers assumed authority around 1800, they set up hospitals to isolate the newly inoculated and natural victims. The first vaccine arrived in 1802, and the 1805 peace with the island's Kandy Kingdom led to the vaccination of all residents, a task accomplished by 1818. Colonial authorities believed endemic smallpox had disappeared by about 1821. Fresh importation of the disease caused outbreaks (in the absence of the needed booster shot) in 1819, 1830–1831 (1,000 cases with 257 deaths), and 1836–1837 (303 deaths). By the 1890s, however, smallpox deaths averaged only about 81 per year in a population of 4 million.

Australia and the Pacific.   The dense Asian–African trade network that kept smallpox circulating in the Indian Ocean did not extend to the isolated islands of the South Pacific, leaving them "virgin soil" for the disease. The British First Fleet entered Australia's Sydney Harbor in 1788 with some 1,000 colonists. Several months later, a disease—thought by many to be smallpox—began its inexorable destruction of the aboriginal population along the continent's coast and up the major rivers. As in other "virgin-soil" epidemics, people fled the wretched and pustule-covered victims, often carrying the highly contagious disease with them into other fresh populations. Many were left to die unattended, lacking even the strength to feed themselves, and many ended up in mass graves. Tens, perhaps hundreds, of thousands who had never seen a European suffered and died from their "dibble-dibble" in the continent's greatest demographic catastrophe. It may be the case that only the interior and northwestern areas of Australia were spared.

Aborigines and some Europeans suffered again in 1829–1830 and the 1860s, whereas European colonists in Melbourne were struck when smallpox accompanied the *Commodore Perry* from Liverpool in 1857. Up to the year 1900, nine more imported cases broke out in Australia, despite **quarantine** policies and widely applied vaccinations that began shortly after 1800. Between May 1881 and January 1882, Sydney suffered 154 reported cases and 40 deaths, mostly among inner-city residents. The number is probably rather low because many were afraid to report for fear of quarantine and eviction from their residences. A quarantine station was established at North Head, and in December 1881 an isolation **hospital** began operation. In all, some 900 underwent quarantine or isolation. Many of these were Chinese, whose community was boycotted and who were forcibly vaccinated. Indeed, the outbreak led to the Chinese Restrictions Bill, which forced quarantine on, and limited the flow of, all new Chinese immigrants. More reasonably, it also led to the provision of a Board of Health, mandatory reporting procedures, and an Ambulance Corps. In 1886 the smallpox-stricken ship *Preussen*, which sailed from Port Said, Egypt, and landed at Adelaide, Melbourne, and Sydney, had its 112 victims successfully isolated, dropping some at each stop. A stringent program of vaccination from 1900 eliminated *Variola major* smallpox from Australia by

1903, but the much less deadly *V. minor* strain arrived from the United States in 1913. Over four years, there were 2,400 cases but only 4 deaths.

French Polynesia suffered its first outbreak of smallpox in 1841 when introduced by a U.S. ship sailing between Valparaiso, Chile, and Hawaii. Six had died on board, but with no obvious cases active, the vessel was allowed to anchor without quarantine in Matavai Bay, Tahiti. The disease spread rapidly among the islanders, but another American ship that had vaccine material arrived soon after, and a program of vaccination was quickly carried out. Though 200 died, smallpox was confined to the northwest portion of Tahiti. Nonetheless, when the King of Moorea visited Tahiti for treatment by colonial doctors, he contracted smallpox and brought it back to his island, resulting in 57 cases and 29 deaths among the natives. Many islands decided to close themselves to any outside traffic until the outbreaks ceased.

Peruvian slavers carried away some 1,000 islanders in a raid in 1862. Once they landed on the continent, the highly susceptible newcomers contracted smallpox, and many died. The remaining 470 were packed back on a ship and sent home. During the journey, all but 15 died, and these brought the horrors of smallpox to their friends and family. By 1870 a scant 111 people remained on the island, of an estimated 4,500 in 1860.

The Portuguese Ferdinand Magellan (1480–1521) staked the Spanish claim to the Philippine Islands in 1520, but a Jesuit priest reported the first incidence of smallpox in the colony only in 1591. A Spanish ship, the *Nao de la China*, sailing from Mexico is credited with the introduction of the disease that reportedly infected one-third of the Batanga tribe and inflicted a high mortality rate, especially among the older members. Soon the disease was associated with demons, a belief that later made colonial medical intervention difficult. Whether imported from Asia, America, or Europe, inoculation became a popular response by the mid-eighteenth century. Though Spanish colonial authorities in the nineteenth century championed vaccination of the indigenous peoples, a lack of resources, poor quality vaccines and personnel, difficulty in travel, native resistance, and a lack of official compulsion resulted in ineffective efforts. Smallpox claimed annual death tolls around 40,000, as well as causing thousands of cases of residual blindness. After becoming a U.S. territory in the wake of the Spanish-American War (1898), The Philippines underwent an aggressive, military-led vaccination program and the strict banning of inoculation. By 1914, 10 million had been vaccinated, and the death toll had dropped to 700. A year later, only 276 died, but after Filipinos assumed control, the incidence spiked, and in 1918–1919, 64,000 deaths were reported (though many were no doubt related to the **influenza pandemic of 1918–1919**). U.S. intervention and new dried vaccine reduced the death toll to 367 by 1929. The last case considered epidemic occurred in 1931, making The Philippines the first Asian-Region country to eliminate the disease.

Africa.   Smallpox arrived in Africa long before Europeans did. At least one Egyptian pharaoh died of it, and Muslim armies and merchants spread it along with the Koran across North Africa and south along the Sahara caravan routes, and along the continent's east coast south of Egypt. Outside of urbanized areas like the Lower Nile, African population densities remained low, and, except along the coasts or established caravan routes, travel and interaction of peoples remained limited. Much of Africa, especially in the south, remained virgin soil even after Muslim traders and slavers in the east and interior and European slavers and colonists along the west and south coastal regions had introduced the disease.

When Portuguese slavers first began collecting and shipping coastal West Africans to the American colonies, they were skimming along the western edge of a region whose interior had long been in regular contact with Arab merchants, who had moved westward across Central Africa, and with North African caravans, which brought the Mediterranean's goods across the Sahara to trade for gold and black **slaves**. Regular visits by the Portuguese no doubt sparked epidemics, especially in those areas that remained "virgin," and scholars tend to agree that slaves rather than European colonists first brought the pox to the Caribbean. On the long, wretched voyages, victims who showed any signs of smallpox were tossed overboard in the hope of stunting an epidemic. That any Africans survived such trips suggests that they had been naturally immunized by exposure in their home communities. Even so, low populations and population densities meant that smallpox was probably never endemic and that the dislocations caused by European colonization and slaving spread the disease and accounted for a terrible toll.

The relative isolation of southern Africa kept it free of smallpox until rather late. The Portuguese colony established at Luanda in 1484 may have introduced the disease into Angola and the southern Congo, though the earliest clear evidence for smallpox in the region is 1620. By the 1680s the area was being ravaged by wars and the disease. Rampant smallpox prompted the region's Brazilian slavers to suspend their activities in 1687.

The Dutch first arrived at Capetown, South Africa, in 1652, but the young colony avoided smallpox for six decades. In 1713 a Dutch ship with East Indian passengers dropped anchor in Cape Colony's Table Bay. Laundry contaminated with smallpox was unwittingly given to local Khoi slaves of the Dutch East India Company who began to fall ill and die. By the epidemic's end, whole villages had been emptied, and 15 percent of the white population was dead. In 1755, 2,100 (nearly half white) died in the Cape over six months after a Dutch ship from Ceylon unloaded its deadly cargo. Again the native people suffered worst, and the region's first segregated hospitals were erected. Fleeing natives spread the disease as far north as modern southern Namibia. The effect on the indigenous societies was so profound that tribal identities were eroded or destroyed in favor of the generic "Hottentot." Passengers or cargo in a Danish ship touched off a two-year outbreak in 1767 that killed 179 whites and 440 slaves. This episode saw the first application of arm-to-arm inoculation in South Africa, though whether it derived from a European or an African Bantu source remains unclear.

After the British captured the Cape in 1795, and again in 1815, the largely agrarian Dutch *Volk* migrated inland. British colonists and troops began arriving in large numbers during the 1820s, spreading out from the Cape. Discovery of diamonds at Kimberley, some 400 miles inland, and of gold along the Witwatersrand ridge fueled a rush to South Africa and to these spots in particular. Europeans, Asians, and foreign Africans surged in. Interdicting illegal slave ships could also create problems, as in 1840, when the east African *Escarpao* was seized by the Royal Navy and taken into the Cape's Simon's Bay. Before the ensuing smallpox epidemic died out, some 2,300 Cape residents had succumbed. When smallpox broke out in Cape Town in 1882, Kimberley carefully guarded its southern approaches with a *cordon sanitaire* and a quarantine station 30 miles out, requiring proof of vaccination and burning sulphur fumigation of goods or a six-week quarantine. But when smallpox entered via African migrants from Portuguese territory in 1884, the authorities dismissed the reports or declared the disease chickenpox, rather than generate flight or alienate recruits for the mines. After a three-year bout, 2,300 were infected, and 700—mostly Bantus—died. The epidemic spawned the Cape Colony's 1883 Public Health Act, which mandated vaccination and notification of smallpox cases to medical authorities.

Further north and east, the expanding Ashanti people had their southerly-routed armies stopped by smallpox in 1824, in the 1860s, and in the winter of 1873. Their problems probably arose when smallpox carriers mixed with nonimmune comrades in the early stages of mobilization. Still further north, among the Muslim populations and their neighbors, the annual Hajj **pilgrimage** to Mecca was a consistent source of population mixing and smallpox contagion.

The nineteenth-century European "scramble for Africa" brought the Belgians, French, Germans, and Italians onto the continent and pushed the European presence—and the accompanying native dislocations—further inland than ever before. Otherwise isolated peoples met smallpox, among other diseases, for the first time. The early penetration of railroads made new inroads for disease (the Mombasa to Uganda line stopped short of Masaai territory, but between 1896 and 1899, the rinderpest-weakened warrior tribes lost 75 percent of their population to smallpox). Flight and the sporadic African practice of inoculation spread the disease like a shadow preceding the Europeans' appearance. Colonial wars also mixed populations and drew smallpox across the countryside sparking outbreaks as it went. Portuguese West Africa suffered 25,000 dead of smallpox in 1864–1865 when it raced through the colony, disrupting the mines' production and trade routes and destroying villages wholesale. In Dahomey the god of smallpox was Sakpata, and ritualized native inoculation continued to be practiced after its ban by colonial authorities. During the Franco-Dahomean War of 1892, smallpox played a significant role in weakening the native army and ensuring its defeat.

Vaccinations began early, but were treated as personal rather than public health prophylaxis. Some mistakenly perceived the procedure to be as dangerous as inoculation. South Africa introduced it before 1812, and it was being employed widely by the 1840s, at least among whites. Madagascar saw its use as early as 1818, and Sierra Leone in 1859. In Egypt and the Sudan, vaccination was compulsory by the early 1820s. But booster shots were needed, and the heat and distances weakened the material until the 1920s, when dried vaccine was made available. Even before then, however, the appearance of *Variola minor*, with its low virulence and immunizing effect, began a natural immunizing process. European colonial troops were usually vaccinated upon induction and again before their theater assignment. But both natural and artificial immunization was sporadic, and large populations remained susceptible. Major outbreaks continued throughout the continent until the concerted efforts to eradicate the disease from the 1960s. Madagascar was the first African region to eliminate the disease, around 1922, but the continent's incidence rate spiked two decades later when 99,000 cases were reported in 1944–1945, during the crucial stages of World War II. As African states gained their independence from the late 1950s, many underwent political upheavals that created resurgences of smallpox and other diseases as a result of violence, social disruptions, and shifts in resource allocation. *See also* Colonialism and Epidemic Disease; Smallpox Eradication; Smallpox in Premodern Europe.

Further Reading

Arnold, David. *Colonizing the Body: State Medicine and Epidemic Disease in Nineteenth-Century India.* Berkeley: University of California Press, 1993.

———. *Imperial Medicine and Indigenous Societies.* New York: Manchester University Press, 1988.

Curson, P. H. *Times of Crisis: Epidemics in Sydney, 1788–1900.* Sydney: Sydney University Press, 1985.

De Bevoise Ken. *Agents of the Apocalypse: Epidemic Disease in the Colonial Philippines*. Princeton: Princeton University Press, 1995.

Hartwig, Gerald W., and K. David Patterson. *Disease in African History*. Durham, NC: Duke University Press, 1978.

Hopkins, Donald R. *The Greatest Killer: Smallpox in History*. Chicago: University of Chicago Press, 1983.

Reynolds, Henry. *Aborigines and Settlers: The Australian Experience, 1788–1939*. North Melbourne: Cassell Australia, 1972.

JOSEPH P. BYRNE

SMALLPOX IN PREMODERN EUROPE.   From the fall of the Roman Empire (c. 476) to the French Revolution at the end of the eighteenth century, **smallpox** gradually emerged to become one of the most significant and deadliest diseases in European history. Smallpox is the common name of the disease in the English-speaking world, derived from the Old English *pocc*, meaning a "pustule." The prefix "small" was added after the 1490s to differentiate it from the great pox, **syphilis**. Alternative early modern (c. 1500–1800) names of the disease in various European languages include *la petite vérole* (French), *Blättern* (German), and *kinderenpocken* (Dutch).

Smallpox spread throughout the whole of premodern Europe, although the severity and frequency of outbreaks varied widely. These depended primarily upon the size, density, and previous exposure to the disease of the population at risk. In large towns by the seventeenth century, smallpox was endemic, afflicting mainly **children** and leaving survivors immunized. Smallpox could account for up to 10 percent of total deaths. In smaller and sparsely populated settlements, the disease was **epidemic**, with infrequent outbreaks that attacked adults as well as children. People of all social classes succumbed to smallpox, from the lowliest paupers to European royalty. The case fatality rate for the strain of smallpox most likely prevalent in early modern Europe, *Variola major*, was around 25 percent: one in four people infected with smallpox died. Of those who survived the disease, there was a high chance of pockmarks causing permanent disfigurement. Further possible consequences of smallpox included blindness and male infertility.

Regarding changes over the premodern period, the sources indicate an increase in the incidence and mortality of the disease around the seventeenth century with a peak in the eighteenth. Historians have generally accounted for this perceived increase in the virulence of smallpox by either a mutation of the **virus** or the introduction of a new and more virulent strain of *variola* into Europe. Alternative explanations emphasize the changing social and economic conditions of early modern Europe—particularly, the rise in population, **urbanization**, and migration—that led to a disease environment more conducive for smallpox. The eighteenth century saw the dissemination of **inoculation**: a practice that conferred lifelong **immunity** upon the recipient and paved the way for the introduction of **vaccination** (c. 1800).

Historical Evidence.   The evidence available for smallpox in medieval Europe (c. 500–1500) is meager and often ambiguous. As with **smallpox in the ancient world**, the first problem is the relative paucity of *all* written records, which were either not created in a largely illiterate society or have not survived to the present day. Secondly, the unspecific nature of disease classification in earlier periods makes identification difficult. To identify a particular disease, therefore, emphasis must be placed upon the descriptions of symptoms and distinctive epidemiological characteristics. Records improve in the early modern period, although regions of Europe—mainly rural areas—remain either undocumented or underresearched by historians. Evidence for smallpox can be found in a wide variety of sources, including medical treatises, burial registers, legal records, parish account books, and personal documents (e.g., diaries and letters), along with plays, novels, and poems. Quantitative evidence on smallpox mortality is rare and is largely restricted to towns from the early modern period onward: for example, the burial registers in Geneva state the cause of death from 1580, those of London from 1629, and those of Moscow from 1680. Quantitative morbidity data—the number of people who were sick—in this period is almost nonexistent.

Medieval Europe.   Two probable smallpox epidemics are documented in the late sixth century. In 573 Bishop Marius of Avenches (Switzerland, c. 530–593) described an epidemic of *Variola* in southern Europe. Seven years later, Bishop Gregory of Tours (France, 538–594) witnessed a fatal disease that struck across northern Italy and southern France. No disease name is recorded, but the detailed description of the symptoms closely resembles that of smallpox. For the next few centuries, very little evidence of the disease exists. It is possible that the Islamic armies of the seventh and eighth centuries spread smallpox into Europe. By the tenth century, a physician-monk called Notkerus, from Switzerland, is reported to have been able to diagnose the disease even before the rash appeared, suggesting familiarity with smallpox. An Anglo-Saxon manuscript from this time contains a prayer to St. Nicaise to defend the suppliant from the disease: Nicaise was the Bishop of Rheims (France) in the fifth century who became the patron saint of smallpox victims.

Into the second millennium, there is the possibility that the Christian armies of the Crusades in the twelfth and thirteenth centuries spread smallpox from the Middle East into Europe. Descriptions of the disease in medical treatises began to appear from this time. For example, Gilbert (fl. 1250), an English physician, compiled a *Compendium Medicinae* (c. 1240) that included an account of smallpox. By the fourteenth century, a number of smallpox epidemics were recorded in Italian cities: Florence (1335), Naples (1336), Siena (1363), Vicenza (1386), and Bologna (1393). In France, King Charles V (1338–1380) caught and survived an attack of smallpox. By the end of the medieval period, smallpox appears to have spread throughout Europe. However, when compared with those of later centuries, medieval sources give the impression of a relatively mild form of the disease. It is possible that the form of smallpox prevalent at this time was of similar virulence to the *Variola minor* strain of the disease, with a case fatality rate of 1 percent, identified in the late nineteenth century. But this must remain a hypothesis that cannot be verified from the limited historical record.

Early Modern Europe.   In Europe and in her colonies around the world, smallpox made the greatest demographic impact during the early modern period. With the rise in urbanization, as more people lived in close proximity to one another, a highly contagious disease like smallpox was able to thrive and survive continually amongst the urban populace. In London by the mid-seventeenth century (population of 400,000), smallpox was an endemic disease, although its death toll continued to fluctuate with epidemic peaks every few years. Smallpox was regularly killing over a thousand Londoners per year, and this increased to a few thousand (or 10 percent of total deaths) at the height of the disease in the mid- to late eighteenth century. Most of the victims were children, because the majority of adults would already have caught smallpox and were thus immunized from future attacks. This pattern of age-specificity is seen in other European cities. Between 1580 and 1760, nearly half of all smallpox deaths in Geneva were of infants under two years old, and four fifths of victims were under five years of age.

In rural and isolated regions of Europe—where the majority of people lived—the epidemiological characteristics of smallpox were noticeably different. When smallpox could not maintain itself endemically, many years could pass between outbreaks. If it then spread among a population where few people had previously caught the disease, the attack rate would be especially high, affecting adults and children. An extreme example of this occurrence was in Iceland in 1707 when almost all the 50,000 inhabitants of the island caught the disease, and 16,000 to18,000 died.

Sometimes smallpox epidemics were isolated in time and place, but the disease could also erupt into European-wide pandemics. In 1614, the disease spread throughout France, Germany, Italy, England, Poland, Flanders, Crete, and Turkey. The prevalence and severity of smallpox across Europe is well illustrated in the number of royalty who either survived or succumbed to the disease. In France, King Louis XIV (1638–1715) caught and survived an attack of smallpox in 1647. His great-grandson, who became Louis XV (1710–1774), was not so lucky and died from smallpox in 1774 at the age of 64. Joseph I Habsburg (1678–1711), Holy Roman Emperor and King of Austria and Hungary, died of smallpox. In Britain, King Charles II (1630–1685) survived an attack of the disease, but he lost two siblings, Prince Henry (1640–1660) and Princess Mary (1631–1660) in 1660. England's Queen Mary II (1662–1694) died of smallpox on December 28, 1694, at the age of 32.

Determinants of Smallpox.   As a contagious disease that only existed within a human host and had no animal reservoir, smallpox's epidemiology was intimately associated with people's movements and migrational patterns. This applies on a global scale—as in the case of **smallpox in colonial Latin America**—and right down to the local level, as rural–urban migrants had a high chance of catching smallpox the moment they arrived in the city. Factors that encouraged migration therefore helped spread the disease. These included migrants forced to travel for want of food but also those attracted to new areas because of better employment opportunities. **Warfare**, involving the movements of numerous troops, aided the spread of smallpox. The **Thirty Years' War** (1618–1648), in which most of the major European countries played a part, is one such example. Peaks in smallpox mortality have also been correlated with the end of wars, when thousands of soldiers and sailors were demobilized and descended upon friendly cities, either bringing the disease with them or being susceptible to it upon arriving.

Modern clinical evidence suggests that **diet** did not affect an individual's chance of catching smallpox. However, there is an indirect link: inadequate nutrition in pregnancy is known to cause low birth weights in infants and a corresponding increased susceptibility to infectious diseases, including smallpox. The virus is also known to do better in relatively low temperatures and humidity, thereby increasing the likelihood of spreading from one person to the next. In early modern London, there was a slight correlation between smallpox epidemics and low winter temperatures, although the seasonality of the disease remained concentrated in the summer and fall.

Reactions and Responses.   Smallpox induced great fear—not only as a cause of death, but also and perhaps more significantly because of the horrific symptoms of the disease and possible permanent disfigurement. Both men and women were pockmarked, but for the latter there was the added dimension of their diminished attractiveness affecting their chances of marriage. Hence, smallpox discourse in the eighteenth century was partly gendered: for men, the disease spoke of the danger to their lives; for women, it was a danger to their beauty. Specific concoctions aimed at reducing and concealing the scarring appear in numerous early modern recipe books and women's domestic manuals.

Running alongside this fear, however, was a certain degree of acceptance of smallpox—an expectation, especially in towns, that the disease was unavoidable and therefore a rite of passage that all children must endure. Consequently, the flight response to smallpox was mixed: some people hastily left the region during an epidemic, but others stayed. This stands in contrast to **bubonic plague** epidemics, for which the general consensus was to flee if at all possible. Similarly, when compared with plague victims, smallpox patients were rarely quarantined. This was to change with the introduction of inoculation in the eighteenth century, when **quarantine** could be part of the treatment regime.

Physicians treated smallpox patients based upon practices that had developed out of the **Greco-Roman medical** tradition: predominantly alterations in diet and a combination of induced bleeding, purging, vomiting, and sweating to balance the humors. Debates within this tradition included the most appropriate time to bleed the patient, what quantity of blood should be extracted, whether to purge or vomit, and whether to keep the patient hot or cold. One of the most magical treatments of smallpox was the use of red objects, the perceived curative powers being based on color sympathy. This treatment persisted through premodern Europe and around the world, appearing, for example, in Japan. Queen Elizabeth I of England (1533–1603) was wrapped in a red cloth when she caught smallpox in 1562. Because the disease could necessitate intensive nursing, women played an important role in the medical care of smallpox patients. Although vilified in medical treatises for their lack of theoretical knowledge, the **nurses'** depth of practical experience with the disease meant they were arguably more helpful to the smallpox patient than the university-trained male physicians. The theories of smallpox causation ranged from bad **air** (*miasmas*), to various forms of contagion, to the disease being an innate condition derived from menstrual blood.

Inoculation. The most important medical and public health development in the history of premodern smallpox came in the eighteenth century, with the development and wide dissemination of inoculation. Also called variolation or ingrafting, the practice in Europe was to make an incision in the arm of the person to be inoculated and then insert some matter taken from the pustules of an active smallpox case. The inoculee would then develop smallpox, but a considerably milder case than that acquired naturally, while still gaining immunity from future attacks. The origins of inoculation are obscure and developed out of **folk medicine**. Lady Mary Wortley Montagu (1689–1762), the wife of the British ambassador to Turkey, observed the local women carrying out the practice, and is famously attributed with popularizing it in England. She had Charles Maitland (1677–1748), an English physician, successfully inoculate her son and daughter: the latter instance, in 1721, was the first time this practice was carried out in England by a member of the medical profession. Opposition to the controversial practice was vociferous. Religious concerns were raised over interfering with divine providence. People also died from acquiring inoculated smallpox: early statistics were as high as 1 in 60, but this fell to 1 in thousands. Despite the early resistance, confidence in inoculation grew as people accepted the much better odds of surviving inoculated versus naturally acquired smallpox. In England the practice was widespread from the mid-eighteenth century onward: consequently, by curtailing smallpox mortality, inoculation might have contributed to population growth at this time. Adoption across the European continent was piecemeal. The French and German medical professions, for example, took longer to accept inoculation than the English. But by the last third of the eighteenth century, it was common practice across Europe, eventually being supplanted by vaccination from the early nineteenth century. *See also* Diagnosis of Historical Diseases; Disease, Social Construction of; Jenner, Edward; Latin America, Colonial: Demographic Effects of Imported Diseases; Smallpox and the American Revolution; Smallpox in Colonial North America; Smallpox in European Non-American Colonies; Syphilis in Sixteenth-Century Europe.

Further Reading

Carmichael, Ann G., and Arthur M. Silverstein. "Smallpox in Europe before the Seventeenth Century: Virulent Killer or Benign Disease?" *Journal of the History of Medicine and Allied Sciences* 42 (1987): 147–168.

Glynn, Ian, and Jennifer Glynn. *The Life and Death of Smallpox.* London: Profile Books, 2004.

Grundy, Isobel. "Medical Advance and Female Fame: Inoculation and its After-Effects" *Lumen* 13 (1994): 13–42.

Hopkins, Donald R. *The Greatest Killer: Smallpox in History, with a New Introduction.* Chicago: University of Chicago Press, 2002.

Landers, John. *Death and the Metropolis: Studies in the Demographic History of London 1670–1830.* New York: Cambridge University Press, 1993.

Lindemann, Mary. *Health and Healing in Eighteenth-Century Germany.* Baltimore: Johns Hopkins University Press, 1996.

Razzell, Peter. *The Conquest of Smallpox: the Impact of Inoculation on Smallpox Mortality in Eighteenth Century Britain.* Firle, UK: Caliban Books, 1977.

Scott, Susan, and Christopher J. Duncan. *Human Demography and Disease.* New York: Cambridge University Press, 1998.

HENRY MEIER

SMALLPOX IN THE ANCIENT WORLD.   Because **smallpox** is caused by a **virus** that induces long-lasting **immunity** in survivors, it required human populations of a certain size (100,000 to 200,000 people) to survive. Consequently it probably did not exist before the development of agriculture in the **Neolithic** period. Research in molecular evolution indicates that within the *Orthopoxvirus* genus the variola virus that causes smallpox is most closely related to the camelpox virus. The variola and camelpox viruses diverged from a common ancestor approximately 6,000 years ago. One scenario for the evolution of smallpox as a human disease is that it was associated with camel domestication in the Bronze Age (c. 3000–1000 BCE) in the Near East or Central Asia. However other scenarios can also be imagined. Smallpox and camelpox may simply share a common ancestor, but the camel need not be the direct source of the human disease. Because the evolution of smallpox was associated with **animal** domestication in Asia during the Neolithic and the Bronze Age, after the migrations to North America, smallpox did not exist in the Western Hemisphere before Columbus.

Ancient Near East and Egypt.   The early history of smallpox is shrouded in obscurity, but there are tentative signs that smallpox was present in the civilizations of the ancient Near East. It has been claimed that smallpox is described in the Ebers Papyrus (c. 1500 BCE) from Egypt, but most medical historians do not accept this. The rash of elevated pustules observed on the skin of three mummies dating to the periods of the XVIII and XX Dynasties in the second millennium BCE (including the mummy of the Pharaoh Ramses V, who died c. 1157 BCE) does resemble the rash of smallpox. Unfortunately, the retrospective diagnosis is not absolutely certain because it was not possible to examine the palms of the hands or the soles of the feet, where the rash would be highly diagnostic of smallpox. Smallpox has also been identified in cuneiform texts from Mari in Upper Mesopotamia dating to the first half of the second millennium BCE. The consistent association of the symptoms described with simultaneous epizootics, however, casts some doubt upon the identification, because by then smallpox had evolved into a purely human disease with no known animal reservoirs—a fact that facilitated its **eradication** in the twentieth century CE.

China.   The philosopher and medical writer Ge Hong (283–343 CE) made the first detailed description of the symptoms of smallpox in China in 342. He attributed the disease to bad **air**. Several other early sources suggest that smallpox first reached China in the second half of the third century BCE. It is said to have been introduced to the country by invading nomadic tribes from Central Asia. The movements of armies and merchants often spread early epidemics of smallpox in China. Smallpox has a long incubation period (7 to 17 days), facilitating its spread by people moving around after infection but before clinical symptoms appear. Sometime during the period of the Tang dynasty (618–907), a Chinese physician named Zhao discovered the technique of **inoculation** or variolation, a technique for immunizing people against smallpox that preceded the modern **vaccination** technique. Four different methods of inoculation were devised in China: 1) making a person wear a garment that had previously been used by a sufferer from mild smallpox; 2) introducing into the nose a piece of cotton cloth with fluid from smallpox blisters; 3) blowing dried powder from smallpox scabs into the nose through a blowpipe; 4) drinking water containing dried powder from smallpox scabs.

India and Japan.   The classic ancient Indian **Ayurvedic** medical text *Susruta Samhita* gives a very clear description of smallpox. Unfortunately, early Sanskrit texts are difficult to date, but it is likely that smallpox was present in India by at least the second century CE, by which time it had definitely reached both the Near East to the west and China to the east. Eventually India acquired a goddess specifically devoted to smallpox, namely Sitala (the cool one). Having smallpox was interpreted as being possessed by the goddess. Smallpox was introduced to Japan from Korea or China in the sixth century CE along with Buddhism. The new **religion** was initially blamed for the appearance of a new disease, although Buddhism managed to survive in Japan. Over the next few centuries, periodic reintroductions of smallpox caused a series of major epidemics in Japan, because the human population density was not high enough at first for smallpox to become permanently endemic in the country.

The Ancient Greek and Roman Worlds.   There is no clear description of smallpox in the texts of the Hippocratic corpus, which pay little attention to epidemic disease in general. Smallpox is one of the more plausible candidates for the identity of the pathogen that caused the **plague of Athens** (430–426 BCE), but there are numerous other theories as well. Moving forward in time, Philo of Alexandria (20 BCE–50 CE) in the first century CE described a **biblical plague** in a way that suggests familiarity with smallpox. However, it is not until the **Antonine "plague"** in the second century CE that the presence of smallpox in the classical world becomes absolutely certain. The Antonine plague started among the soldiers of the Roman army who spent the winter of 165–166 at Seleucia in Mesopotamia during the campaign of Lucius Verus (d. 169) against the Parthians.

According to legend, the epidemic commenced when a demon was released from a golden casket in the temple of Apollo at Seleucia. The disease was then carried back to Rome in 166 by the Roman army. The contemporary physician **Galen** is our main source for the Antonine plague; he observed its effects on a unit of Roman soldiers at Aquileia in Italy in 168–169. The importance of armies for the dissemination of smallpox has already been noted in the case of China. The Antonine plague lasted until about 180, and there was another major epidemic in 189 at Rome described by Dio Cassius (c. 160–229) that might have been another outbreak of the same disease. The historian Ammianus Marcellinus (c. 325–391) stated that the Antonine plague reached Gaul and Germany. Galen described the symptoms of the disease and attempts at treatment in a rather unsystematic manner. The symptoms of the Antonine plague included the characteristic exanthemata, which frequently turned black. Survivors' scabs eventually dropped off the ulcers. Galen's evidence suggests a high frequency of the very dangerous hemorrhagic form of smallpox during the Antonine plague. He also mentions as symptoms upset stomach and diarrhea, followed by black stools in survivors, very strong internal fever (although the skin of patients was cool to touch), vomiting, bad breath, catarrh, and internal ulcerations. The economic and demographic effects of the Antonine plague are the subjects of intense controversy among historians. Unfortunately, the whole period is poorly documented.

Late Antiquity. In late antiquity there are several brief reports of epidemics that resemble smallpox. In 302 Eusebius of Caesarea (275–339) described an epidemic in Syria characterized by a skin rash that spread over the whole body and often resulted in death, or in blindness among survivors. In 451 the invading Huns killed the bishop of Rheims in France. He later became St. Nicaise, the patron saint of smallpox, because he had suffered from the disease the year before his death. Gregory, historian and bishop of Tours (538–594), clearly described smallpox in Italy and France in 580–581. A few years before, Marius (530–594), bishop of Avenches in Switzerland, became the first extant source to use the word "variola" to describe an epidemic disease. Unfortunately he did not describe its symptoms. Such references suggest that during the first few centuries CE, smallpox established itself as an endemic disease in Europe, with periodic epidemics as pools of susceptible individuals gradually accumulated. The patchy record for smallpox across antiquity as a whole may well be a consequence of the inadequacies of the documentary record. However, it may also indicate that smallpox was originally a mild disease, as it is described by **Rhazes** in the tenth century CE, perhaps with the spread of more virulent genotypes from time to time. Research in molecular evolution has shown that the acquisition of immune system genes from their hosts by horizontal transfer has been an important feature of the evolution of poxviruses in general. Consequently, smallpox may originally have been a mild disease, like cowpox, and it may have taken some time to acquire the genes to make it more virulent. *See also* Animal Diseases (Zoonoses) and Epidemic Disease; Chinese Disease Theory and Medicine; Corpses and Epidemic Disease; Diagnosis of Historical Diseases; Greco-Roman Medical Theory and Practice; Hippocrates; Historical Epidemiology; Paleopathology; Plagues of the Roman Empire; Smallpox in Premodern Europe; Trade, Travel, and Epidemic Disease; War, the Military, and Epidemic Disease.

Further Reading

Duncan-Jones, Richard. "The Impact of the Antonine Plague." *Journal of Roman Archaeology* 9 (1996): 108–136.

Gourevitch, Danielle. "The Galenic Plague: A Breakdown of the Imperial Pathocoenosis." *History and Philosophy of the Life Sciences* 27 (2005): 57–69.

Hopkins, Donald. *Princes and Peasants: Smallpox in History.* Chicago: University of Chicago Press, 1983.

Littman, Robert, and M. Littman. "Galen and the Antonine Plague." *American Journal of Philology* 94 (1973): 243–255.

ROBERT SALLARES

SNOW, JOHN (1813–1858).   Among **physicians** John Snow is best remembered as a pioneer in anesthesiology and the author of an early textbook on the subject in the 1840s. His enduring fame, however, is based on two landmark studies of **cholera** in London undertaken in the 1850s. Born and raised in a working-class slum in York, England, Snow was aided by a wealthy uncle who placed him as an apprentice with a **surgeon** in London. After two more apprenticeships with **apothecaries** in Newcastle-on-Tyne he returned to study medicine at the Hunterian School in London and the University of London, from which he earned his M.D.

In one of his cholera studies, the Broad Street Study, Snow described a ferocious but localized cholera outbreak in the St. James, Westminster, area of Soho in London, England. The second was carried out simultaneously, and published concurrently, with a more ambitious attempt to determine the cause of cholera in a general **epidemic** in South London. The first stemmed from a single local **water** source, the Broad Street pump, Snow argued. The source of the second was polluted water from the Thames River. In the twentieth century, Snow's cholera studies were lauded as the very essence of the "epidemiological imagination" and the beginning of modern epidemiology, medical geography, and public health.

Cholera is an epidemic disease whose multiple occurrences in the nineteenth century made it the focus of intense study by medical researchers. At that time, most researchers advanced a **miasmatic** theory of disease, believing that epidemic (and some endemic) conditions were generated in the foul airs of the city. Snow, on the other hand, argued that cholera, and by extension other apparently communicable diseases, were water- rather than airborne. Snow first made his argument in an 1849 pamphlet, *On the Mode of Communication of Cholera.* He tested his theory in both the 1854 St. James neighborhood outbreak and, concurrently, the South London registration districts most affected by the epidemic, publishing the results in 1855.

The map Snow drew of the St. James outbreak has become a central icon in both medical geography and cartography. In it, the density of cases proved to be clustered around a single water source, the Broad Street pump. Snow argued this proved a causal relationship between the single water source and the disease. Snow's map of the localized Broad Street epidemic has come to serve as a symbol for a concrete, cartographic approach to the spatial study of disease incidence. For epidemiologists and public health experts, admiration today is focused on Snow's more ambitious (if less conclusive) study of the effect of metropolitan water supplies on the 1854 cholera epidemic in South London.

Although few of Snow's contemporaries accepted his argument as conclusive, in 1883 **Robert Koch** identified the bacterium responsible for cholera as the waterborne *vibrio cholera.* In the twentieth century, Snow's work became a symbol of an approach to disease studies based on a study of the intensity of disease and the location of disease clusters to potential contaminants. *See also* Farr, William; Cholera: First through Third Pandemics, 1816–1861; Demographic Data Collection and Analysis, History of; Sanitation Movement of the Nineteenth Century; Water and Epidemic Diseases.

Further Reading

Hempel, Sandra. *The Strange Case of the Broad Street Pump: John Snow and the Mystery of Cholera.* Berkeley: University of California Pres, 2007.

Koch, Tom. *Cartographies of Disease: Maps, Mapping, and Medicine.* Redlands, CA: ESRI Press, 2005.

Vinten-Johansen, Peter, et al. *Cholera, Chloroform, and the Science of Medicine: A Life of John Snow.* New York: Oxford University Press, 2003.

TOM KOCH

SOCIAL CONSTRUCTION OF DISEASE.   *See* Disease, Social Construction of.

SOCIAL PSYCHOLOGICAL EPIDEMICS.   A variety of social psychological **epidemics** have been recorded since antiquity. The phenomenon is generally defined as the rapid spread of illness signs and symptoms affecting members of a cohesive group; these unconsciously exhibited physical complaints have no known corresponding organic etiology. Episodes range from examples as diverse as **St. Vitus' dance** mania and Italian tarantism (frenetic dancing thought to be caused by a tarantula bite) during the late Middle Ages to cases of sick building syndrome and **bioterrorism** panics today.

Many agents—demons, **viruses**, witches, chemical toxins, and even society itself—have been attributed as causes of the epidemics. Outbreaks have been viewed as symptomatic of social oppression historically linked to religious persecution, political unrest, cultural intolerance, and economic crisis. Generally, the type of manifestation is contingent upon the cultural preoccupations of certain historical periods, suggesting that outbreaks are socially produced. Episodes thus represent historically specific cultural anxieties.

The first indication of an episode is the collective manifestation of physical complaints without any evident cause. Outbreaks are characterized by medically unexplained physical symptoms such as stomach cramping, dry mouth, uncontrollable twitching or trembling, mild convulsion, irrepressible laughter, or temporary paralysis. They typically occur in small groups situated in enclosed settings such as mills, factories, army barracks, convents, hospitals, prisons, office buildings, and schools. Episodes can last three days to two months.

Little scientific consensus exists on conceptual frameworks and terminology. For example, although the phenomenon has most commonly been referred to as "somatization," "mass hysteria," "mass sociogenic illness," "hysterical contagion," "epidemic hysteria," or "mass psychogenic illness," over 70 synonyms have been identified in the literature. Etiological and epidemiological frameworks are likewise varied and remain inconclusive. Shifting conceptualizations and different historical manifestations make the phenomenon particularly challenging to understand and explain.

Psychological approaches have attributed the occurrence to low IQ scores, childhood trauma, or cognitive dysfunction, whereas other studies suggest a higher preponderance among females and personality types classified as neurotic, extroverted, or paranoid. More recent studies, however, demonstrate neither: given the right set of social conditions, no population is immune; the phenomenon is not correlated to, or caused by, personality or psychological factors. Sociological research suggests that high levels of stress, imitative behavior, or other social strain may be the cause of involuntary psychosomatic reactions within the affected group.

The American Psychiatric Association's (APA) *Diagnostic and Statistical Manual IV* (*DSM IV*) includes this phenomenon as an hysterical neurosis under the category of Somatoform Disorders subcategory Conversion Disorder. The psychiatric assessment is based on the absence rather than presence of physical causes making it a diagnosis of exclusion. Contagious psychopathology, fantasy, and mimesis (imitation) have also been hypothesized as psychiatric cause. The term "hysteria," with its root in the Greek word for uterus (as in "hysterectomy"), has been abandoned for its negative denotation of females as essentially overly emotional, irrational, abnormal, or otherwise deviant.

Although many cases can be shown to have been prompted by actual events, some can arise from rumor of the presence of a **contagion** or other immanent threat. Odor, or the perception of odor, is a common trigger for those situations relating to water, smog, nuclear accidents, or chemical exposure. The fear of **environmental** contagions such as toxic gas from **bioterrorism** or industrial pollution have been known to elicit symptoms such as headache, nausea, breathlessness, weakness, and lightheadedness. The lack of etiological certainty, however, does not detract from the reality of the afflicted, whose complaints should be addressed promptly by health professionals and social authorities.

A thorough investigation upon complaint is imperative to rule out all possible causes to prevent unnecessary social panic and confusion. Environmental analysis and medical tests should be conducted. Occasionally the agent is identified; other times attempts by health authorities to locate and eliminate the source of the problem have failed. Past investigations have been closed prematurely, only to be reopened later upon discovery of causal factors. When all physical explanations are ruled out, investigators may resort to psychological explanations to account for the outbreak and rise in number of cases often leading to resentment amongst the sufferers. Furthermore, economic pressures to reduce emergency services and to resume the work schedule may prevent the exploration of all possible causes and the performance of an exhaustive investigation.

In the heightened "post-9/11" climate, it is highly probable that panic created about bioterrorism may be more dangerous than the actual threat it poses. The consequences of such a panic may result in gross human rights violations. The fear of a threatening agent, increasing numbers of complaints, popular media spectacles and reports, and the legitimating actions of authorities all contribute to tension and thus to the increased probability of symptoms being experienced and reported. All of these factors must be taken into consideration when investigating the source.

Public access to reliable and accurate information is necessary to ensure an educated populace and to avoid widespread social paranoia about unfounded anxieties. Exaggerated media representations and opportunistic government hyperbole, in particular, may contribute to and exacerbate a crisis. Managing the situation thus requires special collaborative efforts by public authorities, health professionals, social experts, and the media.

Psychological epidemics are currently poorly understood. Diagnoses have been—and continue to be—contentious and problematic as a result of classificatory ambiguity, lack of physical/organic evidence, and the highly subjective nature of notions such as threat and risk. The long and controversial history of the concept of hysteria, the lack of theoretical and disciplinary consensus on the mind-body relationship, the political history of its use and implications, the etiological uncertainty, and inconclusive empirical data render the phenomenon a problematic scientific category requiring further attention and research. *See also* Black Death, Flagellants, and Jews; Disease, Social Construction of; Personal Hygiene and Epidemic Disease; Personal Liberties and Epidemic Disease; Poison Libels and Epidemic Disease; Poliomyelitis and American Popular Culture; Religion and Epidemic Disease; Scapegoats and Epidemic Disease.

Further Readings

Balaratnasingam, Sivasankaren, and Aleksandar Janca. "Mass Hysteria Revisited." *Current Opinion in Psychiatry* 19 (2006): 171–174.

Bartholomew, Robert E., and Simon Wessely. "Protean Nature of Mass Sociogenic Illness: From Possessed Nuns to Chemical and Biological Terrorism Fears." *British Journal of Psychiatry* 180 (2002): 300–306.

Boss, Leslie P. "Epidemic Hysteria: A Review of the Published Literature." *Epidemiologic Reviews* 19 (1997): 233–243.

Showalter, Elaine. *Hystories: Hysterical Epidemics and Modern Culture.* London: Picador, 1997.

Wessely, Simon. "Responding to Mass Psychogenic Illness." *The New England Journal of Medicine* 342 (2000): 129–130.

HEIDI M. RIMKE

SPANISH INFLUENZA.   *See* Influenza.

SULFA DRUGS.   The term sulfa drugs (aka sulfonamides) is a generic term for derivatives of the chemical para-aminobenzenesulfonamide (sulfanilamide). Sulfa drugs act by interfering with the incorporation of para-aminobenzoic acid into the vitamin folic acid, thus inhibiting the growth of susceptible **bacteria**. Organisms that do not require folic acid or that obtain it preformed in their **diet**, such as humans, are not affected by this process.

The discovery of Salvarsan for the treatment of **syphilis** by **Paul Ehrlich** in the first decade of the twentieth century stimulated a search for other chemical agents to combat infectious diseases. Despite some modest successes, progress was slow. By 1930 many investigators were especially troubled by the failure to develop chemotherapeutic agents against the bacteria that were the major cause of disease in nontropical countries. The announcement in 1935 of a chemical agent effective against infections caused by streptococcal bacteria was thus greeted with great enthusiasm.

The German pharmaceutical firm I. G. Farben introduced the compound, a dye named Prontosil. An extensive screening program led by German pathologist Gerhard Domagk (1895–1964) first demonstrated its efficacy against deadly hemolytic streptococci in mice in December 1932. Clinical trials began in the following year, and by early 1935 evidence had accumulated that Prontosil was effective against scarlet fever, childbed fever, and a variety of other streptococcal infections. Dogmagk personally confirmed Prontosil's value in December 1935, when he used the drug to cure his daughter of a serious streptococcal infection following a wound.

Domagk was aware that Prontosil did not kill bacteria in the test tube but worked only in the organism. Researchers at Paris's Pasteur Institute suspected that Prontosil itself was not the active drug, but that it was broken down in the body to produce an antibacterial molecule. They demonstrated in late 1935 that Prontosil was indeed decomposed in the organism, and that one of the resulting products, sulfanilamide, was the active drug. Unlike Prontosil, sulfanilamide was not covered by a patent, and eventually it largely replaced the earlier drug. Both drugs were used together to cure Amercan President Franklin Roosevelt's (1882–1945) son of a life-threatening streptococcal infection in December 1936, an event that helped bring these medicines to the attention of the American public.

It was soon discovered that sulfanilamide could be modified by the addition of various chemical groups to produce a whole series of compounds known as sulfonamides or sulfa drugs. A number of these substances, such as sulfapyridine and sulfathiazole, proved to be effective against such diseases as bacterial pneumonia and **meningitis**. One of these drugs may have saved the life of British Prime Minster Winston Churchill (1874–1965) when he was suffering from pneumonia in late 1943. Domagk was awarded the 1939 Nobel Prize in Medicine or Physiology for his discovery of Prontosil.

Although viewed as miracle drugs at the time, sulfa drugs were largely supplanted by more effective and less toxic **antibiotics** over the next few decades. These historically important drugs still have a small place in therapy today, especially in the treatment of urinary tract infections. *See also* Pharmaceutical Industry.

Further Reading

Hager, Thomas. *The Demon under the Microscope.* New York: Harmony, 2006.

Lesch, John E. "Chemistry and Biomedicine in an Industrial Setting: The Invention of the Sulfa Drugs." In *Chemical Sciences in the Modern World*, edited by Seymour H. Mauskopf, pp. 158–215. Philadelphia: University of Pennsylvania Press, 1993.

———. *The First Miracle Drugs: How the Sulfa Drugs Transformed Medicine*. New York: Oxford University Press, 2007.

JOHN PARASCANDOLA

SURGEON.   The role of the surgeon was to treat external diseases and injuries, and the most common treatments in use were bloodletting, tooth pulling, and the cauterizing of wounds and sores. Surgeons performed three major procedures: broken bone setting, limb amputation, and "cutting for stone," which involved slicing into the bladder. Surgeons were not gentlemen, and until the end of the seventeenth century, surgeons in Western Europe were widely seen to be inferior to **physicians**. Like carpenters or barbers, they worked with their hands and sold their services for money. They were generally not university-educated and thus thought to possess no theoretical knowledge of **humoral theory**—the hallmark of intellectual medical authority in this period. Most of all, their trade carried overtones of butchery and torture.

From the early eighteenth century, however, the status of surgery began to rise. Individual surgeons were keen to acquire the social and intellectual eminence of physicians. They began to promote surgery based on new anatomical research of the **Scientific Revolution** rather than on empirical tradition. Innovations in surgical instruments and technique were reflected in the idea of "conservative" surgery, which tried to preserve the function of an injured limb rather than resort to amputation. For the first time, surgeons could become gentlemen and even celebrities. The Scots surgeon William Hunter (1718–1783), for example, opened a private medical anatomy school in London, which became not only a center of surgical teaching and research but also a fashionable place to be seen. In 1745 a group of London surgeons founded a College of Surgeons. In so doing, they made a bid for the same kind of power and prominence as the older Royal College of Physicians.

Developments in medical practice reinforced the new status of surgery. The growth of hospital medical schools in the late eighteenth century brought medical students and apprentice surgeons together, with both "walking the wards" to get experience. Following the upheavals of the French revolution in the 1790s, a new style of medicine began to be practiced in the large municipal hospitals of Paris. Physicians began to move away from the Classical view of the body, in which disease was seen as a functional problem, treated by restoring the balance of the four humors. They embraced a new model of disease as a localized structural defect, one that could be addressed by physical treatments and surgery.

In the first half of the nineteenth century, surgeons consolidated their power in **hospitals**. By the 1850s they had achieved broadly equal status with physicians, and in the next hundred years the status of surgery rose even higher. Two major developments—anesthesia and the "antiseptic method"—dominated surgical practice in the second half of the nineteenth century. Both have become part of surgical mythology, but both were consequences, rather than causes, of the new status and authority of nineteenth-century surgeons. Anesthesia initially emerged in the United States in the 1840s. Agents such as ether, chloroform, and nitrous oxide were initially used in dentistry but rapidly moved into surgery and obstetrics. Surgical practice was already highly invasive before the advent of anesthesia, and its introduction initially made surgery more dangerous as surgeons attempted these ambitious procedures more frequently.

The antiseptic method, meanwhile, was a response to public health reformers, who challenged the new status of hospitals as centers of surgical expertise. By the 1850s most European cities had large hospitals for the poor, and most suffered epidemics of fever and gangrene, known as "hospitalism." In Britain, sanitary reformers such as **Edwin Chadwick** and Florence Nightingale (1820–1910) argued that large hospitals were inherently unhealthy and should be replaced by smaller, rural institutions under the supervision of public health agencies. Surgeons began to look for a scientific response to hospitalism. They hoped to prove conclusively that hospitals were not inherently unhealthy, and in so doing, to preserve and strengthen their intellectual authority.

In 1867 Joseph Lister (1827–1912), Professor of Surgery at Glasgow University, began to dress surgical wounds with bandages soaked in carbolic acid. He found that this simple technique slashed the rate of gangrene and fevers. Lister's work was based on the "germ theory" of the French chemist **Louis Pasteur**. He presented his work as a scientific response to the problem of hospitalism, based on the latest concepts in experimental medicine. Over the next decade Lister expanded his work into an "antiseptic method" of surgery, intended to kill all germs in the operating environment. This included a steam-powered spray to cover patient, surgeon, and nurses in carbolic acid during surgery. In the 1880s and 1890s, the German "aseptic method," based on the idea of excluding **bacteria** from the surgical environment, gradually replaced Lister's complex and demanding technique. But Lister's reputation continued to grow, and in 1900 he became the first British surgeon to be made a lord. Two further technical developments in the 1890s—X-ray diagnosis and blood transfusions—contributed to the eminence of surgery. The surgeon as "hero" had arrived.

By 1900 surgeons were beginning to operate on the brain and abdomen—areas that even a few decades before had been seen as too delicate for surgery. But if surgery grew up in the nineteenth-century hospital, it came of age on the battlefields of the twentieth century. Many of the surgical specialties established by the 1950s—orthopedics, trauma surgery, neurosurgery—had emerged in military hospitals during the First and Second World Wars. With this specialization came even greater reputation. Even in the early twenty-first century, when many aspects of medicine are challenged and contested, surgery has managed to retain its aura of heroism and expertise. *See also* Corpses and

Epidemic Disease; Disinfection and Fumigation; Hospitals and Medical Education in Britain and the United States; Hospitals in the West to 1900; Hospitals since 1900; Medical Education in the West, 1500–1900.

Further Reading

Bynum, W. F., et al. *The Western Medical Tradition, 1800–2000*. New York: Cambridge University Press, 2006.

Lawrence, Christopher, and Richard Dixey. "Practicing on Principle: Joseph Lister and the Germ Theories of Disease." In *Medical Theory, Surgical Practice: Studies in the History of Surgery*, edited by Christopher Lawrence, pp. 153–215. New York: Routledge, 1992.

Worboys, Michael. *Spreading Germs: Disease Theories and Medical Practice in Britain, 1865–1900*. New York: Cambridge University Press, 2000.

RICHARD BARNETT

SWEATING SICKNESS. Commonly referred to as the "English Sweat"—Sudor Anglicanus—this mystery disease struck England in 1485, 1508, 1517, 1528, and 1551. The first outbreak of the sweating sickness was coupled with Henry VII Tudor's (1457–1509) invasion of England in August 1485, leading some commentators to argue that the disease was imported from France. There also appears to have been a widespread but short-lived outbreak on the continent, most notably a two-week visitation in Germany in July 1529. At Marburg it interrupted the Colloquy between Reformation leaders Martin Luther (1483–1546) and Huldrych Zwingli (1484–1531) and left 500 dead in Amsterdam and 1,000 to 2,000 in Hamburg.

This disease illustrates the hazards of diagnosing diseases in the past based on symptoms alone, as it has been diagnosed as several different ailments by modern scholars, and by none convincingly. John Caius (1510–1573), the noted English **physician**, provided the best description of the disease's symptoms in 1552, based on his observation of the 1551 outbreak. The sweating sickness had a sudden onset and ran a 3- to 14-day course. It was characterized by symptoms reputedly more severe than those of **bubonic plague** with a high fever, pain in the extremities and back, vomiting, bleeding, and diarrhea, and it might include multiple organ failure. Most reports of the disease occurred during the summer and early autumn. "The sweat" generally started in rural areas, especially the west of England, but produced higher death rates when it arrived in London and other cities. The disease respected no social class, and nobles as well as peasants died from the sweat. The suddenness of the onset of the disease often led to immediate death, a characteristic described by Caius in *A Boke or Counseill Against the Disease Called the Sweate* (10): "But that immediately killed some in opening their windows, some in playing with children in their street doors, some in one hour, many in two it destroyed." Those who survived the initial onset of the disease could expect a long convalescence. In sum, contemporaries viewed the sweating sickness as often a killer, feared by all.

The English Sweat has been diagnosed as **influenza, typhus, Hantavirus,** and spring-summer **encephalitis** among others. A new leading candidate emerged in 1999—Crimean Congo hemorrhagic fever (CCHF)—but it, too, is subject to challenge. CCHF is caused by a **virus,** but other potential diagnoses have **bacterial** agents, and one interesting possibility—**Babesia**—is a **protozoan** disease. From its symptoms, it appears that the sweating sickness is a vector-borne disease rather than one passed directly from one person to another. The sweating sickness remains a mystery disease with no clearly identified agent of disease, no sure reason for its onset in 1485, and no explanation as to why it vanished in 1551. *See also* Diagnosis of Historical Diseases; Hemorrhagic Fevers; Historical Epidemiology; Plague in Britain, 1500–1647.

Further Reading

Caius, John. "A Boke or Counseill Against the Disease Commonly Called the Sweate." In *The Works of John Caius, M.D.*, edited by E. S. Roberts. Cambridge: Cambridge University Press, 1912.

Carlton, J. R., and P. W. Hammond. "The English Sweating Sickness: A New Perspective on Disease Etiology." *Journal of the History of Medicine and Allied Sciences* 54 (1999): 23–54.

Dyer, Alan. "The English Sweating Sickness of 1551: An Epidemic Anatomized." *Medical History* 41 (1997): 362–384.

Slack, Paul. "Mortality Crises and Epidemic Disease in England, 1485–1610." In *Health and Mortality in the Sixteenth Century*, edited by Charles Webster, pp. 9–59. New York: Cambridge University Press, 1979.

Taviner, M., et al. "The English Sweating Sickness, 1485–1551: A Viral Pulmonary Disease?" *Medical History* 42 (1998): 96–98.

JOHN M. THEILMANN

SYDENHAM, THOMAS (1624–1689). Known as the English **Hippocrates**, Thomas Sydenham was the greatest medical practitioner of his day. A close friend of the **physician** and empirical philosopher John Locke, Sydenham rejected traditional medical practice in favor of firsthand observation and description of suffering patients. Although an avid classifier of diseases, in the spirit of the **Scientific Revolution**, he avoided discussion of ultimate causes of disease and accepted **humoral theory**. He did, however, note that a given disease is the same in "a Socrates or a simpleton" and is not particular to an individual.

The son of a country gentleman, Thomas studied medicine sporadically at Oxford, between hitches with the Parliamentarian cavalry during the English Civil War. He was rewarded with a fellowship at All Souls College, which he abandoned in 1655 when he married. Settling in London, he conducted a medical practice among the poor, during which he carefully compiled his observations of symptoms and the courses of illnesses. He fled London during the Great Plague of 1665, though not before observing a case of plague in Westminster, and published his *Method of Curing Fevers* the following year. A second edition, including a section on plague, appeared in 1668, and a greatly expanded version, titled *Medical Observations*, was released in 1676. This earned him a medical doctorate from Cambridge University, though he was never a full member of the College of Physicians or Royal Society, both of which privileged theory over practice and traditional credentials. Sydenham had little use for either, stressing in his works the importance of abandoning incorrect descriptive models for more accurate ones built up from actual experience.

Just as scientists were developing classification systems for rocks and plants, Sydenham sought to differentiate diseases as carefully as possible. This would, he believed, lead to far more effective treatments. He distinguished continual fevers such as **typhus** and **typhoid** from intermittent fevers like **malaria** and from the diseases whose symptoms included high fevers, plague and **smallpox**. He further distinguished smallpox into two types: the milder "distinct pox" and the very dangerous "flux pox." His erroneous notion that during an epidemic all other diseases convert to or develop into the epidemic disease, however, retarded advances in epidemiological thought until the development of germ theory in the later nineteenth century. In shorter published letters, he described and made recommendations for treating **measles, syphilis**, smallpox, and rheumatic fever. He also updated his *Observations* to include **epidemics** in London from 1675 to 1680.

Despite, or perhaps because of his rudimentary theoretical education in medicine, Sydenham rejected current practices such as medical **astrology** and dependence upon examination of urine and other human waste material, in favor of close attention to the sick human body itself. His descriptions of the symptomatic courses of diseases are thus highly detailed and unambiguous and provide his readers with clear guidelines for diagnosis. His disinterest in theory, however, left him with the **Galenic** model of the human humors, and most of his prescriptions—usually bleeding and inducing vomiting and defecation—directly reflect the limitations of that model. He also ignored the recent advances in human physiology, often made by men he knew. *See also* Plague in Britain, 1500–1647.

Further Reading

Dewhurst, Kenneth. *Dr. Thomas Sydenham: His Life and Original Writings.* Berkeley: University of California, 1966.
Meynell G. G. *Thomas Sydenham's Methodus Curandi Febres Propriis Observationibus Superstructura* [*Method of Treating Fevers*, with English translation]. Folkstone, UK: Winterdown Books, 1987.
———. "Sydenham, Locke, and Sydenham's *De peste sive febre pestilentiali*." *Medical History* 37 (1993): 330–332.

JOSEPH P. BYRNE

SYPHILIS.   Syphilis is caused by the **bacterium** *Treponema pallidum*. The infection occurs during vaginal, oral, or anal sexual intercourse with an infected person. The disease is characterized by three stages. The primary infection begins with a painless sore at the site of infection, usually the genital area. If left untreated, the sore heals within a few weeks, and the disease continues into a secondary stage. At this stage, it can mimic a lot of other diseases, which is why it has been nicknamed "The Great Imitator." After around one to three months, the symptoms usually disappear, and the further course is clinically quiescent. This so-called "latent" stage, during which the infection can only be detected by blood tests, can last a lifetime or, after decades, enter the final, tertiary stage with symptoms appearing on the skin and the in central nervous system, the so called "neurosyphilis."

Treatment for syphilis is simple. Depending on the stage, one to three shots of the **antibiotic penicillin** are sufficient. Infusions of penicillin are required in every stage whenever the central nervous system is affected.

Biological Agent and Its Effects on the Human Body.   Syphilis is caused by *Treponema pallidum*, a spiral-shaped bacterium of the genus *Spirochetae*. It was identified microscopically as the causative agent in 1905 by two Germans, the dermatologist Erich Hoffmann (1868–1959) and the zoologist **Fritz Richard Schaudinn**. The complete genetic code was sequenced and published in 1998 in the journal *Science*.

The disease is characterized by three distinct stages. After an asymptomatic period of about 21 days, the primary chancre, an almost painless sore, appears at the site of infection and heals spontaneously even when left untreated. A classic chancre is only seen in 60 percent of patients. It is usually located in the genital area, but it may also occur at other sites like the mouth.

In 70 to 80 percent of primary cases of syphilis, the lymph nodes of the groin are enlarged, though usually only on one side. At this stage, an examination in a special dark-field **microscope** can directly prove the presence of the bacteria, which are very motile and characterized by extreme bending in the middle. Blood investigations may yield negative results.

Six to twelve weeks after the onset of the primary chancre the patient enters the secondary stage. At that time, *Treponema pallidum* has been disseminated via the blood stream, and any organ can be affected. The secondary stage usually recedes in 4 to 12 weeks, even without treatment. Almost 60 percent of patients with latent or late syphilis deny a history of secondary disease, as the signs, unless severe, are easily overlooked and forgotten. The skin manifestations are termed "syphilids" and are observed in 80 to 95 percent of patients in the secondary stage. The skin rash, which usually occurs on the trunk, may have different patterns (e.g., spots, nodules, with or without scales). Spots and nodules on the palms and soles are very characteristic and strongly suggestive of syphilis. The face can be involved, especially the mid-face and the hairline, giving a crown-like pattern. Hair loss includes two types: hair thinning throughout the scalp and patchy, so-called moth-eaten, alopecia. Another skin sign is the so-called Condylomata lata in 20 to 70 percent of patients in the secondary stage. They are moist, flesh-colored nodules of the genital and anal area, full of *Treponema* bacteria and extremely infectious. In the mouth, flat sores may appear, and the patient can suffer from a sore throat. In over 85 percent of cases, the lymph nodes of the neck, axles, and groin are swollen.

Nearly all organs can be involved during secondary syphilis (e.g., mild swelling of the spleen, reduction of red blood cells, and acute inflammation of the kidneys, liver, and gut with bellyache); acute vision and hearing complications are typical clinical signs for the involvement of the central nervous system. Even bone and muscular symptoms are described.

Most of our knowledge of the natural course of syphilis is derived from the classical Oslo study, which was carried out in the pre-antibiotic era. It was conducted in Oslo, Norway, between 1891 and 1910, when 2,181 cases of syphilis were left untreated and the records of almost 1,000 patients were traced, analyzed, and reported in 1955. According to this study, an untreated patient usually becomes noninfectious as early as six months after the disease has been contracted.

If untreated, the asymptomatic latent stage follows the secondary stage in which the infection can only be proven by positive blood tests. This stage is called late latent syphilis and may continue for the rest of the lifetime in an asymptomatic form in about two-thirds of untreated patients. The other third develops tertiary syphilis, which becomes manifest as skin granulomas (called "gummas") (16 percent), or heart (9.6 percent) or central nervous system (6.5 percent) disease. The last is termed "neurosyphilis"

Transmission.   *Treponema pallidum* is transmitted by an infected person via vaginal, oral, or anal sexual intercourse. If the sore occurs in the mouth, transmission by open mouth kissing is possible. In rare cases, it may be transmitted by nonsexual contact in communities living under conditions of poor **personal hygiene**. Importantly, *Treponema* bacteria are very fragile, and infection can only occur through direct body contact and not by daily activities (e.g., touching toilet seats, using hot tubs, sharing cutlery).

A very special situation is the primarily infected pregnant woman in whom the *Treponema* bacteria can cross the placenta to infect the unborn child. **Children** born with "congenital syphilis" suffer from severe mental and physical disabilities, which is the reason why all pregnant women need to be screened for syphilis infection. A coinfection with other genital diseases such as genital cold sores eases and therefore may mask the discomfort associated with undiagnosed syphilis.

Epidemiology.   Though it first appeared in Western Europe in the later 1490s, syphilis is not only a disease of historical interest. Over the past 60 years, syphilis infection has fluctuated in the United States, as in other developed countries. Syphilis rates peaked during World **War** II, followed by a dramatic decrease, particularly as a result of the introduction of penicillin. Syphilis has been regarded as a typical example of a sexually transmitted infection that can be controlled by public health measures. There are several characteristics of *T. pallidum* that enhance prospects for control and eventual regional elimination: *T. pallidum* is an exclusively human pathogen and has no animal reservoir, and penicillin is still the treatment of choice without problems of antimicrobial resistance. Worldwide, penicillin mass treatment programs in most "hot spots" in the 1950s and 1960s were some of the most successful health programs of the **World Health Organization** (WHO).

However, syphilis remains a public health problem worldwide, and the WHO estimates that 12 million new cases of venereal syphilis occur worldwide annually, mainly in the developing countries, but also in the major urban areas of the United States and western Europe. In the latter, the infections have shifted to particular risk groups (e.g., outbreaks among male homosexuals and abusers of illegal drugs). In Russia and in much of eastern Europe, the reemergence of syphilis is contributing to the **HIV/AIDS epidemics**. Syphilis infection facilitates acquisition and transmission of the human immunodeficiency virus (HIV).

Control of the Disease.   Blood tests are carried out for screening in asymptomatic individuals as well as in patients with clinical symptoms to prove syphilis infection (e.g., in the second and third stages). A presumptive **diagnosis** is possible with the use of two types of blood tests for syphilis. The first is a nontreponemal test, which detects the patient's immune response (antibodies directed against the bacteria's membrane) and are used for monitoring syphilis activity and treatment response. These tests have their limitations because they may yield false positive results in patients not infected with *T. pallidum*. The second type of test, a treponemal specific test, provides evidence of infection.

There is no vaccine for the prevention of syphilis infection. Therefore, the disease has to be treated whenever it is diagnosed. Penicillin is the preferred drug for treatment of all stages of syphilis. Primary and early secondary syphilis is treated with one shot; latent syphilis and tertiary syphilis are treated with three shots of penicillin. Whenever the nervous system is involved, penicillin infusions for 10 to 14 days are required.

Current State of the Disease.   As infection rates in the developed world have been low for decades, most physicians in the developed world are no longer familiar with the symptoms of syphilis. The recent outbreaks of syphilis in urban areas in the United States and western Europe since the beginning of the millennium have completely changed the situation. Awareness in the medical community as well as the public about the possibility of infection with *Treponema pallidum* has had to be reestablished through education and health campaigns. In patients with symptoms pointing at treponemal infection, blood tests for syphilis should be performed deliberately. Screening schedules for syphilis in asymptomatic patients should be maintained and reestablished, respectively. Risk groups at focus are HIV-positive men who have sex with men, prostitutes, and illegal drug abusers.

Because of limited financial resources, there is a different attitude and medical approach in the developing world, where most new infections occur. Screening in these countries can only be focused on the identification of newly infected patients in the primary and secondary stages of syphilis, who can transmit the disease to their sexual partners and, in the case of pregnancy, to unborn children. In these countries, routine screening with at least a non-treponemal test that is cheap but unspecific for syphilis should be performed on a wide scale. *See also* Disease in the Pre-Columbian Americas; Fracastoro, Girolamo; Gonorrhea and Chlamydia; Human Immunity and Resistance to Disease; Paracelsus; Sexual Revolution; Syphilis in Sixteenth-Century Europe; Venereal Disease and Social Reform in Progressive-Era America.

Further Reading

Centers for Disease Control and Prevention. *Syphilis*. http://www.cdc.gov/std/syphilis/default.htm

Clancy, Neil, University of Florida. http://medinfo.ufl.edu/other/histmed/clancy/

Harvard University Library. *Contagion*. http://ocp.hul.harvard.edu/contagion/syphilis.htm

Hayden, Deborah. *Pox: Genius, Madness, and the Mysteries of Syphilis*. New York: Basic Books, 2004.

Holmes, King K., et al. *Sexually Transmitted Diseases*, 4th edition. Columbus, OH: McGraw-Hill, 2007.

Mayo Clinic. *Syphilis*. http://www.mayoclinic.com/health/syphilis/DS00374

Quétel, Claude. *History of Syphilis*. Baltimore: Johns Hopkins University Press, 1990.

Shmaefsky, Brian. *Syphilis*. Philadelphia: Chelsea House, 2003.

Wöhrl, Stefan, and Alexandra Geusau. "Clinical Update: Syphilis in Adults." *Lancet* 369 (June 9, 2007): 1912–1914.

World Health Organization. *Syphilis*. http://www.who.int/reproductive-health/publications/rtis_gep/syphilis.htm

STEFAN WÖHRL AND ALEXANDRA GEUSAU

SYPHILIS IN SIXTEENTH-CENTURY EUROPE.   The virulent irruption of previously unknown **syphilis** in Europe at the end of the fifteenth century introduced a very significant health problem. This was the first known epidemic of a sexually transmitted disease in the West, though there is no consensus on the reasons for its surge at this time.

At the end of the fifteenth century, several authors from Germany, Italy, and Spain discussed a strange, new disease. The German Joseph Grünpeck (c. 1473–1532) published his *Treatise on the Flowing Pestilence, or the French Disease* (Augsburg, 1496) in both Latin and German. In it he explained the emergence of this **epidemic** as a function of celestial causes, as a divine punishment against an immoral world carried out through means of an adverse celestial conjunction. This conjunction of planets, he believed, provoked the pestilential corruption of **air** that poisoned its victims. In this and other ways the era's **physicians** followed the pattern set for explaining and dealing with the plague. The physician Niccolò Leoniceno (1428–1524) participated in the medical dispute at the court of Ferrara, Italy, in the spring of 1497 over the nature of this mysterious sickness. He claimed that syphilis was not new but had been known to and described by classical medical writers. He published his thesis in *Booklet on the Epidemic that Is Commonly Called the French Disease* (Venice, 1497), but despite thorough research, he was not able to prove this assertion.

Avoiding **astrology** and humanism, Spanish physician to the Papal Court Gaspar Torrella (1452–1520) approached the novel disease in a more clinical way. He composed the *Treatise with Advice Against "Pudendagram" or the French Disease* (Rome, 1497). Torrella based his book on a study of 16 case histories, revealing the fruits of careful observations of the pathologic phenomenon but staying within the traditional framework of medical interpretation and explanation. Another Spanish doctor, Francisco López de Villalobos (1473–1549), published *A Summa on Medicine, with a Treatise on the "Bubas" Pestilence* (pox) (Salamanca, 1498). The appended treatise on pox (syphilis) is considered one of the best of all works on the subject in the fifteenth and sixteenth centuries.

Several books written during the first third of the sixteenth century contain carefully drawn verbal pictures of the effects of syphilis. One example is Grünpeck's second book, *Booklet on Mentulagra, Otherwise Known as the French Disease* (1503). Another is the text of German Ulrich von Hutten (1488–1523; *On the Medicine Guaiacum and the French Disease, Book One* [Mainz, 1503]), in which he recorded the benefits he personally received from the use of the new drug guaiacum—derived from South American trees. In a similar vein, the Spaniard Francisco Delicado (c. 1475–1535) wrote *How to Use the Wood of the West Indies: A Healthful Remedy for Every Injury and Incurable Illness* (Rome, 1525).

Undoubtedly, the best work on syphilis, because of its clinical excellence and its literary quality, is the poem *Syphilis, or the French Disease* (Verona, 1530), by the famed Italian physician **Girolamo Fracastoro**. Originally a pastoral character in this work, Syphilis soon became synonymous with the disease itself. In poetic form, Fracastoro summarized his era's knowledge of the disease and imputed sexual transmission to syphilis ("most obscene," he says). In the first of the poem's three books, Fracastoro describes a terrible and new malady that is the result of a fatal conjunction of the planets Jupiter, Mars, and Saturn (a specific conjunction elsewhere blamed for plague). He also links the appearance of the disease in Italy to the French invasion of the 1490s and later military campaigns—from which it received its original popular name, the "French disease." The second book deals with treatment. He prescribed a classical regimen of health and medication but also praised the curative properties of mercury. A good humanist, Fracastoro wraps this in a fable of one Ilceus, on whom Apollo inflicted this disease. The lad is thrice dipped in a stream of mercury ("living silver") by a wood nymph and cured. In the third, Fracastoro praises the glory of the transoceanic discoveries and presents another myth. In the New World, a Spanish army discovers a village of natives whose skins are covered by disgusting ulcers. Their chief explains that the shepherd Syphilis abandoned worship of the sun and received this tremendous scourge from on high, as will all infidels thereafter. The helpful nymph America, however, transplants to this land the beneficent tree, the guaiacus, which will heal them (as it did Von Hutten).

Though modern specialists still argue about the ultimate source of syphilis, most early German, Italian, and Spanish writers blamed its origins and spread on the French, during whose aggression in Italy the disease first clearly appeared. By the 1520s, however, the idea of an American origin emerged, as reflected in Fracastoro's poem. Gonzalo Fernández de Oviedo (1478–1557) clearly sustains this opinion in his *Summary of the Natural History of the Indies* (1526). The first doctor who supported this idea with data was Rodrigo Ruiz Díaz de Isla (1462–1542), in his *Treatise on the "serpentine" disease* (Seville, 1539; composed in 1520). This surgeon explained that an unknown disease, neither seen nor described before, had its origin in Haiti and appeared in Barcelona in 1493. Chroniclers claimed that syphilis was a very common, light, benign, and cutaneous affliction in Indians that caused severe problems for the Spaniards. The "American thesis" explains that the infection was brought back to Spain by Columbus's crews and carried to Italy by Spanish troops. During the siege of Naples, the disease was transmitted to French soldiers of Charles VIII: hence the French name, *mal de Naples*. When the war ended, the troops went back to their respective countries spreading the disease.

But there is **paleopathological** evidence suggesting the existence of syphilis in Europe before Columbus's voyage. Current epidemiological theories maintain that the disease was in existence on all continents before 1492, and certain changes in conditions provoked an increase in the severity of syphilis at roughly that time.

The symptoms of syphilis were acute and dramatic: rashes, eruptions, and ulcers of the skin and mucous membrane of the pharynx, complete alopecia, severe articular pain, and quick organic consumption. From the beginning, its contagious character was patent, but doctors discovered only belatedly its venereal origin. Therefore, the preventive measures were generally those for the plague (**personal hygiene** and appropriate **diet**, public sanitation and **quarantine**). Special preparations of mercury, however, were soon employed as a specific and useful treatment. Though highly toxic to the body as well as to the pathogen, its successes supported the new, iatrochemical approaches of **Paracelsus** and the **Paracelsians**. Another medication also appeared in the epidemic's early stages: the ingestion of large quantities of the decoction of the American guaiacum wood (*Guaiacum officinale*). Though it had little effect, doctors believed the treatment for a disease was to be found naturally in the disease's place of origin.

Both medications were expensive, and the social problem was how to attend to all poor victims of the disease. Special **hospitals** for this duty were set up in Italy during the sixteenth century: the *incurabili* (incurables) hospitals. The Genoese Hospital of the Ridotto is probably one example. The Ridotto accepted the syphilitic poor because they were rejected by the other hospitals because of their incurable disease. Bologna and Ferrara established hospitals for the treatment of syphilis, and in Milan and Orvieto portions of the general hospitals were devoted to syphilitic patients. During the 10 years between 1515 and 1526, another seven incurabili hospitals were founded, and three more included special wards in existing hospitals in several Italian cities. *See also* Astrology and Medicine; Colonialism and Epidemic Disease; Contagion Theory of Disease, Premodern; Diagnosis of Historical Diseases; Disease in the Pre-Columbian Americas; Historical Epidemiology; Humoral Theory; Medical Education in the West, 1100–1500; Plague and Developments in Public Health, 1348–1600; Plague in Europe, 1500–1770s; Poverty, Wealth, and Epidemic Disease; Religion and Epidemic Disease; Sexuality, Gender, and Epidemic Disease; War, the Military, and Epidemic Disease

Further Reading

Allen, Peter Lewis. "The Just Rewards of Unbridled Lust: Syphilis in Early Modern Europe." In *The Wages of Sin: Sex and Disease, Past and Present*, edited by Peter Lewis Allen, pp. 41–60. Chicago: University of Chicago Press, 2000.

Amundsen, Darrel W. "The Moral Stance of the Earilest Syphilographers, 1495–1505." In *Medicine, Society, and Faith in the Ancient and Medieval Worlds*, edited by Darrel W. Amundsen, pp. 310–372. Baltimore: Johns Hopkins University Press, 1996.

Arrizabalaga, Jon, John Henderson, and Roger French. *The Great Pox: The French Disease in Renaissance Europe*. New Haven: Yale University Press, 1997.

Eamon, W. "Cannibalism and Contagion: Framing Syphilis in Counter-Reformation Italy." *Early Science and Medicine* 3 (1998): 1–31.

Fabricius, Johannes. *Syphilis in Shakespeare's England*. London: Kingsley, 1994.

Foa, Anna. "The New and the Old: The Spread of Syphilis (1494–1530)." In *Sex and Gender in Historical Perspective*, edited by Edward Muir and Guido Ruggiero, pp. 26–45. Baltimore: Johns Hopkins University Press, 1990.

McGough, Laura J. "Demons, Nature, or God? Witchcraft Accusations and the French Disease in Early Modern Venice." *Bulletin of History of Medicine* 80 (2006): 219–246.

Quétel, Claude. *History of Syphilis*. Baltimore: John Hopkins University Press, 1990.

Siena, Kevin, ed. *Sins of the Flesh: Responding to Sexual Disease in Early Modern Europe*. Toronto: Centre for Reformation and Renaissance Studies, 2005.

Stein, Claudia. "The Meaning of Signs: Diagnosing the French Pox in Early Modern Ausburg." *Bulletin of the History of Medicine* 80 (2006): 617–648.

JUSTO HERNÁNDEZ

T

TB. *See* Tuberculosis.

THEILER, MAX (1899–1972).   Epidemiologist Max Theiler is best known for developing the first **vaccinations** that could immunize humans against **yellow fever**. He received the Nobel Prize for Physiology or Medicine in recognition of this achievement in 1951.

Theiler was born in Pretoria, South Africa, the son of Sir Arnold Theiler (1867–1936), a veterinary scientist who did research in veterinary **immunology**. Max began his medical education at the University of Cape Town Medical School, but in 1918 he transferred to London to study at St. Thomas Hospital and the London School of Tropical Medicine. He received his medical degree in 1922 and became a Licentiate of the Royal College of Physicians and a Member of the Royal College of Surgeons. After graduation, Theiler took a post in the Department of Tropical Medicine at the Harvard Medical School in Boston, Massachusetts, where he studied a number of infectious diseases, including amoebic **dysentery**, rat bite fever, and yellow fever. In 1930 he joined the International Health Division of the **Rockefeller Foundation** in New York City, where he continued his research on yellow fever. He accepted a position as professor of **epidemiology** and microbiology at Yale University in 1964 and remained there until his retirement in 1967.

In the 1920s, scientists sought to identify the specific factor that caused yellow fever. By 1927 Theiler had proven that the disease was caused not by a **bacterium** but by a filterable **virus** that he hoped to cultivate in the laboratory. At the time, rhesus monkeys were the only animals known to be susceptible to yellow fever, but they were expensive as laboratory animals, so Theiler searched for a less expensive alternative. By 1930 he discovered a means of infecting mice with the yellow fever virus by injecting pieces of infected monkey liver into their heads. Using this procedure, Theiler isolated a strain of the virus that was extremely deadly in mice but that would barely produce a fever when injected into monkeys. Furthermore, he proved that when this strain, which was attenuated, or weakened, in monkeys, was introduced under the skin of humans, it provided immunity to the disease. There were complications associated with this early **vaccination** in some patients, however, so Theiler tried to isolate a safer strain to use in a vaccine. In a new series of experiments, he cultivated the yellow fever virus in chick embryos and by 1937 had managed to develop a safer attenuated virus, named "17D," which was more suitable for use as a vaccine. Thereafter, the Rockefeller Foundation mass-produced 17D vaccine and distributed it without cost to 33 tropical countries from 1940 to 1947. *See also* Yellow Fever in Latin America and the Caribbean, 1830–1940.

Further Reading

Norrby, E. "Yellow Fever and Max Theiler: The Only Nobel Prize for a Virus Vaccine." *Journal of Experimental Medicine* 204 (2007): 2779–2784.

Theiler, Max. "The Development of Vaccines against Yellow Fever." In *Physiology or Medicine: Nobel Lectures Including Presentation Speeches and Laureate's Biographies*, Nobel Foundation, volume 3 (Amsterdam: Elsevier Publishing Company, 1964) pp. 351–359.

Williams, Greer. *The Plague Killers*. New York: Charles Scribner's Sons, 1969.

WILLIAM H. YORK

THIRD PLAGUE PANDEMIC.   *See* Bubonic Plague in the United States; Plague in Africa: Third Pandemic; Plague in China; Plague in East Asia: Third Pandemic; Plague in India and Oceania: Third Pandemic; Plague in San Francisco, 1900–1908.

THIRTY YEARS' WAR.   The Thirty Years' War (1618–1648), fought in the area of modern Germany and its neighbors, is the classic example of a "military mortality crisis," in which war drives a dramatic increase in civilian mortality.

The war was, on one level, a conflict between Catholics and Protestants. As it proceeded, however, almost every major European power, from Spain to Sweden, became involved at one stage or another, and the war became a struggle for European hegemony in which religious differences were secondary. It evolved into the largest war that had been seen in continental Europe since at least Roman times.

The epidemic disease environment of the time was hostile. **Bubonic plague** was an ordinary hazard of life; the major German city of Augsburg had suffered plague in 17 of the 100 years prior to the outbreak of the war. Reports of significant epidemics of other diseases such as **typhus**, dysentery, and **smallpox** were comparatively rare, however. Dearths and famines caused by adverse weather conditions were by no means unknown; there was a sequence of poor harvests in Germany between 1622 and 1628, and a Europe-wide harvest failure occurred in 1635.

During the Thirty Years' War, the population of Germany declined by perhaps a third in urban areas and 40 percent in rural areas. Because the urban population was very small, the key figure is the latter. Although a decline in the birth rate and net emigration played a part in this decline, the major factor was an increase in mortality caused largely by plague and starvation. The classical view is that the exceptional mortality was caused by an unusually rapid geographical spread of epidemic disease, itself caused by troop movements and civilian **flight** from areas affected by war, and by nutritional stress caused by troops who requisitioned and plundered food from the peasantry.

Recent research has deepened this account, emphasizing the "socioeconomic relations of warfare." It focuses on the nature of the relationship between soldiers and the civilians on whom they depended for food, fodder, and shelter. In the Thirty Years' War these relationships gradually became marked by disorder, wanton destruction, violence, and atrocity. By the mid-1620s in some areas, and the 1630s in others, civilians had learned to dread the soldiery and to flee their villages at the first sign of the soldiers' approach. It was these hostile and highly violent relations between the soldiery and civilians that undermined the ability of civilians to feed themselves and led to the frequent and widespread civilian flight of the classical account. *See also* Diet, Nutrition, and Epidemic Disease; Plague in Europe, 1500–1770s; Religion and Epidemic Disease; Typhus and War; War, the Military, and Epidemic Disease.

Further Reading

Asch, Ronald. *The Thirty Years War: The Holy Roman Empire and Europe, 1618–1648.* Basingstoke: Macmillan, 1997.

Outram, Quentin. "The Socio-Economic Relations of Warfare and the Military Mortality Crises of the Thirty Years' War." *Social Science History* 45 (2001): 151–184.

Parker, Geoffrey, ed. *The Thirty Years' War.* London: Routledge, 1997.

QUENTIN OUTRAM

TRADE, TRAVEL, AND EPIDEMIC DISEASE.   The role of trade and travel in the spread of infectious diseases is an ancient one. Wherever humans travel, microbes accompany them. The mobility of humans, ground **animals**, birds, and **insects** has been a continuing influence on patterns of infectious disease occurrence. The speed, volume, and reach of today's trade and travel are unprecedented in human history and offer multiple potential routes for microbial spread around the globe. **HIV/AIDS**, with its primate origins in central Africa, has spread quickly around the world in the past quarter-century. In 2003, **severe acute respiratory syndrome** (SARS) migrated out of the Chinese mainland and then radiated rapidly from Hong Kong to Vietnam, Europe, and Canada.

Vectors such as mosquitoes can travel with trade and transport. In the past several decades, a major mosquito vector for the **Dengue** fever **virus**, *Aedes albopictus* (the "Asian tiger mosquito"), has greatly increased its geographic range between continents. This has occurred, particularly, via the inadvertent intercontinental exportation of mosquito eggs in used car tires into Africa and the Americas. There have been countless other such episodes of geographic spread via trade and travel, over many centuries. The **Black Death** of the fourteenth century, which killed around one-third of the European population, is a well-known example. This dreaded bacterial infection, **bubonic plague**, entered Europe via infected black rats that had spread from the Asian steppes and then westward along the traders' Silk Road toward the Black Sea, an eastern portal to Europe, where it unleashed its devastation over the ensuing half-decade. Recurrences of plague in the European and Islamic worlds are often attributed to humans carrying the necessary rats and fleas along communication routes from reservoirs of endemic plague.

Historically, there were great equilibrations between the regional infectious disease pools across Eurasia during the millennia immediately before and after the time of Jesus Christ. These exchanges of microbes, often with devastating **epidemic** consequences, resulted from the various forms of intensified human contact—trade, travel, military incursions, and conflict. For example, the bubonic plague **bacterium**, *Yersinia pestis*, apparently accompanied Roman legions returning to Constantinople from the Middle East. Indeed, this mirrored the dissemination of the respiratory infection, **tuberculosis**, by Roman legions as they fanned out around the Roman Empire.

Trade. Advances in the ease and speed of transportation, first at sea and then on the land, created new and tighter networks of contact that widened and quickened the spread of epidemic disease and prompted new thinking about it. In mid-nineteenth-century London, Dr. **John Snow** noted that epidemics of cholera followed major routes of commerce between Asia and Europe, consistently appearing first at seaports when entering a new region. Outbreaks of cholera occasionally appeared beyond its natural "homeland." Although this occurred on a localized scale several times during the seventeenth century, it did so more substantively in 1817 as British military and colonial activity in India increased. In 1854 Snow observed that "cholera began to spread to an extent not before known; and, in the course of seven years, it reached, eastward, to China and the Philippine Islands; southward to Mauritius and Bourbon; and to the northwest as far as Persia and Turkey. Its approach towards our own country [England], after it entered Europe, was watched with more intense anxiety than its progress in other directions."

Indeed, cholera provides an excellent example of the role of travel, trade, and human migration (including troop movements) in the localized and, then, distant spread of infectious disease. The disease appears be ancient: descriptions in ancient Hindu, Chinese, and Greek texts from 2,000 to 3,000 years ago refer to severe outbreaks of cholera-like dehydrating diarrheal diseases. Cholera's ancestral homeland appears to have been along rivers and estuaries in India, particularly in the populous basins of the Ganges and Brahmaputra rivers. Cholera epidemics, however, appeared outside south and east Asia with the acceleration of trade and European colonization in the region during the nineteenth century. Discrete epidemic waves over the course of the century challenged early epidemiologists to identify the spatial and temporal factors connected to epidemics, and led to International Sanitary Congresses in which national delegates debated the best ways of containing epidemics without undermining trade.

In the twentieth century, advances in epidemiology have accompanied the even more dramatic evolution in transportation and continue to clarify the relationship of human movement and disease. The still-continuing seventh pandemic of cholera is the largest and longest ever. It began in 1961 and has engulfed Southeast Asia, the Middle East, Russia, Europe, much of Africa (where it has now become endemic for the first time), and the Americas. In 1991 it entered Latin America, where it subsequently caused over 1 million cases and around 12,000 deaths. This distant spread has been attributed to the dumping of cholera-contaminated ship's ballast water off the Peruvian coast—and that at a time when coastal waters were unusually warm (during an El Niño meteorological event) and conducive to the amplification of the cholera *Vibrio* in plankton and its subsequent entry into the local marine food chain, leading to human consumption.

Inadvertent epidemic-related biological introductions through trade also underscored the importance of surveillance of nonhuman activity. The vector mosquito of African **malaria**, *Anopheles gambiae*, entered Brazil for the first time in 1937. The mosquito migrated on the mail boats from western Africa that crossed the Atlantic in just three to four days. This same mosquito species then spread along the Brazilian coastal region and inland and caused up to 50,000 malaria deaths. Fortunately, an extraordinary campaign, led by the American Fred Soper (1893–1977), eliminated this mosquito species from Brazil in the early 1940s.

In recent times, the globalization of food production and distribution has amplified the movement of pathogens from one region to another. For example, an outbreak of cholera in the 1990s in Maryland was traced to the importation of contaminated frozen coconut milk. Alfalfa sprouts grown from contaminated seeds sent to a Dutch grower-and-shipper led to outbreaks of Salmonella food poisoning in both the United States and Finland.

Regional free trade agreements have both caused and brought to light various examples of how intensified, deregulated market competition can heighten the risks of infectious diseases in disempowered and poorly educated workers. For example, in the 1990s there were several outbreaks of **hepatitis** A and cyclosporiasis (a protozoan infection) in the United States caused by fecally contaminated strawberries and raspberries imported from Central America. The North American Free Trade Agreement had eroded environmental and labor standards (such as providing toilet facilities for workers) in the face of the demands of open competition and profitability. This, plus modern rapid air-transport, meant that within two days of the berries being picked, upmarket diners in New York would acquire the same fecally transmitted infections as the dispossessed farm workers in Guatemala.

Travel.   From its points of origin in central and western Africa, **HIV/AIDS** burst on the world scene in the 1980s. Long-distance travel had a great deal to do with its rapid spread. It is widely thought that Cuban troops sent by Fidel Castro to Africa, to assist the quelling of a local conflict, acquired this sexually transmitted disease and took it back to the Caribbean, from whence its subsequent spread was aided particularly by gay sex tourism. In the last 50 years, soldiers, tourists, businesspeople, and even **pilgrims** have all unwittingly contributed to the spread of infectious disease. *Neisseria meningitides* is a pathogen that has long caused seasonal epidemics of **meningitis** in parts of Africa: the so-called "meningitis belt." The disease has recently spread more widely. Studies with molecular markers have shown how Muslim pilgrims who brought an epidemic strain of *N. meningitides* from southern Asia to Mecca in 1987 then passed it on to pilgrims from Sub-Saharan Africa—who, after returning home, were the cause of strain-specific epidemic outbreaks in 1988 and 1989.

West Nile Virus disease (WNV), newly introduced to North America, further illustrates the impact of long-distance trade and travel. The disease has its origins in Africa, and it occurs sporadically in the Middle East and parts of Europe. It was unknown in North America until it arrived in New York in 1999, via an infected *Culex* mosquito on an airplane. There were apparently favorable conditions for the virus to survive and spread within New York City. Early season rain and summer drought provided ideal conditions for *Culex* mosquitoes. July 1999 was the hottest July on record for New York City. Suburban/urban ecosystems supported high numbers of select avian host and mosquito vector species adapted to those conditions. Furthermore, large populations of susceptible bird species existed, especially crows. Suburban/urban ecosystems were conducive for close interactions among mosquitoes, birds, and humans.

West Nile Virus affected birds first; then, as temperature and rainfall changed, the birds left town, and humans became the preferred target for the vector mosquitoes. The disease subsequently spread across the United States and established itself as an endemic virus in a majority of states, harbored by animals (including birds and horses) and transmitted via culicine mosquitoes. There was a marked increase in the number of human cases of

WNV disease during 2002–2003, involving many U.S. states. Today, the disease is well established in a majority of U.S. states.

In July 2003, Mexico declared a state of emergency when West Nile Virus arrived in that country. There had been concern that the disease could spread more rapidly in Central and South America than in North America. Latin American countries could be ideal breeding grounds because of their warmer climate, large bird populations, and year-round mosquito activity. Ecologists have anticipated an increasing range of adverse affects of the WNV infection on domesticated horses and on the diverse animal and bird life in the tropics.

Trade and Travel Combined: Severe Acute Respiratory Syndrome.   SARS emerged from Guangzhong Province in southern China in late 2002, and by year's end, 25 persons in the capital Guanghzou had developed this severe respiratory disease. Soon the disease reached adjoining Hong Kong, where both hospital "super-spreading" and defective sewerage design in high-rise housing amplified the spread. By March–April 2003, cases began to be reported more widely, especially from Canada. Propelled by modern air travel, SARS extended to all continents and 31 countries. Its rapid dissemination to dozens of countries in the first half of 2003, infecting over 8,000 persons and killing one-tenth of them, and its ominous pandemic potential, captured headlines for months.

The actual zoonotic source of the SARS coronavirus, for a while uncertain, is now thought to be a rainforest bat. The evidence suggests that, from this natural animal source, the virus reached humans via the long-distance trading of live wild animals, themselves incidentally infected by the bat virus. Infection of palm civet cats with the SARS virus has been reported. Surveys have shown that the live markets and restaurants in Guangzhong sold various species of small carnivores (e.g., civet cat, raccoon dog, and ferret badger) that were captured in China, Laos, Vietnam, and Thailand, transported to markets (often across national borders), and thereby brought into close proximity with one another.

This type of unregulated trade, and the conditions of the wet markets with live animals for sale, means that infectious agents have great opportunities to move between edible species. Further, the recent popularization and intensification of what was previously a restricted and local practice has escalated urban demand for exotic animal foods in Southern China, and this has greatly amplified the health risks of what previously were localized cultural practices in rural settings.

Dengue Fever.   Dengue fever is numerically the most important vector-borne viral disease of humans. The Dengue virus causes almost 100 million cases of infection each year, with high fatality rate in young **children**. This **hemorrhagic fever** is a good example of how patterns of trade, travel, and settlement can all influence infectious diseases.

Dengue evolved as a specialized human infectious disease sometime during the past three centuries in Asia, apparently from a progenitor zoonotic (animal-to-human) virus that had originated in Africa. The disease then spread in a leisurely fashion between continents. Although details are not known, four different strains of the virus subsequently evolved, in relatively separate geographic regions.

Although Dengue, by its origins, is primarily a tropical disease, its extension in recent decades into various temperate countries reflects both the introduction of the disease's main mosquito vector species, *Aedes aegypti* (which is behaviorally adaptable to both a cooler climate and to an urbanized **environment**), and the increase in imported cases of Dengue resulting from increased travel. The disease was brought under substantial control in the 1930s and 1940s, via mosquito spraying programs, but reestablished itself widely after World War II with the aid of troop movements, increases in travel and trade, and premature relaxation of control programs. This increase in the range of Dengue also reflects the distinctive capacity for rapid evolutionary adjustment of the *Aedes aegypti* mosquito species to coexistence with urban-dwelling humans, having originated in the forests of Africa. Indeed, this mosquito species has followed humankind on its migrations around the world.

Conclusion.   As the diversity and intensity of human activities increases, with the growth of human numbers and wealth, so is there the likelihood that travel and trade will continue to fuel the emergence and spread of infectious diseases. The microbial world is protean in its diversity, strategies, and genetic flexibility, and this, in conjunction with continual changes in human ecology and behavior, ensures that there will be continuing unexpected infectious disease outbreaks. A recent example from the escalating international trade in exotic pets is illustrative: the monkey pox virus was recently introduced into the United States in imported African rodents, bought as illicit pets, with subsequent transmission of the virus to prairie dogs—some of which were then sold in pet shops; from them the virus passed to other pets and to their human owners.

There are, of course, many other permutations to these patterns and determinants of ever-changing infectious disease risks and ecological relationships. One important consideration is that the cross-species transmission of microorganisms can operate in both directions. That is, it can also entail nonhuman primate species and other wildlife being infected by human pathogens. There is speculation, for example, that the demise of the great mammoths of northern America around 13,000 years ago could have been, in part, a result of their infection by germs introduced by the newly arrived proto-Amerindians or their dogs. In modern times, the enteric pathogen, *Giardia* has been inadvertently introduced into the Ugandan mountain gorilla population by humans via contacts that have occurred during ecotourism and conservation activities. Similarly, nonhuman primates have acquired **measles** from ecotourists.

The grand and colorful narrative of microbial traffic among species continues. Indeed, it does so at an ever-faster pace, in a world in which human numbers are growing and human activities are intensifying. *See also* Animal Diseases (Zoonoses) and Epidemic Disease; Black Death, Flagellants, and Jews; Cholera: First through Third Pandemics, 1816–1861; Cholera: Fourth through Sixth Pandemics, 1862–1947; Cholera: Seventh Pandemic, 1961–Present; Colonialism and Epidemic Disease; Contagion and Transmission; Cordon Sanitaire; Early Humans, Infectious Diseases in; Epidemiology; Flight; Geopolitics, International Relations, and Epidemic Disease; Irish Potato Famine and Epidemic Disease, 1845–1850; Latin America, Colonial: Demographic Effects of Imported Diseases; Personal Liberties and Epidemic Disease; Plague: End of the Second Pandemic; Public Health Agencies, U.S. Federal; Quarantine; Slavery and Epidemic Disease; War, the Military, and Epidemic Disease.

Further Reading

Cohn, Samuel. *The Black Death Transformed: Disease and Culture in Early Renaissance Europe.* London: Edward Arnold Publishers, 2002.

McLean, Angela, et al., eds. *SARS: A Case Study in Emerging Infections.* New York: Oxford University Press, 2005.

McMichael, Anthony. *Human Frontiers, Environments and Disease: Past Patterns, Uncertain Futures.* New York: Cambridge University Press, 2001.

McNeill, William. *Plagues and Peoples.* New York: Penguin Books, 1994.

Sleigh, Adrian, et al., eds. *Population Dynamics and Infectious Diseases in Asia.* London: World Scientific, 2006.

Walters, Mark. *Six Modern Plagues, and How We Are Causing Them.* Washington, DC: Island Press, 2003.

Weiss, Robin, and Anthony McMichael. "Social and Environmental Risk Factors in the Emergence of Infectious Disease." *Nature Medicine* 10 (2004): 570–576.

ANTHONY MCMICHAEL

TRANSMISSION OF DISEASE.   *See* Contagion and Transmission.

TRAVEL.   *See* Trade, Travel, and Epidemic Disease.

TRYPANOSOMIASIS.   *See* Sleeping Sickness.

TUBERCULOSIS.   Tuberculosis (TB) is a very contagious, often lethal, bacterial disease resulting from the infection of the lungs and other tissues by the bacillus *Mycobacterium tuberculosis.* Mummified human remains found in both Egypt and Peru demonstrate that tuberculosis has been afflicting humankind for at least several thousand years. Over its history, the illness has been known by the Greek term *phthisis* (pronounced tee-sis) as well as the more general term "consumption," both of which refer to the way that tuberculosis victims seem to waste away, or be "consumed" by the illness. Its highly contagious nature makes tuberculosis an **epidemic** disease in industrializing societies where populations are densely packed and live in poor sanitary conditions. Currently, it is among the most widely spread microbial diseases in the developing world, infecting an estimated one-third of the world's population (more than 2 billion people) and causing between 2 and 3 million deaths per year. Strains of tuberculosis **bacteria** that are resistant to many, if not all, forms of **antibiotic** treatment are becoming more common—a fact which greatly complicates treatment. Overall, tuberculosis presents one of the greatest infectious disease challenges affecting humankind today.

Agent and Effects.   *Mycobacterium tuberculosis* is a rod shaped, Gram-positive bacillus that grows in a highly oxygenated (aerobic) environment. For this reason it grows preferentially in the lungs, but in about 15 percent of cases it infects other tissues such as the bones and lymph nodes, resulting in different disease symptoms. Tuberculosis infections begin when airborne bacteria contact the tissue of the lungs and are engulfed by macrophages (white blood cells). The bacteria have a waxy coating that resists digestion, allowing them to replicate inside the macrophages. More and more macrophages respond to the infection and are themselves infected, resulting in a hard lump of bacteria and dead tissue, called a tubercle (lump or knot), from which the disease takes its modern name. In most cases, the disease is halted at this stage and lies latent, with patients suffering few ill effects, although they will carry the bacteria with them for the rest of their lives. Such latent carriers of tuberculosis are always at risk of the disease becoming active. In approximately 5 to 10 percent of infections, the disease progresses to active tuberculosis, destroying the lungs through the creation of more tubercles and spreading throughout the body in a manner similar to the metastasis of cancer. Patients become weak and waste away; they cough severely, putting those around them at risk for infection. When tubercles form near blood vessels, the result is hemorrhaging in the lungs, causing the patient to cough up blood. Prior to antibiotic treatment, more than half of active tuberculosis cases resulted in death within five years.

Transmission.   Although it takes only a small amount of bacteria to lead to infection, in reality, prolonged exposure to a patient with active tuberculosis is usually necessary for transmission. Numerous variables including age, health, **nutrition**, and **environmental** conditions determine the overall susceptibility of an individual. **Heredity** also seems to play a role in individual susceptibility to tuberculosis. The overcrowded, unsanitary conditions of industrializing cities and prisons were ideal breeding grounds for tuberculosis in eighteenth- and nineteenth-century Europe and America; in England, mortality peaked in 1780 at 1.25 percent of the entire population per year. These conditions prevail in the expanding cities and badly managed prisons of poorer nations today, so that there are more people, in absolute numbers, sick and dying from tuberculosis in the twenty-first century than at any time in the past.

Tuberculosis and Society.   Inevitably, tuberculosis claimed the lives of many of the literary and artistic elite of industrial Europe and America. Among nineteenth-century victims, perhaps the most famous is the poet John Keats, who died of the illness at the age of only 26, but tuberculosis also ended the lives of American author Henry David Thoreau (1817–1862), Russian novelist Fyodor Dostoyevsky (1821–1881), the Polish composer Frédéric Chopin (1810–1849), and several members of the Brontë family. Notable twentieth-century victims include Russian author Anton Chekhov (1860–1904), Czech writer Franz Kafka (1883–1924), and English novelist George Orwell (1903–1950). Brilliant youth cut down in the prime of life is a theme that easily lent itself to drama and Romantic tragedy, and consequently tuberculosis became a fixture in literature and the theater in the nineteenth century. The romanticizing of tuberculosis was taken to such extremes that the physical appearance of individuals in the later stages of the disease— gaunt, pale, delicate—was celebrated as the aesthetic ideal for feminine beauty.

Research and Treatment.   In 1882 the German **physician Robert Koch** definitively identified *Mycobacterium tuberculosis* as the causal agent for consumption (for years thereafter, the bacillus was referred to as Koch's bacillus). This still ranks as one of the most profound achievements in the history of medicine, for not only did it provide a unifying theory and explanation for the various forms of tuberculosis, but it also helped usher in the **germ theory** of disease more generally and helped to establish a path toward more effective treatment.

Prior to Koch's work, the treatment of tuberculosis was a chronicle of applied superstition. For example, scrofula, a form of the disease in which the bacteria infect the lymph nodes of the neck, was believed to be curable by a touch from royalty; English monarchs upheld this tradition until the early 1700s. By the mid-nineteenth century, rest and fresh air were commonly prescribed, leading to the creation of **sanatoria** for the treatment of tuberculosis. Often built in isolated locales, sanatoria offered a retreat where the tubercular patient could partake of rest and fresh air while under the strict supervision of a medical staff. The association between tuberculosis and rest was carried to the tissues of the lung themselves; for years, physicians believed that "relaxation" of the lung was also an effective form of therapy. This relaxation of the tissue was achieved surgically, by collapsing one of the lungs. Today, surgery is sometimes used to remove portions (or all) of a tubercular lung in cases in which the disease is extremely advanced and aggressive.

The most effective treatment for tuberculosis is the use of antibiotics, but even this form of treatment is problematic. The tuberculosis bacillus replicates very slowly; because antibiotics affect bacteria during replication, it takes a very long time to treat

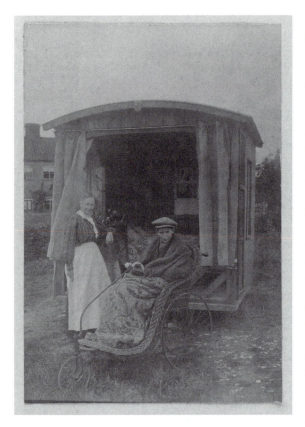

A boy or young man, suffering from pulmonary tuberculosis, sits in a Bath chair in front of his chalet, accompanied by a woman (presumably his mother). The chalet contains a bed and a chair, and is open, possibly to allow fresh air to circulate for the benefit of the inhabitant. Wellcome Library, London.

a tubercular patient. Therefore, antibiotic therapy ordinarily requires six months of disciplined and regular medication. In addition, tuberculosis can go dormant or remain inaccessible to drug treatment deep within diseased tissues. Patients often feel better and end their drug routines prematurely, contributing to the emergence of antibiotic resistant strains of the disease. Because tuberculosis is such a challenge, the **World Health Organization** currently recommends a comprehensive treatment strategy called Directly Observed Therapy (DOTS), which consists of a treatment regimen composed of several different drugs as well as outpatient care and observation to ensure patient compliance.

Vaccination. Since the 1920s, a vaccine for tuberculosis, called Bacille Calmette-Guérin (BCG) vaccine, named after its developers, has been available, but its effectiveness is still unclear. In the production of the vaccine, multiple strains of bacteria were used, resulting in inconsistent results. Many vaccine trials also suffered from a lack of rigor—in some, patients were not screened for latent tuberculosis before receiving the vaccine, and overall the dosage of the vaccine varied from trial to trial. It appears as though the vaccine is effective in preventing some of the more severe forms of the illness and is effective in protecting certain age groups, such as very young children. In other age groups, it seems to offer no protection at all.

Complicating matters is the fact that usage of the vaccine on a large scale makes diagnosis more challenging. Exposure to tuberculosis is usually determined by reaction to a test in which a protein derivative of the bacillus is injected under the skin. A positive reaction indicates infection, either latent or active. However, all patients who receive the BCG vaccine respond positively to the skin test, making it ineffective as a diagnostic tool. This undesirable side effect, coupled with the vaccine's general unreliability, has led the United States to reject the BCG vaccine as a preventive measure. After World War II, combinations of streptomycin, isoniazid, and para-aminosalicilic acid (PAS) proved so successful as an outpatient treatment that most sanatoria worldwide closed down by the 1980s. More recently, isoniazid has been coupled with rifampin and fluoroquinolones, but new challenges have emerged.

Future Research. Improved **diagnostic** tools are very badly needed, especially those that would allow physicians to distinguish quickly whether or not a patient is infected with drug-resistant strains of the bacillus. Here, rapid identification of specific genetic sequences via the technique known as polymerase chain reaction (PCR) is very promising. New drugs are needed as well, for two major reasons. The first is to combat extremely resilient forms of the bacillus. There are currently stains of tuberculosis known as XDR-TB (extremely drug-resistant) that defy treatment with virtually all known antibiotics. These strains have established themselves in vulnerable populations, such as those with **HIV/AIDS**, and are a serious threat to tuberculosis control. The second reason is to shorten treatment times. If new, more effective drugs can be developed that cut treatment time down from six months, patient compliance is likely to increase, improving the overall success rate of the therapy, reducing costs, and lowering the chances for the emergence of resistant strains. Research also continues on a more effective, consistent vaccine. *See also* Air and Epidemic Diseases; Contagion and Transmission; Drug Resistance in Microorganisms; Industrialization and Epidemic Disease; Industrial Revolution; Tuberculosis and Romanticism; Tuberculosis in England since 1500; Tuberculosis in North America since 1800; Tuberculosis in the Contemporary World; Urbanization and Epidemic Disease; Vaccination and Inoculation; War, the Military, and Epidemic Disease.

Further Reading

Centers for Disease Control and Prevention. *TB Introduction*. http://www.cdcnpin.org/scripts/tb/index.asp

Daniel, Thomas M. *Captain of Death: The Story of Tuberculosis*. Rochester, NY: University of Rochester Press, 1997.

Dormandy, Thomas. *The White Death: A History of Tuberculosis*. New York: New York University Press, 1999.

Dubos, René, and Jean Dubos. *The White Plague: Tuberculosis, Man, and Society*. New Brunswick, NJ: Rutgers University Press, 1987.

Markel, Howard. *When Germs Travel: Six Epidemics that Have Invaded America since 1900 and the Fears They Have Unleashed*. New York: Pantheon Books, 2004.

Mayo Clinic. *Tuberculosis*. http://www.mayoclinic.com/health/tuberculosis/DS00372

Reichmann, Lee B., with Janice Hopkins Tanne. *Timebomb: The Global Epidemic of Multi-Drug Resistant Tuberculosis*. New York: McGraw Hill, 2002.

World Health Organization. *Tuberculosis*. http://www.who.int/topics/tuberculosis/en/

JEFFREY LEWIS

TUBERCULOSIS AND ROMANTICISM.   **Tuberculosis** had long been prominent among Europe's poor and displaced, but as the eighteenth century drew to a close, a mushrooming **urbanization** brought about by the **Industrial Revolution** created an **epidemic** within Europe's upper and middle classes. Among the victims were some of the most creative figures of the Romantic era—writers John Keats (1795–1821), Percy Shelley (1792–1822), Emily (1818–1848) and Anne (1820–1849) Brontë, Branko Radečević (1824–1853), Johann Wolfgang von Goethe (1749–1832), Novalis (Friedrich Leopold von Hardenberg, 1772–1801), and Friedrich von Schiller (1759–1805); painters Franz Pforr (1788–1812) and Philippe Otto Runge (1777–1810); and musicians Frédéric Chopin (1810–1849), Niccolo Paganini (1782–1840), and Carl Maria von Weber (1786–1826). The unbridled passion these writers and musicians brought to their art in spite of their physical limitations soon led to the notion that the disease bestowed a heightened spiritual awareness and creative energy to its sufferers. The Romantic Movement to which these artists belonged was a revolt against the formal and rigid aesthetic standards of the period and emphasized a brooding quest for artistic inspiration, a reckless engagement with life, and an idyllic pursuit of the natural world. The idea that aesthetic genius could literally drain the life from an artist was just one more facet in the movement's understanding of the artistic enterprise. Over time, in spite of the vast number of **poverty**-stricken people who suffered from the disease, tuberculosis came to be considered a disease primarily of the upper and middle classes and of sensitive types such as writers and musicians, giving the disease an air of fashion during this period.

Limited scientific knowledge regarding disease pathology opened the door to inductive speculation that tuberculosis might be caused directly or indirectly by the emotion, imagination, and creativity so obvious in its most famous victims. Tuberculosis was the most common of many serious lung diseases called "consumption" for its capacity to emaciate and waste away its victims. That consuming quality of the disease served as a physical manifestation of the psychological and emotional exhaustion associated at that time with creative activity. Keats, who studied medicine before turning to poetry and soon thereafter succumbed to consumption, assumed such a connection when he wrote: "I feel from my employment that I shall never be again secure in robustness." Romantics, like many in the medical community of the time, considered disease to be a part of the process of life itself, an internal quality of the individual, so a predisposition to tuberculosis—called "consumptive diathesis"—might well be indicated by other traits such as artistic talent or romantic sentimentality. Samuel Taylor Coleridge (1772–1834) claimed to have felt Keats's tuberculosis in a handshake long before the disease manifested itself. Prevention and, if necessary, treatment consisted of attempting to moderate or even avoid items or behaviors that could inflame the dormant disease, such as "bad air," crowds, a poor **diet**, sexual desire and sexual activity, and occupations that would accentuate an individual's emotional sensitivity—lawyer, minister, teacher, musician, poet. In his elegy on Keats's death, *Adonais* (1821), Shelley suggested even that the despondency and stress brought on by a harsh review of Keats's poem *Endymion* (1818) contributed to his death. Treatment strategies were complicated by unpredictable relapses, which served as a reminder of how little control sufferers had over the disease. Chopin exhibited such frustration when he wrote from Majorca of his prolonged infirmity in spite of the warm weather, a generous supply of tropical fruits, and the close attention of three famous **physicians**, all of whom disagreed on his prognosis.

The perceived link between tuberculosis and genius led not only to speculation that creative activity might bring on the disease, but also the inverse: that the disease gave its victims an enhanced sense of artistic passion and creative talent. Artists of the Romantic era generally believed that consumption stimulated the brain in much the same manner as opium or alcohol. Later attempts to explain the increased artistic insight and creative output of Romantic writers and musicians, however, have focused on the possibility that such artists acquired a new and profound understanding of life in the face of impending death, accentuated by a physical debilitation that forced the victims to spend more time inside their own imaginations. Certainly, writers from the Romantic era exhibited a deep fascination with life and death, evidenced perhaps most pointedly by Edward John Trelawney's (1792–1881) description of Shelley's cremation. The reverential account ends in Trelawney's stunning confession to finding Shelley's heart untouched by the flames and surreptitiously removing it as a keepsake. On the other hand, the beauty and insight of Romantic poetry was not simply the result of idle time and a sense of desperation. Poems such as Shelley's "Ozymandias" (1817), Keats's "Ode on a Grecian Urn" (1819), and Lord Byron's (1788–1824) "And Thou art Dead, as Young and Fair" (1812) demonstrate a profound concern with the fragile nature of life, as well as the power of artistic achievements to survive centuries after their creators have died. When Keats described his tuberculosis to friends and family, he spoke in terms of a heightened psychological and emotional capability, writing at one point that his imagination had grown to such a degree that he no longer lived in just one world, but a thousand. He left no doubt, as well, of his belief that his creativity was killing him, telling a friend that his life was but a choice between two poisons—spending a few years in India or spending a "feverous life alone" writing poetry.

In spite of Keats's reference to India as a poison, consumptives of the Romantic era traveled widely in search of improved health. Their belief in "balance" as a source of vitality—an outgrowth of **humoral theory**—led them to consider both tropical and bleak wintry climates especially dangerous, but the temperate climes and curative "sea-air" of the Mediterranean made Italy, Majorca, and the Greek islands inviting destinations for those seeking relief. Throughout Italy and the Mediterranean, where draconian administrative measures for isolating **bubonic plague** victims had been in place as early as the fourteenth century, attitudes regarding tuberculosis proved to be dramatically different from those across northern Europe—fearful, judgmental, hysterical—and in spite of their renown, the artists quickly became pariahs. People would refuse to enter carriages in which they had ridden, Paganini was thrown out of his house in Naples, Keats's Italian landlady was afraid to be in his presence, and Chopin was shunned during his stay in Majorca. By contrast, Chopin was greeted personally by Queen Victoria (1819–1901) on a trip to England (though the weather had a devastating effect on his health), and Weber was mobbed and embraced by adoring European crowds, even though both were in the final stages of their diseases. Forced to choose between returning home to a climate thought to be destructive to their health or living with the rejection and isolation their disease brought them in the more temperate locales, most preferred the comfort of home and friends. As a result, Romantics often spent extended periods in the English and European countryside as refugees from the city and its "foul air," as with Chopin's summers at George Sand's (1804–1876) home in Nohant.

Consumption was often used in Romantic literature and beyond as a metaphor for the melancholia and consuming romantic passion so prevalent during the period. Keats's poetry played perhaps the most significant role in fostering the romantic sentimentalism through which tuberculosis came to be viewed. His poems "Ode to a Nightingale" and "La Belle Dame Sans Merci" are particularly effective in romanticizing the connections between consumptive illness, love, and death. By the emergence of Victorian literature around the middle of the nineteenth century, tubercular characters began to appear regularly in novels and dramas, frequently possessing qualities associated with eroticism, beauty, and mystery, as in Henri Murger's (1822–1861) *Scenes of the Bohemian Life* (1848), and later Giacomo Puccini's (1858–1924) *La Bohème* (1896), Charles Dickens's (1812–1870) *David Copperfield* (1849–1850), Victor Hugo's (1802–1885) *Les Misérables* (1862), Alexandre Dumas fils's (1824–1895) *The Lady of the Camellias* (1848), and Giuseppe Verdi's (1813–1901) *La Traviata* (1853). Around the same period, Pre-Raphaelite painters became known for the moody medieval eroticism in their works, achieved through an exaggerated paleness and thinness in their female subjects, for which they hired tubercular models. One such model, Elizabeth Siddal (1829–1862), later even

ENCOUNTERING TUBERCULOSIS IN THE ROMANTIC AGE

. . . [Jean Valjean, known as M. Madeleine] entered Fantine's chamber, approached the bed, and drew aside the curtains. She was asleep.

Her breath issued from her breast with that tragic sound which is peculiar to those maladies, and which breaks the hearts of mothers when they are watching through the night beside their sleeping child who is condemned to death. But this painful respiration hardly troubled a sort of ineffable serenity which overspread her countenance, and which transfigured her in her sleep.

Her pallor had become whiteness; her cheeks were crimson; her long golden lashes, the only beauty of her youth and her virginity which remained to her, palpitated, though they remained closed and drooping. Her whole person was trembling with an indescribable unfolding of wings, all ready to open wide and bear her away, which could be felt as they rustled, though they could not be seen.

To see her thus, one would never have dreamed that she was an invalid whose life was almost despaired of. She resembled rather something on the point of soaring away than something on the point of dying.

The branch trembles when a hand approaches it to pluck a flower, and seems to both withdraw and to offer itself at one and the same time.

The human body has something of this tremor when the instant arrives in which the mysterious fingers of Death are about to pluck the soul.

M. Madeleine remained for some time motionless beside that bed, gazing in turn upon the sick woman and the crucifix, as he had done two months before, on the day when he had come for the first time to see her in that asylum. They were both still there in the same attitude—she sleeping, he praying; only now, after the lapse of two months, her hair was gray and his was white.

From Episode 1, Book 8 of *Les Misérables*, by Victor Hugo.

became the wife of prominent Pre-Raphaelite artist Dante Gabriel Rosetti (1828–1882). Over time, consumption became so fashionable that women began to wear whitening powder rather than rouge and white muslin clothing designed to make them appear more emaciated.

By the end of the nineteenth century, after the **epidemiology** of the disease had been discovered, tuberculosis came to be considered a result of individual degeneracy and social conditions, and perhaps as a consequence of that, associated with ethnic and racial minorities. Nevertheless, the Romantic idea that tuberculosis endowed writers, artists, and musicians with extraordinary creativity lingered well into the twentieth century. This was fueled by a steady stream of creative artists from the late nineteenth and early twentieth centuries who continued to suffer from the disease, including Robert Louis Stevenson (1850–1894), Thomas Mann (1875–1955), and Franz Kafka (1883–1924). Psychologist Havelock Ellis (1859–1939) noted in *A Study of British Genius* (1904) that 40 of his subjects suffered from tuberculosis, and psychologist Arthur Jacobson (1872–1958) wrote in *Genius: Some Revaluations* (1926) that a sure recipe for producing the highest form of the creative mind was to combine a spark of genius with tuberculosis. In fact, Jacobson considered the creative influence of tuberculosis on the human brain to have a biological connection. Such a position was not inconsistent with broader medical opinion at the time. A 1932 article in the *Journal of the American Medical Association* reported that toxins from tuberculosis stimulated the brains of patients so as to produce restlessness, apprehension about death, and general agitation, which, given the limited physical capabilities of the patients, led to an enhanced mental development. In the twenty-first century, with tuberculosis still one of the world's most virulent diseases and no reliable empirical evidence of its connection to genius or creativity, the Romantic views of the disease have largely been relegated to mere historical interest. *See also* AIDS, Literature, and the Arts in the United States; Cinema and Epidemic Disease; Disease, Social Construction of; Literature, Disease in Modern; Plague Literature and Art, Early Modern European; Popular Media and Epidemic Disease: Recent Trends; Sanatorium; Tuberculosis in England since 1500.

Further Reading

Bewell, Alan. *Romanticism and Colonial Disease*. Baltimore: Johns Hopkins University Press, 2000.

Dubos, René, and Jean Dubos. *The White Plague: Tuberculosis, Man, and Society*. New Brunswick, NJ: Rutgers University Press, 1987.

Lawlor, Clark. *Consumption and Literature: The Making of the Romantic Disease*. New York: Palgrave Macmillan, 2007.

Moorman, Lewis J. *Tuberculosis and Genius*. Chicago: University of Chicago Press, 1940.

Ott, Katherine. *Fevered Lives: Tuberculosis in American Culture since 1870*. Cambridge, MA: Harvard University Press, 1996.

Schenk, H. G. *The Mind of the European Romantics: An Essay in Cultural History*. New York: Frederick Ungar, 1967.

DEVON BOAN

TUBERCULOSIS IN ENGLAND SINCE 1500.   Tuberculosis (TB) is an infectious disease caused primarily by *Mycobacterium tuberculosis*, a bacillus discovered in 1882 by the German bacteriologist **Robert Koch**. The disease has been associated with various names such as scrofula or struma indicating swellings of the neck glands, phthisis, or consumption for tuberculosis of the lungs; Pott's disease for spinal infection; and lupus vulgaris for TB of the skin. In the 1930s it was shown that tuberculosis is mainly transmitted by airborne particles (droplets) during talking, coughing, sneezing, and so forth. The exception is *Mycobacterium bovis*, the only **animal** tuberculosis able to infect humans. Here, the bacillus is usually transmitted by ingesting infected milk or meat.

During the sixteenth century, deaths from tuberculosis increased considerably in countries undergoing **urbanization** because the disease is associated with poor and overcrowded living conditions. In England, it caused about 20 percent of all deaths at midcentury, but the greatest concentration of tuberculosis was in London. The London Bills of Mortality, recorded from 1562–1837, show high death rates from consumption, especially in the seventeenth century. Richard Morton (1637–1698), a London **physician**, published the first Western medical text on tuberculosis, entitled *Phthisiologia: or, a Treatise of Consumptions* (1689). Consumption, typified by fever and weight loss, was generally an adult disease, whereas scrofula commonly afflicted children. Scrofulous glands, which sometimes subsided spontaneously, were nevertheless believed to be cured by a monarch's touch through God's grace rather than by medical treatment, and the disease was known as the "King's Evil." Royal touching, instigated by thirteenth-century French and English kings, was particularly revived by Tudor monarchs as a symbol of their divine right to rule. Applicants, vetted by court physicians, were ceremoniously touched during a church service, after which they received gold tokens. Mary I (1553–1558), Elizabeth I (1558–1603), and James I (1603–1625) all touched for the King's Evil. The last monarch to perform the ceremony was Queen Anne (1702–1714). The writer Samuel Johnson (1709–1784) was touched by her in about 1712 but was not cured. On the Hanoverian succession in 1714, the practice was scorned as medieval and superstitious.

Epidemics of tuberculosis during the eighteenth century were associated with the **Industrial Revolution** and its occupations such as coal and tin mining, iron smelting, textile production, and pottery manufacture. Autopsies on Londoners revealed that most had developed TB during their lives, though they might have died of something else. Victims were fearful of tuberculosis and clamored for cures. Resins such as amber and myrrh formed bases for TB medicines, as did turpentine, gold, copper, and phosphorous. Lungwort (*Pulmonaria officinalis*), a plant with leaves similar in appearance to tuberculous lungs, was a specific herbal remedy. Physicians such as **Thomas Sydenham** and George Bodington (1799–1882) recommended fresh air, country living, and horseback riding. Explanations of the disease's cause were rooted in **humoral theory**, which related individual constitution to lifestyle and environment. Later, as tuberculosis developed its own mythology, medical practitioners constructed the "TB diathesis," whereby a tuberculous "taint" was inherited and then brought to fruition through exposure to a cold damp climate, dusty trades, **poverty**, improper **diet**, and so forth. Its stigma was such that family physicians often refrained from diagnosing tuberculosis because of social and employment consequences to patients and their families. Sufferers did not seek treatment for the same reasons. As late as 1912, a prominent English lung specialist, Herbert de Carle Woodcock, described it as a coarse, common disease, attacking failures, the depressed, alcoholics, and lunatics. In this context, he was arguing against the nineteenth-century portrayal of consumption as romantic or "poetic." In truth, it *was* a common disease, and it carried off many young talented individuals including the English poets Lord Byron (1788–1824), John Keats (1795–1821), and Percy Shelley (1892–22), and writers Anne (1820–1849) and Emily Brontë (1818–1848), Robert Louis Stevenson (1850–1894), and D. H. Lawrence (1885–1930).

During the nineteenth century, tuberculosis killed more people, especially young adults, than any other disease, depriving the economy of a labor force at its most productive age. Thirteen percent of all deaths in England and Wales from 1851 to 1910 were from TB, but of those aged 20 to 24, almost half died of the disease. Consumption accounted for 60 to 80 percent of TB deaths. The disease claimed a larger proportion of women's than men's lives at mid-century, partly because of pregnancy and inferior nutrition in cases in which working men in poor households were given the best food. England's worst areas for tuberculosis were the northern and midland industrial-urban areas of Lancashire, the West Riding of Yorkshire, Northumberland, and Birmingham. Despite these shocking statistics, a steady fall in TB deaths was established by 1870, which coincided with a rise in real wages and improvements in housing, hygiene, and diet. People lived longer with the disease, and others seemed able to overcome initial infection.

After Koch's discovery of the bacillus, procedures to deal with tuberculosis as an infectious disease were established. The National Association for the Prevention of Tuberculosis was founded in 1898 to educate the public in preventive measures, to promote the establishment of **sanatoria**, and to campaign for elimination of the disease from cattle. Tuberculosis had been described in slaughterhouse cattle from the early 1800s, but the discovery, in 1890, that 87 percent of Queen Victoria's (1819–1901) cows were infected with *Mycobacterium bovis* was a sharp indicator of its prevalence. In Manchester, for example,

18 percent of the milk supply from local herds was infected, yet it was not until 1929 that the danger of animal-to-human transmission of tuberculosis received government debate. By 1931 over 1,000 children under the age of 15 were dying of bovine TB in England and Wales each year. During the 1930s, tuberculin testing (for TB) was introduced in British cattle, and 40 percent were found to be reactors. Pasteurization, introduced initially to preserve milk, helped control the transmission of bovine disease to humans, resulting in a decline in deaths from 1931 to 1937. However, it was 1960 before all British milk was required to be pasteurized. In Britain, the real battle for tuberculosis control in the animal world is in its transmission from wildlife, principally badgers, to cattle. By 1986 TB had infected 88 herds, but in 2005 over 5,500 herds carried M. *bovis*. Similarly, the incidence in culled badgers rose from 5 percent in 1972 to about 38 percent in 2002–2004. In 2004 there were only 22 identified cases of bovine TB in humans, yet during the following year, 30,000 cattle were slaughtered to prevent the risk of transmission, causing significant economic harm to many farmers.

Tuberculosis bacteria are destroyed by ultraviolet light, a discovery that inspired the Danish physician Niels Ryberg Finsen (1860–1904) to treat TB of the skin with light therapy. During the 1890s, he constructed a powerful carbon arc electric lamp containing rock crystal lenses to focus ultraviolet rays. Finsen's success in treating this disfiguring condition, commonly affecting the face, earned him a Nobel Prize (1903). In 1898 Alexandra (1844–1925), Princess of Wales, who was Danish by birth, donated a Finsen Lamp to the London Hospital. Nurses, wearing dark protective glasses, held rock crystal against the patient's skin to ensure sufficient light penetration. By 1908 the hospital had 13 lamps treating over 1,000 patients a week, and hospitals throughout the country established light therapy departments, which were important up to the 1930s.

The sanatorium movement, based on open-air treatment and education in self-care, was well established by the beginning of the twentieth century. By 1920 there were 176 sanatoria in England. One of the most interesting was Papworth Village Settlement near Cambridge, founded in 1917 by Dr. (later Sir) Pendrill Varrier-Jones (1883–1941). Varrier-Jones believed that TB was incurable, and so his institution was committed to permanent holistic treatment. Papworth was a traditional sanatorium where patients in all stages of tuberculosis were received, but it also included a "settlement" where selected ex-patients (mostly male) were employed and lived with their families in a self-supporting rural community. Papworth Industries, which included cabinet-making, luggage manufacture, printing, poultry farming, and horticulture, was a successful commercial enterprise, expanding from a turnover of £410 in 1918 to over £100,000 by 1938 with about 300 workers. The total population at Papworth in 1938 was 1,000, including staff, 400 patients, and 142 families with 368 children. It was, nevertheless, an institution in an isolated part of the countryside where entertainment and social activities were supervised. Settlers did not rebel. They were generally grateful to be there during years of economic slump.

The results of sanatorium treatment were generally poor. For example, of the 3,000 patients discharged from London County Council sanatoria in 1927, only 24 percent were still alive by 1932. The 1930s and 1940s witnessed the routine use of surgical therapies such as artificial pneumothorax, whereby the diseased lung was collapsed for a period of rest and healing, and thoracoplasty, which collapsed it permanently. There is little evidence that surgical procedures influenced survival rates and, indeed, before the advent of

antibiotics, the course of the disease was totally unpredictable. Furthermore, by 1948 mass miniature radiography of 3 million people had revealed an active-case rate of 4 per 1,000 among those previously unsuspected of having tuberculosis. This created additional pressures on institutional accommodation and required the services of 2,900 more nurses.

Streptomycin, isolated by Selman Waksman (1888–1973) in 1943 in the United States and marketed in 1946, seemed to be the first real hope of a cure for tuberculosis. Postwar Britain could only afford to purchase 50 kilograms, enough to treat about 200 people. Professor (later Sir) Austin Bradford Hill (1897–1991), at the Medical Research Council, designed a fair test by randomly allocating patients to receive some of the limited supply of streptomycin. The results were impressive with 51 percent of the streptomycin patients improving by the end of six months compared to 8 percent of the controls. The problem of streptomycin resistance was solved by combining it with another new drug, para-aminosalicylic acid (PAS). By the 1960s, standard treatment for TB consisted of strepto-mycin for three months, followed by PAS and isoniazid (discovered in 1952) for up to two years. At the end of the 1970s, a multidrug regimen for eight months had become accepted. The Bacille Calmette-Guérin (BCG) vaccine, developed in 1920 by Albert Calmette (1863–1933) and Camille Guérin (1872–1961) in France, was not assessed in England until 1959, but by 1963 it was said to offer 79 percent protection against the infection.

During the 1960s and 1970s, tuberculosis in England came largely under control after centuries of being a major killer. However, since the mid-1980s, there has been a world-wide increase in TB of about 1 percent per year. In the United Kingdom, the increase has been nearer to 2 percent. Tuberculosis in England increased by 25 percent from 1994 to 2004 and continues to rise. Two out of five cases of TB are in London. The incidence in one London borough exceeds 80 per 100,000 a year, comparable to that of a developing country. Three-quarters of people with tuberculosis in England come from an ethnic minority, mainly the Indian Subcontinent and Sub-Saharan Africa. At least 3 percent of people with TB are estimated to be **HIV** positive, although the number is higher in London. About 350 people die of tuberculosis each year. In 2004 the Chief Medical Officer, Sir Liam Donaldson, produced an action plan for stopping tuberculosis in England, which some tuberculosis experts consider impossible to implement because of a lack of resources. See also Tuberculosis and Romanticism; Tuberculosis in North America since 1800; Tuberculosis in the Contemporary World; Vaccination and Inoculation.

Further Reading

Bloch, Marc. *The Royal Touch: Sacred Monarchy and Scrofula in England and France.* Translated by J. E. Anderson. New York: Routledge & Kegan Paul, 1973.

Bryder, Linda. *Below the Magic Mountain: A Social History of Tuberculosis in Twentieth-century Britain.* Oxford: Clarendon Press, 1988.

Dormandy, Thomas. *The White Death: A History of Tuberculosis.* London: Hambledon Press, 1999.

Hardy, Anne. "Reframing Disease: Changing Perceptions of Tuberculosis in England and Wales, 1938–70." *Historical Research: the Bulletin of the Institute of Historical Research* 76 (2003): 535–556.

Waddington, Keir. *The Bovine Scourge: Meat, Tuberculosis and Public Health, 1850–1914.* Rochester, NY: Boydell Press, 2006.

CAROLE REEVES

TUBERCULOSIS IN NORTH AMERICA SINCE 1800. **Tuberculosis** is a chronic, infectious disease, transmitted by **bacteria** called tubercle bacilli and *Mycobacterium tuberculosis*. Tuberculosis was the leading cause of death among North Americans for most of the nineteenth century. The epidemic is believed to have peaked there in the 1850s. In 1839 the German physician Johann Lukas Schönlein (1793–1864) coined the term "tuberculosis," but the disease was more commonly known as "consumption" or "phthisis" throughout the nineteenth century. Tuberculosis afflicted all socioeconomic classes. Nevertheless, nineteenth-century **urbanization** and **industrialization** produced crowded living and working conditions that particularly fostered the spread of disease among the poor. In 1882 the German bacteriologist **Robert Koch** discovered the bacteria responsible for tuberculosis's transmission. His theories challenged previous medical understanding, which conceived of **environment** and **heredity** as underlying causes. In the late 1800s, North American voluntary **Non-Governmental Organizations (NGOs)** and governments intensified tuberculosis control and prevention. **Sanatoria**, or rest hospitals, became a common therapy for middle and upper classes, whereas visiting nurses and outpatient dispensaries offered care to the urban working class. Even with increased public health interventions, tuberculosis killed approximately one in seven North Americans by 1900. Although the Bacille Calmette-Guérin (BCG) **vaccination** helped prevent tuberculosis in Canada, it was not until the Second World War that reliable pharmaceutical cures were discovered. The North American tuberculosis death rate fell dramatically after the 1940s but resurged in the mid-1980s, thanks in part to **drug resistance** among certain strains.

Before 1882. In the nineteenth century, **physicians** and civilians understood consumption as unavoidable, the result of an individual's constitutional weaknesses. Although the causative bacterial agent was unknown until 1882, diagnostic and therapeutic innovations in the early nineteenth century affected patients' experiences.

Clinical diagnosis of consumption became easier in the 1820s and 1830s, when the French pathologist Rene Laennec (1781–1826) published descriptions of its characteristic lesions and symptoms. Laennec introduced the concept of consumption as a specific disease. He also pioneered the method of auscultation of the lungs with the stethoscope, simplifying physical diagnosis. Many North American physicians studied medicine in Paris in the early nineteenth century and brought Laennec's methods home.

Laennec doubted that consumption was contagious, and many North Americans agreed with him. Massachusetts doctor Henry I. Bowditch (1808–1892), for example, understood consumption as primarily hereditary in nature. Such beliefs relied on empirical observations of the disease. From physicians such as Pierre Louis (1787–1872) in Paris and sanitary reformers such as England's **Edwin Chadwick**, North American doctors became acquainted with clinical and **demographic** statistics in the 1830s. These armed physicians with quantitative methods to analyze tuberculosis's incidence.

As diagnostic and observational methods changed, new public health responses and therapies emerged. Consistent statistical collections revealed the extent of tuberculosis and helped to generate demands for reform. Many North Americans supported a **sanitation movement** that encouraged the ventilation of homes, slum clearance, and urban cleanups. Sanitarians also advocated for behavioral changes, including looser clothing for women, exercise, and temperance. Cities and states established permanent boards of health, beginning with the New York City Metropolitan Board of Health in 1866 and the

Massachusetts State Board of Health in 1869. Although all of these responses focused on public health more generally, tuberculosis was of particular concern.

More specific therapies included changes in climate, rest, fresh air, and hardy **diets**. Florida and Cuba attracted many North Americans in the earlier part of the nineteenth century. Dry climates such as Minnesota, Colorado, and the U.S. Southwest began to draw consumptives later. Some physicians used drugs such as iodine or creosote, but most favored behavioral change and physical improvement.

In 1865 the French physician Jean-Antoine Villemin (1827–1892) demonstrated the transmission of tuberculosis and argued that it was contagious. However, many North American physicians disputed his findings and clung to hereditary, behavioral, or environmental explanations.

1882–1943. Biomedical understandings of tuberculosis changed substantially in 1882, when Robert Koch identified its causative microorganism. Koch experimentally inoculated lab animals with material cultured from established tuberculosis cases. He also stained the tissues, making the disease's rod-shaped bacilli visible. His published results announced to the world what some physicians already suspected: tuberculosis was a contagious disease, transmissible between people. The cause and nature of tuberculosis would be reconceptualized according to this **germ theory of disease**.

Koch's ideas spread rapidly to North America but did not win immediate acceptance. Physicians and public health professionals debated how contagious tuberculosis really was. It did not appear as communicable as other infectious diseases. Some medical professionals recognized the obvious correlations between **poverty** and working conditions and tuberculosis incidence, and believed that environment must play at least a complementary role in infection. Theories of tuberculosis's hereditary nature also continued to influence medical professionals. By the early twentieth century, many North American **physicians** began to incorporate newer germ theories with older understandings of consumption. Although they admitted its infectious nature, for example, they argued that some individuals were predisposed by **heredity** to infection.

Tuberculosis's infectious nature raised questions about prevention. Incorporating new ideas about biological inheritance popularized by the period's eugenics movement, some medical professionals saw tuberculosis as linked to poor breeding. Some eugenicists argued that the state could slow transmission by restricting marriage between infected individuals. Others promoted more positive solutions, such as improved maternal and child health programs.

Starting in the late nineteenth century, many cities passed legislation against behaviors believed to facilitate tuberculosis's transmission. Public health leaders such as Hermann M. Biggs (1859–1923), a major figure in the New York City and State Boards of Health, attacked tuberculosis aggressively and demanded greater power to control it. Municipalities demanded that landlords clean up tenements and ventilate buildings and established new offices to inspect milk and meat for tuberculosis. By the 1910s, many health departments required physicians to report tuberculosis cases. New laws increasingly targeted individuals. Many North Americans were forbidden from spitting in public, for example. Advocates for anti-tuberculosis legislation thus prioritized public health over **personal liberties**.

Newly established voluntary associations supported the campaigns for increased interventions. In 1892 Doctor Lawrence Flick (1856–1938) organized the Pennsylvania Society for the Prevention of Tuberculosis, the first such **private agency** in the United States. Medical professionals and interested citizens established many similar associations at the city and state level. In 1900 the Canadian Tuberculosis Association was established, followed by the U.S. National Association for the Study and Prevention of Tuberculosis in 1904. These associations promoted education about tuberculosis transmission and prevention. They also raised funds and awareness.

Public understanding of tuberculosis and its infectious nature increased by the early twentieth century, but the disease continued to infect many. By 1900 approximately one in seven North Americans died from tuberculosis, second only to pneumonia and **influenza**. The search for effective therapies remained important.

Climate and physical improvement continued to influence treatment. These methods were institutionalized in the late 1800s in sanatoriums, specialized hospitals that treated tuberculosis with rest, diet, fresh air, medical supervision, and education. Edward L. Trudeau (1848–1915), a physician and consumptive himself, became interested in them after recuperating in the Adirondacks. Influenced by German sanatorium models and methods, Trudeau opened the Adirondack Cottage Sanatorium in Saranac Lake, New York. Trudeau's institution gained national attention and established an example for others. Trudeau and other sanatorium directors required patients to spend most of their time outdoors or in open buildings, even in winter. The standard treatment included both prolonged rest and guided exercise. Generous diets rounded out the regime, with patients fed large quantities of eggs and whole milk to regain strength. Whereas proponents of sanatoriums argued that they offered genuine cures, some critics saw them as merely a way to isolate infected individuals.

The sanatorium movement grew quickly in North America. The first Canadian institution opened in 1897. Because treatment was expensive, patients tended to belong to the middle and upper classes. In 1905, however, the Canadian Senate and House of Commons passed legislation for the construction of public sanatoriums in each province. The same year, Hermann Biggs established the first public municipal tuberculosis sanatorium in the United States, in Otisville, New York.

State support increased the number of beds available, but many patients continued to recuperate in their homes. At the turn of the century, visiting nurses and tuberculosis dispensaries supplemented home care. Both of these strategies targeted indigent populations, educated patients about transmission and prevention, and registered new cases. Visiting nurses taught patients how to change their behaviors, and encouraged families to isolate tubercular members and to ventilate their homes.

Many scientists also experimented with biomedical therapies. An early hope for a tuberculosis cure materialized with Robert Koch's 1890 development of tuberculin, a substance made of sterilized culture in which tubercle bacilli had grown. Koch's experiments with tuberculin on guinea pigs and humans elicited a physiological reaction, which he hoped demonstrated tuberculin's potential as a treatment. In spite of early excitement and testing, tuberculin failed to cure. Nevertheless, the tuberculin reaction did represent an important phenomenon—a positive reaction to the injection of tuberculin indicated tubercular infection. In 1907 the Austrian physician Clemens von Pirquet (1874–1929) presented his research on the tuberculin skin test, offering medical professionals a more exact diagnostic procedure.

In 1908 the French bacteriologist Albert Calmette (1863–1933) and the veterinarian Camille Guérin (1872–1961) began to experiment with a vaccination created from a weakened strain of M. *bovis*, the bovine form of tuberculosis. The pair spent years at the Pasteur Institute in Paris cultivating a strain of bacilli that were not virulent enough to infect humans but that would confer immunity. After refining their inoculation on animals, Calmette and Guérin tested it on humans in 1921 and produced the BCG vaccine. International acceptance was initially slow. In North America, the Canadian National Research Council first experimented with BCG in 1925 and tested it extensively over the next two decades. The majority concluded that the vaccine was safe and fairly effective, providing immunity in approximately 80 percent of cases. In the United States, physicians proved more skeptical of BCG and doubted its safety and efficacy. Through the 1930s and 1940s, the U.S. Public Health Service instead invested in hygiene reform and the development of pharmaceutical cures.

By the 1920s, tuberculosis had waned among North Americans, in spite of the lack of effective therapies. In the 1920s and 1930s, surgical treatment offered some hope. Physicians in both Canada and the United States experimented with pneumothorax, a procedure in which physicians collapsed a patient's lungs and pumped air into the chest cavity. Others preferred thoracoplasty, a surgery that involved removing ribs to give the lung more space. Both procedures were supposed to let the lung rest and repair. Although surgeries increased in the 1930s, they involved many hazards and their efficacy remained debatable. The brief surgical era in tuberculosis treatment declined with the introduction of effective chemotherapies after World War II.

1943–Present.   The Second World War marked a turning point in tuberculosis management in North America. With the introduction of antibiotics, sanatoria and surgical treatments declined. However, the early faith in pharmaceutical eradication would prove premature by the century's end.

In the early 1940s, tuberculosis rates continued to decline in North America, but at a slower rate than previously. In the United States, the physical examinations required of military recruits revealed that a significant proportion of American men had latent or active tuberculosis. This generated a demand for greater federal government involvement. In 1944 the U.S. Public Health Service established a Tuberculosis Control Division, which adopted **vaccination** with BCG on a wider scale.

Biomedical developments offered new cures. In 1943 Selman Waksman (1888–1973), a microbiologist at Rutgers University, identified an organism named *Streptomyces griseus*. From it, he and his graduate students isolated a potent antibiotic, which they named streptomycin. Streptomycin proved remarkably effective at killing tubercle bacilli. Waksman's research caught the attention of researchers at Minnesota's Mayo Clinic, who experimented with the drug on humans in 1944.

Streptomycin was effective, but many patients relapsed and developed resistance. In the 1950s, researchers in Germany and the United States discovered an antimicrobial drug, named isoniazid, which surpassed streptomycin in its effectiveness. By the late 1950s, the United States and Canada had largely adopted the two-drug regimen, given to most patients for 18 months to two years.

The rise of antibiotic therapy stimulated the decline of older strategies. Saranac Lake closed in 1954, symbolizing the end of the sanatorium era. While the number of sanatorium beds in Canada actually peaked in 1953, the number had declined by half 10 years later. More patients remained at home for treatment. Voluntary associations changed their missions as tuberculosis cases dropped. The U.S. National Tuberculosis Association became the American Lung Association in 1973, shifting its emphasis to all lung disorders.

The seeming triumph over tuberculosis masked its persistence in certain populations. Tuberculosis continued to plague patients without access to regular medical care, such as chronic alcoholics, immigrants, and the urban poor. The decline in state and voluntary commitment to tuberculosis control eroded the social services available to tubercular patients. The perception that it had disappeared in North America led many to disregard it globally.

North America's indifference to tuberculosis unraveled in the 1980s with the appearance of **HIV/AIDS** and multidrug-resistant strains of tuberculosis (MDR-TB). These health issues led to an upsurge in tuberculosis cases. In 1985, the first time that century, the United States recorded a national *increase* in cases. In 1990 MDR-TB appeared in New York. Simultaneously, HIV case rates soared, and researchers recognized tuberculosis as a common AIDS complication. The growing visibility of tuberculosis as a national and international health problem led to renewed public interest. New strategies such as Directly Observed Therapy (DOTS) programs combined drug regimens with regular patient visits to ensure that patients completed the course of pharmaceutical treatment. In 2002 the **World Health Organization** adopted this strategy as a global treatment paradigm.

At the start of the twenty-first century, it became clear that tuberculosis was not an historic ailment, but a very contemporary problem. Tuberculosis was no longer a North American disease, but rather a global **pandemic** that required international efforts to combat. *See also* Human Immunity and Resistance to Disease; Tuberculosis and Romanticism; Tuberculosis in England since 1500; Tuberculosis in the Contemporary World.

Further Reading

Bates, Barbara. *Bargaining for Life: A Social History of Tuberculosis, 1876–1938.* Philadelphia: University of Pennsylvania Press, 1992.

Caldwell, Mark. *The Last Crusade: The War on Consumption, 1862–1954.* New York: Atheneum, 1998.

Dubos, René, and Jean Dubos. *The White Plague: Tuberculosis, Man, and Society.* Boston: Little, Brown, and Company, 1952.

Farmer, Paul. *Infections and Inequalities: The Modern Plagues.* Berkeley: University of California Press, 2001.

Feldberg, Georgina. *Disease and Class: Tuberculosis and the Shaping of North American Society.* New Brunswick, NJ: Rutgers University Press, 1995.

Harvard University Library. *Contagion.* http://ocp.hul.harvard.edu/contagion/tuberculosis.html

Lerner, Barron. *Contagion and Confinement: Controlling Tuberculosis along the Skid Row.* Baltimore: The Johns Hopkins University Press, 1998.

Ott, Katherine. *Fevered Lives: Tuberculosis in American Culture since 1870.* Cambridge, MA: Harvard University Press, 1996.

Ryan, Frank. *The Forgotten Plague: How the Battle Against Tuberculosis Was Won—and Lost.* Boston: Little, Brown, and Company, 1992.

Taylor, Robert. *Saranac: America's Magic Mountain.* Boston: Houghton Mifflin Company, 1986.

Teller, Michael E. *The Tuberculosis Movement: A Public Health Campaign in the Progressive Era.* Westport, CT: Greenwood Press, 1988.

JULIA F. IRWIN

TUBERCULOSIS IN THE CONTEMPORARY WORLD.   The **antibiotic** revolution of the 1940s and 1950s led a range of leading public health campaigners, scientists, and **physicians** confidently to predict the eradication of **tuberculosis** by the year 2000. By the early 1980s, TB appeared to be largely a disease of historical interest in the West, a consensus that indicated a dangerous complacency in the face of the continuing high prevalence of the disease in many developing countries. As recently as 1987, for example, the *Oxford Textbook of Medicine* predicted the virtual eradication of tuberculosis in "most technically advanced countries" before the year 2050. Yet those who considered TB in a global context—especially in impoverished parts of the global South or among the rising homeless populations of the global North—were far less optimistic.

The turning point in global efforts to control TB can be traced to the United States in the mid-1980s. There, a sudden increase in cases was observed in urban areas: between 1985 and 1992 there was a rise in TB cases of over 20 percent. Cities such as New York faced a rapid and unexpected spread of TB that quickly escalated into a public health emergency. This surge in reported cases can be attributed to increases in **poverty** and homelessness during the 1980s combined with the effects of **HIV** infection and the spread of TB strains showing **drug resistance**. The emerging public health crisis facing deprived inner-city neighborhoods represented a microcosm of the changing global incidence of the disease. It soon became apparent that the problems facing inner-city America were surfacing on a global scale in response to the combined effects of drug resistance, HIV, and poverty.

The development of drug resistance is thought to be responsible for around 10 percent of new TB cases worldwide. The problem of drug resistance was encountered soon after the discovery of streptomycin and other anti-TB drugs and led to the gradual emergence of multidrug treatment programs. Factors involved in the emergence of drug resistance include the poor supervision of therapy, the use of badly prepared combination preparations, the existence of inconsistent prescribing practices, the problem of erratic drug supplies, and the lack of regulation of over-the-counter sales of drugs. The most commonly encountered resistance in a microorganism is to a single drug, usually streptomycin or isoniazid, and most TB bacteria with such resistance respond adequately to a multidrug treatment program. The emergence of resistance to rifampicin is much more serious, however, as this is the most powerful anti-tuberculosis drug, with the ability to sterilize lesions by destroying near-dormant "persister" bacilli. Furthermore, most rifampicin-resistant strains are also resistant to isoniazid; by convention, a case of tuberculosis that results from strains resistant to these two agents, with or without additional resistances, is said to be multidrug-resistant. The use of standard short-course treatment becomes not only ineffectual but may even be harmful, as resistance to other drugs such as pyrazinamide and ethambutol also develops as part of the so-called "amplifier effect." In Russia and other states of the former Soviet Union, mutant forms of TB, variously referred to as multidrug-resistant tuberculosis (MDR-TB), have been rapidly spreading in response to chronic overcrowding in the prison system and severe cutbacks in primary health care. The problems and costs of managing each case of MDR-TB are enormous. Successful therapy requires prolonged courses of less effective, more expensive, and more toxic drugs, under long-term supervision. In the case of New York, the spread of MDR-TB was facilitated by reductions in public health expenditures during the 1980s, but the city ended up having to spend 10 times more than it saved in order to bring TB under control. And more recently, the spread of extensively drug-resistant TB (XDR-TB), which is even more virulent than MDR-TB, threatens to disrupt all current efforts to contain the disease: in poorer countries with high proportions of immuno-suppressed individuals, the impact of XDR-TB is potentially lethal. A recent survey reveals that XDR-TB is now present in 17 countries worldwide, and the absence of a coordinated health-care strategy could lead to a shift into the "post-antibi-otic era" of TB control.

The AIDS **pandemic** is now estimated to contribute around 10 percent of TB cases worldwide. In Africa, however, HIV is responsible for at least 20 percent of TB cases. Given that one-third of the world's population carries quiescent TB infection, the effects of immune system damage can be expected to have devastating consequences. For example, the most recent data suggest that in parts of Sub-Saharan Africa, more than one-quarter of the adult population is now infected with HIV, and rates of infection are now rising quickly in South Asia and many other regions. Infection by HIV is currently the most important predisposing factor for the development of overt TB in those infected before or after becoming HIV positive. By the late 1990s, there were estimates of at least 10 million coinfected persons. The increasing recognition of links between TB and HIV among patients has had the adverse effect of adding to the stigma of TB symptoms and has hindered cooperation among patients, health-care workers, and local communities. The return of tuberculosis has also exposed tensions between different conceptions of medicine and **personal liberty**. In the United States, for example, the threat of MDR-TB and coinfection with HIV has led to calls for punitive public health strategies based on mandatory screening and treatment, case notification to public agencies, aggressive contact tracing, and the use of **quarantine**. Such measures are reminiscent of early twentieth-century approaches to public health. They are in conflict with contemporary conceptions of individual liberty, though the recent emergence of new "bio-security" agendas, sometimes linked with reactionary political programs, may alter the direction of public health policies.

A further dimension to the contemporary resurgence of TB is the effects of global social and economic change. Mass movements of people in response to **war**, increased economic insecurity, community breakdown, and other factors have been involved in the spread of TB and other infectious diseases associated with overcrowding, makeshift housing, and poor public sanitation and **personal hygiene**. In London, for example, the overcrowding and stress experienced by recently arrived immigrants have contributed to the spread of the disease, though media reports often misleadingly claim that the disease is being spread by the migrants themselves. In addition to short-term disruption, it is important to consider the longer-term social and economic shifts that have emerged since the early 1970s. There is now increasing evidence that growing poverty, infrastructural decay, and declining health services have facilitated the spread of TB, **diphtheria, sleeping sickness**, and other preventable diseases. Similarly, the spread of TB and other preventable diseases in the so-called "de-developing enclaves" of urban America and the poverty-stricken cities of the former Soviet Union can only be fully understood with reference to the dynamics of global political and economic change since the Second World War. With the advent of more diffuse patterns of **urbanization** and the greater mobility of capital investment, it has become far easier for public health crises to be effectively ignored where they present no generalized threat to the overall well-being of an increasingly globalized economic system.

Over the last 30 years, the historical synergy between health reform and social justice has been displaced by an increasing emphasis on the individual patient or consumer rather than on the wider social and political context of disease. The profit-driven restructuring of global health care has led to widening health inequalities, as the world's poor find themselves unable to benefit from the latest biomedical advances. In comparison with other major health afflictions, TB remains relatively neglected, and most **pharmaceutical** research is devoted to the more lucrative markets for drugs in developed economies rather than to providing remedies for diseases of the less developed global South. Research is also being skewed by the current emphasis on **bioterrorism** and the planning for hypothetical scenarios rather than existing health conditions. Although new scientific advances may play a useful role in the treatment of TB, the eventual eradication of the disease will rest on a political commitment to tackle problems of poverty, inequality, and inadequate access to health care. *See also* AIDS in Africa; Capitalism and Epidemic Disease; Human Immunity and Resistance to Disease; Medical Ethics and Epidemic Disease; Popular Media and Epidemic Disease: Recent Trends; Public Health Agencies, U.S. Federal; Tuberculosis in England since 1500; Tuberculosis in North America since 1800.

Further Reading

Bayer, Ronald. "Public Health Policy and Tuberculosis." *Journal of Health Politics, Policy and Law* 19 (1994): 49–54.

Brudney, Karen, and Jay Dobkin. "Resurgent Tuberculosis in New York City: Human Immunodeficiency Virus, Homelessness, and the Decline of Tuberculosis Control Programs." *American Review of Respiratory Disease* 144 (1991): 745–749.

Coker, Richard J. *From Chaos to Coercion: Detention and the Control of Tuberculosis.* New York: St Martin's Press, 2000.

Farmer, Paul. 'Social Scientists and the New Tuberculosis.' *Social Science and Medicine* 44 (1997): 347–358.

Gandy, Matthew, and Alimuddin Zumla. *The Return of the White Plague: Global Poverty and the "New" Tuberculosis.* New York: Verso, 2003.

Naterop, Eric, and Ivan Wolffers. "The Role of the Privatization Process on Tuberculosis Control in Ho Chi Minh City Province, Vietnam." *Social Science and Medicine* 48 (1999): 1589–1598.

Raviglione, Mario. "XDR-TB: Entering the Post-antibiotic Era?" *International Journal of Tuberculosis and Lung Disease* 10 (2006): 1185–1187.

Van Cleef, M., and H. J. Chum. "The Proportion of Tuberculosis Cases in Tanzania Attributable to Human Immunodeficiency Virus." *International Journal of Epidemiology* 24 (1995): 637–642.

MATTHEW GANDY

TYPHOID FEVER. *See* Enteric Fevers.

TYPHOID FEVER IN THE WEST SINCE 1800. For centuries, fevers were regarded as natural disease processes resulting from humoral imbalances, were treated according to the principles of **humoral theory**, and were classified according to seasonality, severity, and duration. By the early nineteenth century, however, most British physicians followed the view of William Cullen (1710–1790), that fever was a general disease showing a range of inflammatory complications. In France, where pathological anatomy was pioneered, Pierre Bretonneau (1798–1862) identified characteristic intestinal lesions in those who died during an 1816 "continued fever" **epidemic**. These lesions were also seen by Pierre Louis (1787–1872), who published a study of 138 cases in 1829. The disease observed by Bretonneau and Louis, known as dothiénenteritis or **typhoid fever**, was assumed to be similar to British **typhus**. It typically attacked young migrants to Paris and lasted 28 days. Louis's American students were able to identify typhoid when they returned home, among cases formerly diagnosed as "autumnal" or "remittent" fever, but by 1835 one student, William Wood Gerhard (1809–1872), had clearly distinguished between typhoid and typhus. The latter was of shorter duration, displayed no intestinal abnormalities, and was accompanied by a distinctive rash.

The differences between typhoid and typhus, however, were not generally accepted until William Jenner (1815–1898) published his studies of cases at the London Fever **Hospital** in 1849. He reasoned that if the diseases were distinct, they must have specific causes, and the identity of those causes was of great concern. According to one estimate, each year 20,000 people died of typhoid in Britain, and 100,000 survived the disease. From 1856 William Budd (1811–1880), another student of Louis, argued that drinking **water** contaminated by sewage containing an infective agent was the means of transmission, an idea repeatedly reinforced by outbreak studies during the 1860s and 1870s. Epidemics spread by milk were also described, usually involving impure water used for washing dairy equipment. In 1880 Carl Eberth (1835–1926) described a bacillus found in typhoid, which was named *Eberthella typhosa*. Also known as *Bacillus typhosus* and later as *Salmonella typhi*, it was obtained in pure culture in 1884. Given the impossibility of **animal research** (typhoid only infects humans) it was difficult to prove that the bacillus *caused* typhoid, but in 1896 it was shown that that serum from typhoid patients caused the clumping and precipitation of the bacillus in broth cultures, the basis of a test devised by Fernand Widal (1862–1929).

Typhoid affected all classes and occurred sporadically or as small epidemics in villages and towns as well as cities, arising most regularly in late summer. One famous victim was the father of U.S. president Herbert Hoover (1874–1964), a blacksmith, who died in 1880. Another death ascribed to typhoid was that of Prince Albert (b. 1819), husband of Great Britain's Queen Victoria (1819–1901), who died in 1861, although the diagnosis has recently been challenged.

The decline in typhoid correlates broadly with sanitary reform and improvements in plumbing. In 1880 there were 261 deaths from typhoid per million of population in England and Wales, and 358 in Scotland, where the pace of **sanitation** reform was slower. By 1940 there were only three deaths per million in both countries. Hospitalization in fever hospitals, recognition of the role of carriers, and chlorination of water all played important roles. In 1897–1898, Almroth Wright (1861–1947) developed a vaccine, which was first deployed on a mass scale by the British Army First World **War**. Although the efficacy of the **vaccinations** has been questioned, the British anti-typhoid measures were altogether remarkably effective. Typhoid became an almost negligible problem, whereas, during the South African (Boer) War (1899–1901) there had been 59,750 cases among the British and, during the Spanish-American War (1898), 20,926 cases among the Americans.

As sanitary reform reduced waterborne typhoid, epidemiological interest shifted toward foodborne typhoid, especially shellfish, but the realization that outbreaks were often caused by healthy carriers dominated policy in some countries in the early twentieth century. In 1902 **Robert Koch** published a paper on typhoid carriers and began a campaign to prevent typhoid in southwestern Germany. It seemed that 2 percent of infected individuals became carriers. In the United States, the theory was confirmed dramatically in 1906, when a family outbreak in Oyster Bay, near New York, was traced to the cook **Mary Mallon**, who was shown to be linked with outbreaks in seven homes in which she had worked previously. She was also responsible for later outbreaks, despite promising not to take further employment handling food, and was subsequently detained for the rest of her life. The "Typhoid Mary" affair had a profound impact upon American public health, shifting the focus from the environment toward the control of dangerous individuals. Apart from restrictions on employment and, as a last resort, incarceration, surgical treatments for typhoid carriers were also devised, usually involving the removal of the gall bladder, the usual site of continued infection.

In Britain the carrier theory was less influential. The identification of carriers was less proactive, and the powers given to public health officials less extensive. Typhoid had ceased to be endemic, and outbreaks were generally blamed on temporary loss of vigilance with regard to traditional public health measures. Some officials began to consider typhoid a disease of the past. But this view came under strain in the light of the milk-borne Bournemouth outbreak (1936) and the waterborne Croydon outbreak (1937). The former resulted from cows drinking from a river containing sewage from a cottage of a carrier, whereas the latter was probably linked to a carrier among the workmen who repaired a well while chlorination was suspended. Senior British health officials, however, continued to stress sanitation, rather than focusing on carriers as the key to prevention, the chief lesson taken from Croydon being the need for universal chlorination.

During the 1930s there were important developments in the science of typhoid. Arthur Felix (1887–1956), in England, devised a modified Widal test, for an antibody to a particular *Salmonella typhi* antigen, the V_i or "virulence" antigen, which he had discovered in 1934. This led to a new "improved" vaccine (which was later shown to be useless) but, importantly, to phage typing, which was devised by James Craigie (1899–1978) and a colleague in Canada. During the Second World War, the value of phage typing was demonstrated, allowing, for example, sporadic cases to be traced to sources many miles away.

After the war, the British Emergency Public Health Laboratory Service became permanent, with Felix as director of its Central Enteric Reference Laboratory. In 1947 Felix and Craigie published a standardized method of phage typing, and the International Congress for Microbiology recommended that it be adopted universally. An International Committee for Enteric Phage Typing was formed, and Felix's laboratory became the international reference facility. The laboratory supported investigations of outbreaks. Phage typing became the basis of many remarkable detective stories. Notifications of typhoid dropped from 396 in 1948 to 90 in 1960 in England and Wales. For the remaining cases, an effective **antibiotic**, chloramphenicol, become available in 1950; it reduced the mortality rate to around 1 percent. Trials of the drug in the treatment of carriers, however, were inconclusive.

Compared to most other European counties, Britain had the advantage of not having been occupied during the war, facilitating postwar progress in controlling the threat of typhoid. Soon, a large proportion of the remaining cases in Britain were contracted abroad, mainly in continental Europe or on the Indian subcontinent. The hazards of overseas travel were dramatically illustrated in 1963 by the large waterborne outbreak at the ski resort of Zermatt, Switzerland, which led to cases among vacationers from many countries, including the United Kingdom. The large outbreak of typhoid in Aberdeen, Scotland, the following year, which hospitalized over 500 people, was also the result of imported infection, in this case via a surprising route: in a large can of corned beef. An official enquiry concluded that the infection had entered through a defect in the can during manufacture in Argentina using unchlorinated cooling water. The role of overseas **trade and travel** as the source of the majority of the remaining typhoid cases in Western countries reflects the continued prevalence of the disease in less developed regions. *See* *also* Contagion and Transmission; Diet, Nutrition, and Epidemic Disease; Disinfection and Fumigation; Enteric Fevers; Personal Hygiene and Epidemic Disease; Public Health Agencies in Britain since 1800.

Further Reading

Huckstep, R. L. *Typhoid Fever and Other Salmonella Infections*. Edinburgh: Livingstone, 1962.

Mendelson, J. Andrew. "'Typhoid Mary' Strikes Again: The Social and the Scientific in the Making of Modern Public Health." *ISIS* 86 (1995): 268–277.

Mermin, Jonathan H., et al. "Typhoid Fever in the United States, 1985–1994." *Archives of Internal Medicine* 158 (1998): 633–638.

Smith, David F., et al. *Food Poisoning, Policy and Politics: Corned Beef and Typhoid in the 1960s*. London: Boydell and Brewer, 2005.

Wilson, L. G. "Fevers and Science in Early Nineteenth-century Medicine." *Journal of the History of Medicine and Allied Sciences* 33 (1978): 386–407.

DAVID F. SMITH

TYPHOID MARY.   *See* Mallon, Mary.

TYPHUS.   Typhus, from the Greek word for "smoky" or "hazy," which describes neurological symptoms of the disease, is the designation for an illness caused by infection with rickettsial organisms and characterized by a fever and a rash. Typhus is usually divided into two major categories: classic **epidemic** typhus and its recurring form known as "Brill-Zinsser disease," and murine typhus or "tabridillo."

Biological Agent and Its Effects on the Human Body.   Both types of typhus are caused by rickettsiae, very small bacterial organisms that share with **viruses** the habit of living inside the cells of the infected host. Because they exhibit characteristics of both **bacteria** and viruses, they were for some years thought to be a separate category of infectious microorganism, but in the late 1960s, they were demonstrated to be true bacteria. The name "rickettsiae" for these organisms was derived from Howard Taylor Ricketts (1871–1910), a **physician** who lost his life to typhus in 1910 while conducting some of the earliest studies on these pathogens.

Epidemic typhus is caused by *Rickettsia prowazekii*, and murine typhus by *Rickettsia typhi*. Both epidemic and murine typhus exhibit an incubation period varying from 5 to 15 days, after which the onset of the disease is abrupt. A rapidly rising fever is accompanied by headache, loss of appetite, and general malaise. Chills, nausea, and prostration may ensue during the first week. After the fourth day, a widespread noneruptive rash appears under the skin. After a week, the fever usually subsides, and recovery is rapid. In fatal cases, however, prostration becomes more marked, with increasingly severe neurological symptoms including deafness, stupor, delirium, and symptoms of circulatory collapse preceding death. For classic epidemic typhus, the death rate in untreated cases usually varies from 5 to 25 percent and occasionally reaches 40 percent. In cases of murine typhus, the disease is almost never fatal, with a mortality rate of only about 2 percent.

Since the introduction of broad-spectrum **antibiotics** in the late 1940s, death need not result from either form of typhus if the disease is recognized early and treated promptly. A case of typhus produces a long **immunity**, but under certain circumstances, epidemic typhus may recur. The observation of typhus-like symptoms without the existence of an epidemic was originally noted in 1910 by Nathan Brill (1860–1925) and hypothesized in 1934 by Hans Zinsser (1878–1940) to be a recurrence of typhus in persons who had suffered a previous attack. When experiments in the 1950s confirmed that typhus could recur years after the initial infection, the condition was named Brill-Zinsser disease.

Transmission.   *Rickettisa prowazekii* is transmitted by an insect, the human body louse *Pediculus humanus corporis*. The body louse spends its entire lifetime in the clothes of humans. Lice take four to six blood meals a day from hosts, and human blood constitutes their only food. *R. prowazekii* in the blood of an infected person are ingested by feeding lice and multiply rapidly in louse intestines. They are secreted in the feces of infected lice and transmitted to new hosts by contact of infected louse feces with skin abrasions caused when the human host scratches the unpleasant itch caused by the lice as they feed. The vector louse also dies from its infection with *R. prowazekii*.

Rickettsia typhi is a natural infection of rats and is transmitted by the rat flea, *Xenopsylla cheopis*. The name "murine typhus" reflects the disease's relation to rats, and humans living in areas where rats are abundant are most susceptible. Like epidemic typhus, murine typhus is transmitted when a human host rubs infected rat feces into the abrasion caused by a flea bite. Neither the rat nor the rat flea suffers ill effects from the infection.

Epidemiology with Specific Factors.   Classic, epidemic typhus has long been known as a disease of cold weather and of crowds. Its various names—jail distemper, ship fever, camp fever, famine fever—suggest the poor hygienic conditions characteristic of groups of people confined to close quarters in cold weather without access to clean clothes or bathing facilities. Epidemics peak in winter and taper off in the spring.

Murine typhus, in contrast, is more often associated with warmer climates and human living conditions where rats are abundant. Local names for the disease reflect the human-rat **environmental** connection: shop typhus, urban typhus, and "tabridillo" in Mexico.

History.   The first account of typhus by a contemporary described a disease that occurred during the 1489–1490 **wars** in Granada, Spain. It killed 17,000 Spanish soldiers—six times the number killed in combat. In the early sixteenth century, another typhus epidemic may have altered European history. The French army was at the point of a decisive victory over the Italians and Spaniards in Naples when the disease struck down 30,000 French soldiers, forcing a withdrawal of the troops that ended the French threat. In 1548 **Girolamo Fracastoro**, who had observed this epidemic in Italy, published the first clear description of what he termed a "lenticular or punctate or petechial" fever. By the end of the sixteenth century, typhus—presumably epidemic typhus introduced by Europeans—was also recorded in Mexico, where it killed over 2 million Native Americans.

In the nineteenth century, the incidence of typhus increased dramatically. In 1812 typhus plagued Napoleon's (1769–1821) invasion of Russia. Between 1816 and 1819, a great epidemic struck 700,000 people in Ireland. Confusion of typhus with **typhoid**, which also produces a rash, muddled the clinical understanding of the disease. In 1837 William Gerhard (1809–1872) described specific intestinal lesions that characterized typhoid but not typhus. Gerhard's work, however, was not immediately accepted. Even into the twentieth century, some confusion continued in nomenclature between typhus and typhoid. In 1848 European revolutions spawned typhus epidemics. A particularly severe outbreak in Silesia prompted German physician **Rudolf Virchow** to observe that typhus primarily afflicted the poor, the uneducated, and the unclean. He

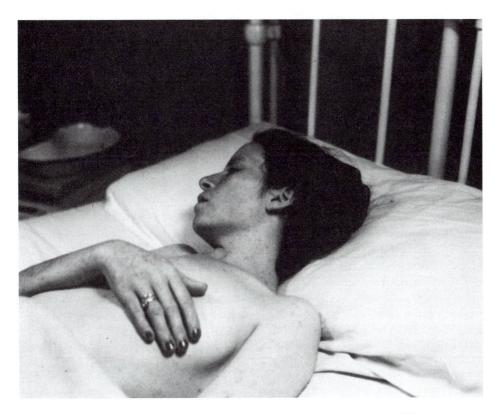

Typhus rash on the face and neck of a woman in the Fever Hospital, Abbassia, Egypt, 1943. Courtesy of the National Library of Medicine.

called for democracy, education, and public health measures as proper "treatment" for the epidemic.

During the last quarter of the nineteenth century, the advent of the **germ theory** of infectious disease led bacteriologists to search for a microbial cause of typhus. In 1909, **Charles Nicolle**, director of the Institut Pasteur in Tunis, Tunisia, demonstrated that the body louse transmitted typhus. In 1910 Howard Taylor Ricketts, working in Mexico City, described tiny microorganisms in the blood of typhus victims, in infected lice, and in lice feces. Before he could confirm his observations, however, he became infected with typhus and died. In 1916 Brazilian Henrique da Roca Lima (1879–1956) described similar organisms, which he named *Rickettsia prowazekii* after Ricketts and Stanislaus von Prowazek (1875–1915), a researcher who had also died from a laboratory-acquired typhus infection.

In the 1920s, American epidemiologist Kenneth Maxcy (1889–1966) described a widespread form of typhus fever that was endemic. He postulated that some **ectoparasite** of the rat was its vector. By 1931 infected fleas had been found in nature that confirmed Maxcy's hypothesis. In 1932 the Swiss pathologist Herman Mooser (1891–1971) proposed the name "murine typhus" for the disease to indicate its relationship with the rat. Mooser also distinguished in the laboratory the causative organism *Rickettsia typhi* from *Rickettsia prowazekii*.

Research, Prevention, and Therapeutic Efforts.   After rickettsiae were identified as the causative agents of typhus, many paths were explored to prevent or treat the infections. During World War I, the only effective approach was vigilance in keeping soldiers and civilian populations free from body lice. This was accomplished largely through showers for people and steam-cleaning of clothing. The result was not highly effective.

During the interwar period, a number of candidate **vaccines** against *R. prowazekii* were developed. The most promising grew the large concentrations of rickettsiae needed for vaccine production in the yolk sacs of fertile hens' eggs. The yolk sac typhus vaccine was administered to all U.S. servicemen at the beginning of World War II, but it was never completely evaluated. The reason for this was the development of the highly effective **insecticide** dichloro-diphenyl-trichloroethane (DDT). A "blowing machine" was developed to blow DDT under clothes so that people did not have to disrobe to be treated. When a typhus epidemic struck Naples, Italy, in the winter of 1943–1944, the outbreak collapsed with astonishing speed once DDT was brought into use. Within two decades, however, the adaptive resistance of lice to DDT was documented, and its ecological hazards were documented so that is no longer widely used.

In 1948 broad-spectrum **antibiotics** were discovered to be effective treatments for all rickettsial diseases. Since then, little research has been conducted on vaccines to prevent typhus. Civilian and military physicians have relied almost completely on the use of antibiotics to cure rickettsial diseases.

Current State of the Disease.   In the twenty-first century, typhus poses little threat in populations in which Western medicine makes antibiotics widely available to treat infections. The principal locales where *R. prowazekii* is still likely to be contracted because of infestations of body lice in local populations are the cool, mountainous regions of Africa, Asia, and Central and South America. In addition, recent molecular and genetic screening techniques have shown that fleas that live on flying squirrels can transmit *R. prowazekii*. Campers, inhabitants of wooded areas, and wildlife workers may be vulnerable to typhus if they come in close contact with flying squirrels, their ectoparasites, or their nests. Murine typhus still exists worldwide and may be contracted anywhere rats are prevalent and humans may be bitten by their fleas. *See also* Colonialism and Epidemic Disease; Insects, Other Arthropods, and Epidemic Disease; Irish Potato Famine and Epidemic Disease, 1845–1850; Personal Hygiene and Epidemic Disease; Poverty, Wealth, and Epidemic Disease; Typhus and Poverty in the Modern World; Typhus and War; War, the Military, and Epidemic Disease.

Further Reading

Centers for Disease Control and Prevention. *Typhus.* http://www.cdc.gov/ncidod/diseases/submenus/sub_typhus.htm

Harden, Victoria A. *Rocky Mountain Spotted Fever: History of a Twentieth-Century Disease.* Baltimore: Johns Hopkins University Press, 1990. (See especially chapters 6, 9, and 10.)

National Library of Medicine. *MedLine+.* http://www.nlm.nih.gov/medlineplus/ency/article/001363.htm

Pelis, Kim. *Charles Nicolle, Pasteur's Imperial Missionary: Typhus and Tunisia.* Rochester, NY: University of Rochester Press, 2006.

Zinsser, Hans. *Rats, Lice, and History*, revised edition. Edison, NJ: Transaction Publishers, 2007.

VICTORIA A. HARDEN

TYPHUS AND POVERTY IN THE MODERN WORLD. "The history of typhus," wrote German **physician** August Hirsch (1817–1894) in his classic nineteenth-century study of disease, "is written in those dark pages of the world's story which tell of the grievous visitations of mankind by **war**, famine, and misery of every kind" (1883; p. 35). Hirsch's formulation is a poetic shorthand for the past, present, and, most probably, future, of a particularly dreaded disease. For there is a repetitive quality among typhus stories, each of which seemingly takes Hirsch's formula of "war, famine, and misery" as a guiding theme, masking—at least from a distance—the distinctiveness of individual outbreaks and personal suffering. Whether we are visiting instances of "war," "jail," "ship," or "spotted" fever in the sixteenth to eighteenth centuries, "hunger" fever in the nineteenth, or "typhus fever" as presently defined, we witness similar stories of human suffering. No wonder, then, that many a student of typhus has come to see the disease as a kind of moral barometer of civilization.

It should be noted that these stricken civilizations tended to dwell in temperate zones. Similar living conditions in more tropical climes might set the stage for the free play of a host of other diseases—but not of typhus. This geographic constraint was well known, long before it could be effectively explained. It was one of the disease's great mysteries.

Origins. Mystery has similarly shrouded typhus's origins. There are those who believe that the unknown **epidemic** (430–426 BCE) known as the **Plague of Athens** was typhus. Of course, efforts to diagnose early epidemics are notoriously difficult. Earlier diagnosticians classified diseases in different ways. Moreover, "typhus" was only clearly differentiated from "typhoid" in the nineteenth century—and, from "murine" typhus in the 1930s. Despite these redefinitions, historians of disease generally agree that classic typhus was striking down Europeans by the latter part of fifteenth century. Thereafter, great numbers of individuals displayed its characteristic fever, rash, searing headache, and delirium. Typhus followed the ever-present course of military conflict over the next couple of centuries, spreading throughout Europe and into North Africa and remaining long after those wars had ended. (It even, as Hans Zinsser [1878–1940] demonstrated, influenced the outcome of more than one of those conflicts.) It also struck residents of the "New World."

Nineteenth-Century Patterns. After the **Napoleonic Wars** ended, typhus began to settle among populations already suffering from the darker side of the **Industrial Revolution**. Consequently, those studying the conditions of the laboring poor began to study typhus more closely. **Rudolf Virchow**'s celebrated examination of the typhus epidemic in Upper Silesia (1848) was in fact preceded by investigations into the connections of **poverty** and disease by men such as Scotland's William Pulteney Alison (1790–1859). Alison, a politically and philosophically inclined professor at Edinburgh's medical school, argued in 1841 that pauperism was the "great and general disease of the body politic"—and that the causal chain leading from economic hardship to deprivation to disease was evident. Typhus, which persisted in poorer sections of Scotland and Ireland even when it was growing less common in more opulent locales, offered an illustrative example. (Still, Alison believed that typhus was caused by particular morbid agents.) The apparent pervasiveness of typhus during the **Irish Potato Famine** of 1846–1849 lent further credit to his arguments. Virchow noted the influence of Alison and others on his interpretation of the Silesian outbreak.

At the time typhus struck in 1847, Upper Silesia, an area now split between Poland and the Czech Republic, was an economically depressed province of Prussia with a large

Catholic Polish population. According to Virchow's later report (1848), the Prussian government had essentially ignored the growing epidemic—and the locally influential Catholic clergy were inclined to preach that the people's wretchedness was a means of their salvation. Virchow was finally sent to the typhus-ridden area in February 1848. There, he quickly compiled materials for his classic study. Relying on the case histories and autopsy records of doctors—who played the forward-thinking heroes (and, more than occasionally, martyrs) in his narrative to the villainous forces of church and state, Virchow presented a striking and moralizing picture of typhus. Typhus was, fundamentally, the product of the near-feudal state that persisted in Upper Silesia. The rich were no longer bound by an older mentality of *noblesse oblige* and instead "indulge[d] in the luxury and the follies of the court, the army and the cities." The poor, on the other hand, were kept in their poverty by ignorance and neglect. Whatever the specific causes of typhus, its cure could only be found in the overturn of feudal oppression by "full and unlimited democracy" (pp. 89–90). The synchronicity of Virchow's conclusions with Karl Marx (1818–1883) and Friedrich Engels's (1820–1895) *Communist Manifesto* (1848) was no coincidence—despite distinct differences in their ideologies.

The broad outlines of misery that shaped Virchow's typhus story were also evident in any number of mid-century typhus epidemics. In many of these instances, misery had opened the door to typhus, but what followed *after* typhus often had regionally specific, and occasionally broadly national, consequences. The effects of Ireland's mid-century famine tend to be well known. Disease and hunger combined to provide a strong motive for mass emigration. A number of those immigrants took ship for America, arriving in eastern port cities that in turn became (relatively circumscribed) hubs of typhus. The impact of typhus in Tunisia is less well known. During the nineteenth century, Tunisia's leaders had made a number of questionable financial decisions, largely in an effort to keep up with their Western neighbors to the north. Then, in the 1860s, the already-burdened country was plagued by drought, crop failure, and two "classic" plagues: **cholera** and typhus. By 1869 the country was officially declared bankrupt, and, with that, the stage was set for its eventual appropriation by France as a "protectorate."

Still, when August Hirsch wrote his revised disease geography in the early 1880s, "typhus" was being written on far fewer of western Europe's "dark pages." Hirsch was not the only doctor to be perplexed by the disease's sudden retreat. By the century's end, typhus had been constrained to a veritable "ring" around the United States and western Europe: in Eastern Europe, North Africa, and Mexico (with occasional incursions into American seaports and more persistent outbreaks in Ireland). It seemed to have been domesticated. Yet in this ring around the West, it continued to be perceived as a threat—and as a mystery.

The Twentieth Century: Explaining Mysteries.   By the start of the twentieth century, much had been learned about the cause and spread of many diseases. The so-called **germ theory** of disease—roughly, that one specific microbe caused one specific disease—had been effectively demonstrated and disseminated as the new bacteriological gospel. Knowledge of the microbial causes of such diseases as cholera, **tuberculosis**, and **bubonic plague** was in hand; the complications caused by "vectors," such as mosquitoes for **malaria**, were also understood. Laboratory studies had been central to these successes. Typhus proved resistant to the prying of laboratory methods. Consequently, neither the disease's causal agent nor its mode of human-to-human transmission had been identified. Without a known microbial agent, diagnosis, too, remained difficult. In 1898 one of America's top diagnosticians, Nathan Brill (1860–1925), published a paper on an apparent "typhoid fever" epidemic among recent immigrants into New York. Only when he returned to the problem over a decade later did he determine that his patients had been suffering from typhus, not typhoid. In 1900 typhus remained, as Hirsch had described it, a mysterious disease of human misery. Ultimately, its connection to human misery helped guide efforts to unravel those mysteries.

In the first decade of the twentieth century, French researchers in Tunisia and American researchers in Mexico, began to make progress in the longstanding effort to understand the disease. The "answer" was first demonstrated in Tunis—earning **Charles Nicolle** the Nobel Prize (1928) and relegating the Americans in Mexico to the role of providing confirming evidence. Nicolle was well familiar with the history and reputation of typhus, but, until he moved from France to Tunisia, he had not encountered the disease in a patient. As director of Tunisia's Pasteur Institute, Nicolle was soon faced with a typhus epidemic that took the lives of the two doctors with whom he had intended to visit patients. During subsequent outbreaks, Nicolle set his colleague, Ernest Conseil (1879–1930), to work on the disease's epidemiology. Conseil followed outbreaks back to laborers in the countryside, who moved to the city in early spring to find work. Their numbers increased dramatically in years of drought—such as 1909—when they could find no agricultural work. In the city, they lived in squalor. Conseil discovered that the epidemic tended to spread only to those in close proximity to them: innkeepers, doctors, and others who cared for them in the hospital. Later, Nicolle would describe his discovery of typhus transmission as a "eureka moment" arising from Conseil's Hirschean observations. Typhus, he reasoned, must be spread by something close to the body: something that was removed by a thorough scrubbing and change of clothes: "It could only be the louse!" Nicolle quickly turned to the laboratory to demonstrate his hypothesis.

Longstanding mysteries of typhus had been illuminated. Why did typhus follow human misery and movement? Why did it shun areas that were either too frigid or too hot? The louse provided the answer. Where the body louse thrived, typhus could take root. Yet even this new insight did not dispel all the mystery or overturn all the moral judgments attached to the disease. The perception of lice as filthy creatures would have done little to overthrow these assumptions. Indeed, the association of typhus with lice made the tragedy of its continued existence more dramatic still. Typhus could—should—be controlled; but it was not. As Nicolle's good friend Hans Zinsser wrote, "Typhus is not dead. It will live on for centuries, and it will continue to break into the open whenever human stupidity and brutality give it a chance, as most likely they occasionally will" (1963, p. 301).

In the meantime, typhus, in its classic, louse-borne form, continued to be further differentiated from disease varieties once thought identical to it. Typhus outbreaks in Mexico during the late 1920s and early 1930s attracted researchers from around the world. They determined that the typhus of Mexico was different. Maintained in rats and transmitted to humans by fleas, it was milder than the epidemic variety—and was evolutionarily distinct. (This realization led Nicolle, Zinsser, and others to press for further study of the evolution of infectious diseases.) With this knowledge, Zinsser returned to study Nathan Brill's mildly ailing immigrant population. Strangely, most of these patients had been in the United States for decades, safely outside active typhus centers. Zinsser determined that the immunity conferred by typhus was durable, but not absolute. Decades after a typhus victim had recovered, the disease could reappear—or, "recrudesce." If conditions were right—that is, if body lice were abundant—typhus might erupt.

The discovery that the louse acted as a necessary link between human misery and typhus encouraged an all-out war on the louse. That lice tended, particularly as the twentieth century progressed, to be found on the poor certainly did little to discourage the aggressiveness of those campaigns. Whether among laborers at the border of the United States and Mexico, black populations in South Africa, or nomadic laborers (or colonial troops) in North Africa, typhus was kept away from more affluent neighbors by aggressive attacks on lice. It can hardly be surprising that these campaigns often seemed to shade imperceptibly into campaigns against the poor people harboring the lice.

The Persistence of Typhus.   Typhus epidemics appear far less frequently today. This is, in part, the result of developments in vaccines and **antibiotics** from the mid-twentieth century. Despite these advances, however, the story continues. In the 1990s, for example, typhus ravaged the higher and relatively cool regions of Burundi in Africa, underscoring the misery that had resulted from civil war, mass dislocation, and relocation in refugee camps.

The persistence of typhus and its continued coupling with human misery despite the advances of science and the efforts of global health workers support history's judgment of the disease as a window onto the often-tragic "health" of civilization. As Nicolle noted in *Naissance, Vie, et Mort des Maladies Infectieuses* (1930; pp. 195–196):

> Typhus presents itself to us as both a plague and a moral lesson. It tells us that man has only recently emerged from barbarity, that he still carries on his skin a disgraceful parasite such as brutes themselves carry, and that, when man conducts himself like a brute, this parasite . . . will prove, in effect, that he is merely a brute. The disappearance of typhus will only be possible on that day when, wars having disappeared, the work of a collective hygiene will suppress the louse. Humanity will only know this immense progress when it merits it. Will we ever merit it?

See also Diagnosis of Historical Diseases; Ectoparasites; Environment, Ecology, and Epidemic Disease; Historical Epidemiology; Insects, Other Arthropods, and Epidemic Disease; Personal Hygiene and Epidemic Disease; Pesticides; Sanitation Movement of the Nineteenth Century; Typhus and War.

Further Reading

Andersson, Jan O., and Siv G. E. Andersson. "A Century of Typhus, Lice and Rickettsia." *Research in Microbiology* 151 (2000): 143–150.

Hamlin, Christopher. "William Pulteney Alison, the Scottish Philosophy, and the Making of a Political Medicine." *Journal of the History of Medicine and Allied Sciences* 61 (2005): 144–186.

Hirsch, August. *Handbook of Geographical and Historical Pathology*, volume 1. Translated by Charles Creighton. London: The New Sydenham Society, 1883.

Humphreys, Margaret. "A Stranger to Our Camps: Typhus in American History." *Bulletin of the History of Medicine* 80 (2006): 269–290.

Markel, Howard. *Quarantine! East European Jewish Immigrants and the New York City Epidemics of 1892*. Baltimore: Johns Hopkins University Press, 1997.

Virchow, Rudolf. "Report on the Typhus Epidemic in Upper Silesia." *Social Medicine* 1 (2006): 11–98.

Zinsser, Hans. *Rats, Lice and History*. Boston: Little, Brown, 1963.

KIM PELIS

TYPHUS AND WAR.   Since at least the sixteenth century, epidemic **typhus** has been one of the most common and deadly **epidemic** diseases to accompany armies on campaign. Typhus in general is caused by **bacteria**-like microorganisms known as rickettsia, which are spread by wingless body lice, rodent fleas, mites, or ticks. There are three variants of typhus: flea-borne endemic (murine), louse-borne epidemic, and mite-borne scrub. Researchers developed vaccines against endemic and epidemic typhus in the early 1930s, but none yet exists for scrub. Early typhus symptoms include headache, acute fever, and small pink spots on the skin; vomiting and prostration may follow.

Louse-borne Epidemic Typhus.   In epidemic typhus—also known as **war** fever, ship fever, camp fever, jail fever, and the Hungarian disease—delirium and deafness often precede the final stage of circulatory collapse (toxemia) that brings on death in anywhere from 5 to 40 percent of untreated cases. Full recovery confers limited **immunity**. The body louse *Pediculus humanus corporis* that transmits the pathogenic *Rickettsia prowazeki* lives in human clothing and feeds on human blood. The pathogenic bacteria are deposited on the victim's skin in powdery louse feces and enter when the skin is abraded by the victim's scratching. Lice will migrate from one human to another, thus spreading the rickettsia from dying or immune hosts, but they thrive on bodies whose clothing is undisturbed and unlaundered for long periods. Low levels of **personal hygiene**, so common in pre-contemporary armies, were the louse's best friend. When combined with cold-weather campaigning, exposure to the elements, forced exertion, and poor **diet**, the infected louse and its tiny parasite could cripple the most valorous of soldiers and the greatest of history's armies. Before the twentieth century, disease—especially typhus—invariably killed more soldiers than action in battle, sometimes four or five times as many. The 1906 Russo-Japanese War was the first major conflict whose battle casualties outnumbered those from disease.

Early Appearances.   Typhus symptoms are close enough to those of **measles**, **malaria**, and **typhoid fever** to make undoubted **historical diagnoses** a real problem. Medical pioneer Hans Zinsser (1878–1940) noted that murine typhus was known to Western medicine since at least the eleventh century CE, though the early sixteenth-century Italian physician **Girolamo Fracastoro** considered epidemic typhus a new disease (though louse transmission was not discovered until 1909 by **Charles Nicolle**). The earliest clearly recorded military outbreak was during the last phase of the five-century *Reconquista*, the Christian Spanish siege of Muslim Granada during the winter of 1489–1490. Fracastoro echoed contemporary claims that the disease had been brought into Iberia by Spanish soldiers who had been fighting alongside the Venetians against the Turks in Cyprus. At Granada, epidemic typhus is said to have accounted for 17,000 of the Spanish casualties, whereas the Moors accounted for 3,000. Final Christian victory was postponed until the fateful year 1492.

Fracastoro noted cases in Spanish-dominated southern Italy as early as 1505, but its earliest Italian outbreak was at the French siege of Naples in 1528, in the midst of the Habsburg-Valois Wars. Typhus, plague, and desertion had cut Emperor Charles V's (1500–1558) Spanish and German garrison down to around 11,000 disheartened men who found themselves surrounded by a proud French army of some 28,000. In early July, disease began to pick off the French, soldier and commander alike. Typhus is considered to have been the principal killer, as disease reached deadly epidemic levels. With much of his army sickly or expired, the new French commander, the young Marquis de Saluzzo (1490–1533), raised the siege on August 29 and began the long march back north. Imperial troops and allies harried the slow-moving columns mercilessly, and Charles's victory was complete. Twenty-four years later his fortunes were reversed, however, when his army of Spaniards, Germans, and Italians besieged the well-defended, French-held fortress city of Metz. This was to be the first step in a final, victorious Habsburg counteroffensive against his perennial enemy. Ill-advisedly opening the siege in October, in a single month he lost 10,000 of his 75,000 men to typhus (and other diseases including **dysentery**), which then spread across the countryside. Charles raised the siege in January, and his defeat helped persuade him to retire as Emperor in favor of his brother Ferdinand (1503–1564).

Typhus had checked an Imperial army a decade earlier, in 1542, when Joachim II Hektor von Brandenburg (1505–1571) organized an international force against the Turks who had just occupied the Hungarian city of Buda (Budapest). In his history of the campaign, surgeon Thomas Jordanus von Klausenburg (1540–1585) left a clear picture of the effects of the Christian army's lack of good food, water, and beer, and of the filth and heat of the march. Dysentery, enteric fevers, and, above all, typhus dissolved away the war machine even before it reached the city. The resulting peace left the Muslim Ottomans in command of the Hungarian Plain.

Early Modern Trends and Examples. Seventeenth-century armies fighting the **Thirty Years' War** (1618–1648) and the English Civil War (1642–1648) were no cleaner or better fed, and thus no less susceptible to lice and rickettsia than their predecessors. Whether Catholic Imperial, Protestant German, French, Spanish, Danish, English, or Swedish, soldiers shared typhus among themselves and the civilian populations through whose countryside and city streets they trudged. Armies marched, countermarched, and fought relatively rarely, spending much of their time foraging for food and needed supplies. Germany provided most of the battlefields and foreign armies with little concern for the local civilians spread disease with abandon. Reinforcements, new recruits, and fresh national armies kept the fires of war and pestilence stoked, whereas the disease-ridden were often taken in by, or forced upon, local households. Rural refugees crowded besieged cities and suffered from typhus alongside defenders, further blurring distinctions between soldier and civilian. As the Swedes approached Nuremberg in the summer of 1632, Imperial Habsburg forces interposed themselves, remaining outside the city. By September scurvy and typhus had ravaged both armies, and both moved on, littering their paths with the sick, dying, and newly infected. By war's end, typhus may have killed more than 10 percent of the total German population, and disease in general accounted for 90 percent of Europe's casualties. Peace treaties led to demobilization, first in 1635 and finally in 1648: troops returning home took typhus with them in every direction. Thereafter, as biologist R. S. Bray put it, "Typhus went on to affect the outcome of every war on the European continent up until the Second World War."

During the early stages of the English Civil War, the Parliamentary army led by the Earl of Essex marched toward Royalist Oxford. In mid-April 1643, his 18,000 men stopped and surrounded the town of Reading for two weeks in mid-April. In an odd reversal, townspeople transmitted typhus to the Roundheads, who broke camp and quickly relocated to Buckinghamshire. Though no record of casualties exists, the toll was enough to dissuade Essex from attacking Oxford, which was well enough, because the King's army was in the process of rapidly passing the disease along to Oxford's residents and to the villagers beyond. The following July, Essex and his men marched west and occupied Tiverton, Devonshire, which raised the townspeople's mortality rate by nearly 10 times normal according to burial records. Though less spectacularly, this pattern of typhus dissemination continued for much of the war.

The eighteenth century produced few peaceful years, and national armies became larger than ever before. The aggressive and protracted territorial wars of France's Louis XIV and Frederick the Great of Prussia, and then the French Revolutionary and counter-Revolutionary campaigns of the 1790s, mobilized hundreds of thousands of men and sent them streaming across Europe time and again. Central Europe north of the Alps and from the Rhine to Silesia (modern western Poland) hosted most of the military activity and suffered most from the diseases it spread. In every army, typhus took its inevitable toll among the ranks, and every army spread the disease as it marched and foraged. Conditions in sedentary army camps grew especially squalid, and cities and fortresses were often targets. Burdened with refugees, defending garrisons, and enemy troops, towns became focal points for typhus outbreaks. During the War of Spanish Succession (1702–1714), Bavarian Augsburg suffered in 1703–1704, first when occupied by friendly French and Bavarian troops and then when captured by the English and Austrians. Burial records show interments more than tripling between 1702 and 1704, and returning to normal in 1705. Dresden was wracked twice during the Seven Years' War (1756–1763), in 1757 and 1760, and in 1758 Breslau in Silesia matched 9,000 local military deaths from typhus and related diseases with those of 9,000 of its own citizens.

The Modern Era.   The **Napoleonic Wars** between 1796 and 1815 dwarfed those of earlier rulers, as did Napoleon's armies and those sent against him. After the Battle of Austerlitz in December 1805, Napoleon left 48,000 wounded French and allied troops in various forms of shelter in Brno. Of these, 12,000 died of typhus. In June 1812, Napoleon led 650,000 French and allied troops into Russia. Thanks to typhus exposure as they crossed Polish territory, only 130,000 remained fit to fight at Borodino (September 7), and fewer than that entered Moscow a week later. The horrors of the French midwinter retreat resulted in fewer than 40,000 reentering Central Europe in 1813. Nevertheless, Napoleon returned to France and raised another army of half a million men. Of these 105,000 were lost in battle in Germany (Dresden and Leipzig) in August and October 1813, but an estimated 219,000 died of disease within less than a year.

In spring 1813, Bavarian authorities wisely established sanitary stations along their eastern border to intercept French stragglers from the Russian campaign. Those who were diseased, generally with typhus, were isolated in lazarettos or other isolation facilities such as military hospitals. This kept the region free of epidemic typhus until October brought the new French army, its diseased troops, and its battle casualties. The diseased and wounded, prisoners and the abandoned, and, increasingly, diseased civilians flooded **hospitals** and other care facilities. These were transformed into filthy hellholes reminiscent of the worst medieval **pest houses**. According to Bavarian records, between October 1813 and June 1814, civilians suffered 18,427 cases of typhus, of which 3,084 were fatal, numbers that are undoubtedly very low given the chaotic conditions. The retreating French army continued to fill hospitals with its diseased and dying, but by June or July the typhus epidemic in Germany had ended.

Nineteenth-century wars tended to be on a smaller scale and more quickly decided than those of the previous century. This generally meant fewer potential typhus carriers, less time on campaign, and less impact on civilian populations. The American Civil War (1861–1865) seems to have produced very few cases of typhus. When France and Britain sent armies to aid the Ottoman Turks against the Russians in the Crimean War (1854–1856), they were repeating an old pattern. The allies bottled up the Russians at Sevastopol in September 1854 and established siege camps around the city. Cholera, dysentery, and typhoid established themselves and horrified the early newspaper war correspondents and their readers. British reformers, including the nurse Florence Nightingale, saw to it that British conditions were improved, including the regular laundering of clothing, which helped discourage the body louse. When the French contracted typhus in the fall of 1855, suffering over 17,000 deaths, the British remained largely unaffected, with only 62 fatalities. At war's end, soldiers spread both typhus and **cholera** outward from the battleground. The French took the precaution of quarantining returning troops—primarily on the Isles d'Hyere near Toulon—who thus carried neither disease home. British military leaders, however, allowed unfettered return, which resulted in local epidemics back home.

At the southern tip of the Ottoman Empire, Egyptian troops with Sudanese allies invaded Ethiopia in 1876 and promptly contracted typhus. Attempts to isolate cases merely resulted in the spread of the disease to military camps and other Egyptian units. Ethiopian units also caught typhus—some thought from Egyptian **corpses**, others from the **miasma** that had rendered the corpse—and carried it into their towns, such as Aduwa, which lost over 60 percent of its people.

Nicolle's 1909 discovery of the role of lice prompted the use of hot baths and steam cleansing of clothing as prophylactics by some armies in World War I (1914–1918). The realities of the front, however, made such niceties rare. When Austrian troops invaded Serbia in late 1914, many contracted typhus, and huge losses forced their early withdrawal. They left behind some 60,000 prisoners, most of whom were diseased. The Serbs spread these about the countryside in camps, and typhus spread with them. A third of Serbia's 350 physicians succumbed to the fever, as did fully half of the Austrian POWs. Though typhus was rare in the Western trenches, perhaps as a result of cross-immunization by the common rickettsial trench fever, it swept through armies on the Eastern Front. During the seven years between 1916 and the end of the Civil War, an estimated 30 million Russian soldiers and civilians suffered from typhus, and 10 percent of these died. About 1930, Austrian-born Pole Rudolf Weigl (1883–1957) developed the earliest typhus vaccine.

Though military personnel during World War II (1939–1945) generally went on campaign having been vaccinated against epidemic typhus, civilians whose environments were disrupted by the war often suffered. In Poland typhus was nearing elimination (between 2,000 and 4,000 annual cases) when the German army invaded in September 1939. Nevertheless, the Nazi authorities began rounding up Polish Jews under the false pretext that they were carriers of exanthematous typhus whose relocation aided public health. In fact, the horrendous conditions of the Nazi death camps only fostered disease among the living. Destructive Nazi policies and activities also led to malnutrition and reduced levels of health care and hygiene in conquered Jewish communities throughout occupied Europe, which led to outbreaks of typhus and its spread through mass resettlement.

With the German conquest of France in 1940, life in French Algeria and Morocco underwent rapid and jarring change, including shortages of soap, insecticides, and new clothing. In 1942 the disruption was accelerated, and epidemic typhus appeared among the native Arab and Berber peoples as well as European civilians and refugees. Dissemination was widest and fastest in more densely populated areas including major cities. A larger percentage of native North Africans than Europeans contracted typhus, though death rates were much higher among the less naturally immune Europeans. Moroccan authorities acted quickly to immunize and to isolate known cases, which helped reduce the annual number of cases from 25,000 in 1942 to 4,000 the following year. Cases spiked again in 1945, but with ample use of DDT—first developed as an insecticide in 1939—they fell to 126 in 1947. All told, at least 50,000 and perhaps a quarter-million Algerian residents fell ill, and 12,840 died between early 1942 and mid-1944; from 1942 to 1945, an estimated 40,200 Moroccans fell ill of typhus, and 8,040 died.

In British-controlled Egypt, the war effort required the **migration** of workers from typhus-ridden areas to northern cities such as Cairo and Alexandria. Incidence rates rose dramatically, and by war's end, authorities recorded an additional 110,000 typhus cases and 20,000 fatalities. Imperial Japan's occupation of Korea resulted in many typhus-carrying Korean laborers being shipped to wartime Japan, reintroducing the disease for the first time since 1914. When the war ended, many of these laborers were repatriated to Korea, bringing their disease with them. Many Japanese returning home from Korea also carried typhus, sparking epidemic outbreaks in Osaka, Tokyo, and Yamagata. In Algeria, Egypt, and Korea, late- or postwar immunizations and extensive use of the **pesticide** DDT for fumigation brought the epidemics to a close.

Allied occupiers paid less attention to typhus cases in Japan. Immunizations for scrub typhus have never been developed, and both Japanese and Allied forces fighting in the Southwest Pacific islands and in Ceylon and Burma suffered from the harvest mite-borne disease. Whereas no Japanese figures are available, an estimated 18,000 Allied troops came down with the disease and a few percent died of it. Careful ground-clearing at new facilities sites and application of pesticides on clothing and blankets tended to keep the mites at bay.

Though typhus is rarely encountered today, African civil and regional wars still spawn sporadic reports of the disease from isolated refugee camps, or more widely as in war-ravaged Burundi in 1997 (24,000 cases reported). It has also been reported that typhus has been weaponized into an aerosol biological warfare agent. Though rickettsiae are in some ways perfect candidates for this use, it is very difficult to maintain virulence during production, and the disease is not directly passed on by human contact. *See also* Diagnosis of Historical Diseases; Historical Epidemiology; Napoleonic Wars; Thirty Years' War; Typhus and Poverty in the Modern World.

Further Reading

Azad, A. F. "Pathogenic Rickettsiae as Bioterrorism Agents." *Clinical Infectious Diseases* 45 Suppl. (2007): 52–55.

Baumslag, Naomi. *Murderous Medicine: Nazi Doctors, Human Experimentation, and Typhus.* Westport, CT: Praeger, 2005.

Humphries, Margaret. "A Stranger to Our Camps: Typhus in American History." *Bulletin of the History of Medicine* 80 (2006): 269–290.

Prinzing, Friedrich. *Epidemics Resulting from Wars.* Oxford: The Clarendon Press, 1916.

Sherman, Irwin W. *The Power of Plagues.* Washington, DC: ASM Press, 2006.

Zinsser, Hans. *Rats, Lice, and History*, revised first edition. Edison, NJ: Transaction Publishers, 2007.

JOSEPH P. BYRNE

U

URBANIZATION AND EPIDEMIC DISEASE. The origins of city development date back to the late **Neolithic** period. The adoption of agriculture and the advent of sedentary living led to worldwide population increase and settlements of ever-higher density. Human susceptibility to **epidemics** of infectious diseases has its origins among the dense populations of the earliest cities. Some diseases—for example **schistosomiasis** and **malaria**—are transmitted to humans via an animal vector, whereas others are passed by human-to-human **transmission**. The latter—for example **typhoid fever, leprosy,** or amoebic **dysentery**—may be caused by a microorganism that renders the host infective for a prolonged period of time, thus enabling its survival even in smaller communities. However, the most rapidly spreading acute infections, such as **cholera, smallpox,** mumps, **measles** (rubeola/rubella), and chickenpox, rely on large concentrations of people available for infection.

The Beginnings. Our nomadic ancestors did not settle down long enough in one place to suffer the ill effects of pollution, for example by contaminating **water** sources with human and animal wastes. Nor did they come into close and prolonged contact with animals, and thus they were spared the zoonotic diseases picked up by their sedentary successors. As a result of the more abundant food supplies agriculturalists enjoyed, their populations increased rapidly when compared to the smaller bands of hunter-gatherers. On the other hand, the diet of sedentary populations would have been less varied, with heavy reliance on cereals. In years of crop failure or animal diseases, famine was an unavoidable reality. It can be assumed that zoonotic diseases were contracted through close contact with domesticated animals, such as dogs, goats, and cattle, but another source of infectious diseases was rodents and insects attracted by accumulating waste and stored foodstuffs in permanently settled habitations. Because these settlements were usually situated along watercourses, waterborne diseases such as schistosomiasis (bilharzia), a disease that is still prevalent today throughout the Nile valley, could have established themselves among these sedentary populations. Another waterborne disease, typhoid fever, might also have originated in these early settlements. Population numbers were probably not large enough, however, to sustain the ravaging epidemics experienced in the centuries leading up to the modern era. In addition, many survivors of illnesses would have built up temporary or permanent **immunity**, and many infectious diseases might have become less virulent over time and eventually have become endemic, minimizing the chances of epidemic outbreaks among early urban populations.

Early Cities.   During the later part of the Neolithic period (c. 5000–3000 BCE), the Bronze Age (c. 3000–1000 BCE), and the subsequent Iron Age, increasing population numbers and advances in technology led to the foundation of new urban centers and the enlargement of existing cities in Egypt, Mesopotamia, South Asia, China, and South America. Hand in hand with an increase in populations, food demands increased, and many of these settlements thrived because of innovations such as irrigation systems. They also domesticated a wider range of **animals** and increased the possibility of the transmission of new zoonotic diseases. Egyptian medical papyri of the second millennium BCE and texts found in the capital of the Hittite empire (modern Turkey) describe epidemic outbreaks, though of which diseases remains unclear. Viral diseases such as smallpox and measles possibly originated in these densely populated cities, but the scientific evidence is inconclusive. The skin lesions observed in the mummified remains of Pharaoh Ramses V, who died in 1157 BCE, are often attributed to smallpox, but a number of other diseases are equally likely, and analysis of ancient DNA has thus far not confirmed the diagnosis. Other clues come from the writings of Mesopotamia and China, as well as the recorded **biblical plagues**.

A number of factors made early cities the perfect places for epidemics: high population density; crowded and often squalid living conditions; poor public sanitation; water supplies of questionable purity; food supplies that attracted rodents and other disease vectors; regular trade connections with other cities and the regular arrivals of travelers and merchants, especially by ship; **war**; and the housing of refugees. Greek historian Thucydides (460–395 BCE) survived and described in detail what is now regarded as the first recorded epidemic in antiquity, the **Plague of Athens**. In 430 BCE, at the outset of the Peloponnesian War, an outbreak of an infectious disease hit the city-state of Athens. The Athenian army and inhabitants of the city and the surrounding countryside were sheltering behind the city walls, and this concentration of people provided the necessary number of hosts for the unidentified disease to spread and kill at least one-third of Athenians. Further epidemics occurred in the following years, also afflicting the enemy city-state of Sparta, as well as the eastern Mediterranean more widely. The Plague of Athens has been attributed to **bubonic plague**, measles, smallpox, and **hemorrhagic fevers**, among others, but recent ancient DNA analysis of teeth from putative victims of the epidemic has identified the causative agent as typhoid fever. According to historical accounts, the disease spread from Ethiopia to Egypt and Libya, and it probably arrived by ship in the harbor of Athens before it spread through the overcrowded city.

Though lagging behind the Greek city-states in urban development, Rome, capital of the Roman Republic and later Empire, housed enough people to sustain epidemic diseases from early in its history. From 165–166 to 185 CE, Rome and other Roman cities were ravaged by an epidemic outbreak brought back to the capital by troops returning from Northern Mesopotamia. Named the **Antonine Plague** after the Roman emperor who fell victim to the disease, its signs and symptoms were described by the Greek physician

Galen, and it appears that it may have been smallpox. From 251 to 266, Rome was again the scene of a devastating disease outbreak, known as the Plague of Cyprian, after the bishop of Carthage, whose city was equally affected by the epidemic, with thousands of people dying each day. The Plague of Cyprian has been tentatively identified as measles. The high number of deaths during these outbreaks might indicate that there had been no prior exposure to this disease or to the previous Antonine plague. It also attests that population numbers were large enough to sustain epidemic outbreaks of infectious diseases.

Although previously described epidemics claimed large numbers of lives much worse was to come. The Byzantine Empire and its capital, Constantinople, were hit by what is known as the first plague pandemic, the **Plague of Justinian**. The origins of the disease have been traced to Egypt, from whence it was transported to Constantinople by ships delivering grain to the metropolis in 541–542 CE. Rats living in large granaries within the city could have easily spread the disease identified as bubonic plague from contemporary descriptions—a disease that recurred regularly over the next 200 years, spreading throughout the Byzantine Empire and well beyond and killing probably more than half of the entire population.

The Era of the Black Death.   Although urban life had remained vital throughout the Middle Ages in the Islamic world and what remained of the Byzantine Empire, the Latin West was underdeveloped until the later thirteenth and fourteenth centuries. Rising populations everywhere fed burgeoning cities that offered new occupational opportunities and freedoms. Wealthy classes independent of the older nobility and church built trading networks and rudimentary industrial concerns. These same classes established independent or semi-independent civic governments following the ancient Roman Law, seizing, buying, or negotiating their freedom of action from their sovereign lords. Cities were crowded warrens where rich and poor lived cheek-by-jowl and little effort was directed to sanitation. Drains were choked with refuse and rivers served as sewers. Ships plied ancient coastal routes, and powerful port cities like Genoa and Venice stretched trading tentacles as far as the Crimea. It was along these trade routes and into these urban centers that plague rats traveled in the later 1340s, bringing a scythe-like pestilence for which no one was prepared. From towns and cities, the disease moved outward into rural areas as people fled the horrors so graphically depicted by the literate urban classes. Returning in 10-year and then longer cycles, the plague eventually settled in cities, the brisk commercial traffic of which refreshed the supply of infected rodents, and the filth of which promised a large reservoir of native rats.

Though populations dropped throughout the West, by the sixteenth century many cities had either reemerged or had grown up to house high concentrations of people and had begun to serve as links in maritime chains that stretched ever further across the globe. Older diseases like measles and smallpox became endemic amid population concentrations heavy enough to sustain them. New ones like **syphilis** and **yellow fever** found "virgin soil" in densely packed port cities and military camps. Because no Christian, Muslim, nor Jew understood the microscopic pathogens that caused these maladies, neither physicians nor public health efforts were of much value. Some measures, like **quarantine** and *cordons sanitaires*, could limit exposure at least somewhat, but most efforts were in vain.

European Expansions and Early Modern Cities.   With the activities of European explorers and colonists Old World diseases were unintentionally introduced to the Americas. Tenochtitlán, present day Mexico City, was an enormous urban center and capital of the Aztec Empire. Within a few years of the arrival of the first Spanish ships in 1521, however, the city's inhabitants were massacred by smallpox, enabling the Spanish conquistador Hernándo Cortés (1485–1547) to conquer the Aztec Empire. Further smallpox outbreaks occurred in the Incan Empire of modern Peru, killing most of the native inhabitants of the capital Cuzco. Other new diseases such as measles, typhoid, and **influenza** swept colonial cities of both urban natives and native-born colonists.

As in the Old World, urbanized civilizations like those of Peru and Mexico featured cities in which concentrations of people fed the epidemics, which then spread into the countryside and from region to region along trade routes linking these centers. Because the civilizations' economy, culture, and political life were focused on the cities, they became the target of European predation. With populations and garrisons weakened by disease, the Spaniards had little trouble seizing control, especially when they were immune.

In both Europe and the colonial world, cities grew in size and importance. Sanitation and water supply remained problems, and travel and trade continued to introduce and reintroduce dangerous pathogens. Personal cleanliness was rare, so fleas, ticks, lice, and mites found comfortable homes on human bodies. As administrative centers, cities invited foreigners and natives to mix and mingle with the capitals' citizens. Increasingly industrialized towns and cities brought folks from the countryside into the wretched and growing slums—people who then added to the filth and demand for water. Close quarters meant easy transmission of pulmonary diseases. Plague slowly disappeared giving way to smallpox in the eighteenth century and then cholera and **tuberculosis** in the nineteenth. Yet smallpox prompted **inoculation** early in the century and **vaccination** later on, and worldwide cholera pandemics in the 1839s and 1840s spawned new and very fruitful thinking and action regarding urban sanitation and general cleanliness. The **Sanitation Movement of the nineteenth century** was an urban movement dedicated to cleaner living and fresher water. Tubercular patients were removed to sanatoria from pollution-hazed cities, and municipal water supplies were separated from polluted upstream sources. Urban **hospitals** began to provide more sophisticated treatments, and the emerging acceptance of **germ theory** from the 1870s meant a growing number of effective treatments developed using the new science of bacteriology. New understandings of **insect** vectors revealed that plague could be limited by killing rats and their fleas, and that drainage could control the yellow fever that scourged American cities and the malaria that killed in Europe and Africa.

Reemerging and New Diseases of the Modern World.   Although modern medicine enables most of the world's population to lead relatively healthy and long lives, reemerging and new infectious diseases present an increasing threat. This is especially true in the huge cities of the developing countries in Asia, Africa, and South America. As centuries before in Europe, the large cities and suburbs of the modern world attract uneducated and unskilled newcomers seeking accommodation, work, and food, leading to the development of largely unsanitary and crowded areas where the economically less successful congregate. The constant influx of new residents into cities and suburbs across the globe taxes infrastructures such as water and sewer provision and can also introduce both new and old diseases, whereas spreading urban development opens previously uninhabited areas and can bring people into contact with new diseases. The reemergence of tuberculosis (TB) is a good example of the return of an old infectious disease. By the mid-twentieth century, TB was considered nearly eradicated, but recently the disease has been making a comeback in the troubling form of new drug-resistant strains. New cases are reported on a regular basis, and it is the large metropolitan areas that are most affected. Furthermore, the **Human**

Immunodeficiency Virus (HIV/AIDS), an infection of epidemic proportions since its emergence in the United States in the 1980s, is largely transmitted within the male homosexual and drug cultures of large cities. In addition, the rise and spread of prostitution and the practice of casual sexual encounters within urbanized areas throughout the world helps to spread the virus. Other sexually transmitted diseases such as syphilis and **gonorrhea** are also once again on the increase. Reemerging infectious diseases include urban yellow fever, which occurs in the cities of South America and Africa, where the mosquito vector has adapted to breed in water containers, discarded car tires, open sewers, and flower pots. **Dengue** hemorrhagic fever is also reaching epidemic proportions in the cities of Southeast Asia and South America.

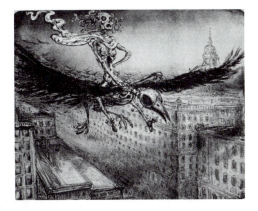

Disease, in the form of a skeleton on a skeleton crow, flies into a city, threatening death. Early twentieth-century drawing. Courtesy of the National Library of Medicine.

Childhood diseases, such as measles and **diphtheria**, which were once well controlled by immunization programs, are also returning. With the decline in vaccination programs and the availability of large numbers of susceptible people, cities are a major resource for these reemerging viruses. Furthermore, air travel enables infectious diseases to cover vast distances, moving from city to city, emerging in unlikely parts of the world.

In 2003, **Severe Acute Respiratory Syndrome** (SARS), caused by a highly infective pneumonia **virus**, was stopped short of becoming a major threat after it spread from southeastern China to Hong Kong, Beijing, and eventually Toronto, Canada. Live animals kept in crowded conditions and close contacts between humans and animals may enable viruses to jump the species barrier. The **Avian influenza** virus, which first reemerged in birds in the Far East in 2004, is feared to cross the animal-human border eventually because of its ability to change genetically, and human deaths caused by the virus have already been reported worldwide. However, if the virus is able to pass from human to human, a major pandemic outbreak is likely, which could spread rapidly within cities and from one urban center to the next. *See also* Colonialism and Epidemic Disease; Contagion and Transmission; Diagnosis of Historical Diseases; Disease in the Pre-Columbian Americas; Drug Resistance in Microorganisms; Environment, Ecology, and Epidemic Disease; Historical Epidemiology; Hospitals and Medical Education in Britain and the United States; Industrialization and Epidemic Disease; Personal Hygiene and Epidemic Disease; Plague in Britain, 1500–1647; Plague in Europe, 1500–1770s; Plague in San Francisco, 1900–1908; Plagues of the Roman Empire; Plagues of the Roman Republic; Poverty, Wealth, and Epidemic Disease; Religion and Epidemic Disease; Sexual Revolution; Yellow Fever in North America to 1810; Yellow Fever in the American South, 1810–1905.

Further Reading

Barnes, Ethne. *Diseases and Human Evolution*. Albuquerque: University of New Mexico Press, 2005.

Byrne, Joseph P. *Daily Life during the Black Death*. Westport: Greenwood Press, 2006.

Cliff, Andrew, Peter Haggett, and Matthew Smallman-Raynor. *Deciphering Global Epidemics: Analytical Approaches to the Disease Record of World Cities, 1888–1912*. New York: Cambridge University Press, 1998.

Greenblatt, Charles, and Mark Spigelman, eds. *Emerging Pathogens: Archaeology, Ecology and Evolution of Infectious Disease*. New York: Oxford University Press, 2003.

King, Helen, ed. *Health in Antiquity*. New York: Routledge, 2005.

Kiple, Kenneth F., ed. *Plague, Pox and Pestilence*. London: Weidenfeld and Nicolson, 1997.

———, ed. *The Cambridge World History of Human Disease*. New York: Cambridge University Press, 1993.

McNeill, William H. *Plagues and Peoples*. Harmondsworth: Penguin Books, 1994.

Scott, Susan, and Christopher J. Duncan. *Biology of Plagues: Evidence from Historical Populations*. New York: Cambridge University Press, 2001.

Watts, Sheldon. *Epidemics and History: Disease, Power and Imperialism*. New Haven: Yale University Press, 1997.

TINA JAKOB

V

VACCINATION AND INOCULATION. Inoculation and the later practice of vaccination entail the introduction of disease-related biological material under the skin in order to produce an immunizing reaction in the human body. The term inoculation comes from the Latin word *inoculatio* (*in:* into; *oculus:* bud), and it means to graft. In the field of medicine, inoculation is the introduction of microorganisms, disease agents, infective material, serum, and other substances into tissues of living plants, animals, people, or culture media.

Because the smallpox (*variola*) virus was involved in one of the first inoculations of a European, the procedure is also called variolization. It had long been known in the East Asia, having been employed in China from the tenth century by means of introducing into the nose dust of variolic scrapings. From the time of the seventeenth-century emperor K'ang (1654–1722), the Chinese used the practice very widely, especially on soldiers and children. In the twentieth century, this practice was still being used in some regions of China. Indians also practiced variolization from ancient times. They would puncture the distal part of the deltoides muscle with a needle moistened in variolic pus. The technique spread as far as Istanbul, Turkey.

In 1714 the Greek doctor Emmanuel Timonis, who lived in Istanbul, presented an article outlining his success with variolization to the Royal Society in London. This was published in the Society's *Philosophical Transactions*. The scientific community did not acknowledge Timonis's findings immediately, but the intervention of Lady Mary Wortley Montague (1689–1762) proved invaluable. She arrived in Turkey in 1717 with her husband, who had been appointed ambassador. She had suffered with smallpox in the past, and as soon as she learned of the technique, she ordered her son to be variolized by the ambassador's physician, Dr. Charles Maitland (1677–1748). After the family's return to Britain in 1717, Lady Montague spread the news of the value of inoculation. Because several epidemics of smallpox had occurred during those years, people willingly followed Lady Montague's advice, and

ON EARLY ATTEMPTS TO INOCULATE FOR MEASLES (1774)

Attempts have been made to communicate the measles, as well as the small-pox, by inoculation, and we make no doubt but in time the practice may succeed. Dr. Home of Edinburgh says, he communicated the disease by the blood. Others have tried this method, and have not found it [to] succeed. Some think the disease would be more certainly communicated by rubbing the skin of a patient who has the measles with cotton, and afterwards applying the cotton to a wound, as in the small-pox; while others recommend a bit of flannel which had been applied to the patient's skin, at the time of the disease, to be afterwards laid upon the arm or leg of the person to whom the infection is to be communicated. There is no doubt but this disease, as well as the small-pox, may be communicated various ways; the most probable, however, is either from cotton rubbed upon the skin, as mentioned above, or by introducing a little of the sharp humour which distils from the eyes of the patient into the blood. It is agreed on all hands that such patients as have been inoculated had the disease very mildly; we therefore wish the practice were more general, as the measles have of late become very fatal.

From *Domestic medicine; or, The family physician: being an attempt to render the medical art more generally useful, by shewing people what is their own power both with respect to the prevention and cure of diseases. Chiefly calculated to recommend a proper attention to regimen and simple medicines.* By William Buchan, M.D. of the Royal College of Physicians, Edinburgh . . . *The second American edition, with considerable additions, by the author.* Philadelphia: Printed by Joseph Crukshank, for R. Aitken, at his book-store, opposite the London Coffee-House, in Front-Street., MDCCLXXIV. [1774]

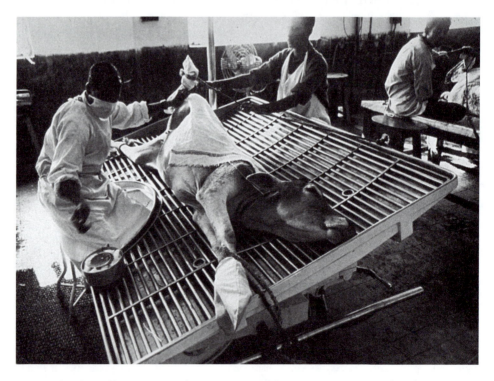

Freeze-dried smallpox vaccine being prepared from virus grown on the skin of a calf in Bangladesh. WHO photo. Courtesy of the National Library of Medicine.

in 1721 and 1722 a significant number were inoculated.

The Scots **surgeon** John Hunter (1728–1793), pioneer in experimental surgery, carried out the first self-inoculation of pus from a patient suffering with venereal disease in 1767. Hunter intended to determine whether **syphilis** and **gonorrhea** were the same disease. But the patient had both syphilis and gonorrhea, and Hunter was convinced that it was the same disease.

The English surgeon **Edward Jenner** coined the term *vaccination* in 1798 for his technique of producing in human beings the disease called cowpox (*Variolae vaccinae*). After observing carefully and proving that people who had suffered from cowpox never contracted smallpox, he concluded that artificially inducing a mild variety of *Variolae* through vaccination was a way to protect against the far more deadly **smallpox**. Jenner's technique was based on a **folk** practice that he experimentally confirmed but could not fully explain. Now we know that the smallpox **virus** (*Variola virus*) is genetically related to the cowpox virus (*Cowpox virus*). Due to this genetic resemblance, each is able to produce a cross-defense against the other in the human body.

> **SOME EARLY SUCCESSFUL VACCINATIONS, BY DISEASE**
>
> **1796: Smallpox**, by English physician **Edward Jenner**
>
> **1897: Bubonic Plague**, by the Russian doctor **Waldemar Mordechai Haffkine**.
>
> **1912: Pertussis**, by the Belgian doctors Jules Bordet (1870–1961) and Octave Gengou (1875–1957).
>
> **1923: Diphtheria**, by the French doctor Gaston Léon Ramon (1886–1963).
>
> **1927: Tuberculosis** (BCG: Bacillus Calmette-Guérin), by the French veterinaries Léon Calmette (1863–1933) and Camille Guérin (1872–1961).
>
> **1927:** Tetanus, by the French doctor Gaston Léon Ramon (1886–1963).
>
> **1935: Yellow Fever**, by South African doctor **Max Theiler**.
>
> **1955:** Injectable **Polio** Vaccine (IPV), by the American doctor **Jonas Edward Salk**.
>
> **1961:** Oral Polio Vaccine (OPV), by the Polish-born American doctor **Albert Bruce Sabin**.
>
> **1964: Measles**, by the American doctor **John Franklin Enders**.
>
> **1967:** Mumps, by the American doctor Maurice Ralph Hilleman (1919–2005).
>
> **1970:** Rubella, by the American doctors Stanley A. Plotkin (1932–) and colleagues
>
> **1981: Hepatitis** B, by the French doctor Philippe Maupas (1939–) and the American doctor Maurice Ralph Hilleman (1919–2005).

In 1877 the French chemist **Louis Pasteur** broadened the definition of vaccination to include any medical procedure using a vaccine—a small amount of attenuated or dead pathogen agents that cause a certain disease—to induce in people protection against diseases. Through **animal research**, he discovered that by gradually giving animals small doses of the germ of a specific disease, he could make them immune to that disease. He started by administering doses of weak germs, followed by more active germs, and finally one dose of the most active ones. After the full course, the animal was protected against that disease.

The Spanish doctor Jaime Ferrán (1851–1929) was the first to use a vaccine against a bacterial infection in human beings in 1885, during a severe **epidemic** of **bacterial cholera** in Valencia, Spain. The vaccine, which included dead germs of cholera, proved to be effective. Three months later, Pasteur successfully employed a vaccine against rabies. It was the first time a killed-pathogen vaccine was used against a viral disease. During the following years, several vaccines were developed.

During research on the vector of **yellow fever**, in the first years of the twentieth century, several volunteers allowed themselves to be bitten by the *Aëdes aegypti* mosquito, which they thought was the carrier of the causal agent of yellow fever. Because they developed the disease, they proved it was the vector of yellow fever, but unfortunately, some of them died. Because vaccination introduces pathogens—whether living or dead—into the human body, there was both professional and popular resistance to its use at various points in its development. This was especially true when the popular media reported experiments on large numbers of people that resulted in many contracting the disease. This occurred after 1902 in the Indian Punjab with a **bubonic plague** vaccine, and in the United States following the development of the live **polio** vaccine.

By the twenty-first century, safe and effective vaccines have been developed for a wide range of diseases, and these have proven to be invaluable tools in the medical battle against epidemic disease. *See also* Chinese Disease Theory and Medicine; Pharmaceutical Industry; Plague in India and Oceania: Third Pandemic; Poliomyelitis, Campaign Against; Sabin, Albert; Salk, Jonas E.

Further Reading

Allen, Arthur. *Vaccine: The Controversial Story of Medicine's Greatest Lifesaver.* New York: Norton, 2007.

Colgrove, James. *State of Immunity: The Politics of Vaccination in Twentieth-Century America.* Berkeley: University of California Press, 2006.

Durbach, Najda. *Bodily Matters: The Anti-Vaccination Movement in England, 1853–1907.* Durham, NC: Duke University Press, 2005.

Farmer, Laurence. "The Smallpox Inoculation Controversy and the Boston Press, 1721–1722." *Bulletin of the New York Academy of Medicine* 34, 9 (1958): 599–608.

Harvard University Library. *Contagion.* http://ocp.hul.harvard.edu/contagion/vaccination.html

Jenner, Edward. *Vaccination against Smallpox.* Amherst, NY: Prometheus Books, 1996.

Link, Kurt. *The Vaccine Controversy: The History, Use, and Safety of Vaccinations.* New York: Praeger, 2005.

JUSTO HERNÁNDEZ

VENEREAL DISEASE AND SOCIAL REFORM IN PROGRESSIVE-ERA AMERICA.   The early twentieth century is frequently referred to as the Progressive Era in America. In reaction to changes brought about by industrial **capitalism**, Progressive reformers wanted government to intervene more than ever before in American economic and social life. Under President Theodore Roosevelt (1858–1919), Progressives undertook national efforts to break up large trusts, regulate railways, ensure pure foods and drugs, and enact various other political and economic reforms. The Progressive movement, however, was as much a cultural, and even a religious, phenomenon as a political one. Early on and for several distinct reasons, reformers tackled the sex trade and its role in spreading the social ill of sexually transmitted diseases.

Progressive leaders, who largely represented the middle class, were as concerned as many other middle-class Americans about the changes that immigration and **industrialization** were effecting on the nation, resulting in a more diverse culture. Moralism was an important part of their agenda. Progressives tended to be especially concerned about the leisure patterns and morals of the working class. Men of the working class were often viewed by the reformers as sexually lascivious and uncontrolled. Working-class women were sometimes stereotyped as being ignorant and promiscuous.

Issues of sexual morality easily fit within the Progressive framework. Some reformers preached education as the means to slow the spread of sexual vice and disease, whereas others called for repressive measures, such as the eradication of prostitution. There was, however, a continued hesitancy to discuss sexual matters in the early twentieth century, as reflected in the terminology used in newspapers and other popular media. For example, the term "social evil" was consistently used in reference to prostitution, which is generally not mentioned by name. Similarly, **syphilis** and **gonorrhea** were referred to as "social diseases." And the effort to combat these problems was referred to as the "social hygiene" movement.

Prince Morrow (1846–1913), a New York **physician**, is generally regarded as the "Father of Social Hygiene." Morrow was born in Kentucky and received his medical training in Europe. In 1901 Morrow chaired the Committee of Seven of the New York County Medical Society on venereal disease. It was apparently his attendance in 1902 as a U. S. delegate at the International Conference on Prophylaxis of Syphilis and Venereal Disease in Brussels, however, that stimulated him to become a crusader against venereal disease. Upon returning from this meeting, he immediately began to speak and write on the subject.

In 1904 Morrow published a book on *Social Disease and Marriage*, in which he emphasized the toll that syphilis and gonorrhea took on marriage and family life. He told of sterility among women, congenital blindness in infants, insanity, and other problems that these infections could introduce into the family. He spoke of the "innocent victims," the wives and unborn children, who might contract the disease because of the indiscretion of the husband and father. And he traced these infections ultimately back to prostitution. Morrow agreed, however, with a group of nineteenth-century reformers who had placed the blame on the male client rather than the female prostitute, who had usually been viewed as the main culprit.

Morrow also opposed the "conspiracy of silence" about venereal disease, believing that ignorance and prudishness were responsible for the high incidence of syphilis and gonorrhea. He complained that social sentiment held that it was a greater impropriety to mention venereal disease publicly than to contract it privately. The New York physician also argued that the public should be made fully aware of the consequences of contracting a venereal infection.

Convinced that there was a need for an organization to deal with the problems of prostitution and venereal disease, Morrow formed the American Society for Sanitary and Moral Prophylaxis in 1905. The professed aim of the Society was to prevent the spread of diseases that had their origin in the "social evil." Twenty-five physicians attended the organizational meeting at the New York Academy of Medicine. Believing that venereal disease was not strictly a medical issue, Morrow soon reached out to clergy, educators, journalists, and others to expand his organization, which grew to a membership of nearly 700 by 1910. In that same year, similar groups that had been founded in a number of cities, such as Philadelphia and Detroit, came together with Morrow's organization and under his leadership to establish the American Federation for Sex Hygiene.

At about this time, most large American cities had also begun to organize vice commissions to combat prostitution. These commissions emphasized that prostitution was a particular problem in cities. Young men looking for work migrated to urban areas, where they were away from the watchful eyes of family and neighbors and were often lonely. The cost of living was high, and wages were low, and so young bachelors frequently postponed marriage. The cities also offered more opportunities for social contacts between the **sexes**, at dance halls, movie theaters, and other amusement venues. As more women entered the workplace, the vice commissions noted, social contacts between the sexes also increased. Some observers pointed out that women who had to earn their living sometimes turned to prostitution because it offered more lucrative earnings than many low-wage jobs. And single young women who lived apart from their families were subject to the same loneliness and temptations as young men in that position.

Although most social reformers agreed on a strategy of combating prostitution through education or through repression, there were still advocates of the view that prostitution would never be eliminated and that it was therefore best for the state to regulate it. Some physicians, in particular, continued to argue that licensing and inspecting prostitutes were the only sure means of controlling venereal disease. In 1910 the debate reached a climax when the State Legislature of New York passed the act popularly known as the Page Law. The act established a night court for women, required the fingerprinting of convicted prostitutes, and provided for the medical inspection of prostitutes. If a woman was found to be infected with a venereal disease, she could be detained for treatment. Opponents were outraged, as they believed the law essentially established state-regulated prostitution. The New York Court of Appeals ended the debate over the law in 1911 when it found the section dealing with medical inspection and detention of prostitutes to be unconstitutional because it violated due process by making the diagnosis of the physician binding on the court.

The battle over the Page Law seems to have served to unite the various social hygiene and anti-vice groups. Social hygienists tended to believe that sex education and public enlightenment were the best strategies for dealing with the problems of prostitution and venereal disease. They were especially concerned with the health aspects of the problem. The anti-vice organizations, on the other hand, focused more on so-called white slavery (forcing women into prostitution) and the repression of prostitution. Although Morrow recognized the advantages of combining forces, it was not until after his death in 1913 that these forces came together. Before his death, however, Morrow had persuaded a leading philanthropist to raise most of the funds needed to form a federation.

Several months after Morrow's death, leaders of his American Federation for Sex Hygiene and of the American Vigilance Association, an organization formed in 1912 that focused on eliminating the traffic in women, met in Buffalo to discuss a merger. The representatives voted to consolidate as the American Social Hygiene Association. John D. Rockefeller Jr. (1874–1960), who attended the Buffalo meeting, provided the greatest financial assistance to the new organization in its early years. In the previous year, Rockefeller himself had created a Bureau of Social Hygiene for the scientific study of prostitution and venereal disease. Charles W. Eliot (1834–1926), President Emeritus of Harvard University, agreed to serve as the first president of the American Social Hygiene Association. Operation began on January 21, 1914, with the responsibility for management of the Association initially shared by James Bronson Reynolds (1861–1924), an attorney experienced in vice investigations, and physician William Freeman Snow (d. 1950), a professor at Stanford University and a California public health official. The Association's office was at first located in New York City.

Snow, who soon became the Association's first executive director, discussed the origin and meaning of the phrase "social hygiene" in a 1916 report. He related that the term apparently originated in 1907 with the Chicago Society for Social Hygiene, a group that at the time was primarily concerned with sex education. He went on to define the term as follows: "Its present meaning is largely due to the necessity for some descriptive activities directed toward sex education, the reduction of venereal disease, and the repression of prostitution." Thus, the new Association's name and its goals incorporated the concerns of the different groups of reformers that came together to found it. *See also* Disease, Social Construction of; Non-Governmental Organizations (NGOs) and Epidemic Disease; Personal Hygiene and Epidemic Disease; Personal Liberties and Epidemic Disease; Public Health Agencies, U.S. Federal; Religion and Epidemic Disease; Sanitation Movement of the Nineteenth Century; Scapegoats and Epidemic Disease; Sexuality, Gender, and Epidemic Disease.

Further Reading

Alexander, Ruth. *The "Girl Problem": Female Sexual Delinquency in New York, 1900–1930.* Ithaca: Cornell University Press, 1995.

Brandt, Allan M. *No Magic Bullet: A Social History of Venereal Disease in the United States since 1880,* expanded first edition. New York: Oxford University Press, 1987.

Bristow, Nancy K. *Making Men Moral: Social Engineering during the Great War.* New York: New York University Press, 1996.

D'Emilio, John, and Estelle B. Freedman. *Intimate Matters: A History of Sexuality in America,* 2nd edition. Chicago: University of Chicago Press, 1997.

Hobson, Barbara Meil. *Uneasy Virtue: The Politics of Prostitution and the American Reform Tradition.* New York: Basic Books, 1987.

Snow, William F. "Progress, 1900–1915." *Social Hygiene* 2 (1916): 37–47.

JOHN PARASCANDOLA

VIRCHOW, RUDOLF (1821–1902).   Prussian **physician** Rudolf Virchow, the father of cellular pathology and a critical researcher on social determinants of disease, was born in 1821 in Pomerania. A leading figure in the Revolution of 1848, he made singular contributions to clinical medicine, medical theory, and theories of the social context of disease.

After receiving his medical degree in 1843, Virchow served as an intern at Berlin's Charité Hospital where he worked under pathologist Robert Froriep (1804–1861). There he became the first to describe leukemia (1845) and, in 1846, to detail the process by which blood clots cause thrombosis and embolism. Also in 1846, Virchow literally redefined health and disease. Most believed sickness was a condition foreign to normal tissues, a type of parasite on the healthy body. Virchow argued that disease resulted when healthy tissues were transformed by disease, their functions impaired as a result. Health was the absence of disease, disease the transformation of healthy tissue.

With others of his era—such as **Edwin Chadwick** in Great Britain—Virchow was a leader in describing the social context in which disease took hold. In 1848 the Prussian government sent Virchow to investigate a violent **typhus** epidemic in Upper Silesia, an area undergoing a famine. His report publicly blamed the government for the social realities he argued created an environment in which the **epidemic** could flourish. "It was a failure by the government to allow autonomous self-rule, to provide proper roads, agricultural improvements, and support of industry that had led to present conditions," Virchow argued. The root cause of the typhus epidemic, in other words, lay in the conditions of systemic poverty, social degradation, and a lack of adequate sanitation. What made Virchow's argument unique, and uniquely powerful, was its combination of the clinical, including autopsy, and the social into a single argument.

When a series of popular uprisings for social change swept across much of Europe in 1848, Virchow proved to be a firebrand as a public speaker arguing for political change that many believed would result in better social conditions. Briefly disciplined by the government, Virchow was later named to a chair in pathology at the University of Würzburg where he wrote the landmark text *Cellular Pathology* (1859). That work focused disease studies on the chemical and physical events occurring at the cellular level. Virchow's interests in physical anthropology and archeology led him to form the German Society for Anthropology, Ethnology, and Prehistory in 1869. He remained a publicist for public medical matters, founding and/or editing *Reform of Medicine* (*Mediscinische Reform*), *Archive for Pathological Anatomy and for Clinical Medicine*, *Journal of Ethnology*, and *Virchows Archiv*. Virchow was a member of the German Reichstag from 1890 to 1893 and functioned as a liberal critic of Chancellor Otto von Bismarck (1815–1898), who challenged him to a duel. Nonetheless, Virchow's renown as a researcher of infectious diseases and pathology garnered him the presidency of the First International Congress on Leprosy, held in Berlin in 1897.

Twentieth-century social epidemiologists best remember Virchow as the founder of cellular pathology and for his argument that the state is responsible for conditions that promote epidemic diseases. Ever since, proponents of social medicine and social reformers have invoked his name in arguing that social factors such as **poverty**, poor sanitation, and inadequate medical infrastructure contribute to epidemic and endemic disease. See also Contagion Theory of Disease, Premodern; Demographic Data Collection and Analysis, History of; Environment, Ecology, and Epidemic Disease; Epidemiology, History of; Sanitation Movement of the Nineteenth Century.

Further Reading

Ackerknecht, Erwin H. *Rudolf Virchow*. New York: Arno Press, 1981.

Krieger, Nancy. "Comment: A Vision of Social Justice as the Foundation of Public Health: Commemorating 150 Years of the Spirit of 1848." *American Journal of Public Health* 88, 11 (1998): 1603–1606.

McNeely, Ian F. "*Medicine on a Grand Scale*": Rudolf Virchow, Liberalism, and the Public Health. London: Wellcome Trust, 2002.

Nuland, Sherwin. B. *Doctors: The Biography of Medicine*. New York: Vintage Books, 1995.

Rosen, George. *History of Public Health*. Expanded Edition. Baltimore: Johns Hopkins University Press, 1993.

Virchow, Rudolf. "Report on the Typhus Epidemic in Upper Silesia." *Social Medicine* 1 (2006): 11–98.

TOM KOCH

VIRUS.   Prior to the 1930s, "virus" was general term for any microbial agent of infectious disease. Since then, however, the term has been restricted to such agents that pass through filters that retain **bacteria** and other larger microbes, appropriately called "filterable viruses." The simple term "virus" is now used.

Viruses are obligate intracellular parasites that can exist as potentially active but inert entities outside of cells. Viruses can infect many animal, plant, and protist cells with effects ranging from unapparent infection to lethality. All virus infections have an entry phase; an intracellular phase of multiplication, integration, or latency formation; a virus release phase; and usually some type of host response. These host responses usually appear as signs and symptoms of the infection. Well-known virus diseases include **measles**, chicken pox, rabies, **hepatitis**, the common cold, **influenza, yellow fever**, and **AIDS**.

Initial Entry and Local Virus Multiplication.   All viruses have some structural features in common: a core of nucleic acid (either RNA or DNA) that acts as the viral genome and encodes the viral functions, and a coat of protein that may or may not be surrounded by a lipid membrane. At the cellular level, a virus first must enter the cell, often by adsorption or attachment to a specific receptor on the surface of the target cell. A virus receptor may be a molecule or group of molecules that the cell uses for other purposes; for example, one of the lymphocyte cell recognition molecules is used by the human immunodeficiency virus (HIV) as its attachment and entry site. In some cases, only the viral nucleic acid enters the cell, but in other cases, the entire virus is taken into the cell, and the viral genome is exposed after a process of "uncoating." If virus proteins enter along with the genome, the proteins often regulate expression and replication of the viral genes. Some viral proteins may function to suppress host gene expression to help the virus subvert cellular processes to its own advantage. Some genes of the virus are expressed immediately after infection, and their translation into proteins starts the intracellular virus replication phase. Once a large number of viral genomes have been produced, and a sufficiently large pool of virus structural proteins has accumulated, virus assembly takes place.

The Virus Release and Viremic Phase.   The cell then ruptures or is lysed from within by specific enzymes. Hundreds to thousands of new infectious virus particles burst forth from each infected cell, each one available to spread the infection. Some viruses, however, do not undergo this "lytic cycle" but have evolved a symbiotic relationship with the host cell. They integrate their genomes into the host cell chromosome in a "repressed" or latent state by a complex process that differs for RNA- and DNA-containing viruses.

Common routes of infection of **animals** are through the respiratory tract, the gastrointestinal tract, directly into the blood stream, by sexual contact, or by the bite of an infected insect vector. After the local infection of susceptible cells, the initial viremia (virus in the blood) transports the progeny virus to target cells or tissues in the body where the virus may replicate further, adding more virus to the blood (secondary viremia). Often, the immunological responses of the individual are provoked only by the secondary viremia because the primary viremia may be inadequate in duration or intensity to do so.

Immunological Responses in the Host.   Most virus infections are asymptomatic or, at most, cause such common and inconsequential symptoms that the infection passes unnoticed. Analysis of the antibodies in normal human serum shows that we have many antiviral antibodies that indicate a history of prior unrecognized encounters with many viruses.

The viremic phase of infection allows the cells of the immune system to respond to the presence of virus. If the virus is sufficiently immunogenic, a primary antibody response occurs in about a week. This response results in the production of long-lasting memory–B cells that can be activated later by subsequent exposure to the same virus to provide a rapid and intense secondary immune response. This immunological memory is the primary reason for lifelong immunity once a person has survived a particular viral infection.

The specific antibodies produced by the primary immune response can combine with the virus in the blood and result in circulating immune complexes that facilitate the destruction and clearance of the virus from the body, but also result in activation of some processes such as the production of fever.

Some viruses that enter into a latent or symbiotic state within the host cell can provoke abnormal cell behavior. Many such viruses carry extra genes that regulate cell division and can result in the malignant transformation of the cell to produce a cancer.

These cancer-causing (oncogenic) viruses are a special group of viruses that are of great current interest because of both their special biology and their practical importance.

Effects on the Host. The usual outcome of a viral infection is recovery of the organism with long-lasting immunity. After the initial local virus multiplication, viremic phase, and immunological responses, the virus is eliminated from the body. The immune memory cells provide for long-term protection against another infection. If this sort of immunity is produced by deliberate infection, usually with a weakened strain of virus, the process is called **vaccination** (more accurately, immunization). If, however, the immune system is compromised, if the virus replication overwhelms the immune system, or if the virus enters cells or tissues that are hidden from the immune system, the virus may destroy critical tissues or organs and result in illness or death.

The classic mode of prevention of viral diseases is by artificial immunization with whole attenuated viruses or parts of virus particles. This approach was first used in the case of **smallpox** when it was observed that infection with viral material from a mild case often resulted in a mild case of smallpox (so-called inoculation or variolation) that then conveyed lifelong immunity. Later, a related but nonlethal virus, the cowpox virus was used to induce immunity to smallpox.

Some viruses, after the primary infection, enter into a latent form and remain asymptomatic until later reactivation. The herpes group of viruses is especially prone to such latent infections. Initial infection, for example, with the chicken pox virus (actually a member of the herpes group) produces viremia and generalized skin rash. The virus then latently infects the dorsal root ganglia of the spinal cord and later, at times of lowered immunity, the virus reactivates producing skin lesions along the distribution of the spinal nerve, resulting in a case of "shingles." Chicken pox and shingles are different manifestations of the varicella-zoster virus. A few viruses (e.g., HIV) are known to replicate at such a low level and to remain relatively benign initially, yet to escape the immune system and establish a true persistent infection.

Host cell proliferation may result from latent virus infections resulting in local, limited growths such as viral warts and the small skin lesions caused by the virus of *molluscum contagiosum*. Other latent infections can lead, in ways not yet fully understood, to malignant diseases such as Burkitt's lymphoma, nasopharyngeal carcinoma, Kaposi's sarcoma, and **cervical cancer**.

Virulence and Transmission. Viruses are called virulent if they have a high propensity to cause disease or other evidence of infection. This principle has been widely exploited to produce vaccine strains of viruses. Virulence may be related to the interaction of essential viral functions with related host cellular functions. In certain cases, the virulence genes of the virus can be deleted or modified to make avirulent variants. A virus strain may be virulent for one host species and avirulent for another. Repeated selection for virulence in one host species may select for mutations that render the virus less virulent (attenuated) in another. The transmissibility of the virus is an important factor in the spread of infections and is often a genetic property of a specific viral strain. Highly transmissible strains of the influenza virus and of the common cold virus are much more likely to cause epidemic outbreaks than virus strains of lower transmissibility.

Because viruses are intracellular parasites that depend on many cellular processes for their growth and replication, there are few unique, virus-specific pathways that can be targeted with antiviral drugs without interfering with the uninfected host cells. The very simplicity of viruses and their nearly total dependence on cellular functions have been major reasons why there are few effective antiviral drugs and why viral chemotherapy remains a stubborn challenge. *See also* Contagion and Transmission; Hemorrhagic Fevers; Human Immunity and Resistance to Disease; Human Papilloma Virus and Cervical Cancer; Immunology; Poliomyelitis.

Further Reading

Acheson, Nicholas H. *Fundamentals of Molecular Virology*. Hoboken, NJ: Wiley, 2007.

Crawford, Dorothy H. *The Invisible Enemy: A Natural History of Viruses*. New York: Oxford University Press, 2002.

Fields, B. N, D. M. Knipe, and P. N. Howley, eds. *Fields' Virology*, 3rd edition. Philadelphia: Lippincott-Raven, 1996.

Levy, J. A., H. Fraenkel-Conrat, and R. A. Owens, eds. *Virology*, 4th edition. Engelwood Cliffs, NJ: Prentice Hall, 1994.

Oldstone, Michael B. A. *Viruses, Plagues, and History*. New York: Oxford University Press, 1998.

WILLIAM C. SUMMERS

W

WAR, THE MILITARY, AND EPIDEMIC DISEASE. The relationship between military activity and **epidemic** disease is an ancient and complicated one. Disease is met with at every stage of an army's life: its formation from raw recruits, its training, its off-duty pleasures, its encampments, its travel through its own territory and then the enemy's, its engagements with the enemy, its treatment of the wounded, its advance after victory or retreat after defeat, its ravaging of the enemy's countryside and towns between battles, its sieges, its transport and housing of prisoners, and its return home and demobilization.

Wars have involved thousands, tens, and even hundreds of thousands of soldiers at a time. Recruits from distinct disease ecologies intermingle and share their diseases and those of their new home until they are "seasoned." On campaign, soldiers bring their own diseases and encounter new ones. Fatigue, malnutrition, wounds, and stress lower immune responses, whereas camp life in crowded and unsanitary conditions encourages the spread of contagious diseases and creates ideal ecological niches for both native and imported parasites. Civilians also play various roles in these processes as sources of disease, victims of diseased soldiers and their parasites, healers and caregivers, medical researchers and innovators, and refugees. War disrupts societies in manifold ways, from forced quartering to destruction of homes and hospitals, from sparking local and regional epidemics to the voluntary and forcible displacement of large populations whose squalid new living conditions invite wholesale death by disease. This entry presents a few contemporary and historical examples of the many ways in which war and disease intersect.

Mobilization and Training of U.S. Armed Forces. Though an army may be gathered only from among local populations, as when city-states fought one another in ancient Greece or medieval Italy, armies have historically brought men together from near and far. Pathogens of many types arrived at camp with them, and many of these could spread quickly, especially among those who had never encountered them before.

Prior to the U.S.-Mexican War (1846–1848) and Europe's Crimean War (1853–1856) few armies kept records that fully detail personnel deaths. During America's Civil War (1861–1865), many Confederate records were lost when Richmond was burned, but Federal (U.S.) records remain intact. They show that recruiting in 1861 and 1862 brought urban and rural men, often from far-flung regions, together in very close quarters for training, and that this led to an immediate spike among them of the typically childhood diseases of **smallpox**, scarlet fever, erysipelas, and **measles**. The last was especially contagious, striking a third to a half of recruits in epidemics lasting as long as two months. When African Americans were first inducted in 1863, the effects of congregating were even greater, though the initial high incidence of diseases slid downward very rapidly.

In April and May 1898, 150,000 American men were recruited to serve in the Spanish-American War. Many volunteers battled measles, mumps, and even **meningitis**, but **typhoid fever** struck most widely and severely. Because survivors gained immunity, typhoid struck hardest at induction and training camps. Endemic in much of the United States, *typhi* bacilli were deposited by carriers in their feces. This material was then spread by incidental contact or by houseflies that were attracted to feces, horse manure, and other organic material. Flies walked and fed on contaminated waste, then landed or defecated on people, food, and other objects commonly handled. At a large camp, a million or more flies could hatch daily. Eventually, 24,000 cases resulted in 2,000 deaths, peaking in late August and early September. Men were first brought together in state basic training camps, then concentrated in four so-called national camps that brought men from across America together. The mixing of these men with those from other camps, and the continued routing of the volunteers among camps, served to spread the disease even more widely, accounting for fully half of the typhoid cases.

This experience, the research into typhoid by **Walter Reed** and the Typhoid Board, and the conclusions made by the Dodge Commission, led to routine typhoid vaccination of U.S. recruits from 1911 and to much greater attention being paid to camp sanitation and **personal hygiene**. Between America's entry into World War I (1914–1918) in April 1917 and December 1918, 3,700,000 recruits underwent training in camps that ranged in quality from long-established bases to tent cities. Although only 244 contracted typhoid fever, over 92,000 suffered from mumps, almost 61,000 from measles, 16,236 from **tuberculosis**, and 15,488 from rubella, scarlet fever, or meningitis. As during the Civil War, most cases occurred early in the mobilization process. The huge exception was the "Spanish" **influenza**, which struck U.S. camps in September and October 1918 with 327,480 cases.

A range of immunizations, several of which had been developed by the military, was available to the World War II inductees. Only after the war, however, was a full range of **vaccinations** developed. The vaccines currently given to U.S. trainees include measles, mumps, rubella; **hepatitis** A; hepatitis B; influenza vaccine; polio vaccine; **diphtheria**, acellular pertussis, tetanus; meningococcal conjugate vaccine; and, if warranted, varicella and **yellow fever** vaccine. Still others are provided if deployment is into disease-ridden environments.

Camp Conditions and Life. A study published in 2005 theorized that the great **influenza pandemic of 1918–1919**—which killed an estimated 40,000,000 people—had its origin in a huge rear area British military camp in northern France (Etaples) in the winter of 1917–1918. The authors note that this installation contained dangerous toxic gas supplies that were mutagenic, as well as large numbers of swine, fowl, and horses—all associated with **animal** forms of influenza. Typically 100,000 men were housed here, but turnover was great as they transited to and from the frontlines and back and forth from Britain. Leakage of gas could have altered swine, avian, or equine flu **viruses**, allowing them to lodge with the hoards of transient soldiers and spread to friend and foe alike. If true, then this is certainly the most egregious example of unsanitary camp conditions affecting the history of human disease.

Troops barracked at home also suffered from the influenza. Fort Riley, Kansas, has the distinction of being the known point of origin of the pandemic in the United States (March 1918), and the flu clearly spread through the network of military bases and camps and to the neighboring communities and beyond. These installations suffered one death per hour at the pandemic's height, or about 200 per week, whereas British home camps lost 2,000 per week. Despite good sanitation and nutritious food, living conditions were still crowded and allowed the virus free reign. Though an extreme case, this was by no means a unique experience: in 1950, a modern Israeli military facility near Tel Aviv suffered a bout of **West Nile Fever**, for which 636 of the resident 1,000 soldiers had to undergo treatment.

Before the advent of germ theory and the emphasis on sanitation, military camps, bases, and forts tolerated poor quality food and **water**, lax standards for waste removal, and substandard personal hygiene—all of which fostered the growth and spread of pathogens and disease. For military personnel, flight was not an option, unless insightful commanders took the lead. When **bubonic plague** struck the enormous Russian Black Sea fortress of Ochakov in the spring of 1739, the Russian commander eventually decided to relocate the garrison to Ukraine, but not before some 30,000 had fallen victim. **Cholera**, too, could sweep through military bases, as it did in July1830 at the Russian Caspian Sea port city of Astrakhan. Because of the regular relationships, commercial and otherwise, between soldiers and civilians, the disease spread quickly through the city of 37,320, causing 3,633 cases with a mortality rate of 91 percent. At the same time, Moscow lost 3,102 to cholera, its garrison taking a quarter of the fatalities. But progressive commanders who sought to stanch the epidemic sometimes paid a price, as when Russian Novgorod's barracks erupted in riot against harsh sanitation measures being implemented at the base.

With the development of European **colonialism** in the eighteenth and nineteenth centuries, European troops and sailors often found themselves in tropical ports and bases where local diseases could—and did—run rampant. The British military first encountered endemic cholera in the early 1780s in Ganjam, India, when 1,143 soldiers in a garrison of 5,000 fell ill. Another thousand cases soon weakened the Madras garrison, and the disease spread to Britain's Indian allies. The origins of the first cholera pandemic are also found among the British in northwest India, in 1817. An especially virulent epidemic in 1861 in Delhi and Lahore, in which 457 cases resulted in 261 deaths over 10 days, threatened to topple the regime and prompted the imperial government immediately to establish the Indian Sanitary Commission.

Africa earned its nickname as the white man's grave. Military occupation of ports and forts always accompanied colonization, and troops sent to serve needed several weeks—sometimes more—to acclimate their bodies to the weather and disease **environment**. Yet even the best "seasoning" might not prepare a unit, as in 1778 at the Senegalese Fort St. Louis. Apparently Senegal had not known yellow fever, but it arrived with a slave ship from Sierra Leone, where, as elsewhere, it had long been endemic. The British colonists and soldiers as well as local natives dropped from the disease, suffering a mortality rate of

60 percent in what some consider Africa's first epidemic of yellow fever. It continued to affect colonial armies in much of West Africa, and Sierra Leone itself suffered 15 epidemics between 1815 and 1885. In similar ways, European and U.S. colonial armies in the Caribbean, Southeast Asia, and the Philippines suffered far more from disease than hostile action.

The First Gulf War (1990–1991): Protecting Coalition Troops against Disease. In the summer and fall of 1990, over half a million Coalition troops from 40 countries shipped out to Saudi Arabia and other friendly nearby states to force Iraqi dictator Saddam Hussein (1937–2006) to abandon his military occupation of Kuwait. Coalition war planners expected to encounter the diseases and perhaps case rates experienced in the region during World War II. The predominant participants—U.S., British, and Canadian soldiers and marines—were carefully vaccinated against childhood diseases such as diphtheria and **polio**, as well as influenza, yellow fever, hepatitis A, and tetanus, and many were also vaccinated against anthrax and plague. Military planners employed a sophisticated regimen of prophylaxis to insure that serious infectious diseases remained in check. Desert camps and staging areas were kept sanitary, ample potable water was provided, and food was continually inspected for tainting or parasites. **Insecticides** and repellents were applied lavishly, inspection and surveillance for disease was constant and careful, and an infectious disease diagnostic laboratory was included along with state-of-the-art field medical facilities. Along with standard theater diseases, planners feared Iraqi biological weapons use. During the build up from July 1990 to January 1991, 60 percent of U.S. service personnel experienced predictable and nonacute gastrointestinal ailments such as diarrhea and mild colds and other respiratory ailments that accompany close living quarters. They reported only 32 cases of leishmaniasis (caused by a **protozoon** carried by sandflies), 7 cases of **malaria**, and 1 of West Nile fever. Only one U.S. serviceman died of an infectious disease, a case of meningococcal meningitis. Very limited contact with local residents and general lack of privacy kept rates of venereal disease far below the norm for troops in theater. Many veterans of the nine-month campaign have long complained of a variety of chronic ailments generically labeled Gulf War Syndrome, though no single cause has been widely accepted.

Disease and Military Opportunism. An outbreak of epidemic disease may so debilitate a military force that its misfortune tempts its enemies. The **Plague of Justinian** that began in the sixth century CE so weakened both the Persian and Byzantine empires and their armies that the upstart Muslim forces from Arabia had little trouble conquering the first and devouring much of the second in the middle of the seventh century. When the English army positioned in southern Scotland near Selkirk contracted the plague in 1349, the Scots thought that their hour had arrived. In the course of their advance, the clansmen shared the English fate, and before long 5,000 Scots had succumbed to the Black Death. In the Western Hemisphere the diseases that accompanied the Europeans and Africans from the late fifteenth century mowed down the indigenous peoples and opened doors for conquest. The Aztec capital of Tenochtitlán, praised for its size and wealth by the Spaniards who first encountered it, lost half of its population to smallpox and lay prostrate before the victorious Spanish conquistador Hernán Cortés (1485–1547) in 1521. Within only a few years the disease had penetrated to Peru and killed the Inca emperor Huayna Capac (1464–1527) and his wife, an event that precipitated a civil war. The Incan losses to both violence and imported disease opened the door to Spain's Francisco Pizarro (1471–1541), who smashed the Incan empire in 1532. In 1706 an outbreak of yellow fever in English Charleston, South Carolina, tempted the French and Spanish naval squadron in

St. Augustine, Florida, to sail north to make an easy conquest. The colonial militia, which had stayed outside the fevered city, remained healthy and staved off the small fleet, which retired to its base.

Disease on Campaign.   Epidemic outbreaks rarely started or ended conflicts, but, as at Selkirk, they often played roles in determining battles and even campaigns. Debilitating diseases did not have to kill combatants to cripple an army; they could simply take so many off active duty as to blunt its effective force. Early in the American Civil War, the Confederate forces in western Virginia were halted (September 13, 1861) during an otherwise successful campaign when a combination of measles, dysentery, typhoid fever, and pneumonia struck the men with a biblical fury. In 1722 Czar Peter the Great of Russia (1672–1725) was forced to halt his campaign of expansion in the Caucasus during the Russo-Persian War because of **ergot**-tainted rye bread. It was said he lost 20,000 men to the disease. In the later sixth century CE, the Christian Ethiopian prince Abraha (r. c. 525–553) controlled a considerable portion of the Arabia Peninsula. The prince's military campaign to convert Arabians to Christianity in 569–571 was halted abruptly when smallpox or measles broke out among his troops as they approached the important trading center of Mecca. So weakened were the Ethiopians that they lost what they had controlled in Arabia, an event celebrated in the Koran's Sura 105. Had Mecca been converted, the life story of Muhammad (579–632), Prophet of Islam, might have been very different. The Black Death brought hostilities between France and England to a standstill in 1349; in 1691 yellow fever felled 3,100 British sailors on 18 British warships bound from Barbados to French Martinique, forcing the fleet to return to England, and it was probably malaria that forced Attila the Hun (406–453) to halt his horde's advance through Italy to Rome in 452. Tropical campaigns could be especially deadly before troops could undergo vaccination.

But armies were not merely victims of disease: they were often responsible for spreading it, among enemy as well as friendly populations, and sometimes at long distances. In 1643 English Royalists were engaged in civil war with Parliament's army, and both were maneuvering across the English landscape. The problem was that both armies were suffering from typhus, and both spread it liberally among the people along their routes. During the cholera pandemic of 1831, the Czar sent Russian troops into Russian Poland from Volhynia to confront revolutionary students and other liberals. The freedom-loving Poles were met not only with Russian bayonets but also with the cholera that accompanied the regiment. The Boer War in South Africa broke out in the early stages of the Third Plague Pandemic. Between 1899 and 1902, British cargo vessels bringing military supplies from ports in South America brought plague to South African ports, and from there, military transport trains carried it inland, where it readily spread among the civilian population. In 1936 smallpox broke out among unvaccinated Ethiopians who were fighting Benito Mussolini's (1883–1945) Italian army in Somalia. Somali nomad tribes came into contact with the Ethiopians, and over a six-week period 1,142 cases developed among civilians, with 471 fatalities. During the early stages of American involvement in the Vietnam War, bubonic plague broke out in several South China Sea provinces. It moved along the coast and then inland. U.S. military activity in the region disrupted the rodent populations—largely bandicoots—among which the *Xenopsylla cheopis* flea made its home. Average annual reported cases of plague among the South Vietnamese were 15 from 1956–1960 and 4,000 from 1965–1970. After the U.S. military withdrawal, annual cases dropped to around 2,500. During the War, 25,000 cases of plague were reported, though estimates run as high as 250,000 throughout Vietnam. Unreported cases probably meant untreated cases, which would have meant a very high mortality rate.

Siege.   Siege warfare entailed one army surrounding a second army or garrison within a city or other well-fortified defensive position. Given the stagnant nature of a siege, living conditions in both the attackers' camp and the defensive position would deteriorate as weeks and often months would pass. Food and clean water were vital for both parties, and though the besieged were often in the worse position, the attackers were often little better off. Typhus, dysentery, and venereal diseases could run rampant through either or both armies. During the supposedly "bloodless" Glorious Revolution in 1688–1689 King James II's (1633–1701) troops besieged a Protestant garrison in the northern Irish city of Derry. Troops and civilians numbering 37,000 suffered a 105-day siege and 10,000 deaths largely as a result of typhus and dysentery. James's Catholic army suffered also, however, from dysentery and typhus as well as syphilis, and the siege was broken. The famous **Plague of Athens** occurred as the Spartan army hemmed the city in. As was often the case with sieges, many people from the countryside had flooded into the city, putting a greater strain on food supplies and other necessities and creating the kind of crowded conditions in which epidemics can thrive.

Armed Forces, War, and Venereal Diseases.   Traditionally all-male organizations, armies have contracted and spread venereal diseases such as syphilis and gonorrhea in numerous ways. During training or while barracked at home, soldiers may have access to prostitutes or other willing sex partners, including one another. "Camp followers," who included prostitutes (Union Civil War General Joe Hooker's [1814–1879] "hookers"), often trailed premodern armies on campaign, and while on duty in foreign noncombat zones or on leave from an active zone, military personnel may take advantage of local sex professionals. In cities such as Saigon during the Vietnam War, Paris during World War II, or Tokyo during the Korean War, many sex workers were displaced young women, often from rural areas and with little or no access to health care or physical protection. Although modern armies have long provided "hygiene" education to enlighten the unsophisticated recruit, drugs, alcohol, peer pressure, loneliness, and the stress of battle may override even the most graphic warnings. Finally, venereal diseases may be contracted or spread during rapes, which may occur in the wake of battle or in the depths of boredom accompanying a campaign in or occupation of enemy territory. Rape is far from unknown as a means of degrading a defeated enemy population or venting frustration by brutalizing the enemy's women sexually. This was especially feared by German civilians as Soviet troops approached Adolf Hitler's (1889–1945) Reich in early 1945. Before and during World War II the Japanese armed forces compelled thousands of Korean women into sexual service as military prostitutes, effectively institutionalizing their continuous rape.

Napoleon Bonaparte (1769–1821) mandated licensing and medical examination of French prostitutes, and those in British naval ports were subjected to the Contagious Diseases Acts of the1860s, which also required regular screening for venereal diseases. In Australia during World War II, press and civic groups such as the Women's Christian Temperance Movement and the newly formed Australian Society for the Eradication of Venereal Diseases unduly whipped up popular opinion against women who entered the wartime workforce and the contrived epidemic of sexually transmitted diseases (STDs) that accompanied it. Public voices flatly blamed and stigmatized liberated women— their healthy inhibitions dulled by "strong drink"—for catering to servicemen's lusts (including those of 1 million transiting American GIs). City governments hired additional policewomen to handle the supposed influx of "promiscuous amateurs" who needed to be screened for disease for the public's and military's protection. Though during World War I, 1 in 10 Australian soldiers contracted an STD, in the early 1940s, only 1 percent did.

In the United States, mobilization in 1942 prompted a coordinated state, local, and federal Public Health Service effort to deal with the potential problem. Like the Australian programs, it targeted women. Within two years, 47 "rapid treatment centers" had been established to isolate women (and some men) who had venereal diseases and were thus deemed public health threats. Military authorities also created prostitute-free zones around military bases and training facilities, an activity sanctioned by the May Act of 1941. The War Department pressured mayors and urban police chiefs to close down brothels, but local interests often outweighed federal influence and threats. The military also tried to reduce the demand for commercial sex: films and posters stressed the horrors of STDs, public relations campaigns enlisted celebrities to extol the virtues of sexual abstinence, and the United Service Organization (USO) worked to entertain and distract troops.

Returning Troops and Refugees.   There are many cases in the historical record of armies or military units returning home and bringing with them diseases of all kinds. As troops are demobilized, they spread their diseases deep into the population of their home states. The **Antonine Plague** of the mid-second century CE that struck the Italian peninsula and western Mediterranean was either smallpox or measles carried by Roman troops returning from duty in Mesopotamia. When the novel disease hit the "virgin soil" in the west, it did tremendous damage. In 570 Byzantine troops on campaign near Mecca (Saudi Arabia) contracted a similar disease and, upon return, spread it about the eastern Mediterranean. As the remnants of Napoleon's Grande Armee completed their retreat from Russia in 1812 and 1813, they carried typhus, dysentery, malaria, and influenza with them. They infected and killed thousands in the German lands they passed through and thousands more in France. At the end of the Crimean War, typhus had been a problem for the British and French armies in the Black Sea region. In 1856 returning French troops were quarantined on an island off the southern French coast, averting any outbreak at home. British troops, on the other hand, returned directly and sparked an outbreak of typhus in the British Isles.

Refugees fleeing a victorious enemy can also spread disease. One of the most significant cases was that of French smallpox carriers fleeing the advancing Prussian army in 1870. Conditions in and around Paris were frantic as new troops were being mustered, existing units repositioned, and thousands packing and fleeing. Smallpox had been rampant in the area since 1868, and it began to spread in every direction. Between 60,000 and 90,000 French are thought to have died in 1870–1871. French prisoners of war (723,500) brought the disease to Germany, and by spreading the prisoners around the new country in 78 prisoner facilities, the military authorities spread the disease. In 1871–1872 an estimated 162,000 were reported dead of the disease. Fleeing French carried smallpox into England (42,000 deaths), Belgium (21,315 deaths) Switzerland, and northwestern Italy, prompting outbreaks, and even New York City suffered 3,084 cases and 805 deaths connected with these refugees. The French army of 1 million had 125,000 cases of smallpox, of whom 23,500 died. The German army, on the other hand, had vaccinated its troops every seven years since 1834, and it only recorded 8,500 cases among its 1.5 million soldiers, of whom 460 died. All told, an estimated 500,000 Europeans—mostly children—succumbed to smallpox. This prompted England and Germany to make vaccination compulsory in 1871 and 1874, respectively.

Contemporary conflicts also produce refugee emergencies, especially in war-torn parts of Africa. In 1994 civil war in Rwanda displaced 1.2 million refugees who established camps outside the Eastern Zaire city of Goma. Living in filth with little or no fresh water, these people suffered greatly from cholera as well as malnutrition. In 1999 Mozambique's civil war sent thousands into northern South Africa, where epidemic malaria quickly broke out. This spread to tourists in the Kruger National Park, and eventually 50,000 cases were reported.

Epidemics in Postwar Conditions.   The social, economic, and physical disruptions caused by war, especially among the defeated, have often left openings for serious outbreaks of deadly diseases. Returning soldiers and prisoners of war, displaced and homeless people, refugees, and occupying soldiers all bring with them their various pathogens. Infrastructural elements such as hospitals, suppliers of medicines, and freshwater delivery systems are often simply gone, as are medical specialists and even primary care providers. The attitude of the victor is often key: if vengeful, it may carry off what it can and damage the ability of the defeated society to care for itself for decades; if magnanimous, it may provide extensive resources to repair, rebuild, and restructure.

Between the 1770s and 1918, Poland had been divided among Germany, Austria-Hungary, and Russia. With the defeat of Germany and Austria and the collapse of Russia in the First World War (1914–1918), international treaties reconstituted Poland as a republic. The country's three regions had been tramped across by armies advancing and retreating, reinforcements traveling to the fronts, prisoners heading to camps, wounded returning for care, demobilized divisions redeploying westward, repatriating Poles, and Russian and Ukrainian refugees first from the War and then from the violent birth pangs of the Soviet state. The new Polish government established a Ministry of Health whose initial duty was to stem the tide of infectious diseases that had been ground into the Polish people. By the summer of 1919, it had established 44 mobile epidemic disease units with 2,400 beds, 103 local hospitals with a total of 4,400 beds, and 35 disinfection units. Twenty-three epidemic medical specialists helped coordinate the efforts of local physicians and other health-care providers. Limited funds, infrastructure, and supplies undermined efforts to tackle the wide array of diseases and huge number of cases encountered.

War and Reemergent Epidemic Disease.   From the early 1990s, wars, civil wars, and endemic regional violence in portions of central Africa have created the social disruption, destruction of medical and public health infrastructure, and forced migration on which epidemic diseases thrive. In war-swept villages and overpopulated refugee camps, poor sanitation, malnutrition, tainted water, stress, and unavailability of needed drugs and other medical supplies affect all involved, but especially the most vulnerable, not least the children. Between 1990 and 1993, crude death rates (CDR) of refugees in countries like Kenya, Ethiopia, and Zimbabwe were 5 to 12 times higher than back home before the violence. Those who were displaced and remained in their home countries fared far worse, with CDRs 12 to 20 times higher those before the disruption. Most common were deaths of infants and children from preventable diseases. A study of Lacor Hospital in war-torn Uganda from 1992 to 2002 demonstrated that almost 80 percent of admissions were of infants, children, and women, and that the most common complaints were typical childhood diseases easily preventable under normal circumstances. Ebola, HIV/AIDS, malaria, and tuberculosis came next, with violence-related injuries and wounds fluctuating with the local level of fighting.

Sleeping sickness is endemic in most of Africa between the Sahara and the southernmost regions and was brought under control by successful efforts to control the tsetse fly vector and livestock infections. These efforts flagged as political turmoil turned to open conflict in Uganda in the mid-1970s. As a result, sleeping sickness rebounded, leading to a reported 40,000 cases over two decades and a suspected number 10 times as high. Treatment is expensive and complicated, but without it, the disease is virtually always fatal. In Sudan, civil war led to sleeping sickness's reemergence in 1997, and soon its prevalence rates in some areas rose to between 20 and 50 percent. By 2007 it ranked beside AIDS as the top regional killer. In Uganda the epidemic occurred when war disrupted living conditions, increased the likelihood of human exposure to the infected tsetse fly, decreased the likelihood that victims would have access to treatment. The cessation of insect control efforts and the movement of displaced people into swampy, fly-infested areas increased transmission rates, while the closure of clinics and blocking of relief efforts denied access to lifesaving services. The Sudanese civil war effectively halted the medical surveillance of populations, especially of refugees, in which the disease was rampant. But even if needful populations had been identified, poor and dangerous transportation infrastructure, roadblocks, official corruption, and the desire of each faction to murder its enemies would have seriously hampered relief efforts.

Military Research on Infectious Disease, Prophylaxis, and Treatment. During World War II, German units serving along the Metaxis Line in Greece and in the southwestern USSR suffered heavily from malaria. Hitler's Army Medical Academy, as well as pharmaceutical companies such as Bayer and I. G. Farben, searched for new malaria drugs and a vaccine and for new means of insect control. Correct dosing of Plasmochine and Atabrine, the two standard drugs, remained elusive, and ruthless experimentation on prisoners and the mentally disabled took many lives. Armies have always had a huge stake in developing the ability to curb the effects of disease, but only since the development of smallpox inoculation in the eighteenth century could they effectively do so. Military researchers, often under combat conditions, have worked diligently to defeat disease, and the ranks of the disease fighters are rife with military careerists. They include the work of Walter Reed and **William Gorgas** in fighting yellow fever, as well as the efforts of **Alphonse Laveran** and **Ronald Ross** to understand malaria and its transmission. The current protocols for treating malaria were developed and tested by U.S. military researchers in Vietnam

Biological or Germ Warfare. From at least 1347, when Mongol warriors hurled bubonic plague corpses into the Christian outpost of Kaffa hoping to spread the pestilence, belligerents have sought to use disease as a means of weakening the enemy forces. Advances in germ theory and microbiology in the later nineteenth and early twentieth century unlocked the secrets of dangerous pathogens, allowing scientists to "weaponize" a range of biological agents. The second Gulf War ignited when Iraqi dictator Saddam Hussein (1937–2006) refused to disavow or allow inspection of biological weapons development sites, and these remain a grave concern to diplomats and military planners worldwide.

In the early 1930s, the Empire of Japan began a concerted effort to develop effective weapons using a score of different pathogens. Though outlawed by the Geneva Convention of 1925 (not ratified by Japan), the program was initiated and led by the racialist microbiologist Dr. Shiro Ishii (1892–1959). As Japanese militarists gained power and influence in the government during the 1930s, they saw the value of germ warfare, and Ishii was provided with laboratory facilities first in Tokyo and then in Manchuria. At Pingfan, near Harbin, Ishii's infamous Unit 731 built a research city housing some 400 human laboratory subjects, including political and military prisoners. By the end of World War II, 20,000 Japanese military and personnel had worked for Unit 731's facilities at Pingfan and scattered across the Empire. Inmates were given many diseases, including anthrax, dysentery, diphtheria, hemorrhagic fevers, smallpox, typhoid, and yellow fever. Autopsies and vivisections were performed, vaccines tested, and the remaining corpses incinerated in crematoria. An estimated 20,000 people died under these conditions. Pathogens in powder form were placed in bombs and shells, and in August of 1942, 80 victims in Jiangshan Province, China, died of purposely cholera-tainted fruits, rice cakes, and well water. At the same time, an estimated 200,000 died of weaponized cholera in Shangdon Province, and an equal number succumbed to the same in Yunnan Province. By the end of 1942, 1,700 Japanese soldiers who had entered contaminated zones had died of these diseases. Between medical experiments and "field tests" perhaps as many as half a million people perished at the hands of Ishii and his scientists. *See also* Cholera: First through Third Pandemics, 1816–1861; Malaria and Modern Military History; Measles in the Colonial Americas; Napoleonic Wars; Poverty, Wealth, and Epidemic Disease; Race, Ethnicity, and Epidemic Disease; Smallpox and the American Revolution; Smallpox in Colonial Latin America; Thirty Years' War; Typhus and War; Yellow Fever Commission, U.S.; Yellow Fever in Latin America and the Caribbean, 1830–1940.

Further Reading

Accorsi, S., et al. "The Disease Profile of Poverty: Morbidity and Mortality in Northern Uganda in the Context of War, Population Displacement and HIV/AIDS." *Transactions of the Royal Society of Tropical Medicine and Hygiene* 99 (2005): 226–233.

Bayne-Jones, Stanhope. *The Evolution of Preventive Medicine in the United States Army, 1607–1939.* Washington, DC: Office of the Surgeon General, 1968.

Byerly, Carol R. *Fever of War: The Influenza Epidemic in the U.S. Army during World War I.* New York: New York University Press, 2005.

Cirillo, Vincent J. *Bullets and Bacilli: The Spanish-American War and Military Medicine.* New Brunswick, NJ: Rutgers University Press, 2004.

Cooter, Roger, et al., eds. *Medicine and Modern War.* Amsterdam: Editions Rodopi, 1999.

Garfield, Richard, and Alfred Neugat. "Epidemiologic Analysis of Warfare: A Historical Review." *Journal of the American Medical Association* 266 (1991): 688–692.

Ghobarah, Hazem Adam, et al. "Civil Wars Maim and Kill People—Long after the Shooting Stops." *American Political Science Review* 97 (2003): 189–202.

Hyams, Kenneth C., et al. "Endemic Infectious Diseases and Biological Warfare during the Gulf War: A Decade of Analysis and Final Concerns." *American Journal of Tropical Medicine and Hygiene* 65 (2001): 664–670.

Kreidberg, M. A., and M. G. Henry. *History of Military Mobilization in the United States Army, 1775–1945.* Westport,CT: Greenwood Press, 1975.

Levy, Barry S., and Victor W. Sidel. *War and Public Health.* Washington, DC: American Public Health Association, 2000.

McLeod, E. Peter. "Microbes and Muskets: Smallpox and the Participation of Amerindian Allies of New France in the Seven Years' War." *Ethnohistory* 39 (1992): 42–64.

Military Medicine 170, 4 Suppl. (April, 2005). (Contains several articles on U.S. military contributions to infectious disease research.)

Pederson, Duncan. "Political Violence, Ethnic Conflict and Contemporary Wars: Broad Implications for Health and Well-Being." *Social Science and Medicine* 55 (2002): 175–190.

Prinzing, Friedrich. *Epidemics Resulting from Wars.* Oxford: Clarendon Press, 1916.

Sartin, Jeffrey S. "Gulf War Syndrome: The Final Chapter?" *Mayo Clinic Proceedings* 81 (2006): 1425–1425.

Shanks, Leslie, and Michael Schull. "Rape in War: The Humanitarian Response." *Journal of the Canadian Medical Association* 163 (October 31, 2000): 1152–1156.

Smallman-Raynor, Matthew, and Andrew D. Cliff. "Civil War and the Spread of AIDS in Central Africa." *Epidemiology and Infection* 107 (1991): 69–80.

———. "Impact of Infectious Diseases on War." *Infectious Disease Clinics of North America* 18 (2004): 341–368.

———. *War Epidemics: An Historical Geography of Infectious Diseases in Military Conflict and Civil Strife, 1850–2000.* New York: Oxford University Press, 2004.

Sturma, Michael. "Public Health and Sexual Morality: Venereal Disease in World War II Australia." *Signs* 13 (1988): 725–740.

Tangermann, R. H., et al. "Eradication of Poliomyelitis in Countries Affected by Conflict." *Bulletin of the World Health Organization* 78 (2000): 330–338.

Valente, F., et al. "Massive Outbreak of Poliomyelitis Caused by Type-3 Wild Poliovirus in Angola in 1999." *Bulletin of the World Health Organization* 78 (2000): 339–346.

Wilensky, Robert J. *Military Medicine to Win Hearts and Minds: Aid to Civilians in the Vietnam War.* Lubbock: Texas Tech University Press, 2004.

JOSEPH P. BYRNE

WATER AND EPIDEMIC DISEASES.   Water plays a vital role in transmitting several deadly **epidemic** diseases, the most notable being **cholera, typhoid**, and **dysentery**. The three main pathogens for these waterborne diseases are *Vibrio*, *Shigella*, and *Salmonella* genera. Epidemics are most apt to spread in urban areas by the contamination of drinking water by human feces that contain the microorganisms of each disease. Waterborne epidemics have played an important part in shaping modern public health policy. The epidemiological link between infected water supply and epidemic disease was first made in mid-nineteenth-century Britain, and projects to reform municipal water supplies have followed since that time. Despite the fact that waterborne epidemics have virtually been eliminated in most Western countries, they continue to threaten widespread disaster among populations whose systems of public sanitation and health remain underdeveloped.

Although waterborne epidemics are a serious threat to human health, a host of other illnesses are water related. Water is a breeding ground for **insects** and other parasites that spread deadly epidemics such as **malaria** and **Dengue**. Other health threats spread by water include intestinal worms, anemia (a nutritional deficiency), schistosomiasis or Bilharzia, leptospirosis (an infection that occurs through direct contact with the urine of infected animals), and **Legionnaires' disease**. Interdisciplinary research on emerging infectious diseases has shown that the variety of water-related microbial diseases is increasing. Since 1970 several new species have been identified, including cryptospordium, *Escherichia coli* 0157, rotavirus, **hepatitis** E and A viruses, and norovirus. Industrial pollution of water with substances such as arsenic and lead also contributes to water-related death tolls, as does the addition of excess fluoride (which can lead to fluorosis). According to the **World Health Organization** (WHO), as of 2004, water-related diseases remained the leading cause of morbidity and mortality worldwide.

Drinking Water, Sanitation, and Waterborne Diseases.   The pollution of drinking water is the principal factor in spreading waterborne disease. Since antiquity there has been a concern for the quality of drinking water. Although there was no direct recognition of the role of water acting as a medium in spreading epidemics, the ancients viewed water as central to individual health. The seminal public health document in the classical Greek **Hippocratic Corpus**, *Airs, Waters, Places*, considered water as a vital component of the maintenance of health and contributor to disease. The Hippocratic author stated, "the effect of water on the health must not be forgotten. Just as it varies in taste and when weighed, so does its effect on the body vary as well." The Hippocratic theory of epidemic disease causation, or miasma theory, had direct implications for public health in the ancient world. Following miasma theory, the ancients believed that epidemics were transmitted through the putrefaction of the **air** by rotting animal or vegetable material. As a result, public health efforts focused on preventing bad smelling air, fumigating unpleasant spaces, and producing general environmental cleanliness. Water only contributed to epidemic disease if it smelled bad and helped corrupt the atmosphere. The importance of water in the ancient world can also be seen in the expansive and intricate water supply for the city of Rome, which began around 313 BCE. The association of epidemics and stagnant water also led the Romans to begin massive drainage projects, which was perhaps the first intervention against vector-borne diseases such as malaria. The ancient Greeks also took great care to obtain clear, fresh water, as they supplemented local city wells with mountain spring water. Although water played a role in distributing disease in the ancient world, historical epidemiologists have not fully examined mortality trends during water-related epidemics.

Throughout the Middle Ages (c. 500 CE–c. 1500 CE) and into the early modern period (c. 1500–1800), the scarcity of water became an important factor in European communal life. In most areas, people spent much of their time gathering water from streams, rivers, and wells. Water continued to be associated with disease, as medieval governments feared that stagnant water and marshes were the source of plagues and fevers. In Valencia, Spain, for example, a law was passed that sentenced any farmer to death who planted rice too close to villages or towns. The deliberate pollution of water in spreading epidemics was also feared. The best example of this is the major epidemic of the **Black Death**, between 1348 and 1352, as social groups such as Jews were accused of **poisoning** wells and were sentenced to death. By the sixteenth and seventeenth centuries, water companies in some European urban centers began to supply water to the houses of private customers. In 1613 wealthy Londoners could be supplied with water from either The London Bridge Water Company or The New River Company. By the end of the seventeenth century, many European cities had followed. The first municipal waterworks supply in the United States was the Fairmount Waterworks Company, which operated in Philadelphia from 1819. However, improved water-related technology still lagged behind the growing problem of up-stream pollution, which was intensified by urbanization and industrialization. In places such as the Ganges River Valley in India, long distance pilgrimages along what has been called the "epidemic highway" clearly fostered the pollution and spread of water-related epidemics. What is clear is that before the twentieth century, the distribution and access to water in households was insufficient and largely uneven. More common sanitary technology consisted of cesspits or chamber pots, where refuse was stored until horse drawn carts would collect the offensive matter. Even costly private water supplies were unpredictable and intermittent. By the early nineteenth century, water filtration became increasingly seen as important to health. The first municipal filtration system was built in Paisley, Scotland, in the early 1830s.

Although water clearly played a role in the distribution of certain diseases throughout history, low population density and inadequate water supply systems probably kept the threat of widespread waterborne epidemics at bay. Intense and rapid **urbanization** and **industrialization** in Europe during the eighteenth and nineteenth centuries increased population densities and environmental pollution, adversely affected living conditions for many, and expanded the threat of disease. Concurrent improvements in water supply exacerbated the threat: once contaminated, pumped and piped water is a highly efficient medium for the transmission of epidemic disease. Indeed, as population densities rose, waterborne epidemics replaced plague as the primary hazard to urban populations. Cholera, **typhoid fever, dysentery**, and various conditions of diarrhea all contributed to the staggering mortality rates witnessed by nineteenth-century populations. The dominance of miasma theory and anticontagionism deflected attention from direct person-to-person spread of disease and further hindered effective responses until the full development of **germ theory**. The medical understanding of the specificity of disease and the role of water in spreading epidemics began to change first with epidemiological and bacteriological studies conducted in western Europe in the second half of the nineteenth century.

Establishing the Link between Water and Epidemics. The London anesthetist and epidemiologist **John Snow** was the first to discover that cholera was a waterborne disease. Conducting epidemiological investigations in London in the 1840s and 1850s at a time when cholera was devastating Europe, Snow argued that cholera was a singular disease with a singular route of transmission. Only a previous case of cholera could give rise to another, and the causative agent had to be introduced into the body by swallowing the dejecta of a previous case. Under Snow's model, water became the central vehicle for transmitting the epidemic over large metropolitan areas. Snow's famous investigation of the relationship of cholera incidence to neighborhood use of the water pump on Broad Street, where cholera had struck particularly hard, led authorities to disable the pump and greatly reduced the disease's local incidence. In a larger metropolitan investigation of two London water companies, Snow mapped the relationship of cholera deaths to water suppliers and demonstrated that the mortality rate for the residents supplied by the Southwark and Vauxhall Company was between eight and nine times greater than for those supplied by the Lambeth Company, which had moved its water source upstream to a less polluted area of the Thames River. Snow's theory of disease transmission was as important as his epidemiological investigations. Although few contemporary physicians and public health reformers believed Snow, his research influenced the direction of public health throughout the second half of the nineteenth century.

Between 1860 and 1880, epidemiological investigations in Britain by John Simon (1816–1904), head of the Medical Department of the Privy Council and Local Government Board, and his inspectors provided the substantial evidence that typhoid, diarrhea, dysentery, and cholera were spread by contaminated water—a conclusion many consider the greatest achievement of nineteenth-century epidemiology. The most important of these epidemiologists were George Buchanan (1831–1895) and John Netten Radcliffe (1826–1884). Radcliffe's studies were particularly significant, especially his investigation of the cholera epidemic in East London in 1866. Here, Radcliffe joined with statistician **William Farr** and chemist Edward Frankland (1825–1899) to demonstrate that the East

London Waterworks Company had been drawing its water from an unfiltered source, thus fostering the spread of the epidemic. By the early twentieth century, the growing discipline of bacteriology had isolated the agents of the major epidemic diseases, thus confirming what half a century of epidemiological work had sought to prove. Once the theory of waterborne transmission was universally accepted, however, private institutions, governments, and scientists constantly argued over the policies needed to reform and safeguard water supplies. What was clear by the twentieth century, however, was that the provision of safe water was the responsibility of government. By the end of the nineteenth century, most Western countries had begun massive projects to construct safe and clean water supply systems.

Throughout the twentieth century, water standards and infrastructure made clear progress in the developed world. Although changes in water supply had clearly been made in most Western countries, the control of standing water as a breeding ground for insects was virtually unresolved. One important example is the experience of the United States in the 1930s and 1940s. The creation of the Tennessee Valley Authority by President Franklin D. Roosevelt (1882–1945) in 1933 marked the beginning of a massive drainage campaign in the southern United States against environments conducive to malaria and **yellow fever**. Although malaria affected around 30 percent of the region's population when the TVA began, by the 1950s, the diseases were virtually eliminated. Worldwide, however, malaria remains the most important parasitic infectious disease. Although the **World Health Organization** (WHO) began a malaria eradication program in 1955, many areas of the world, most notably Sub-Saharan Africa, are still rife with the disease.

Current Problems.   The prevention of water-related disease in developed countries through elaborate systems of water filtration, water analysis, and public health infrastructure has led to dramatic improvements in health. In part because of improved water supply, most western countries have experienced increased life expectancy, lowered infant mortality, and the virtual elimination of the major epidemic waterborne diseases. One recent achievement is the U.S. Safe Drinking Water Act of 1974, through which the federal government regulated drinking water for the first time. However, as a result of ineffective systems of waste disposal and improper hygiene, even in some developed countries access to safe drinking water in low-income communities is still a major threat to health, as the standard of treatment and **disinfection** of drinking water is often inconsistent. In developing countries, waterborne diseases constitute around four-fifths of all illness. The leading cause of childhood death worldwide is infantile diarrhea. Often, the installation of adequate public sewage systems is deterred by political instability and marred by the high cost of such projects. Across the world, the collection of reliable data on water supply and disease is lacking. Furthermore, the detection and epidemiological investigation of water-related epidemics is generally inadequate in most countries worldwide. Statistics gathered by the United States between 1991 and 2000 have shown that the etiological agent of around 40 percent of water-related outbreaks was not identified. Because of different approaches in recording disease outbreaks, the exchange between central and local public authorities, waterworks companies, and international organizations is often poor.

International campaigns to secure clean water are currently being waged. The leader is the JMP (Joint Monitoring Program), a WHO and United Nations Children's Fund (UNICEF) co-sponsored program that has conducted a series of global water-related reports worldwide since 1991. Using national censuses and household surveys, the JMP has made clear that monitoring problems are most acute in urban slums, small towns, and rural areas. In 2002 the JMP reported that about 2.6 billion people live without even the most basic sanitation facilities.

Epidemiological and ecological studies have only recently begun to examine the full picture of the relationship between water and epidemic disease. This relationship involves a complex host of factors, including competitive environmental advantages for hosts and pathogens, host immunity, microbial virulence, and evolution. However, with the emergence of new water-related infectious diseases such as the new strain of cholera, *El Tor* Serotype, and the reemergence of other salmonellas and *E. coli* species, more research is crucially needed. Another example is **schistosomiasis**, a chronic debilitating disease spread by water that affects more than 200 million people worldwide. Cholera epidemics still are prevalent in parts of Africa and India. Millions of people throughout the world are at risk of contracting waterborne epidemics because of limited access to safe water and lack of public health infrastructure.

Victims of waterborne epidemics are usually treated by oral rehydration therapy (ORT), a simple and cost-effective solution. When provided quickly after symptoms appear, ORT virtually eliminates mortality from waterborne pathogens that kill through massive dehydration. The major problem worldwide is access to this therapy, particularly in rural areas. ORT also does not protect sufferers from tissue damage that results from the invasion of waterborne pathogens in the intestinal lining. Clearly, more long-term assessments need to be made both on effective therapies and on changes in the virulence of waterborne pathogens.

The importance of water in the transmission of illness is being continually assessed as new tools become available through advances in science, medicine, technology, and epidemiology. The emergence of new species, as well as the reemergence of previously known pathogens poses continual threats to human health. Universal access to safe drinking water and effective sanitation is of primary concern to public health. The United Nations considers a reliable and clean source of drinking water a fundamental basic human right and argues that it should be the highest priority of any country. If clean water is seen by the international community as a universal right, its provision worldwide is desperately lacking. *See also* Biological Warfare; Bioterrorism; Capitalism and Epidemic Disease; Cholera: First through Third Pandemics, 1816–1861; Cholera: Fourth through Sixth Pandemics, 1862–1947; Cholera: Seventh Pandemic, 1961–Present; Colonialism and Epidemic Disease; Ectoparasites; Environment, Ecology, and Epidemic Disease; Latin America, Colonial: Demographic Effects of Imported Diseases; Malaria in Africa; Malaria in Medieval and Early Modern Europe; Malaria in the Americas; Malaria in the Ancient World; Pesticides; Poison Libels and Epidemic Disease; Poliomyelitis; Poverty, Wealth, and Epidemic Disease; Protozoon, –zoa; Sanitation Movement of the Nineteenth century; Yellow Fever in Colonial Latin America and the Caribbean; Yellow Fever in Latin America and the Caribbean, 1830–1940; Yellow Fever in North America to 1810; Yellow Fever in the American South, 1810–1905.

Further Reading

Duffy, John. *The Sanitarians*. Chicago: University of Illinois Press, 1990.

Ewald, Paul. *Evolution of Infectious Disease*. New York: Oxford University Press, 1994.

Goubert, Jean-Pierre. *The Conquest of Water: The Advent of Health in the Industrial Age*. Translated by Andrew Wilson. Princeton: Princeton University Press, 1989.

Hamlin, Christopher. *A Science of Impurity: Water Analysis in Nineteenth-Century Britain*. Berkeley: University of California Press, 1990.

Hardy, Anne. *The Epidemic Streets*. New York: Oxford University Press, 1994.

Hunter, Paul. *Waterborne Disease: Epidemiology and Ecology*. New York: John Wiley & Sons Press, 1997.

Luckin, William. *Pollution and Control: A Social History of the Thames in the Nineteenth Century*. Boston: Adam Hilger Press, 1986.

JACOB STEERE-WILLIAMS

WEST NILE FEVER.   West Nile **Virus** is transmitted to humans primarily by mosquitoes. For most people the disease is mild, but for some people the disease can cause paralysis, **encephalitis**, or death. In nature, the virus cycles between songbirds and mosquitoes. West Nile Virus is originally from the Old World, but it has become successfully established in the New World.

Biological Agent and its Effects on the Human Body.   West Nile Virus (WNV) is an arbovirus (short for arthropod-borne virus) in the family Flaviviridae, which includes some of the most important arboviruses infecting humans (e.g., **Dengue fever** virus, **yellow fever** virus). WNV resembles a tiny (50-nanometer) sphere with small spikes. WNV contains a single central strand of RNA as its genetic component, surrounded by a protein-containing envelope. When an infective mosquito bites, a highly variable number of virus particles (3 to 200,000) are deposited into the skin along with the mosquito's saliva. It is believed that WNV particles first invade and replicate within dendritic cells (immune cells in the skin), then spread to regional lymph nodes, and finally move into the blood where they are distributed throughout the body. In most people, WNV infections are asymptomatic. However, about 20 percent of people get West Nile fever, accompanied by fatigue, headache, muscle ache, and sometimes a rash. Rapid onset of symptoms occurs within 3 to 14 days after being bitten by a WNV-infected mosquito, and symptoms generally last a few days. In severe cases, symptoms can last up to a month. Recovery is mediated by neutralizing antibodies produced in response to WNV infection. In a small proportion of people (around 1 percent, mostly elderly), antibodies fail to halt the infection, and WNV invades the central nervous system. This is a grave situation and can lead to serious and sometimes fatal **meningitis**, encephalitis, ocular complications, or a flaccid, **polio**-like paralysis. Neurological symptoms persist for months, even for life. There is no cure.

Transmission.   WNV is a zoonotic disease. These are diseases that normally cycle among wildlife but can also infect humans. WNV is primarily a disease of songbirds and is transmitted from bird to bird by mosquitoes, particularly in the genus *Culex*. Songbirds are more important than other types of animals in the **transmission** cycle because songbirds produce very high concentrations of WNV in their blood. This is important because there is a threshold amount of virus (around 10^4 to 10^5 plaque-forming units per milliliter of blood) necessary to infect mosquitoes. Although humans (and horses) may be severely affected by WNV, they are considered "dead-end" hosts because they do not produce enough WNV in their blood to infect mosquitoes and therefore cannot contribute to the transmission cycle. Indeed, WNV levels in some songbird species (e.g., crows) get so high that healthy birds can sometimes contract WNV infections from pecking at sick birds that are shedding lots of WNV from their mouths and cloacae. People contract WNV primarily via mosquito bites. In the early 2000s, however, it was recognized that, as with many other types of blood infections, some people have acquired WNV infections through blood transfusions, organ transplantations, or breastfeeding.

Epidemiology.   Like many arboviral diseases, West Nile fever has a seasonal pattern. Most human cases occur in late summer. At the beginning of each mosquito season, transmission is usually low, and so the risk of being bitten by an infectious mosquito is also low. WNV requires several rounds of mosquito-bird-mosquito transmission in order to gain intensity. This is known as viral amplification. The intensity of WNV amplification within a given locality depends on the local species of birds and mosquitoes present and their respective susceptibilities to WNV. The more susceptible the bird or mosquito species, the greater will be the WNV amplification within that locality. Similarly, the intensity of WNV amplification during a given year depends on local meteorological conditions. More than any other environmental factor, temperature plays a role in driving WNV amplification. Warmer temperatures accelerate both mosquito and virus development. Thus, production of infectious mosquitoes can happen quickly. Cooler temperatures prolong these processes, and the virus has less time to undergo multiple rounds of amplification. Thus, the intensity of WNV amplification (and incidence of human cases) tends to be less when summers are cool.

Because WNV is found in northern latitudes where mosquito activity ceases during the winter months, there is some uncertainty as to how WNV transmission in these areas is reinitiated at the beginning of each mosquito season. Theories include 1) influx of WNV-infected birds migrating northward, 2) influx of WNV-infected mosquitoes blown northward on prevailing winds, and 3) persistence of over-wintering mosquitoes infected with WNV. The last theory has gained support from studies demonstrating that WNV-infected mosquitoes can, at low levels, pass the virus on to their progeny through a process known as transovarial transmission. This is crucial to the "over-wintering mosquito theory" because in temperate latitudes, *Culex* mosquitoes spend the winter hibernating in protected places as mated, non–blood fed females. Because they do not feed on blood before initiating hibernation, the only way that over-wintering *Culex* mosquitoes can be infected with WNV and thus initiate transmission the following spring is through transovarial transmission.

History of Major Outbreaks.   *West Nile Story* is a modern-day classic about how a relatively minor and little-known disease, when introduced into a new **environment**, suddenly erupted into a continent-wide **epidemic**. WNV was first isolated in 1937 from the blood of a febrile patient in the West Nile district of Uganda, Africa. Other isolates were made in the early 1950s from apparently healthy **children** in Egypt. Initially, WNV was considered a minor arbovirus that caused little illness in humans. But that assessment changed when cases of WNV encephalitis in humans and horses appeared in Israel and France during the 1960s. Since then, sporadic outbreaks of encephalitic WNV infections have occurred throughout the Mediterranean region, eastern Europe, India, and Australia. In August 1999, a virulent Middle Eastern strain of WNV caused a sudden outbreak of encephalitis among residents of New York City. How WNV crossed the Atlantic Ocean is unknown; perhaps it arrived via infected mosquitoes in shipping containers or airplanes, or via the importation of infected, exotic birds. WNV first took root in the Bronx Zoo, where zookeepers noticed unusually high sickness and mortality among both captive exotic birds and free-ranging native birds. After some initial confusion, the link was made between bird die-offs in the zoo and the appearance of encephalitis in humans. An intense mosquito control operation was rapidly implemented by New York City to quell the spread of the disease. Despite these efforts, WNV reappeared the following spring, and by the end of summer 2000, it had spread to several mid-Atlantic states. Expansion of WNV during the next three summers was amazing. By the end of 2004, WNV was present in all 48 contiguous states of the United States, in areas of southern Canada, and in parts of the Caribbean and Latin America. As WNV moved across North America, a pattern emerged. During its initial introduction into an area, WNV transmission was generally low. But during the second year, WNV transmission exploded, often producing extensive bird die-offs and high incidences of human disease. By the third year, WNV transmission generally subsided. For many parts of eastern North America, WNV transmission has remained low, perhaps because of the development of immunity in bird populations and the presence of a marginally susceptible urban vector species (*Culex pipiens*). Curiously, WNV transmission has remained intense in the upper Great Plains, despite the short transmission season. Apparently, the ecology of northern prairies, with their large songbird populations and presence of a highly susceptible vector species (*Culex tarsalis*), favors the continued transmission of WNV. Despite fears to the contrary, WNV has not caused major epidemics or bird mortalities in the Caribbean and Mexico.

Current Situation of the Disease.   There is no treatment for WNV disease. Therefore, public health policy has stressed prevention. Prevention can be done in three ways: **vaccination**, traditional mosquito control, and avoidance of mosquito bites. There are two types of WNV vaccines available for horses, and several vaccine candidates for humans are undergoing development. Until these become available, recommendations on WNV prevention focus on community mosquito control and on avoidance of mosquito bites. Peak transmission occurs during late summer, and the primary vectors (*Culex*) are nocturnal. Therefore, it is recommended that during late summer, one should either avoid being outdoors after dark or wear **insect** repellent on skin and clothes when out at night. *See also* Pesticides.

Further Reading

Cann, Alan J. *RNA Viruses: A Practical Approach*. New York: Oxford University Press, 2000.

Centers for Disease Control and Prevention. *West Nile Virus*. http://www.cdc.gov/ncidod/dvbid/westnile/

Despommier, Dickson. *West Nile Story: A New Virus in the New World*. New York: Apple Tree Productions, Inc., 2001.

Hayes, E. B., and D. J. Gubler. "West Nile Virus: Epidemiology and Clinical Features of an Emerging Epidemic in the United States." *Annual Review of Microbiology* 57 (2006): 181–194.

Mayo Clinic. *West Nile Virus*. http://www.mayoclinic.com/health/west-nile-virus/DS00438

Sfakianos, Jeffrey N. *West Nile Virus*. Philadelphia: Chelsea House, 2005.

U.S. Geological Survey Maps. http://westnilemaps.usgs.gov/

World Health Organization. *West Nile Encephalitis*. http://www.who.int/vaccine_research/diseases/west_nile/en/

JEFFERSON VAUGHAN

WHITE PLAGUE.   *See* Tuberculosis.

WHOOPING COUGH.   Whooping cough, also known as pertussis, is a highly contagious and life-threatening respiratory infection. Its common name comes from the most characteristic sign, a prolonged series coughs followed by a loud "whoop" of in-rushing breath. Whooping cough has historically been considered a childhood disease; although its threat is greatest for young children, however, it can occur at any age.

It is possible that a passage by **Avicenna** in 1010 CE may be the first reference to a disease that can be recognized as whooping cough. The initial description of whooping cough is attributed to Guillaume de Baillou (1538–1616), an early epidemiologist and **physician** in Paris, who described the characteristic cough during an **epidemic** in 1578. He likened the cough to a dog's barking, and so the disease was termed "the dog cough." English physician Thomas Willis (1621–1675) provided a more definitive description of the disease in 1675. That same year, **Thomas Sydenham** gave the disease its current common name.

Since its early descriptions, and likely well before that, epidemics of whooping cough have occurred at about three- to five-year intervals. This period of time allows for a new group of susceptible **children** to be born and exposed to scattered individuals in the community who are infected. Currently, about 30 to 50 million cases of pertussis occur per year worldwide. Annually, as many as 300,000 people die from whooping cough. This mortality rate makes pertussis one of the most frequently fatal diseases for which we have a means of prevention by **immunization**. People who recover from pertussis generally have lifelong immunity to reinfection. On the other hand, medical immunization does not provide permanent protection. As a result of decreasing immunity over a person's life, there has been a shift in the age of people affected by pertussis, with increasing numbers of teens and adults and decreasing numbers of younger children becoming infected.

Whooping cough is caused by *Bordetella pertussis*, a Gram-negative coccobacillus. The **bacteria** travel easily in droplets coughed out by infected individuals and inhaled by others nearby. The ease of aerosolizing large numbers of the bacteria during severe coughing spells contributes to the very high degree of **contagion**. When the bacteria are inhaled into the trachea and bronchi, they produce a hemagglutinin that helps them bind to the surface of the epithelial cells that line the airways. As they multiply, the bacteria make and release toxins that contribute to the severity of the infection. Pertussis toxin and tracheal cytotoxin cause destruction of the cilia that propel infected mucus, contributing to additional bacterial growth. These toxins also destroy the epithelial cells lining the airways, leading to the severe cough of pertussis. A related disease, parapertussis, is caused by *B. parapertussis*, which lacks the toxins produced by *B. pertussis*. Because of the lack of destructive bacterial toxins, parapertussis is much less severe and less protracted than pertussis. Both *B. pertussis* and *B. parapertussis* appear to be limited to humans as their hosts. Another related a bacterium, *B. bronchoseptica*, causes pneumonia and other respiratory infections in **animals**, especially dogs, but rarely in humans.

The manifestations of pertussis are most severe in children, especially young infants. In children, the disease typically has three stages: the catarrhal, the paroxysmal, and the convalescent.

The initial, catarrhal, stage begins about seven to ten days after exposure to an infected person, and appears much like a common cold or other mild upper respiratory infection. During this stage the child typically has a runny nose, a mild cough, and little if any fever.

Over the next week or two, the cough gradually grows more severe, and the child develops the typical paroxysmal coughing bouts of pertussis. Each paroxysm consists of a string of 10 to 30 barking, staccato coughs that may last a minute or more. Finally, the child takes a deep breath in, causing the whooping sound that gives the disease its name. These paroxysms are terrifying both to the child who cannot breathe and to bystanders who are powerless to aid the child. During each paroxysm, the child will turn first red, then blue for lack of oxygen; he will stream tears, mucus, and saliva; at the end he will collapse in fatigue and may even have a seizure as a result of lack of oxygen. This will happen as often as 20 times a day and can be precipitated by attempts to eat or drink, or by any activity. As this paroxysmal phase goes on for up to a month, the child can become progressively exhausted and even malnourished because of the inability to eat. Especially in small infants, these paroxysms can cause severe enough respiratory difficulty to cause sudden death.

Finally, after weeks of violent paroxysms of cough, there will be a gradual decrease in the frequency and severity of these episodes as the child enters the convalescent phase. The convalescing child may continue to have coughing spells for as long as six months after the onset of the illness.

Because of the degree of damage done to the cells lining the trachea and bronchi and the compromised nutrition of the child, secondary infections, especially pneumonia, are frequent. The pressure waves of the cough itself can also cause complications, ranging from hernias to pneumothorax (rupture of a lung as a result of over-expansion) to bleeding into the brain or spinal cord. Whether because of this hemorrhage or because of oxygen deprivation to the brain, as many as 1 percent of infants who survive whooping cough have permanent neurologic damage, ranging from seizures to mental handicaps, blindness, deafness, paralysis, or coma.

Pertussis is most hazardous when it occurs during the first six months of age. In young infants, the diameter of the trachea is much smaller, and its cartilage rings are much less stiff than later in life. Because of this, respiratory failure during a paroxysm of cough is much more likely. Younger infants also have a less well-developed immune system and nutritional reserve and so are more likely to develop pneumonia or other secondary infections.

Teens and adults who have pertussis usually have a much milder course of the disease. The catarrhal stage is mistaken for a cold; the paroxysms of cough are usually not as severe as they are in children and are rarely accompanied by the whooping noise. The adult with pertussis will usually seek medical help and finally be diagnosed because the cough lasts for weeks to months without improvement. Despite the less severe nature of the disease in adults, they can also develop secondary infection. During coughing spells, they may faint, pass urine involuntarily, and even cough hard enough to break a rib.

During both the catarrhal and paroxysmal stages, the patient with whooping cough is highly contagious and can easily pass the disease on to others near him. Because of their milder disease and the likelihood that it will not be diagnosed promptly, teens and adults are a more likely source of contagion than young children are.

The **diagnosis** of whooping cough can usually be made easily in children based on the severity and duration of their cough and the absence of fever. In teens and adults, the diagnosis is usually thought of during epidemics of disease in the community or because of the prolonged persistence of the cough. In any age group, the diagnosis is confirmed by culturing B. *pertussis* from secretions obtained by a nasal swab or by examining secretions with immunofluorescent stains. However, these techniques may be positive in as few as 80 percent of cases. Polymerase chain reaction studies may offer a faster and more sensitive way to confirm the diagnosis.

The bacterium that causes pertussis is quite sensitive to erythromycin. Treating a patient with the **antibiotic** erythromycin during the catarrhal phase may shorten and make less severe the paroxysmal phase. Unfortunately, because of the mildness of the catarrhal phase, it is unlikely that a patient will be recognized unless there is a history of recent contact with someone who has active pertussis or there is a community epidemic. Giving antibiotics during the paroxysmal phase is not likely to influence the severity of disease in the patient, but will make him less contagious after about five days of treatment.

Pertussis is a disease that can be prevented by immunization. In the 1940s a combined immunization against **diphtheria**, pertussis, and tetanus (DPT) became widely available. Infants were immunized at two, four, and six months of age, with booster doses before starting school. Prior to the availability of this preventive measure, as many as 147,000 cases of pertussis occurred in the United States annually, and about 8,000 children died of it. The incidence of the disease dropped to only a few thousand per year as a result of immunization. There were side effects associated with the original agent, a derivative of whole bacterial cells. Most children had redness and soreness at the site of injection for a few days; about 1 percent developed fever and irritability. Rarely, some children even developed seizures and other neurologic problems. These severe reactions were estimated to occur about once in 100,000 immunized children. In the 1990s, a more purified acellular product became available that provides the same degree of immunity with far fewer

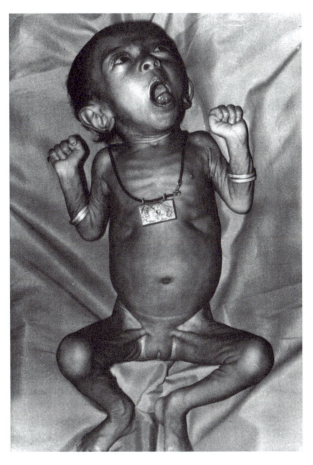

A female Indonesian child suffering from malnutrition and whooping cough. WHO photo. Courtesy of the National Library of Medicine.

side effects. Unfortunately, because of concerns that some parents have about the safety of the immunization, they withhold it from their children. This subjects the children to a much higher risk of complications and even death from the now-preventable disease. *See also* Human Body.

Further Reading

Allen, Arthur. *Vaccine: The Controversial Story of Medicine's Greatest Lifesaver*. New York: W. W. Norton, 2007.

Bell, Louis M., ed. *Guide to Common Childhood Infections*. New York: Macmillan Publishing Company, 1998.

Centers for Disease Control and Prevention. *Whooping Cough/Pertussis*. http://www.cdc.gov/nchs/fastats/whooping.htm

Mayo Clinic. *Whooping Cough*. http://www.mayoclinic.com/health/whooping-cough/DS00445

Pickering, Larry K., ed. *Red Book: 2006 Report of the Committee on Infectious Diseases*, 27th edition. Elk Grove Village, IL: American Academy of Pediatrics; 2006.
World Health Organization. *Pertussis.* http://www.who.int/topics/pertussis/en/

CHARLES V. BENDER

WORLD HEALTH ORGANIZATION. *See* International Health Agencies and Conventions.

WU LIEN TEH (WU LIENDE OR WU LIANDE, 1879–1960). Wu Liende, plague expert and Chinese public health pioneer, was born in Penang in the Straits Settlements (now Malaysia) on March 10, 1879. While at the Penang Free School, Wu decided to become a **physician** because as an Asian he was barred from the civil service but not from a profession such as medicine. He matriculated at Emmanuel College, Cambridge, in 1896 for the natural science course. After his three-year course, he spent the summer of 1899 studying with a prominent English bacteriologist and pathologist, Dr. German Sims Woodhead (1855–1921).

Earning his degree in medicine at St. Mary's Hospital in London, Wu became house physician at the Brompton Hospital for Consumption and Diseases of the Chest to learn more about **tuberculosis**, a major disease in the Straits Settlements. Subsequently he studied with **Ronald Ross** at the new Liverpool School of Tropical Medicine, with Karl Fraenkel (1861–1901; former assistant to **Robert Koch**) in Halle, Germany, and with Ukrainian Elie Metchnikoff (1845–1916) at Paris's Pasteur Institute.

After a short period as a researcher and private practitioner in Penang, he accepted an offer from Yuan Shih-kai (1859–1916), Grand Councillor of China, to become vice-director of the Imperial Medical College in Tientsin, a school recently established to teach Western Medicine.

An outbreak of **plague in China's** region of Manchuria in 1910 gave Wu a new direction in his work. There he investigated the nature of plague, the organism, and its mode of spread. His modern European training provided him with approaches that were universally admired, and for the first time, Western medicine was learning from a Chinese physician about modern medicine.

An International Plague Conference, held in Mukden during April 1911, was the first international scientific meeting held in China. Wu was the president of the conference, the proceedings of which became a major reference on **pneumonic plague**.

Wu did not return to Tientsin but continued to study plague in Harbin. In one of its final acts before the Republican Revolution in October 1911, the Imperial regime established Western medicine as official state policy with the establishment of the North Manchurian Plague Prevention Service under Wu's direction. This service continued until 1931 as China's main defense against plague as well as **cholera**. Wu became *the* authority on pneumonic plague, and his 1926 monograph is still a standard reference.

Wu Liende was an effective organizer and administrator: a founding member of the China Medical Association in 1925 and of its successor, the Chinese Medical Association in 1932, and an advocate for uniform standards in Chinese medical education and health promotion groups such as the National Anti-Tuberculosis Association. Wu had an active interest in the medical culture of China and coauthored *History of Chinese Medicine* (1932, 1936).

As events led up to World War II, Wu resumed general medical practice in Penang after a hiatus of some 30 years. After the War, Wu used his international contacts and stature to advocate for improved public health measures in Malaya. To the end of his life, he worked to end one of Asia's major health problems, opium use and addiction.

Further Reading

Wu, Lien Teh. *Plague Fighter: The Autobiography of a Modern Chinese Physician.* Cambridge: W. Heffer & Sons, 1959.
Wu, Yu-lin. *Memories of Dr. Wu Lien-Teh, Plague Fighter.* Singapore: World Scientific, 1995.

WILLIAM C. SUMMERS

Y

YELLOW FEVER. Yellow fever is an acute, infectious disease characterized by frontal headaches, fever, prostration, muscular pain, proteinuria (excess protein in the urine), jaundice, and, in the final stages, internal bleeding, kidney failure, delirium, and convulsions. Vomiting partly digested blood from stomach hemorrhages—called "black vomit"—is a particularly ominous sign. In the eighteenth and nineteenth centuries, yellow fever's unpredictability, rapid course, and horrifying outcome (death seven to ten days after onset) created mass panic and paralyzed commerce. Even though **typhoid fever** had a higher fatality rate, it failed to arouse a similar public reaction. Yellow fever was indisputably "the single most dreaded disease in the Americas."

Yellow fever was known by 150 synonyms, most of which were based on a single terrifying symptom (*vomito negro*), geographical location (Boullam fever), season of prevalence (autumnal **epidemic** fever), or severity (malignant bilious fever). "Yellow Jack," its most familiar name, originated from the **quarantine** flag that adorned suspect ships in harbor.

Etiology. Yellow fever became the first viral disease experimentally proven to exist in humans when, in October 1901, James Carroll (1854–1907), of the U.S. Army Yellow Fever Board in Cuba, demonstrated that yellow fever was caused by a living organism smaller than any known **bacterium**. Carroll filtered serum from confirmed yellow fever patients through a sterilized porcelain filter, and the bacteria-free filtrate produced the disease when injected into nonimmune volunteers. Importantly, blood taken from yellow fever patients whose illness had been caused by the ultrafiltrate produced the disease in a third individual.

The causative agent, an arbovirus (transmitted by arthropod vectors) of the *flaviviridae* family, which includes the **West Nile** and **Dengue fever** viruses, was isolated in 1927. A decade later, **Max Theiler**, a medical researcher at the **Rockefeller Foundation** Yellow Fever Laboratory in New York City, developed a live, attenuated vaccine derived from the 17D **virus** strain. Mass immunizations of U.S. military personnel in World **War** II

GRIFFITH HUGHES'S DESCRIPTION OF YELLOW FEVER IN BARBADOS (1715)

The Patient is commonly seized with a shivering Fit, as in an Ague, which lasts an Hour or two, more or less; and the Danger is guessed at, according to the Severity and Continuance of the Ague.

After the shivering Fit, a violent Fever comes on, with excessive Pains in the Head, Back, and Limbs, Loss of Strength and Spirits, with great Dejection of Mind, insatiable Thirst and Restlessness, and sometimes too with a Vomiting, attended with pains in the Head, the Eyes being red, and that Redness in a few days turning to Yellowness.

If the Patient turns yellow too soon, he hath scarce a Chance for Life, and the sooner he does so the worse.

The Pain in the Head is often very great, when first seized with this Fever.

After some Days are past, this Pain abates, as well as the Fever; and the Patient falls into a breathing Sweat, and a temperate Heat, so that he appears to be better; but on a narrow [closer] View, a Yellowness appears in his Eyes and Skin, and he is visibly worse.

About this time he sometimes spits Blood, and that by Mouthfuls; as this continues, he grows cold, and his Pulse abates till at last it is quite gone; and the Patient becomes almost as cold as a Stone, and continues in that state with a composed, sedate Mind.

In this Condition he may perhaps live Twelve Hours without any sensible Pulse or heat and then expire.

Such were the Symptoms and Progress of this Fever in the Year 1715 . . .

After Death, the Corps of such appear livid in some Parts or other; or else marked with pestilential Spots, Carbuncles, or Buboes.

From Griffith Hughes, *The Natural History of the Barbados* (London, 1750), p. 38.

(1939–1945) proved the vaccine's benefits: not a single vaccinated serviceman contracted yellow fever during the conflict. The 17D vaccine is still the gold standard and provides decades-long, and possibly lifelong, immunity.

Transmission. In the aftermath of the Spanish-American War (1898), U.S. occupational forces in Cuba faced a more lethal foe than the vanquished Spanish army: yellow fever. In response to this crisis, Army Surgeon General George Sternberg (1838–1915) established the U.S. Army Yellow Fever Board in May 1900 with follow-up instructions to "give special attention to questions relating to the etiology and prevention of yellow fever." In a remarkably short time, the board, headed by Major **Walter Reed** and comprised of contract surgeons (civilian physicians) James Carroll, Jesse Lazear (1866–1900), and Aristides Agramonte (1868–1931), discredited the prevailing etiological theories (bacteria, noxious **air**, filth, soiled clothing/bedding). Their everlasting contribution to modern medical science was the demonstration that yellow fever was not contagious, but was spread from human to human solely by means of the bites of infected female *Aedes aegypti* mosquitoes.

The **insect**-vector theory did not originate with Reed and his coworkers. In 1881, Cuban physician Carlos Finlay (1833–1915) had postulated a relationship between the mosquito now known as *A. aegypti* and yellow fever. He was never able to prove his hypothesis, however, despite carrying out more than 100 mosquito inoculations in 90 subjects over a 20-year period. The Reed board succeeded because it discovered the keys to infectivity that had eluded Finlay. First, the mosquito could acquire the yellow fever germ from a donor only during the first two or three days of the disease, when the virus titer was high in the bloodstream. Second, the imbibed virus needed a two-week incubation period within the mosquito's body before the insect could infect a healthy recipient—a process termed *extrinsic incubation*. During this time, the virus multiplied and traveled from the mosquito's stomach to its salivary glands.

Epidemiology.   Yellow fever evolved first in the swampy and riverine regions of Africa, and natives developed a high tolerance. When Africans were brought to the Americas as slaves, slavers brought the disease with them in shipboard water supplies. In the Western Hemisphere, yellow fever epidemics usually began in July, peaked in September, and ended with the first hard frost. An attack conferred lifetime immunity against the disease. *A. aegypti*, known as the "household" mosquito because of its preference for human habitations, breeds in standing water found in roof gutters, ditches, cisterns (principal foci), horse troughs, tanks, water barrels, and other rainwater receptacles. Swarms of newly hatched mosquitoes, the presence of yellow fever carriers (undiagnosed mild cases) to which these insects had access, and warm and humid conditions combined to provide ideal conditions for the propagation of the disease among a susceptible population. In numerous instances, the seeds of destruction were unwittingly imported into maritime cities in the form of infected newcomers and mosquito-infested cargoes.

From 1702 to 1879, the English colonies and the United States experienced at least 113 yellow fever epidemics. The most notorious outbreaks decimated Philadelphia in 1793 (4,044 deaths, 10 percent of the population), New Orleans in 1853 (about 9,000, 9 percent), and Memphis, Tennessee, in 1878 (5,150, 10 percent). The 1878 epidemic was a stupendous calamity. It started in New Orleans and spread by rivers and railroads to Memphis and to 200 other towns throughout the Mississippi and Ohio River valleys, leaving in its wake an estimated 100,000 cases and 20,000 fatalities. The economic cost to the country ranged up to $200 million. Is it any wonder then that a contemporary Memphis newspaper personified yellow fever as "The King of Terrors"?

Social Impact.   What set yellow fever apart from other diseases was its staggering social impact—most noticeably in the semitropical climate of the American South. Once the disease became entrenched in a community, people shunned others and seemed moved only by the instinct of self-preservation. Those who could afford it fled to safer locations. As the dead piled up, shops, businesses, and trading houses closed. Countless acres of fertile farmland lay idle. The resulting economic disaster fueled public health reform. Whereas northern sanitarians focused on pure food, milk, and drinking water, their southern counterparts formed health departments explicitly to fight yellow fever. Their concern was more with saving business losses than with saving lives. Any lives spared could be attributed to improved sanitation systems (drainage, sewerage, and water) that unintentionally reduced mosquito breeding areas.

The Reed board's findings revealed that yellow fever was not an inscrutable pestilence to be feared, but a comprehensible mosquito-borne disease that could be prevented. Only after laypersons—who lagged behind the medical profession in acceptance of the mosquito menace—understood this, could the blind panic that had been an enduring feature of eighteenth- and nineteenth-century epidemics subside.

Public Health.   Throughout the nineteenth century, yellow fever was central to debates on public health practice. In this regard, the importance of the Reed board's elegant, foolproof discoveries cannot be exaggerated, for they provided a scientific rationale for redirecting yellow fever control efforts. Old approaches included such absurd methods as burning pine tar in the streets to dispel poisonous air; twentieth-century procedures focused on systematically destroying adult mosquitoes and their larvae, eradicating breeding sites, and preventing mosquitoes (netting and screens) from biting anyone with the disease.

By instituting sanitary regulations based exclusively on the mosquito doctrine, Major **William Gorgas**, the chief sanitary officer of Havana, rid the Cuban capital of yellow fever for the first time in two centuries. From 1853 to 1900, there were 36,000 deaths from yellow fever in Havana; by October 1901, not a single case of the disease was reported in the city. This was the first example in history of ending an epidemic by controlling its vector. Applying the same techniques in 1904 that had proven so successful earlier in Havana, Gorgas—now a colonel—and his sanitary team preserved the health of the labor force constructing the Panama Canal. From May 1906 until the canal opened in 1914, there were no cases of yellow fever in the Canal Zone. Gorgas estimated that 71,000 lives were saved in the process.

Current Status.   As we enter the twenty-first century, yellow fever is found only in South America and Africa. Despite the availability of a safe and effective yellow fever vaccine, large populations in these countries remain unvaccinated. In Africa, where only 6 percent of the people have been immunized, yellow fever epidemics have recurred in every decade of the twentieth century, with the most severe in Ethiopia in the 1960s (about 30,000 deaths). Thousands died of the disease in Ghana in the 1970s, Nigeria in the 1980s, and the Sudan in 2003. Smaller outbreaks occurred during the 1990s.

The last yellow fever epidemic in North America occurred in New Orleans in 1905 (3,402 cases; 452 deaths); it was aborted by quick implementation of mosquito suppression measures. Since then, only a handful of unvaccinated U.S. citizens have become yellow fever victims, all having contracted the disease during international travel. *See also* Yellow Fever Commission, U.S.; Yellow Fever in Colonial Latin America and the Caribbean; Yellow Fever in Latin America and the Caribbean, 1830–1940; Yellow Fever in North America to 1810; Yellow Fever in the American South, 1810–1905.

Further Reading

The American Experience: The Great Fever [film]. PBS, 2006.

Bean, William B. *Walter Reed: A Biography.* Charlottesville: University Press of Virginia, 1982.

Bloom, Khaled J. *The Mississippi Valley's Great Yellow Fever Epidemic of 1878.* Baton Rouge: Louisiana State University Press, 1993.

Centers for Disease Control and Prevention. *Yellow Fever.* http://www.cdc.gov/ncidod/dvbid/yellowfever/

Cirillo, Vincent J. *Bullets and Bacilli: The Spanish-American War and Military Medicine*. New Brunswick, NJ: Rutgers University Press, 2004.

Humphreys, Margaret. *Yellow Fever and the South*. New Brunswick, NJ: Rutgers University Press, 1992.

Mayo Clinic. *Yellow Fever*. http://www.mayoclinic.com/health/yellow-fever/DS01011

Philip S. Hench Walter Reed Yellow Fever Collection, University of Virginia. http://yellowfever. lib.virginia.edu/reed/

Pierce, John R., and Jim Writer. *Yellow Jack: How Yellow Fever Ravaged America and Walter Reed Discovered its Deadly Secrets*. Hoboken, NJ: Wiley, 2005.

World Health Organization. *Yellow Fever*. http://www.who.int/csr/disease/yellowfev/en/

VINCENT J. CIRILLO

YELLOW FEVER COMMISSION, U.S.   **Yellow fever** devastated American troops occupying Cuba during and after the Spanish-American War (1896). In May 1900, Army Surgeon General George Sternberg (1838–1915) created a medical board to investigate infectious diseases prevalent on the island, particularly yellow fever. Major **Walter Reed**, a career army **surgeon** then completing a study of **typhoid fever** in U.S. army camps, headed the new Yellow Fever (or Reed) Commission. The three other members of the Commission were temporary wartime surgeons. James Carroll (1854–1907) worked with Reed in army laboratories in Washington, Cuban-born Aristides Agramonte (1868–1931) was an experienced yellow fever investigator, and Jesse Lazear (1866–1900) was a brilliant young researcher from Johns Hopkins Medical School in Baltimore.

The Mosquito Hypothesis.   Assembling in Havana in June 1900, the Commission quickly demonstrated that the **bacterium** *Bacillus icteroides*, suspected by several other researchers, did not cause yellow fever. Two other theories, however, did capture their attention. Havana **physician** Carlos Finlay (1833–1915) was convinced that the female *Culex fasciatus* mosquito (now *Aedes aegypti*) transmitted yellow fever. Despite two decades of experimentation, Finlay never succeeded in transmitting yellow fever to nonimmune immigrants through the bite of infected laboratory mosquitoes. Immigrants, mostly Spanish nationals, had agreed to participate because they fully expected to contract yellow fever naturally after arriving in Cuba. The second theory had been developed by Henry Rose Carter (1852–1925) of the U.S. Public Health Service. In 1898 he analyzed detailed house-by-house and day-by-day observations of a yellow fever outbreak in two isolated towns in Mississippi. He concluded that there was a gap of approximately two weeks—the "extrinsic incubation period"—between the identification of the first case in a community and the appearance of subsequent cases. It was probably Lazear who combined the two theories, hypothesizing that yellow fever was transmitted by a mosquito that had incubated the infectious agent for approximately two weeks.

Human Subjects Experiments.   Commission members agreed that experimentation on human beings, including themselves, was necessary to prove the mosquito hypothesis. Mosquitoes raised in Lazear's laboratory were fed on the blood of active yellow fever cases at the Las Animas Hospital near Havana. After several days, these "loaded" mosquitoes, were allowed to bite military volunteers as well as Carroll and Lazear. Carroll and one soldier developed yellow fever and recovered. Lazear died following a violent attack. Agramonte, assumed to have acquired immunity in childhood, was not an experimental subject. Reed, who had left Cuba temporarily to complete his typhoid report, considered these cases suggestive but not conclusive, because the subjects had not been strictly isolated from sick patients or random mosquitoes.

With Sternberg's approval, Reed designed his now-famous human experiments at a mosquito-free site, named Camp Lazear, near Havana. Subjects were recruited from non-immune Spanish immigrant laborers. Each was offered $100 to participate and an additional $100 plus the best care available from American medical officers if he developed yellow fever. American soldiers also volunteered. Some refused the money, avowing that they volunteered "in the interest of humanity and the cause of science." Reed insisted on written informed consent in English or Spanish from all volunteers, a revolutionary concept in human experimentation.

The experiments were conducted between November 1900 and January 1901. Several carefully isolated volunteers became ill after being bitten by loaded mosquitoes. Reed thus confirmed the mosquito theory. In another experiment, healthy volunteers were housed in a mosquito-free cabin with screened windows. For 20 nights, they slept on bed linens and wore nightclothes soiled with the vomitus and excrement of hospitalized yellow fever victims. Despite the revolting conditions, these men remained well, disproving the popular theory that contaminated nonliving objects (fomites) transmitted yellow fever. A second group stayed in a partitioned cabin with a screened opening between the two rooms. The men in one room were bitten by loaded mosquitoes and some developed yellow fever. The volunteers in the second room remained well, thus disproving the theory that contaminated air in a building transmitted yellow fever.

Application of the Commission's Work.   The usual sanitation and **quarantine** measures had failed to halt yellow fever in Cuba. U.S. army physicians, who followed the Commission's work closely, quickly recognized the importance of destroying mosquitoes and their larvae. Havana sanitary officer, Major **William Gorgas**, despite lingering personal doubts about the mosquito theory, initiated a military-style campaign against the mosquito and the eggs it laid in standing **water**. Gorgas's "mosquito brigades" went house to house, covering or applying a thin layer of oil to cisterns and draining standing water. Within months, Havana was free of yellow fever, a remarkable demonstration of the application of scientific medicine to public health.

Reed returned to Washington and was considered for the post of Army Surgeon General. He died of appendicitis in 1902. Carroll, with Reed's support, returned to Cuba in late 1901, where he demonstrated that yellow fever was caused by an organism smaller than a bacterium. He died in 1907, possibly from cardiac complications of yellow fever. Lazear is remembered as a martyr to medicine. Agramonte continued medical research at the University of Havana and later in New Orleans, dying in 1931. Within a few years, Gorgas successfully applied the mosquito theory to yellow fever (and malaria) as chief medical officer of the Panama Canal project. In the century since the successful work of the Yellow Fever Commission, medical historians and other interested parties have argued over the perceived slighting of Finlay as the discoverer of the mosquito vector of yellow fever, the issue of Walter Reed's failure to participate personally in human experiments, the impression of some participants that Reed received disproportionate acclaim for the Commission's work, and the ethics of medical experimentation on military volunteers. *See also* Colonialism and Epidemic Disease; Environment, Ecology, and Epidemic Disease; Human Subjects Research; Insects, Other Arthropods, and Epidemic Disease; Medical Ethics and Epidemic Disease; War, the Military, and Epidemic Disease; Yellow Fever in Latin America and the Caribbean, 1830–1940; Yellow Fever in the American South, 1810–1905.

Further Reading

Bean, William. *Walter Reed: A Biography*. Charlottesville: University Press of Virginia, 1982.

Bryan, Charles, Sandra Moss, and Richard Kahn. "Yellow Fever in the Americas." *Infectious Disease Clinics of North America* 18 (2004): 275–292.

Philip S. Hench Walter Reed Yellow Fever On-line Collection. http://yellowfever.lib.virginia. edu/reed/

Pierce, John R., and Jim Witter: *Yellow Jack: How Yellow Fever Ravaged America and Walter Reed Discovered Its Deadly Secrets*. Hoboken, NJ: John Wiley and Sons, 2005.

SANDRA W. MOSS

YELLOW FEVER IN COLONIAL LATIN AMERICA AND THE CARIBBEAN.

Yellow Fever or, as it was called by early modern Iberians, *vomito prieto* (black vomit), was one of the most important factors in the shaping of the social, cultural, political, and economic states of the Spanish and Portuguese colonies of the "New World." In the Americas, **epidemics** of yellow fever defeated armies and decimated Indian and European populations, while sparing African slaves. The works of the *flavivirus* causing *vomito prieto* shaped the Latin America that emerged after the European conquest and colonization.

In 1648 yellow fever paid its first recorded visit to the Spanish colonies when epidemics shook Yucatán (Mexico) and Cuba. Three factors explain the relative delay of the appearance of this disease in the Western Hemisphere: the yellow fever **virus's** short life cycle, its endemic state in most of West Africa, and the characteristics of this germ's vector.

Once in a human body, the yellow fever virus's life cycle is particularly short. In seven to ten days the host is either killed or becomes immune to the disease. Yellow fever induces an effective and life-lasting immune response in its victims and runs a relatively mild course when it is first acquired during infancy. Thus, enslaved African Americans, having lived in close contact with the virus since childhood, were ineffective as a means of transport for the virus. Its transfer from the "Old" to the "New" World needed a large nonimmune population; one that would allow for the virus to pass from host to host during the 12-week trip from Africa to the Americas. In addition, like the virus itself, the vector for the **transmission** of yellow fever, the *Aedes* mosquito, adapted to human populations and settlements and breeds, almost exclusively, in shallow clay pots or other containers of undisturbed water, both of which were common elements on slave trading ships.

Although delayed, the arrival of yellow fever on American shores was not silent. Yellow fever quickly presented itself with terrifying epidemics. Thousands of Europeans died in the midst of high fever, palpitations, muscular cramps, exhaustion, and jaundice from liver failure. Victims suffered profuse bleeding from skin wounds and body orifices, including the upper intestinal track, from which digested blood—which turns black—was vomited. This black body emission gave the name to the disease in the Spanish realm, *vomito prieto*.

Colonial Latin American statistics of yellow fever's impact are, at best, unreliable, since only nonimmune guests presented yellow fever's classic symptoms. Mild cases, especially in Africans and **children** of all races, went unrecognized as merely *calenturas* (high fevers). Thus, only severe cases of yellow fever were recorded as such, while mild cases were not accounted for. Such bias explains, at least partially, the high mortality rates (deaths/cases of illness) recorded by chroniclers of the royal Spanish medical corps, the *protomedicato*—rates as high as 70 percent). Modern mortality estimates are around

10 percent. Because yellow fever virus induces a permanent immunity in survivors, it became a disease of the immune-naïve European residents as well as of visitors, foreigners, newcomers, and invaders, such as the 1,500 soldiers sent by France to invade St Lucia in 1655.

"Brazen Jack" (as yellow fever was called by many Britons) also helped Spaniards defend Cartagena de Indias (Colombia) when in 1741 British Admiral Edward Vernon (1684–1757) launched the largest amphibious military assault before the Second World War. Of the 22,000 men assailing Cartagena, at least half died of *vomito prieto* during the unsuccessful three-month campaign.

The disease also played a major role in the fates of the two most powerful armies of the late eighteenth century, when they attempted to invade St. Domingue, the northern portion of the island of Hispaniola (present-day Haiti and the Dominican Republic). By 1775 St. Domingue had grown to be the most lucrative colony in the world, thanks to its sugar plantations. The ubiquitous plantations on the island provided the perfect breeding grounds for *Aedes* mosquitoes and made *vomito prieto* equally omnipresent. After the French Revolution brought turmoil even to the more distant French colonies, the black slaves on St. Domingue armed themselves, ousted the colonial government, and in 1804 established the first free black republic (in the Western Hemisphere second only to the United States in declaring independence). The chain of events that finished in the foundation of Haiti was stalwartly influenced by "Yellow Jack."

With the excuse of preventing further slave rebellions in the rest of the Caribbean, British Prime Minister William Pitt (1759–1806) sent a 20,000-man army to invade St. Domingue. The French were not willing to lose their most precious overseas possessions without a good fight and sent around 35,000 soldiers to subdue both Britons and the rebellious slaves led by Toussaint L'Ouverture (1742–1803). Between 1793 and 1798, both armies arrived in the yellow fever-infested northern portion of Hispaniola. Although some historians refute the number of deaths attributed to yellow fever and malaria in St. Domingue as exaggerated by contemporaries, it is undeniable that yellow fever played a major role in shaping the events in the former French colony. By 1798, 12,500 Britons had died either at the hands of L'Ouverture's followers, or of yellow fever or malaria. The French contingent did not fare much better; only 6,000 of them returned home. Haiti has retained both its liberty and its population of predominantly African extraction.

Brazil received the lion's share of the African diaspora to the Americas. Common sense suggests that the gigantic Portuguese colony should have been the place in which most yellow fever epidemics occurred during Latin America's colonial period. To the contrary, however, after the first big yellow fever epidemics between 1685 and 1696, Brazil did not suffer another bout with the disease until 1845. At this time Europeans were lured to join the predominantly immune African population living in Brazil in "whitening" campaigns carried out by the Creole government. It was only then that the mild variant of yellow fever that had thrived endemic in the Brazilian cities and plantations for two centuries suddenly found plenty of susceptible victims. Yellow fever epidemics struck Salvador, Rio de Janeiro, and other Brazilian cities, killing thousands. Almost all of them were recent immigrants. By 1860, in Rio de Janeiro alone, 60,000 people had died of *vomito prieto*. But, if in Brazil yellow fever's absence in 1807 lured exiled Portuguese King João VI (1767–1826) to establish his court in Rio de Janeiro, after the Napoleonic invasion of Portugal the same year, in Cuba, "Jack's" presence became an irresistible excuse for invasion.

By the late nineteenth century, Cuba was the only remaining Spanish colony in the Western Hemisphere. The United States, however, was interested both in the riches of Cuba's sugar plantations, and in establishing hemispheric hegemony. Americans found in the epidemics that ravaged their southern neighbors the perfect excuse to invade Cuba and put an end to the four-century-long colonial enterprise of Spain in the Americas. American warmongers promoted the Spanish-American War, at least in part, as a way to defend Louisiana and Florida from the successive visits of "Brazen Jack." According to American officials, these epidemics generally originated in Cuba. The U.S. army ousted from Cuba Spanish colonists, the *Aedes* mosquito, and with it yellow fever. All this was to the great amusement of the Cubans, who had become immune to yellow fever thanks to many earlier outbreaks.

Yellow fever killed thousands of French workers struggling to build a canal in Central America in the late nineteenth century and made the French enterprise fail, thus paving the way for American intervention. In the wake of the Spanish-American War Theodore Roosevelt (1858–1919) became president of the United States and successfully secured the secession of Panama from Colombia. The U.S. government effectively controlled mosquito-breeding fields in the Panamanian jungle and avoided the fate of the French. American engineers created the Panama Canal, which would be crucial to the consolidation of U.S. hegemony over the former Iberian colonies and to its rise as a world power. *See also* Latin America, Colonial: Demographic Effects of Imported Diseases; Slavery and Epidemic Disease; War, the Military, and Epidemic Disease; Yellow Fever Commission, U.S.; Yellow Fever in Latin America and the Caribbean, 1830–1940; Yellow Fever in North America to 1810; Yellow Fever in the American South, 1810–1905.

Further Reading

Alchón, Suzanne Austin. *A Pest in the Land: New World Epidemics in a Global Perspective.* Albuquerque: University of New Mexico Press. 2003.

Cook, Noble David. *Born to Die: Disease and New World Conquest 1492–1650.* New York: Cambridge University Press, 1998.

Gehlbach, Stephen H. *American Plagues: Lessons from our Battles with Disease.* New York: McGraw-Hill. 2005.

Kiple, Kenneth F., and Stephen V. Beck. *Biological Consequences of the European Expansion, 1450–1800.* Brookfield, VT: Ashgate/Variorum, 1997.

Watts, Sheldon J. *Epidemics and History: Disease, Power, and Imperialism.* New Haven, CT: Yale University Press. 1997.

Wills, Christopher. *Yellow Fever, Black Goddess: The Coevolution of People and Plagues.* Reading: Addison-Wesley Publishers, 1996.

PABLO F. GOMEZ

YELLOW FEVER IN LATIN AMERICA AND THE CARIBBEAN, 1830–1940.
Yellow fever in postcolonial Latin America and the Caribbean region was largely endemic where present. It presented essentially a mild **childhood** disease, but it could and did flare into **epidemics**, usually because of its importation into port cities by ships from other, infected seaports. It played a part in U.S. southern expansion in 1847, and a half-century later, this latter conflict—the Spanish-American War—led to the research that finally allowed for control of the disease. International concern with yellow fever in the Western Hemisphere also led directly to the formation of organizations that helped to eradicate

smallpox and are still working to eradicate infectious diseases such as **measles** and **tuberculosis**.

The Mexican-American War (1846–1848).   U.S. notions of Manifest Destiny dictated that the young republic seize southern border territories—now Texas, Arizona, Southern California, and New Mexico—from Old Mexico. American strategists envisioned a strike deep into Mexican territory at Mexico City itself, the success of which would provide the leverage necessary to wrench away the northern provinces in a peace treaty. They designed an amphibious landing at Veracruz by General Winfield Scott (1786–1866) and an army of 10,000. Planners were careful to set dates that avoided the area's storms and the mainland's spring yellow fever season, a factor for which Scott had great respect. U.S. plans went awry, however, and the landing took place almost two months late and dangerously close to yellow fever season. The U.S. forces besieged Veracruz as the first cases of yellow fever began to appear. By March 29, the city had surrendered and the Mexican garrison had evacuated. Scott moved in quickly and marched out on April 2 en route to Mexico City via the Sierra Madres and the fever-free zone. He had narrowly bypassed one of the Mexicans' most effective allies, and few U.S. troops had fallen ill to *Il vomito*. Scott's capture of the Halls of Montezuma in September all but ended the conflict. By **war**'s end, over 13,000 U.S. servicemen had been killed, though about seven fell to disease, predominantly yellow fever, for every battle death.

Brazil, Panama, and Cuba to 1903.   Brazil had suffered yellow fever epidemics in the late seventeenth century but was free from major outbreaks until the mid-1800s. An American ship docking at Bahía in the fall of 1849 is said to have carried fresh, infected mosquitoes from New Orleans and Havana. These may have infected Danish crewmen who went ashore in Rio de Janeiro and began spreading the disease through the city as native mosquitoes feasted on their tainted blood. The disease disseminated linearly through the streets until most of the capital was affected, some four months after their arrival. By the end of 1850, 90,658 cases had been reported, of which 4,160 proved fatal. But this was just the beginning. Once reestablished, the fever flared again and again, especially among the newly arrived and the younger whites who had had little or no immunity-conferring exposure. In the 1850s, 10,173 died; in the 1860s, only 1,815. The 1870s saw a resurgence with 13,140 yellow fever deaths. This decade's increase in yellow fever was shared by much of South America. In Argentina, for example, Buenos Aires alone suffered some 15,000 deaths. In the next decade, the toll in Rio dropped to 9,563, though 2,115 died in 1889 alone. The early 1890s doubled that annual rate, and by late 1894 the city had lost 14,944. Another 5,722 died between 1885 and 1900, bringing the toll since 1850 to nearly 60,000. Like much of Africa, Rio gained the reputation of the "white man's grave," and immigration from Europe dropped off. Because of the variety of theories of causation (fomites, **miasma**, insects, interpersonal **contagion**) officials took few actions to address the situation before 1903.

The utility of—indeed the need for—a sea passage across Central America linking the Atlantic and Pacific Oceans had long been recognized. The British held the Isthmus of Panama with a vague plan for shortening the distance between India and England with a canal, but the native mosquitoes and fever finally forced them to relinquish their claims to Colombia. Following their success with the Suez Canal, the French De Lesseps Panama Canal Company obtained rights from Colombia to dig across the 50-mile wide, jungle-encrusted strip of land. Work proceeded from 1882 to 1889; the costs were enormous. The firm went bankrupt because of cost overruns, poor and corrupt management, and yellow fever. Managers maintained a steady flow of nonimmune workers, and the mosquitoes provided a death rate of 176 per 1,000 in 1886. After nearly seven years, some 22,000 laborers and engineers had succumbed to the disease, reflecting mortality rates that fluctuated wildly from 12 to 70 percent depending on the season.

In Cuba, yellow fever may have been endemic as early as the 1760s, and it clearly was in Havana and other coastal cities by the mid-nineteenth century. Yellow fever was endemic in many of the coastal and low-lying regions of the island, but higher, interior areas remained virgin soil. In 1895 a major insurgency broke out, and over the next three years Spain sent thousands of its troops to reinforce the colonial garrisons. Whereas the new forces brought and spread **smallpox**, they contracted yellow fever in epidemic proportions. While on maneuvers against guerrillas in the island's hills, they carried the disease with them, introducing it among the defenseless civilian populations. At the same time, unimmunized Cuban civilians who had been "reconcentrated" by force from the countryside to huge urban camps shared the Spanish soldiers' fate. Overcrowded and unsanitary habitations, barracks, and hospitals facilitated the spread of the fever, along with many other diseases. By the end of the Spanish-American War in 1898, 53,440 Spanish soldiers, or over a quarter of the total Spanish forces, had died of disease, with yellow fever predominating. Over the same four years, over 200,000 Cubans died of smallpox and other illnesses that accompanied the Spanish counter-insurgency and military activities.

Havana suffered an epidemic when victorious but susceptible U.S. troops entered the capital. Chief Sanitary Officer for the U.S. Army **William Gorgas** headed an effort to sanitize the city of filth, removing what were believed to be the sources of the disease. Over a year into the program, the fever was still rampant, well above its usual endemic incidence levels. In 1900 **Walter Reed** and his **Yellow Fever Commission** joined Gorgas and confirmed the theory presented 19 years earlier by U.S.-educated Havana physician Carlos Finlay (1833–1915) that mosquitoes—and neither contagion nor corrupted air—transmitted the responsible microbe. Gorgas again went to work, this time against open and standing water pools in which the mosquitoes bred. Swampy areas were drained, ditches and watercourses screened off, and oil sprayed on still water. The city that had reported 1,400 active cases in the summer of 1900 reported only 37 in 1901 and no cases by the end of summer 1902.

Rio and Panama and after Gorgas's Success. A delegation of French scientists including **Paul-Louis Simond** of the **Pasteur** Institute arrived in Rio in 1900 to study yellow fever *in situ* and to benefit from the recent insights gained by the Americans in Cuba. Over the course of five years, the crew developed important information about the life of the mosquito, transmission of the disease, and means of countering it. In 1903 Rio's young Dr. Oswaldo Cruz (1872–1917) convinced the Brazilian legislature to establish a Yellow Fever Service, despite fervent popular and media skepticism and opposition. Service officers attacked mosquito breeding grounds as Gorgas's men had but concentrated on fumigating against the adults and went beyond them in reporting cases and isolating victims (a major reason for opposition). In less than a year, the Service's efforts had paid off, however, and the incidence of the disease fell off dramatically. Rio eliminated epidemic yellow fever by 1906, and within two or three years the disease itself was eliminated.

Following the Spanish-American War, the U.S. Congress authorized the purchase of the French canal and already-established railroad right-of-way in Panama, but the Colombians balked, refusing to sign the necessary treaty. With French and U.S. support,

Panamanians rebelled and gained their autonomy from Colombia in late 1903. Almost immediately the new government ceded the Canal Zone to the United States with the Hay-Bunau-Varilla Treaty. Gorgas was dispatched to the Zone with the mission of eliminating the mosquitoes and the threat of yellow fever, which he did in about two years; the last death from the disease in the region occurred in 1906. Work on the canal began in 1907 and continued into 1914, unhampered by yellow fever.

In 1913 the American non-governmental **Rockefeller Foundation** established its International Health Commission (IHC) with the goal of eliminating threats to human health in the Western Hemisphere. Yellow fever and malaria were specifically targeted for elimination in 1915. Yellow fever was believed to be a predominantly urban and coastal disease, which meant that depriving the mosquitoes of their breeding grounds in a few highly populated locations would do the trick. Guayaquil, Ecuador, was the first battleground. William Gorgas arrived in 1916 to find that urban environmental factors such as stagnant drinking water sources were directly linked to the mosquito problem, but the IHC wanted nothing to do with improving the infrastructure. U.S. entry into World War I (1914–1918) delayed Gorgas's project, but in November 1918 it began in earnest. Within two years, it had proven successful and was handed over to the Ecuadorian government in 1920. The IHC next targeted towns along the coasts of Mexico and Peru, and between 1921 and 1924 efforts were rewarded with success.

Four coastal regions of Brazil had long been on the IHC list, but as states rather than the federal government controlled Brazilian public health machinery, the Foundation had no leverage. In addition, Oswaldo Cruz had established programs for local **fumigation**, and neither he nor most Brazilians desired foreign intrusion. This changed in 1928 when yellow fever again broke out in Rio de Janeiro, for the first time in two decades. The federal authorities agreed to work with state public health authorities and complemented Cruz's fumigation with Gorgas-style draining and oiling. Results were disappointing, but a change of government in October 1930 meant unhampered federal initiative along IHC lines. This outbreak forced the scientists to realize that there were also rural animal reservoirs of the disease ("jungle yellow fever"-carrying monkeys), and that simply targeting the coastlines would never be enough. The International Health Division (name changed in 1927) shifted its efforts to the development of a vaccine.

Yellow Fever and Hemispheric Health Organization.   The international epidemic of the 1870s that struck Argentina, Brazil, Paraguay, and Uruguay jumped northward by sea into the Mississippi Valley, resulting in a major outbreak of yellow fever in 1878. This prompted the United States to offer to host the Fifth International Sanitary Conference in 1881 in Washington, D.C. The conference was attended largely by diplomats and a few medical specialists, and an attempt was made to organize the kind of international reporting and communication that could stop the cross-border passage of disease. Participants also heard from Dr. Carlos Finlay about his theory of yellow fever's vector. By the end of the decade, the movement for hemispherical cooperation over issues of trade had resulted in the First International Conference of American States, held in Washington, D.C., in 1890. This body created the International Union of American Republics, which later became the Organization of American States. Delegates to the Second International Conference, in Mexico City in 1901, organized the First General International Sanitary Convention of the American Republics (Washington, D.C., 1902), which was to generate "sanitary agreements and regulations" to halt the spread of disease across the hemisphere. Also established was a permanent board for executive oversight, the International Sanitary

Bureau—later the Pan American Health Organization (PAHO)—the world's oldest continuing international health agency. Later in the century, it would be directly involved in the **World Health Organization** disease (smallpox, tuberculosis, measles) eradication programs. Yellow fever remained at the center of concern of these organizations, but by the time the Second International Convention convened, in Washington in 1905, the successes of Reed and Gorgas had borne fruit, and a pattern of international cooperation and action had begun to develop. The Third Convention (Mexico City, 1907) called for organized infectious disease information collection and communication by each member nation to the Bureau and urged the European powers with American colonies to join the Convention's efforts, especially with regard to yellow fever.

The successes of international cooperation and national efforts are evident in such cases as that of Bolivia, which established a Yellow Fever Service only in 1932. Since then about 10,000 cases have been reported, roughly evenly split between mosquito-borne and jungle types. 1936 saw the last mosquito-borne epidemic, and the *Aedes aegypti* mosquito itself was eliminated from the country in 1943. The existence of reservoirs of jungle yellow fever and continuing incursions into the previously undisturbed natural wilderness will ensure a flow of yellow fever cases. *See also* Environment, Ecology, and Epidemic Disease; Latin America, Colonial: Demographic Effects of Imported Diseases; International Health Agencies and Conventions; Sanitation Movement of the Nineteenth Century; Trade, Travel, and Epidemic Disease; Yellow Fever Commission, U.S.; Yellow Fever in Colonial Latin America and the Caribbean; Yellow Fever in the American South, 1810–1905.

Further Reading

Chaves-Carballo, Enrique. "Carlos Finlay and Yellow Fever: Triumph over Adversity." *Military Medicine* 170 (2005): 881–885.

Cueto, Marcus. *The Return of Epidemics: Health and Society in Peru in the Twentieth Century.* Burlington, VT: Ashgate, 2001.

Delaporte, Francois. *The History of Yellow Fever: An Essay on the Birth of Tropical Medicine.* Cambridge, MA: MIT Press, 1991.

Farley, John. *To Cast Out Disease: A History of the International Health Division of the Rockefeller Foundation (1913–1951).* New York: Oxford University Press, 2004.

Harvard University Library. *Contagion.* http://ocp.hul.harvard.edu/contagion/panamacanal.html

McCullough, David. *The Path between the Seas: The Creation of the Panama Canal, 1870–1914.* New York: Simon and Schuster, 1977.

Smallman-Raynor, Matthew, and Andrew D. Cliff. "The Spatial Dynamics of Epidemic Diseases in War and Peace: Cuba and the Insurrection against Spain, 1895–98." *Transactions of the Institute of British Geographers* new series 24 (1999): 331–352.

Ward, James S. *Yellow Fever in Latin America: A Geographical Study.* Liverpool: University of Liverpool Press, 1972.

JOSEPH P. BYRNE

YELLOW FEVER IN NORTH AMERICA TO 1810.   Between 1693 and 1810, **yellow fever** was one of the most dreaded of all **epidemic** diseases to afflict the American colonies and United States. It has not been possible to determine positively that yellow fever was present in this country before 1692. Although **smallpox** and **tuberculosis** had higher death rates, yellow fever struck so quickly and was so devastating that mortality rates from 10 percent to 70 percent were not uncommon during epidemics. These factors and the disease's unknown cause helped spread fear and panic throughout the country. It was not until the beginning of the twentieth century that researchers found the cause to be a **virus** transmitted to humans when bitten by an infected *Aedes aegypti* mosquito. This explained why the disease was not contagious and why it occurred only during the summer months: the mosquito that carries the disease dies when cold weather arrives.

Yellow fever symptoms usually appear within six days of infection and range from very mild to so severe that death results. Classic cases are characterized by fever, headache, yellowish discoloration of the skin and body tissues, and bleeding into the stomach and intestinal tract. Individuals who recover from yellow fever have lifetime **immunity**. Because of the wide range of symptoms, yellow fever has always been difficult to diagnose and has been confused with many other illnesses such as **malaria**, scurvy, **typhoid**, and **typhus**.

The disease has been known by some 150 names. The yellowish color of affected skin caused it to be labeled yellow fever, while other names included "bleeding fever" and "Yellow Jack" (because of the yellow **quarantine** flag flown by ships). The black blood–laden fluids vomited by the victims provided the name "black vomit." It was first identified as "yellow fever" by Griffith Hughes in his *Natural History of Barbados* (1750).

Infected African mosquitoes probably accompanied to the New World ship-borne **slaves** who were immune to the disease's effects. The first recognizable epidemic in the Western Hemisphere struck Barbados in 1647 and then spread to other areas of the Caribbean. By the late 1600s, yellow fever had begun to be reported in the English colonies on the continent, chiefly in the major cities along the east coast that conducted **trade** with the Caribbean.

Charleston, South Carolina.   The first yellow fever epidemic in Charleston began during the late summer of 1699 and killed nearly 200 individuals. The disease afflicted many government officials and caused great concern among the residents. Government and business activity nearly ceased until cold weather came, and the epidemic ended. Although physicians recognized the disease by its symptoms, its cause was not understood, and it was believed to be a contagious disease.

In 1706, French and Spanish armies stationed at St. Augustine, Florida, believed they could seize Charleston because yellow fever was once again ravaging the city. They were unable to overcome Charleston's fortifications and the spirited defense of its militiamen, while the yellow fever killed nearly 5 percent of the city's population of about 1,300 people. This epidemic also created havoc with government and commercial affairs and raged into October. But when cold weather arrived, Charleston was freed from its grip.

The city experienced an epidemic in 1728 and again only four years later. The 1732 epidemic reached its height in July with as many as 12 deaths daily. There were so many funerals each day that the city prohibited the tolling of funeral bells, and wealthier residents fled to country plantations to escape the disease. This epidemic killed 130 individuals, and all government and commercial affairs ceased until the cold winter weather began.

Charleston also experienced major epidemics during 1739, 1745, and 1748. The disease did not reach epidemic proportions again, however, until the summer of 1792 and each summer thereafter from 1794 to 1799.

Because it was believed that yellow fever was a contagious disease, quarantine laws were imposed, and a board of health was established in 1796. As the eighteenth century came to a close, physicians began to realize that the disease was not contagious because those in close contact with yellow fever victims did not get the disease nor did it spread into the countryside.

New Haven, Connecticut.   A severe outbreak of yellow fever occurred at New Haven in 1794 and killed about 70 percent of those who were infected. A ship from the West Indies arrived in June, and within days members of a nearby family came down with the dreaded disease. They had come in contact with clothes belonging to a sailor on the ship who died from yellow fever, and the clothes were thought to have brought the disease to New Haven. Noah Webster (1758–1843), of dictionary fame, observed and wrote about this epidemic. He believed that certain atmospheric conditions, such as the cleanliness of the **air**, determined whether or not the disease would spread in a certain geographical area. In this case, he theorized that some fish cleaned near the family's home may have contaminated the air and caused the family to become ill.

New York City.   Yellow fever struck New York City during the summer of 1702. Twenty people died daily during this outbreak, and the final death toll reached nearly 600 persons or about 10 percent of the estimated population. City authorities spread quicklime and coal dust in the streets and lit bonfires in order to clean and sanitize the supposedly "corrupted" air.

Outbreaks of yellow fever ravaged New York City in 1743 and again in 1745. A 1795 epidemic killed 732 persons of an estimated population of about 50,000. The cause of this epidemic was greatly disputed, but most observers believed that the disease arrived aboard a ship. Another severe epidemic occurred in 1798, causing more than 2,000 deaths.

Philadelphia, Pennsylvania.   The yellow fever epidemic of 1793 infected 17,000 people with 5,000 deaths (10 percent of the population). During the summer of 1793, thousands of French refugees came to Philadelphia from St. Domingue with news of the French Revolution and the yellow fever that raged in the Caribbean islands. The city was also in the grip of a lengthy drought, and the **water** was so low and drainage so poor in the waterways and marshes that rotting animals, dead fish, and sewage caused stagnation and horrible odors. Although unknown to anyone at that time, ideal conditions existed for the mosquito population to expand rapidly and spread the disease.

Philadelphia was then serving as the nation's capital while the city of Washington was being constructed, and the severity of the epidemic caused all government operations to cease. As the deaths began to mount, the mayor of Philadelphia asked the medical community and government officials to consider how the contagion might be controlled. It was at first deduced that hygiene and climate were responsible for causing the disease. Coffee beans brought by a ship from St. Domingue and left to rot on a wharf were also blamed for having caused the epidemic. A controversy about whether the disease was contagious or was caused by bad air added to the city's general fear and panic.

By September, those who could left the city. Among them were George Washington (1732–1799), other government officials, business people, and ordinary citizens. In all, some 12,000 people left the city to escape the dreaded pestilence. However, news of the Philadelphia plague was known throughout the region, and some refugees were robbed whereas others were quarantined at isolated locations. In Philadelphia, victims were often turned out by their own families, and the poor were left to die in the streets. Because the cause of the disease was unknown, all manner of preventive methods were tried, such as bonfires, sprinkling vinegar on clothing and household furnishings, and firing guns so that the smell of gunpowder would permeate the air.

As civil unrest and chaos spread through the city, the mayor was able to enlist volunteers to help run the government and take action to control the disease. **Hospital** care was improved so that people could successfully recover, an orphanage was established, the dead were properly disposed of, and relief was provided for the poor. Their work went so well that donations of money, food, and supplies began arriving. By November the disease had weakened, and the city was returning to normal. *See also* Colonialism and Epidemic Disease; Contagion Theory of Disease, Premodern; Corpses and Epidemic Disease; Disinfection and Fumigation; Environment, Ecology, and Epidemic Disease; Insects, Other Arthropods, and Epidemic Disease; Latin America, Colonial: Demographic Effects of Imported Diseases; Public Health Agencies, U.S. Federal; Rush, Benjamin; Yellow Fever in Colonial Latin America and the Caribbean; Yellow Fever in the American South, 1810–1905.

Further Reading

Duffy, John. *Epidemics in Colonial America.* Baton Rouge: Louisiana State University Press, 1971.

Estes, J. Worth, and Billy G. Smith, eds. *A Melancholy Scene of Devastation: The Public Response to the 1793 Philadelphia Yellow Fever Epidemic.* Canton, MA: Science History Publications, 1997.

Harvard University Library. *Contagion.* http://ocp.hul.harvard.edu/contagion/yellowfever.html

Humphreys, Margaret. *Yellow Fever and the South.* Baltimore: Johns Hopkins University Press, 1999.

Pierce, John R., and Jim Writer. *Yellow Jack.* Hoboken, NJ: Wiley, 2005.

Powell, John Harvey. *Bring Out Your Dead: The Great Plague of Yellow Fever in Philadelphia in 1793.* Philadelphia: University of Pennsylvania Press, 1993.

RICHARD EIMAS

YELLOW FEVER IN THE AMERICAN SOUTH, 1810–1905.   Although **yellow fever** continued to afflict the United States during the 1800s, it was during this period that the disease eventually receded in the central and northern Atlantic coast regions. Nonetheless, it became an increasingly serious problem for the southern states into the early twentieth century.

The last significant yellow fever **epidemics** to strike the northeastern United States were in 1805 when major outbreaks occurred in both Philadelphia and New York. Although the disease appeared infrequently in succeeding years, another epidemic did not occur until 1819, when it struck Baltimore, Philadelphia, and Boston. It lingered for the next three summers in Philadelphia and Baltimore and made one final visit to New York in 1822. After that time, yellow fever was no longer a major problem for the states north of Virginia.

Although infected individuals continued to arrive at northern coastal cities, strict **quarantines** helped keep the disease from spreading. The shorter northern summers also limited the activities of the disease-carrying *Aedes aegypti* mosquito and contributed to the elimination of yellow fever in the central and northern Atlantic coast regions.

As the country grew and expanded south to the Gulf Coast states, profitable **trade** relationships developed with the West Indies, Africa, and South America. Sailing vessels frequently stopped for food and water at ports in the West Indies where yellow fever was common. Disease-carrying mosquitoes as well as infected passengers and crew often arrived on slave or trade ships from Africa or South America. As a result, yellow fever continued to be carried to the southeastern Atlantic coast and along the entire gulf shore from Florida to Texas where the warm, damp climate was an ideal habitat for the *Aedes aegypti* mosquito.

Fortunately, when cooler winter weather arrived in late November or early December the mosquito population was greatly reduced, and yellow fever ended for that particular year. Nonetheless, yellow fever continued to return year after year, and it was rare that more than two or three years passed without a minor outbreak. Periodically the disease assumed major proportions, often destroying from 5 to 10 percent of the population.

Although it is now known that yellow fever is spread by the *Aedes aegypti* mosquito, its cause was still as great a mystery during the 1800s as it had been since it was first encountered 200 years earlier. Yellow fever was difficult to diagnose because early symptoms of the disease could easily be confused with other diseases. The medical community was aware that a diagnosis of yellow fever was certain to cause economic upheaval, possibly lead to panic and mass exodus and cause nearby towns to institute quarantines and blockades against the infected city. Therefore, they seldom dared make this pronouncement without first consulting their colleagues. Even then there was no assurance that the question was settled, for the findings were almost certain to be questioned. As a result, presence of the disease was rarely made public before the situation was beyond control.

As yellow fever became a serious threat to public health, it touched off a decades-long public debate concerning whether or not yellow fever was an imported contagious disease or a noncontagious fever generated in filth and decaying substances. The public tended to believe that it was a contagious disorder, whereas the medical profession generally felt that it was not a contagious disease.

Depending upon the severity of the epidemic, preventive measures included **disinfection** by spreading quicklime in gutters, sewers, and outhouses as well as in the graveyards and on the **corpses** of victims. Rooms and buildings where the sick had died were thoroughly cleaned and fumigated. Cannons were fired at sunrise and sunset, and barrels of tar were placed at street corners and burned during the night to fight the **miasma**. Since the cause of yellow fever was unknown, the effectiveness of these measures was questionable, though fumigants may have kept mosquitoes at bay.

New Orleans.   New Orleans was the largest city on the Gulf Coast in the early 1800s with a population of 10,000. Although the city had experienced mild outbreaks of yellow fever in the late 1700s and early 1800s, it was not until 1811 that a more severe epidemic claimed 500 lives. In 1817 the disease claimed more than 800 victims. There was a minor outbreak the following year followed by a major epidemic in 1819. By 1820 the population exceeded 27,000, and 20 years later the city had over 100,000 inhabitants. Three successive epidemics from 1853 to 1855 claimed 14,000 lives. Following the 1858 epidemic, almost 5,000 yellow fever victims were counted among the dead. New Orleans experienced relatively few cases from 1859 to 1867, in large part because of the Union blockade and martial law during the Civil War. In the latter year, however, a major epidemic took 3,100 lives. A few scattered cases appeared in 1868 and 1869, and in 1870 the disease again flared up in epidemic proportions, killing almost 600 citizens. Throughout the 1870s cases appeared every summer, but only in 1873 and 1878 did the disease reach epidemic proportions. In 1873 the death toll was just over 200, but the 1878 epidemic resulted in over 4,000 deaths.

Although yellow fever cases continued to be diagnosed almost every summer, New Orleans had experienced the last of the great epidemics. The disease flared up once more in 1897, and on this occasion there were about 300 deaths. The disease struck again with epidemic force in 1905. However, by this time, the role of the *Aedes aegypti* mosquito was more clearly understood, an effective program for mosquito **eradication** was implemented, and the epidemic was over before the end of August. Even so, this last outbreak of yellow fever in the United States brought death to 452 residents.

Other Southern Cities before the Civil War. Because of its size and role as the major southern port, New Orleans bore the brunt of these onslaughts, and the pattern established by the disease there was duplicated in dozens of other cities and towns. Charleston, South Carolina, only a third as large as New Orleans, experienced a similar pattern of outbreaks. A series of epidemics arrived in the late 1790s and early 1800s. Major epidemics struck the city again in 1817 and 1819, and after that time there was a succession of epidemics, with the peak being reached during the 1850s.

North Carolina also suffered several outbreaks of yellow fever. Wilmington was afflicted from 1796 to 1862, and New Bern and other towns were also affected. Georgia's major port, Savannah, suffered a series of yellow fever epidemics from 1800 to 1858. Because the Atlantic coast of Florida was sparsely settled and had no major ports, it largely escaped the disease. Even so, St. Augustine and Jacksonville suffered occasional epidemics in the years prior to the Civil War. Key West, off the tip of the Florida peninsula, and Pensacola, on the Gulf Coast, however, were frequently visited by the disease. The history of yellow fever in Pensacola is a repetition, on a smaller scale, of what happened in New Orleans and along the entire Gulf Coast.

In 1839, when yellow fever struck the city of Galveston, Texas, its population was just over 2,000, and the outbreak claimed 200 lives. For the rest of the 1800s, with only a few minor exceptions, whenever a major yellow fever epidemic broke out in New Orleans, it almost always afflicted the cities of Galveston and Houston.

The most northerly ports to suffer from yellow fever epidemics were Norfolk and Portsmouth, Virginia. Norfolk, which bore the brunt of the attacks, endured a series of epidemics starting in the 1790s and then experienced one final devastating blow in 1855. At the time of this epidemic Norfolk and Portsmouth had a combined population of between 25,000 and 30,000, and the number of deaths was close to 3,000.

During and after the Civil War. With some exceptions, yellow fever was not a major problem during the Civil War years 1861 to 1865. The effectiveness of the Northern blockade of Southern ports and the disruption of normal trade relations undoubtedly played a role in keeping yellow fever to a minimum. The chief epidemics of the war years occurred in Charleston, in Wilmington and New Bern, North Carolina, in Pensacola and Key West, Florida, and in Galveston, Texas. Following the war, the disease appeared infrequently during 1866 and then broke out in many places along the Gulf Coast in 1867, one of the major yellow fever years. From Pensacola to Brownsville, Texas, almost every town was affected. After a four-year lull, the pestilence returned in 1871 and again in 1873. In neither of these years, however, was it as widespread or as severe as in 1867.

During the 1870s, cases were reported nearly every summer in many of the Gulf Coast towns, but the disease did not generally become epidemic until the summer of 1878, a momentous year in the annals of yellow fever. The distinguishing characteristic of this outbreak was that it swept far up the Mississippi River. Almost from the beginning of the century, riverboats had carried yellow fever from New Orleans to many river towns in Louisiana and Mississippi. Natchez, Mississippi, more than 200 miles up the river from New Orleans, was first attacked in 1817 and suffered repeatedly in the succeeding years. Vicksburg, Mississippi, further north, witnessed its first outbreak in 1841.

By the 1870s railroad expansion and the development of faster steamboats, coupled with the gradual spread of the *Aedes aegypti*, made it possible for yellow fever to reach as far north as St. Louis. The 1878 epidemic struck first at Baton Rouge and Vicksburg, then at Memphis and Cairo, Illinois, eventually reaching St. Louis. At the same time, the disease moved up the Tennessee River to Chattanooga, Tennessee, and traveled up the Ohio River as far as Louisville, Kentucky. Memphis, Tennessee, which had a population of about 35,000, was hit the hardest with some 15,000 yellow fever cases and about 3,500 deaths. Vicksburg, another town to feel the full impact of the epidemic, reported more than 3,000 cases and over 1,000 deaths in a population of about 12,000.

Although the fever returned to New Orleans, Memphis, and a number of other cities in 1879, no serious epidemics developed. Throughout the 1880s and early 1890s, the United States enjoyed relative freedom from yellow fever. Scattered cases appeared here and there, but with the exception of an outbreak in Florida in 1888, the disease did not reach major epidemic proportions. The Florida epidemic was centered around Jacksonville on the Atlantic Coast and ranged inland as far as Gainesville. Before cool weather halted the disorder, the cases numbered in the thousands, and deaths in the hundreds.

The beginning of the end of yellow fever's seemingly endless attacks on North America came just three years after the disastrous yellow fever year of 1878, when Carlos Finlay y Barres (1833–1915) of Cuba theorized that the *Aedes aegypti* mosquito transmitted the disease. In 1900 the U.S. Army Commission on Yellow Fever in Havana headed by **Walter Reed** confirmed his theory with human volunteers at the cost of three additional lives.

There is no question that yellow fever slowed growth and development throughout the South, but the widespread epidemic of 1878 hastened the development of state and local health boards and was also responsible for the first attempt to create a national health department in the United States. Yellow fever played an important role in focusing attention on public health needs and in bringing pressure to bear upon legislative bodies to institute the necessary reforms to protect the health of its citizens. *See also* Contagion Theory of Disease, Premodern; Corpses and Epidemic Disease; Disinfection and Fumigation; Environment, Ecology, and Epidemic Disease; Insects, Other Arthropods, and Epidemic Disease; Public Health Agencies, U.S. Federal; Rush, Benjamin; Yellow Fever Commission, U.S.; Yellow Fever in Colonial Latin America and the Caribbean; Yellow Fever in Latin America and the Caribbean, 1830–1940; Yellow Fever in North America to 1810.

Further Reading

Crosby, Molly Caldwell. *The American Plague.* New York: Berkley Books, 2006.

Delaporte, Francois. *History of Yellow Fever.* Cambridge, MA: MIT Press, 1991.

Duffy, John. *From Humors to Medical Science: A History of American Medicine.* Urbana: University of Illinois Press, 1993.

Duffy, John. *Sword of Pestilence: The New Orleans Yellow Fever Epidemic of 1853.* Baton Rouge: Louisiana State University Press, 1966.

Humphreys, Margaret. *Yellow Fever and the South.* Baltimore: Johns Hopkins University Press, 1999.

Pierce, John R., and Jim Writer. *Yellow Jack: How Yellow Fever Ravaged America and Walter Reed Discovered Its Deadly Secrets.* Hoboken, NJ: Wiley, 2005.

Public Broadcasting Service. *The Great Fever.* http://www.pbs.org/wgbh/amex/fever/

Trask, Benjamin H. *Fearful Ravages: Yellow Fever in New Orleans, 1796–1905.* Lafayette: Center for Louisiana Studies, University of Louisiana at Lafayette, 2005.

RICHARD EIMAS

YERSIN, ALEXANDRE (1863–1943). Swiss **physician** and microbiologist Alexandre Yersin is credited with having discovered the *Yersinia pestis* plague **bacterium**. He began his medical studies in his native Switzerland at Lausanne, followed by further studies at Marburg, Germany, in 1884, and at the Hôtel Dieu hospital in Paris in 1885–1886. He wrote his medical thesis on **tuberculosis** in 1888 while working on **vaccinations** against rabies at the **Pasteur** Institute in Paris. In the summer of 1889, he completed **Robert Koch's** course in bacteriology in Berlin, giving him exposure to the two leading—and competing—approaches in the new science. Returning to Paris later the same year, he worked with Emile Roux (1853–1933) on **diphtheria** and became a naturalized French citizen.

On the verge of a promising scientific career, the reclusive Yersin in 1890 suddenly fled the Pasteur Institute to travel to Indochina where, in 1892, Albert Calmette (1863–1933) was able to persuade him to join the French colonial health service. When news of the Hong Kong **bubonic plague** outbreak of 1894 reached Saigon, French health officials immediately despatched Yersin to the beleaguered British port.

Yersin arrived three days after a Japanese team headed by **Shibasaburo Kitasato**, who had studied under Koch in Berlin. The two men have been jointly linked to the discovery of the plague bacillus. Yersin, however, was the better scientist, and much later, his more accurate results eventually resulted in the taxonomic naming of the bacillus *Yersinia pestis* after him in 1971. Its earlier denomination had been *Pasteurella pestis*. Yersin's original description of the plague bacillus was concise and correct, whereas Kitasato's contained errors. In addition, only Yersin suggested that rats were a major factor in the **transmission** of the disease. Finally, only Yersin persisted in plague research, returning to Emile Roux's Paris laboratory in 1895 to develop an anti-plague serum from the blood of horses to boost human immune systems. Following his stint in Paris, Yersin returned to Indochina where he also developed a preventative anti-plague vaccine from a live but attenuated organism in 1896. It proved of limited value because it only afforded protection for two weeks. Later that year, Yersin traveled to plague-infected southern China to test the Pasteur Institute's anti-plague serum. In 1897 he appeared in Bombay for the same purpose, but the results in both China and India proved disappointing.

Yersin rarely returned to Europe after 1900. He helped found the Medical School of Hanoi in 1902 and was its first director. He also pioneered in the cultivation of rubber trees imported from Brazil. From 1904 until his death in 1943, he served as Director of the Pasteur Institute at Nhatrang, Vietnam. His burial site there later became a venerated pilgrimage site, and his memory is honored by the Vietnamese state. *See also* Pasteur, Louis; Third Plague Pandemic related articles.

Further Reading

Howard-Jones, Norman. "Kitasato, Yersin and the Plague Bacillus." *Clio Medica* 10 (1975): 23–27.
Marriott, Edward. *Plague: A Story of Science, Rivalry, and the Scourge that Won't Go Away.* New York: Metropolitan, 2002.

MYRON ECHENBERG

Z

ZOONOSIS. *See* Animal Diseases (Zoonoses) and Epidemic Disease.

Glossary

Abscess: An inflammatory, pus-filled pocket created by the immune system to isolate a foreign object; the purpose is to contain the infection in this location and quickly remove the invader

Acute: Proceeding quickly and/or lasting a short time

Adsorption: The attachment of a virus to a cell

Aerosol, -ize: Small particles suspended in the air, such as small drops of liquid; to create small droplets spread into the air (i.e., through sneezing aerosolized droplets containing bacteria)

Agar: A chemical obtained from red algae or seaweed that forms a jelly-like constancy at room temperature; it is often used as a growth medium for bacterial or fungal cultures or as part of a method to separate parts of proteins and DNA

Agent: A substance or organism that has a specific and predictable effect on a cell or organism; an infectious disease used as a biological weapon

Alopecia: Loss of hair as the result of an autoimmune disease in which the body attacks hair follicles, preventing hair growth

Animalcule: An historic term used to describe microscopic organisms (single- or multi-celled)

Anthrax: A bacterium *Bacillus anthracis* which can cause a severe infection and, in some cases, death; transmission usually occurs through spores (the dormant form of the bacterium)

Antibacterial: A chemical applied to living tissue to prevent the growth of bacteria

Antibody: A protein produced by the immune system for the detection, and ultimately destruction, of foreign microbes

Antigen: A molecule (foreign or self) against which the body produces an immune response

Antimicrobial: A chemical that prevents growth of microorganisms, typically disease-causing microbes

Antisepsis, -tic: The use of antimicrobials on tissue to kill bacteria and prevent infection

Antiserum: Fluids passed from one organism to another, containing specific antibodies for the purpose of passing on immunity (i.e., acquired immunity)

Arbovirus: A virus transmitted to humans by an arthropod (short form of "arthropod-borne virus")

Arenavirus: A genus (or large group) of viruses that exist in animals; often they are transmitted to humans by rodents

Armamentarium: The total collection of resources and equipment used by physicians or a hospital

Aseptic: The technique used to prevent contamination by foreign microbes when working with either bacterial cultures or sterile objects

Aspirates: Objects removed by aspiration, or the collection of a sample that has been aspired (suctioned up) into a dispensing tube or pipette

Asymptomatic: Without symptoms of a disease; occasionally a disease is present with no symptoms, hindering diagnosis

Attenuated: Weakened; referring to a less virulent form of a virus used in vaccines to allow for immunological resistance to that virus

Autoimmune: The inability of the immune system to recognize parts of the body as self, resulting in the body attacking itself

Avirulent: Not disease-causing

B cell: A cell of the immune system that produces antibodies

Bacillus (pl. bacilli): A rod-shaped bacterium; a member of the genus Bacillus

Bacteriology, -ist: The study of bacteria and scientific applications; one who studies bacteria

BCG vaccine: Bacille Calmette Guerin vaccine made from a bacterium related to tuberculosis to immunize individuals against the disease

Benign: A disease that is not progressing; a noncancerous tumor

Bezoar Stone: A "stone" found in the intestines made from undigested food, such as salts

Bills of Mortality: Mortality counts reported weekly by causes of death and parishes of Londoners, compiled by local parish officials and published as pamphlets; began in Italian cities in the fifteenth century and in England in the early sixteenth century; lasted into the nineteenth century

Bioinformatics: The study of biology using mathematics and computer science for modeling and organization of molecular biology information

Biopsy: A procedure used to diagnose cancer in which a piece of tissue is removed and examined or analyzed

Biovar: A bacterial strain that differs from others (of the same species) in biochemical or physiological characteristics

Bleeding: Also "bloodletting" or "phlebotomy"; the premodern medical practice of opening a patient's vein with a sharp lancet and letting blood flow in a controlled manner; according to humoral theory, this helps balance the body's humors for good health or healing

Bloodletting: See "bleeding"

Broad-spectrum: Referring to an antibiotic's ability to target a wide range of bacterial classes of pathogens, as compared to narrow spectrum antibiotics

Bubo: A visible swollen lymph node at the armpit or groin, characteristic of the bubonic plague, gonorrhea, syphilis, or tuberculosis

Caravanserai: A stopping place for caravans, usually provided with food, water, shelter, and a wall around the site

Carrier: An individual who has either an infection or genetic trait with the ability to transmit it to another; may not display characteristics

Case fatality rate (CFR): The proportion of individuals who die from a disease

Catarrh: A runny nose; mucus drainage

Cell: The basic unit of life that contains elements necessary to reproduce, metabolize, and maintain homeostasis, or internal consistency; cells can be specialized to form a tissue or they can exist as single-celled organisms

Chemoreceptor: A type of cell that converts a chemical signal (from a protein or other chemical) into an electrical signal within the cell, which allows for fast responses

Chemotherapy: Any treatment for a disease using a chemical, most often refers to treatments for cancer that stop cell multiplication

Chromosome: A compact piece of DNA that forms in a dividing cell; humans have 23 pairs

Chronic: Lasting a long time or recurring frequently

Chronic disease: A long-lasting, continuous disease; typically refers to a disease with symptoms that are apparent for more than three months

Cilium (pl. cilia): An extension of a cell that either provides movement or is used for sensing the environment

Clinical: Referring to the treatment or observation of patients in a controlled setting

Clone: An organism that has the same DNA as another

Commensal, -ism: A type of symbiosis, a relationship between two organisms such that one benefits from the relationship and the other is not significantly affected

Constitution, -al: The total of an individual's physical makeup; relating to an individual's well-being

Culture: n. A mass of microbes; v. To create such a large group of cells by spreading them over agar to allow them to grow quickly—a technique used largely for identification of disease

Dejecta: Feces or excrement

Delirium: A sudden loss of cognition

Demographic: Referring to characteristics of a certain population (e.g., race, age, income)

Dendritic cell: A cell with dendrites, or cellular projections; dendritic cells of the immune system produce antigens (or recognition sites) for T cells

Dermatitis: Inflammation of the skin

Didactic: Performing an educational function

Differential diagnosis: A systematic method of determining the cause of a patient's disease by exploring symptoms, referring to the patient's family, and examining the patient

Diuretic: A drug that increases urine production in the kidneys, causing an increase of water loss from the body

DNA (deoxyribonucleic acid): A double helix found in every organism for the purpose of storage, replication, and expression of cellular information; found in the nucleus of human cells

Dye: Used to stain, or color, specific parts of the cell either to make the cell more visible or to highlight particular parts

Ecology: The patterns of interaction of all various plants and animals within a specific environment

Ectopic: Displacement of a bodily organ, for example, the development of both kidneys on one side of the body

Edema: The swelling of an organ or tissue because of an excess of fluid outside the cells

Electrolyte: Ions (atoms with charges) found in the body used to maintain a charge across the membrane of the cell, particularly in nervous, cardiac, and muscular tissue

Electron Microscope: A microscope with a very high magnification that works by passing electrons through the sample to get a picture

Electuary: A drug made into a paste with sugar or honey to be administered orally

Eliminate: To remove all natural incidence of a disease from a given area

Emergent disease: A disease or variation of a disease that is increasing its presence in human populations for the first time, especially in an endemic or epidemic level

Endemic: Referring to a disease that is maintained in a population over a long period of time; from a certain area or population

Enteric: Referring to the intestines

Enterotoxin: A toxin produced from certain bacteria that affect the digestive system; food poisoning comes from the ingestion of these bacteria, whose toxins are poisonous

Environment: The external conditions in which an organism lives and with which it interacts

Enzootic: An "endemic" disease present in an animal rather than a human population

Enzyme: A protein that speeds up a reaction or process in a living organism

Epiphenomenon (pl. epiphenomena): A byproduct of another event

Epithelial cells: Those cells forming the issue that provides the lining of bodies (i.e. the skin, intestinal lining, respiratory lining, and mucus membranes)

Epizootic: An unusually widespread disease present in an animal population

Eradicate: To "uproot" or eliminate the natural occurrence of a disease completely from the earth; to date only smallpox has been eradicated

Etiology: The cause of a disease

Ex voto: A religious object dedicated to thanking a saint or deity, often for lifting an epidemic

Exanthem (pl. exanthemata): A widespread rash found on an individual; usually caused by a virus or bacterial infection or an allergic reaction to a drug

Excreta: An organism's waste material

Exotoxin: A protein excreted by a microbe that is harmful to the host

Express: To show the characteristics of having a particular gene (e.g., expressing blonde hair as the result of having certain genes)

False positive/false negative: An inaccurate result of a test for the presence of a given disease

Febrile: Relating to a fever; an increase in body temperature

Feudal: Pertaining to the medieval European social and political hierarchy that was based upon the agricultural labor of peasant serfs and noblemen's oaths of homage

Focus: With reference to an epidemic disease, the geographic point of origin or a long-lasting reservoir

Fomite: Any inanimate object that may carry an infectious disease

Genocide: Deliberate destruction of, or attempt to destroy, an ethnic human population

Genome: The whole genetic sequence of an individual, including the coding and noncoding portions of DNA

Genotype: The genetic information stored for an individual, usually describing genes inherited for a particular trait; as compared to phenotype

Genus (pl. genera): The subgroup of organisms under the family; in the scientific name, the genus is the first, capitalized word

Germ: Generic term for a microorganism, usually pathogenic, such as a bacteria or fungus

Gram-positive/Gram-negative: The result of a Gram stain, which produces a purple (positive) or pink (negative) color depending on the composition of the bacteria's cell wall; the Gram stain is a method used to separate bacteria into two major groups

Granuloma: An area of dense inflammatory tissue, often associated with hypersensitivity toward a chronic infection

Hematemesis: Vomiting blood; caused by erosion of the stomach or esophagus as the result of an infection, ulcer, or other disease

Hematuria: Blood in the urine, observable in most conditions only by viewing red blood cells under a microscope

Hemorrhage, -agic: Bleeding, or relating to bleeding

Herd immunity: The theory that vaccinating the majority of the population for a disease will help prevent the rest of the population from acquiring it because of the lower number of carriers

Heterozygote: A person with two different versions of a particular gene

Hominin: A being that is a human or human ancestor, including chimpanzees

Homozygote: A person with two copies of the same version of a particular gene

Horizontal gene transfer: The transfer of genetic information between bacteria that is not from parent to offspring

Host: Any living organism that provides its machinery (reproductive, metabolic) for the use of a virus or parasite

Humor: Fluid in the body; comes from the ancient belief that a disease comes from the four fluids in the body (blood, yellow bile, black bile, and phlegm) being out of balance

Hydronephrosis: Stretching, or distension, of the kidney, as the result of a blockage of the uterine tube causing urine to build up in the kidney

Hyperemia: Increased blood flow to a particular part of the body

Hypodermic: Beneath the skin

Hypotension: Low blood pressure

Hypothesis: The premise that an experiment is designed to test

Iatrochemical: Relating to iatrochemistry, a branch of chemistry from the sixteenth and seventeenth centuries that attempted to find a cure for diseases with chemistry

Immunity: The ability of the body to fight off a disease easily because of previous exposure

Immunogenic: The ability to illicit an immune response

Immuno-suppressed: Having an immune system that is less active, either because of a disease or as the result of certain medical treatments (i.e., chemotherapy)

In utero: In the uterus

In vitro: Occurring in a controlled environment outside a living organism; literally, in glass

In vivo: In a live system

Incidence: The number of new cases of a disease (contraction, death) that develop over a particular period of time

Incubation: The process of disease development between the infection of a person and the first appearance of symptoms

Indian Medical Service: British colonial governmental organization (1886–1947) dedicated to the health care of British military and citizens, and by extension of the native peoples, in India

Indigenous: Native to a particular region or locale

Infarction: The loss of blood supply to part of an organ leading to death of tissue

Infectious: Referring to a disease caused by a microbial agent

Infectious period: Period of time during which an infected person can transmit a given disease to another

Inflammation: A response to an infection or irritant that results in swelling, redness, warmth, and pain

Intracellular: Inside the cell

Laboratory assay: An experiment performed in a laboratory that attempts to quantify a property of a substance

Latent: Present, but hidden; a disease that does not show symptoms for a period of time

Lesion: An abnormality in the tissue of an organ as a result of disease or injury

Lethality: The ability of a disease to cause death

Leukocyte: White blood cell

Lipid: A fat molecule, such as a fatty acid or steroid, that is insoluble in water

Lymphocyte cell: A kind of white blood cell that is involved in the immune response by producing antibodies, allowing for the specificity of the immune system

Lyse: To break open; usually referring to the breaking open of a cell by disruption of the cell membrane

Macrophage: A differentiated white blood cell that ingests dangerous foreign substances, such as bacteria or cancer cells

Macroscopic: Observable with the naked eye, not needing a microscope

Malignant: Referring to a disease that is progressively worsening; commonly referring to cancer that has spread to other parts of the body

Memento mori: A cultural symbol or reminder of human mortality and death

Metabolic: Referring to metabolism or the digestion of nutrients

Miasma: The historic theory that disease is spread through "bad air"

Microbe: A microorganism

Microbiology, -ist: The study of microorganisms, specifically those that are pathogenic, or cause disease; a person who studies microbiology

Microorganism: A microscopic living organism, such as a bacterium, fungus, or protozoon

Mitosis: The process by which cells divide in order to increase number of cells; particularly the dividing of the cell nucleus

Monocyte: A type of white blood cell found in the blood that is part of the immune system and fights bloodborne pathogens

Morbidity: The incidence or prevalence of total and/or new cases of a disease

Mortality: The number of deaths as the result of a disease

Motile: Able to move independently

Mucus: Secretion of the mucus membranes found in the nose, lips, throat, ears, and genitalia, used to collect foreign objects after they have entered the body or as a lubricant for movement such as food down the esophagus

Murine: Referring to rats or mice

Mutate, mutation (genetic): A change in information of DNA, resulting in different characteristics

Neonatal: Relating to a newborn infant, typically within four to six weeks after the child is born

Neurasthenia: A diagnosis made in the late 1800s for individuals expressing symptoms of fatigue, thought to be caused by an urbanized civilization; probably used to describe a wide variety of diseases

Neurologic: Referring to the nervous system; a disease that affects the central nervous system

Neutrophil cell: An immune cell that ingests foreign invaders (bacteria) through phagocytosis and digests them; they contain many sacs of digestive enzymes for this purpose

Niche: The ecological job of an organism in its environment, especially its role in the food chain

Nonspecific: Not specific, used to describe an infection caused by an unknown pathogen

Nosological: Referring to the classification of diseases

Nucleus, -ei: The membrane-bound organelle of the cell that contains genetic material (DNA), found in eukaryotic cells (not present in bacterial cells)

OED: Oxford English Dictionary; a standard source for English word etymology and history

Opportunistic: A disease that infects after another infection has weakened the immune system

Organism: A living being, existing as a single cell, such as a bacterium, or a multi-cellular organism, such as a human being

Outpatient: A patient who does not have to stay in a hospital for treatment; outpatient surgery allows the patient to return home the same day

Papular: Having papules, or raised bumps on the skin

Parasite: An organism that requires the resources of another organism (its host) to live and reproduce

Parasitology, -ist: The study of parasites and their relation to their hosts; one who studies parasites

Paroxysm: A sudden onset of symptoms, usually painful, from a disease

Pathenosis: The concept that in any given time and place a group of diseases exists together, but should one disappear, another will takes its place

Pathogen: Any biological agent that causes disease (bacterium, virus, parasite)

Pathogenic: Capable of causing disease

Pathological: Referring to behaviors that are caused by mental illness or instability, and/or being abnormal or extreme

Pathology, -ist: The study of disease: its causes, development, treatment, and diagnosis

Periodicity: Occurring at discrete and regular intervals, usually time intervals

Petri dish: A shallow dish used to hold small biological samples for observation; may contain agar for bacterial growth

Phage: A virus that attacks a bacterial cell, also bacteriophage

Phage Typing: Using the mode of action of a virus to identify a particular bacterium that the phage specifically attacks; detection is done by staining the viruses prior to infection and identifying the stain following infection

Phagocytosis: The cellular process of ingesting large particles by means of folding the cellular membrane into a pocket that pinches off into the cell to form a vacuole

Pharmacopoeia: A book that contains a list of medicines in wide use as well as information about their preparation

Phenotype: The expressed genetic information for an individual that is visible to an observer; as compared to genotype

Phlebotomy: See "bloodletting"

Physiology, -ist: The study of the ways in which the human body functions; one who studies the body

Placebo: A pill or other medium with no medication given as a control in a study (to see if giving a remedy has an effect without the medication)

Plague/pestilence: Often used generically for epidemic disease outbreaks of various types, including insect infestations (e.g., a plague of locusts); specifically, plague refers to Y *pestis* infection

Plasmid: A circular extra piece of DNA typically found in bacterial cells; scientists alter plasmids, causing bacteria to make desired proteins

Pneumonia: An infection of the lungs in which the oxygen-containing sacs of the lungs become filled with fluid as an immune response to a foreign pathogen

Polydactyly: Having more fingers or toes than normal

Polymorphism: The existence of a variety of forms of gene, or alleles, present in a population

Prevalence rate: A calculated term used to describe how a disease has spread

Prion: a protein that acts as an infections agent causing such diseases as mad cow disease or Creutzfeldt-Jakob disease

Prodromal: period of time during which a disease is taking its course but not manifesting symptoms

Progenitor: An ancestor; a progenitor cell is an undifferentiated cell that can differentiate into specialized cells

Prognosis: A doctor's prediction of the development of a disease in a patient (how long the patient is expected to live)

Prophylaxis, -actic: An attempt to prevent an infection by protecting the body before an exposure to a pathogen; prophylactics are drugs, actions, or other means believed to protect a body or community against disease

Proteinaceous: Made of proteins, or the macromolecule composed of amino acids which act as enzymes, messengers, or antibodies, and also serve many other roles

Proteomics: The study all of the proteins of an organism

Protist: A member of the kingdom Protista, usually a single-celled, prokaryotic organism (a cell that does not have a membrane-bound nucleus)

Pseudopod: Literally, a false foot; an extension of the cellular membrane from an amoeboid cell used for locomotion or for sensing the environment

Public health: The study and practice of preventing and treating community-wide disease; community may be defined from local to global

Pulmonary: Referring to the lungs

Purgative: Causing cleaning or purging, particularly of the bowels; a medicine that does so

Pus: A yellow-white liquid produced as part of an inflammatory response to an infection that includes dead immune cells that have killed the pathogen

Pustule: A collection of pus directly under skin, a pimple made of pus

Putrefaction: (premodern) deterioration of the structure or life force of a person, organ, or other object as a result of the effects of corrupted air or other substance; (modern) the breakdown of tissues before or after death caused mostly by bacterial infections

Quartan fever: A fever that has lasted 72 hours (i.e., into a fourth, *quartus*, day) intermittently; this is indicative of a bacterial infection

Quiescent: Lacking activity, being at rest; a disease causing no symptoms

Receptor (cell wall): A protein found on a cell wall that responds to a specific protein or chemical signal to cause a change within the cell

Reemergent disease: A disease that once affected a particular area or population, was largely eliminated, and then reappeared in endemic or epidemic form

Regimen: A regulated course of action; for example, a schedule of daily antibiotics or a specific diet

Replicate: Making a copy; DNA replication is the method by which DNA duplicates to be passed to two daughter cells during cell division (mitosis)

Reservoir: A host for a pathogen in which the pathogen is often undetected for a long period of time

Resistance: Acquired or evolved ability of an organism to avoid being negatively affected by another organism or drug

Respiratory: Referring to the respiratory system; the organ system that deals with gas exchange in an organism

Retrovirus: A virus that contains RNA (instead of DNA) as its genetic material; these viruses contain proteins to allow the RNA to be copied as DNA and thus to be used by the host cell

RNA (ribonucleic acid): A form of genetic information storage that is mostly used for transmitting information from DNA to making proteins, copied from the DNA template

Sarcoma: A cancer of connective tissue (bone, blood, cartilage), as opposed to epithelial tissue of an organ

Screening: Studying a particular feature or physical trait through examining a large number of individuals

Secondary infection: An infection that occurs during or as a result of another infection

Sepsis: Also known as blood poisoning, an excessive immunological response to an infection, either caused by the infection or by a dysfunction in the immune system, which causes the circulatory system to malfunction and eventually to lead to organ failure

Septicemia: See sepsis

Sequela (pl. sequelae): A continuing pathological condition caused by a previous infection or trauma

Serogroup: A group of microorganisms that have a common antigen

Serological: Pertaining to serology, or the characterization of immunological substances including antibodies and antigens

Seropositive: Having a particular antibody present in the blood; often used to test if an individual has been exposed to a particular infectious agent

Serotype: The testing of a microorganism for the presence of a specific antigen, or a microorganism that has a tested antigen

Serum: Plasma with clotting factors removed

Simian: relating to monkeys, apes, and other nonhuman primates

Species: The smallest classification of organisms in the scientific organization of all organisms, grouping organisms that are the closest related; for example, *Homo sapiens*, is the genus and species name of man

Sporocyst: A sack that encases spores, or the reproductive elements of asexual organisms; the larval form of parasitic worms

Sputum: Mucus or phlegm from the respiratory tract that comes up when coughing

Stain: The coloring of a specific biological element to distinguish it from others; for example, a bacterium can be stained to test if it is Gram-positive or Gram-negative (see definition), or cells and tissues can be stained to visualize a particular component such as nuclei or DNA

Strain: A genetic type or variation of an organism, especially a human pathogen

Sylvatic: Referring to a wild as opposed to a domestic state of animals; pathogen that affects only wild (not domesticated) animals

Symbiotic: A relationship between two organisms of different species in which at least one of the organisms benefits and the other is not harmed

Symptom: A physical or psychological abnormality in a person that suggests the presence of one or more pathogens or disease states

Synchrony: Simultaneous or near simultaneous occurrence of two or more events

Syndrome: The combination of signs and symptoms of a patient's disease; the observable results of a disease that allow for detection

Systemic: Referring to a body system or the body in total

T cell: One type of cell of the immune system that helps to fight against infection by recognizing infection in other cells

Tertian fever: A fever that occurs every third (*tertius*) day (after 48 hours), usually referring to the fevers caused by malaria

Therapeutic: Ability to heal or to benefit the immune system

Therapy: The treatment of an illness or disease

Theriac: A premodern Western general remedy composed by apothecaries of many ingredients including snake flesh

Tissue: A collection of cells that perform a similar function, tissues combine to make organs

Toxin: A chemical that is harmful to an organism produced by living organisms

Transmission rate: Average number of people who catch a disease from an infected person over a given period of time

Unguent: An ointment used to soothe a wound on the surface of the body

Variolation: An outdated method to immunize an individual for smallpox by the controlled infection with the smallpox virus

Vector: An object or organism (often an animal) that does not cause a disease itself but that carries the pathogen from one organism to another

Vernacular: Language of the common people; often as opposed to Latin, Arabic, Sanskrit or other scholarly or literary languages with multicultural audiences

Virgin-soil epidemic: Initial outbreak of an infectious disease previously unknown to or absent from a specific geographical area for many generations

Virology, -ist: The study of viruses and diseases they cause; one who studies viruses and viral diseases

Virulence: A microorganism's level of ability to infect and cause disease

Zoonosis, -tic: A pathogen that is normally spread through animals

Compiled by Rebecca and Elizabeth Repasky

Bibliography

Selected Websites

Centers for Disease Control and Prevention. http://www.cdc.gov/

Doctors without Borders (Médecins sans Frontières). http://www.msf.org/

Harvard University Library. *Contagion: Historical Views of Diseases and Epidemics.* http://ocp.hul.
   harvard.edu/contagion/
   http://ocp.hul.harvard.edu/contagion/generalmaterials.html

Jones, Michael Owen, dir. *Online Archive of American Folk Medicine.* University of California, Los
   Angeles. http://www.folkmed.ucla.edu/index.html.

"The Living City: New York City Project." http://www.tlcarchive.org/htm/home.htm

Modern Languages Association. *History of Health Sciences Links Page.* http://www.mla-hhss.org/
   histlink.htm

National Institutes of Health. http://www.nih.gov/

National Library of Medicine. http://www.nlm.nih.gov/

National Museum of Health and Medicine. http://www.nlm.nih.gov/hmd/medtour/nmhm.html

PubMed Medical Journal Search Engine. http://www.ncbi.nlm.nih.gov/PubMed/

U.S. Public Health Service. http://www.usphs.gov/

Wellcome Trust (UK). http://www.wellcome.ac.uk/

World Health Organization. http://www.who.int/en/

World Health Organization's Weekly Epidemiological Record [updated weekly]. http://www.who.int/
   wer/en/

World Health Organization's Historical Collections [documents, reports, etc.]. http://www.who.int/library/collections/historical/en/

Reference Works

Alexander, Martin, et al. eds. *Encyclopedia of Microbiology*. New York: Academic Press, 2000.

American Medical Association. *American Medical Association Complete Medical Encyclopedia*. New York: Random House, 2003.

Applebaum, Wilbur. *Encyclopedia of the Scientific Revolution*. New York: Routledge, 2008.

Barnard, Alan. *Encyclopedia of Social and Cultural Anthropology*. New York: Routledge, 2002.

Boslaugh, Sarah E., ed. *The Encyclopedia of Epidemiology*. London: SAGE Publications, 2007.

Breslow, Lester. *Encyclopedia of Public Health*, 4 volumes. Farmington Hills, MI: Gale Group, 2002.

Bynum, W. F., and Helen Bynum, eds. *Dictionary of Medical Biography*. Westport, CT: Greenwood, 2006.

Bynum, W. F., and Roy Porter. *Companion Encyclopedia of the History of Medicine*, 2 volumes. New York: Routledge, 1994.

Cancik, Hubert. *Brill's New Pauly: The Ancient World*. Leiden: Brill, 2002.

Davidson, Linda Kay, and David M. Gitlitz. *Pilgrimage: From the Ganges to Graceland, an Encyclopedia*. Santa Barbara: ABC-CLIO, 2002.

Ember, Carol R., and Melvin Ember. *Encyclopedia of Medical Anthropology: Health and Illness in the World's Cultures*. New York: Springer, 2003.

Engs, Ruth C. *The Eugenics Movement: An Encyclopedia*. Westport, CT: Greenwood Press, 2005.

Facts on File. *Encyclopedia of World History*, 7 volumes. New York: Facts on File, 2007.

Faragher, John Mack. *The American Heritage Encyclopedia of American History*. New York: Henry Holt, 1998.

Gao Duo. *Chinese Encyclopedia of Medicine*. London: Carlton Publishing, 2004.

Glick, Thomas F., et al., eds. *Medieval Science, Technology, and Medicine: An Encyclopedia*. New York: Routledge, 2005.

Goldfield, David R. *Encyclopedia of American Urban History*. Thousand Oaks, CA: Sage, 2006.

Gorbach, Sherwood L., et al. *Infectious Diseases*. Philadelphia: Lippincott, 2003.

Handbook of Diseases, 3rd edition. Philadelphia: Lippincott, 2004.

Hatfield, Gabrielle. *Encyclopedia of Folk Medicine: Old World and New World Traditions*. Santa Barbara: ABC-CLIO, 2003.

Heggenhougen, Kris. *International Encyclopedia of Public Health*, 6 volumes. New York: Academic Press, 2008.

Kiple, Kenneth F., ed. *The Cambridge Historical Dictionary of Disease*. New York: Cambridge University Press, 2003.

———. *The Cambridge World History of Human Disease*. New York: Cambridge University Press, 2001.

——, et al., eds. *Plague, Pox and Pestilence: Disease in History.* New York: Marboro Books, 1997.

Kirch, Wilhelm. *Encyclopedia of Public Health.* New York: Springer, 2008.

Kohn, George Childs, ed. *Encyclopedia of Plague and Pestilence from Ancient Times to the Present.* New York: Facts on File, 2001.

Last, John M. *A Dictionary of Epidemiology,* 4th edition. New York: Oxford University Press, 2004.

Longe, Jacqueline L. *The Gale Encyclopedia of Medicine,* 5 volumes. Stamford, CT: Gale, 2006.

McNeill, William H. *Berkshire Encyclopedia of World History.* Great Barrington, MA: Berkshire Publishing, 2005.

Merriam Webster's Medical Dictionary. New York: Merriam Webster, 2007.

Moore, Elaine A., and Lisa Marie Moore. *Encyclopedia of Sexually Transmitted Diseases.* Jefferson, NC: McFarland, 2004.

Pickering, L. K., ed. *Red Book: Report of the Committee on Infectious Diseases,* 27th edition. Elk Grove Village, IL: American Academy of Pediatrics, 2006.

Rashid, Roshdi, ed. *Encyclopedia of the History of Arabic Science,* 3 volumes. New York: Routledge, 1996.

Service, M. W. *The Encyclopedia of Arthropod-transmitted Infections.* Wallingford, UK: CABI Publishing, 2001.

Shoquist, Jennifer, and Diane Stafford. *Encyclopedia of Sexually Transmitted Diseases.* New York: Facts on File, 2003.

Sienkewicz, Thomas J., ed. *Encyclopedia of the Ancient World,* 3 volumes. Pasadena, CA: Salem Press, 2002.

Smith, Raymond. *Encyclopedia of AIDS: A Social, Political, Cultural, and Scientific Record of the HIV Epidemic.* New York: Routledge, 1998.

Snodgrass, Mary Ellen. *Historical Encyclopedia of Nursing.* Santa Barbara, CA: ABC-CLIO, 1999.

——. *World Epidemics: A Cultural Chronology of Disease from Prehistory to the Era of SARS.* Jefferson, NC: McFarlane, 2003.

Strickland, G. T., ed. *Hunter's Tropical Medicine and Emerging Infectious Diseases,* 8th edition. Philadelphia: W B Saunders Co., 2000.

Tibayrenc, Michel. *Encyclopedia of Infectious Diseases: Modern Methodologies.* New York: Wiley, 2007.

Turkington, Carol, and Bonnie Ashby. *The Encyclopedia of Infectious Diseases.* New York: Facts on File, 2007.

Vauchez, Andre. *Encyclopedia of the Middle Ages.* New York: Routledge, 2001.

Venes, Donald. *Taber's Cyclopedic Medical Dictionary,* 20th revised edition. Philadelphia: F. A. Davis, 2005.

World Health Organization. *World Health Statistics, 2007.* Geneva: WHO, 2007.

History of Medicine

Amundsen, Darrel W. *Medicine, Society, and Faith in the Ancient and Medieval Worlds.* Baltimore: Johns Hopkins University Press, 1996.

Barry, Jonathan, and Colin Jones. *Medicine and Charity before the Welfare State*. New York: Routledge, 1991.

Bates, Don. *Knowledge and the Scholarly Medical Traditions*. New York: Cambridge University Press, 1995.

Brockliss, Laurence, and Colin Jones. *The Medical World of Early Modern France*. New York: Oxford University Press, 1997.

Bullough, Vern L. *Universities, Medicine, and Science in the Medieval West*. Burlington, VT: Ashgate, 2004.

Bynum, W. F. *Science and the Practice of Medicine in the Nineteenth Century*. New York: Cambridge University Press, 1994.

Bynum, W. F., Anne Hardy, Stephen Jacyna, Christopher Lawrence, and E. M. Tansey. *The Western Medical Tradition, 1800 to 2000*. New York: Cambridge University Press, 2006.

Bynum, W. F., and Roy Porter. *Medical Fringe & Medical Orthodoxy, 1750–1850*. London: Croom Helm, 1987.

Campbell, Sheila, et al., eds. *Health, Disease and Healing in Medieval Culture*. Toronto: University of Toronto Press, 1992.

Cavallo, Sandra. *Charity and Power in Early Medieval Italy: Benefactors and their Motives in Turin, 1541–1789*. New York: Cambridge University Press, 1995.

Cunningham, Andrew. *The Medical Enlightenment of the Eighteenth Century*. New York: Cambridge University Press, 1990.

Cunningham, Andrew, and Perry Williams. *The Laboratory Revolution in Medicine*. New York: Cambridge University Press, 1992.

Esch, Gerald. *Parasites and Infectious Disease: Discovery by Serendipity and Otherwise*. New York: Cambridge University Press, 2007.

Fábrega, Horacio. *Evolution of Sickness and Healing*. Berkeley: University of California Press, 1997.

Farley, J. Bilharzia. *A History of Tropical Medicine*. New York: Cambridge University Press, 1991.

Fissell, Mary E. *Medicine Before Science: The Business of Medicine from the Middle Ages to the Enlightenment*. New York: Cambridge University Press, 2003.

———. *Patients, Power and the Poor in Eighteenth-Century Bristol*. New York: Cambridge University Press, 1991.

Garcia-Ballester, et al., eds. *Practical Medicine from Salerno to the Black Death*. New York: Cambridge University Press, 1994.

Gentilcore, David. *Healers and Healing in Early Modern Italy*. New York: University of Manchester Press, 1998.

Getz, Faye Marie. *Medicine in the Middle Ages*. Princeton, NJ: Princeton University Press, 1998.

Gray, Alastair. *World Health and Disease*, 3rd edition. Philadelphia: Open University Press, 2001.

Grell, Ole Peter, and Andrew Cunningham, eds. *Medicine and the Reformation*. London: Routledge, 1993.

———. *Religio Medici: Medicine and Religion in Seventeenth-Century England*. Aldershot, UK: Scolar Press, 1996.

Grmek, Mirko. *Western Medical Thought from Antiquity to the Middle Ages*. Cambridge, MA: Harvard University Press, 1998.

Kennedy, Michael T. *A Brief History of Disease, Science and Medicine*. Mission Viejo, CA: Asklepiad Press, 2004.

Lindemann, Mary. *Health and Healing in Eighteenth-Century Germany*. Baltimore: Johns Hopkins University Press, 1996.

———. *Medicine and Society in Early Modern Europe*. New York: Cambridge University Press, 1999.

Lloyd, Geoffrey, and Nathan Sivin. *The Way and the Word: Science and Medicine in Early China and Greece*. New Haven, CT: Yale University Press, 2002.

Loudon, Irvine, ed. *Western Medicine: An Illustrated History*. New York: Oxford University Press, 1997.

Marble, Allen E. *Surgeons, Smallpox, and the Poor: A History of Medicine and Social Conditions in Nova Scotia, 1749–1799*. Montreal: McGill University Press, 1993.

McVaugh, Michael R. *Medicine before the Plague: Practitioners and their Patients in the Crown of Aragon: 1285–1345*. New York: Cambridge University Press, 1993.

Nutton, Vivian. *Ancient Medicine*. New York: Routledge, 2004.

———. *Medicine at the Courts of Europe, 1500–1837*. New York: Routledge, 1990.

O'Boyle, Cornelius. *The Art of Medicine: Medical Teaching at the University of Paris, 1250–1400*. Boston: Brill, 1998.

Pagel, Walter. *Joan Baptista Van Helmont: Reformer of Science and Medicine*. New York: Cambridge Press, 2002.

Park, Katherine. *Doctors and Medicine in Early Renaissance Florence*. Princeton: Princeton University Press, 1985.

Pelling, Margaret. *The Common Lot: Sickness, Medical Occupations and the Urban Poor in Early Modern England*. New York: Longman, 1998.

Pomata, Gianna. *Contracting a Cure: Patients, Healers, and the Law in Early Modern Bologna*. Baltimore: Johns Hopkins University Press, 1998.

Pormann, Peter E., and Emily Savage-Smith. *Medieval Islamic Medicine*. Washington, DC: Georgetown University Press, 2007.

Porter, Roy. *The Greatest Benefit to Mankind: A Medical History of Humanity*. New York: Norton, 1997.

———, ed. *Patients and Practitioners: Lay Perceptions of Medicine in Pre-Industrial Society*. New York: Cambridge University Press, 1985.

Porter, Stephen. *The Popularization of Medicine*. New York: Routledge, 1992.

Rawcliffe, Carole. *Medicine and Society in Later Medieval England*. Stroud, Gloucs, England: Sutton, 1997.

———. *Sources for the History of Medicine in Late Medieval England*. Kalamazoo, MI: Medieval Institute Publications, 1995.

Rothman, David, et al., eds. *Medicine and Western Civilization*. New Brunswick, NJ: Rutgers University Press, 2003.

Selin, Helaine, and Hugh Shapiro, eds. *Medicine across Cultures: History and Practice of Medicine in Non-Western Cultures*. Dordrecht: Kluwer, 2003.

Siraisi, Nancy. *Medieval and Early Renaissance Medicine*. Chicago: University of Chicago Press, 1990.

Starr, Paul. *The Social Transformation of American Medicine: The Rise of a Sovereign Profession and the Making of a Vast Industry*. New York: Basic Books, 1982.

Unschuld, Paul U. *Chinese Medicine*. Brookline, MA: Paradigm, 1998.

———. *Medicine in China: A History of Ideas*. Berkeley: University of California Press, 1988.

———. *Medicine in China: Historical Artifacts and Images*. New York: Prestel, 2000.

Veith, Ilza. *The Yellow Emperor's Classic of Internal Medicine*. Berkeley: University of California Press, 2002.

Wear, Andrew. *Knowledge and Practice in English Medicine, 1550–1680*. New York: Cambridge University Press, 2000.

Westerlund, David. *African Indigenous Religions and Disease Causation: From Spiritual Beings to Living Humans*. Leiden: Brill, 2006.

Wujastyck, Dominik. *The Roots of Ayurveda*. New York: Penguin, 2003.

Zysk, Kenneth. *Asceticism and Healing in Ancient India: Medicine in the Buddhist Monastery*. New York: Oxford University Press, 1991.

Diseases and Epidemics

Crawford, Dorothy H. *The Invisible Enemy: A Natural History of Viruses*. New York: Oxford University Press, 2002.

Frank, Steven A. *Immunology and Evolution of Infectious Disease*. Princeton, NJ: Princeton University Press, 2002.

Gordis, Leon. *Epidemiology*, 2nd edition. New York: Saunders, 2000.

Hagen, Thomas. *The Demon under the Microscope*. New York: Harmony Books, 2006.

Hendrickson, Robert. *More Cunning than Man: A Complete History of the Rat and Its Role in Human Civilization*. New York: Kensington Books, 1983.

Kenrad, Nelson. *Infectious Disease Epidemiology: Theory and Practice*. Boston: Jones and Bartlett, 2006.

Holmes, King K., et al. *Sexually Transmitted Diseases*. 4th edition. Columbus, OH: McGraw-Hill, 2007.

Lashley, Felissa, and Jerry D. Durham, eds. *Emerging Infectious Diseases: Trends and Issues*. New York: Springer, 2007.

McKenna, Maryn. *Beating Back the Devil*. New York: Free Press, 2004.

McMichael, Tony. *Human Frontiers, Environments and Disease*. New York: Cambridge University Press, 2001.

Morabia, Alfredo Morabia, ed. *A History of Epidemiologic Methods and Concepts*. Basel: Birkhauser Verlag, 2004.

National Research Council. *Under the Weather: Climate, Ecosystems, and Infectious Disease*. Washington, DC: National Academies Press, 2001.

Oldstone, Michael B.A. *Viruses, Plagues, and History.* New York: Oxford University Press, 1998.

Rothmna, Kenneth J. *Epidemiology: An Introduction.* New York: Oxford University Press, 2002.

Sauerborn, Rainer, and Louis R. Valérie. *Global Environmental Change and Infectious Diseases: Impacts and Adaptation Strategies.* New York: Springer, 2007.

Stolley, Paul, and Tamar Lasky. *Investigating Disease Patterns: The Science of Epidemiology.* New York: Scientific American Library, 1998.

Torrey, E. Fuller, and Robert H. Yolken. *Beasts of the Earth: Animals, Humans, and Disease.* Piscataway, NJ: Rutgers University Press, 2005.

Walters, Mark J. *Six Modern Plagues and How We Are Causing Them.* Washington, DC: Island Press, 2004.

History of Epidemics (General)

Ackerknecht, Erwin H. *History and Geography of the Most Important Diseases,* revised first edition. Baltimore: Johns Hopkins University Press, 1982.

Alchón, Suzanne Austin. *A Pest in the Land: New World Epidemics in a Global Perspective.* Albuquerque: University of New Mexico Press, 2003.

Altman, Linda J. *Plague and Pestilence: A History of Infectious Disease.* Berkeley Heights, NJ: Enslow Publishers, 1998.

Arnold, David. *Colonizing the Body: State Medicine and Epidemic Disease in Nineteenth-Century India.* Berkeley: University of California Press, 1993.

Bollett, Alfred Jay. *Plagues & Poxes: The Impact of Human History on Epidemic Disease.* New York: Demos Medical Publishing, 2004.

Bourdelais, Patrice. *Epidemics Laid Low: A History of What Happened in Rich Countries.* Baltimore: Johns Hopkins University Press, 2006.

Boyd, Robert T. *The Coming of the Spirit of Pestilence: Introduced Infectious Diseases and Population Decline Among Northwest Coast Indians, 1774–1874.* Seattle: University of Washington Press, 1999.

Bray, R. S. *Armies of Pestilence: The Effects of Pandemics on History.* Cambridge, UK: Lutterworth Press, 1998.

Campbell, Judy. *Invisible Invaders: Smallpox and Other Diseases in Aboriginal Australia 1780–1880.* Melbourne, Australia: Melbourne University Press, 2002.

Champion, Justin A. I., ed. *Epidemic Disease in London.* London: Centre for Metropolitan History Working Papers Series 1, 1993.

Cliff, Andrew, et al. *Deciphering Global Epidemics: Analytical Approaches to the Disease Records of World Cities, 1888–1912.* New York: Cambridge University Press, 1998.

Cook, Noble David. *Born to Die: Disease and New World Conquest, 1492–1650.* New York: Cambridge University Press, 1998.

Cook, Noble David, and W. George Lovell, eds. *"Secret Judgments of God": Old World Disease in Colonial Spanish America.* Norman: University of Oklahoma Press, 1992.

Cooper, Donald B. *Epidemic Diseases in Mexico City, 1761–1813.* Austin: University of Texas Press, 1965.

Cunningham, Andrew, and Ole Peter Grell. *The Four Horsemen of the Apocalypse: Religion, War, Famine and Death in Reformation Europe*. New York: Cambridge University Press, 2000.

De Bevoise, Ken. *Agents of the Apocalypse: Epidemic Disease in the Colonial Philippines*. Princeton, NJ: Princeton University Press, 1995.

De Paolo, Charles. *Epidemic Disease and Human Understanding: A Historical Analysis of Scientific and Other Writings*. Jefferson, NC: McFarland and Co., 2006.

Duffy, John. *Epidemics in Colonial America*. Baton Rouge: Louisiana State University Press, 1971.

Eckert, Edward A. *The Structure of Plagues and Pestilences in Early Modern Europe: Central Europe, 1560–1640*. New York: S. Karger Publishing, 1996.

Epstein, P. R. "Commentary: Pestilence and Poverty—Historical Transitions and the Great Pandemics." *American Journal of Preventive Medicine* 8 (1992): 263–265.

Gehlbach, Stephen H. *American Plagues: Lessons from Our Battles with Disease*. New York: McGraw Hill, 2005.

Giblin, James Cross. *When Plague Strikes: The Black Death, Smallpox, AIDS*. New York: Harper, 1996.

Gottfried, Robert S. *Epidemic Disease in Fifteenth-Century England: The Medical Response and the Demographic Consequences*. New Brunswick, NJ: Rutgers University Press, 1978.

Grob, Gerald N. *The Deadly Truth: A History of Disease in America*. New York: Cambridge University Press, 2002.

Hays, J. N. *The Burden of Disease*. New Brunswick: Rutgers University Press, 1998.

Johns, Alessa, ed. *Dreadful Visitations*. New York: Routledge, 1999.

Jones, David S. *Rationalizing Epidemics: Meanings and Uses of American Indian Mortality since 1600*. Cambridge, MA: Harvard University Press, 2004.

Karlen, Arno. *Man and Microbes: Disease and Plagues in History and Modern Times*. New York: Simon and Schuster, 1995.

———. *Plague's Progress: A Social History of Man and Disease*. London: V. Gollancz, 1996.

Keys, David. *Catastrophe: An Investigation into the Origins of the Modern World*. New York: Ballantine Press, 2000.

Knobler, Stacey, et al., eds. *The Impact of Globalization on Infectious Disease Emergence and Control: Exploring the Consequences and Opportunities*. Washington, DC: National Academies Press, 2006.

Kunitz, Stephen J. *Disease and Social Diversity: The European Impact on the Health of Non-Europeans*. New York: Oxford University Press, 1994.

Ladurie, Emmanuel LeRoy. "A Concept: The Unification of the Globe by Disease (14th to 17th Centuries)." In *The Mind and Method of the Historian*, translated by Siân Reynolds and Ben Reynolds, pp. 28–83. Chicago: University of Chicago, 1981.

Mack, Arien. *In Time of Plague: The History and Social Consequences of Lethal Epidemic Disease*. New York: New York University Press, 1992.

Markel, Howard. *Quarantine! East European Jewish Immigrants and the New York City Epidemics of 1892*. Baltimore: Johns Hopkins University Press, 1999.

———. *When Germs Travel: Six Major Epidemics that Have Invaded America since 1900 and the Fears They Have Unleashed.* New York: Pantheon, 2004.

McBride, David. *From TB to AIDS: Epidemics among Urban Blacks since 1900.* New York: State University of New York Press, 1991.

McKenna, Maryn. *Beating Back the Devil: On the Front Lines with the Disease Detectives of the Epidemic Intelligence Service.* New York: Free Press, 2004.

McNeill, William. *Plagues and Peoples.* Garden City, NJ: Anchor Press, 1975.

Morrison, A. L., Julius Kirschner, and Anthony Molho. "Epidemics in Renaissance Florence." *American Journal of Public Health* 75 (1985): 528–535.

Nikiforuk, Andrew. *The Fourth Horseman: A Short History of Epidemics, Plagues, Famine and Other Scourges.* New York: M. Evans and Co., 1993.

Ranger, Terence, and Paul Slack. *Epidemics and Ideas.* New York: Cambridge University Press, 1992.

Rothberg, Robert I., ed. *Health and Disease in Human History: A Journal of Interdisciplinary History Reader.* Cambridge, MA: MIT Press, 2000.

Schultheiss, E., and L. Tardy. "Short History of Epidemics in Hungary until the Great Cholera Epidemic of 1831." *Centaurus* 11 (1966): 279–301.

Shah, Nayan. *Contagious Divides: Epidemics and Race in San Francisco's Chinatown.* Berkeley: University of California Press, 2001.

Sherman, Irwin W. *The Power of Plague.* Washington, DC: American Society for Microbiology, 2006.

Smallman-Raynor, M. R., and A. D. Cliffs, eds. *War Epidemics: An Historical Geography of Infectious Diseases in Military Conflict and Civil Strife, 1850–2000.* New York: Oxford University Press, 2004.

Stathakopoulos, Dionysios. *Famine and Pestilence in the Late Roman and Early Byzantine Empire: A Systematic Survey of Subsistence Crises and Epidemics.* Burlington, VT: Ashgate Publishing Company, 2004.

Treadwell, Perry. *God's Judgment? Syphilis and AIDS: Comparing the History and Prevention Attempts of Two Epidemics.* Lincoln, NE: Writer's Club Press, 2001.

Twitchett, Denis. "Population and Pestilence in T'ang China." In *Studia Sino-Mongolica*, edited by Wolfgang Bauer (Wiesbaden: Franz Steiner Verlag, 1979) pp. 35–68.

Watts, Sheldon. *Epidemics and History: Disease, Power and Imperialism.* New Haven, CT: Yale University Press, 1997.

Wills, Christopher. *Yellow Fever, Black Goddess: The Co-evolution of People and Plagues.* New York: Helix Books, 1998.

Winslow, Charles-Edward Amory. *The Conquest of Epidemic Disease: A Chapter in the History of Ideas.* Madison: University of Wisconsin Press, 1980.

History of Public Health

Alexander, John T. *Bubonic Plague in Early Modern Russia: Public Health and Urban Disaster.* Baltimore: Johns Hopkins University Press, 1980.

Arnold, David. *Colonizing the Body: State Medicine and Epidemic Disease in Nineteenth-Century India.* Berkeley: University of California Press, 1993.

Baldwin, Peter. *Contagion and the State in Europe, 1830–1930.* New York: Cambridge University Press, 1999.

———. *Disease and Democracy: The Industrialized World Faces AIDS.* Berkeley: University of California Press, 2005.

Christakos, George, et al. *Interdisciplinary Public Health Reasoning and Epistemic Modeling: The Case of the Black Death.* New York: Springer, 2005.

Cipolla, Carlo. *Fighting the Plague in Seventeenth-Century Italy* (Merle Curti Lectures, 1978). Madison: University of Wisconsin Press, 1981.

———. *Miasmas and Disease: Public Health and the Environment in the Pre-industrial Age,* translated by Elizabeth Potter. New Haven: Yale University Press, 1992.

———. *Public Health and the Medical Profession in Renaissance Florence.* Cambridge: Cambridge University Press, 1976.

Dowdle, W. R., and Donald Hopkins, eds. *The Eradication of Infectious Diseases.* New York: Wiley, 1998.

Eyler, John. *Victorian Social Medicine: The Ideas and Methods of William Farr.* Baltimore: Johns Hopkins University Press, 1979.

Farley, John. *To Cast Out Disease: A History of the International Health Division of the Rockefeller Foundation (1913–1951).* New York: Oxford University Press, 2004.

Gilbert, Pamela K. *Mapping the Victorian Social Body.* New York: State University of New York Press, 2004.

Goubert, Jean-Pierre. *The Conquest of Water,* translated by Andrew Wilson. Princeton, NJ: Princeton University Press, 1986.

Hamlin, Christopher. *Public Health and Social Justice in the Age of Chadwick: Britain, 1800–1854.* New York: Cambridge University Press, 1998.

Hardy, Ann. *The Epidemic Streets: Infectious Diseases and the Rise of Preventive Medicine, 1856–1900.* New York: Oxford University Press, 1993.

Harrison, Mark. *Public Health in British India: Anglo-Indian Preventive Medicine 1859–1914.* New York: Cambridge University Press, 1994.

LaBerge, Ann Elizabeth Fowler. *Mission and Method: The Early Nineteenth-Century French Public Health Movement.* New York: Cambridge University Press, 2002.

Packard, Randall, et al., eds. *Emerging Illnesses and Society: Negotiating the Public Health Agenda.* Baltimore: Johns Hopkins University Press, 2004.

Porter, Dorothy. *Health, Civilization and the State: A History of Public Health from Ancient to Modern Times.* New York: Routledge, 1999.

———, ed. *The History of Public Health and the Modern State* (Clio Medica 26). Atlanta: Rodopi, 1994.

Rosen, George. *A History of Public Health.* Expanded Edition. Baltimore: Johns Hopkins University Press, 1993.

Sheard, S., and H. Power, eds. *Body and City: Histories of Urban Public Health.* Burlington, VT: Ashgate, 2000.

Stevens, Rosemary A., et al., eds. *History and Health Policy in the United States: Putting the Past Back In*. New Brunswick, NJ: Rutgers University Press, 2006.

Ward, John W., and Christian Warren. *Silent Victories: The History and Practice of Public Health in Twentieth-Century America*. New York: Oxford University Press, 2007.

Disease, Society and Culture

Aberth, John. *From the Brink of the Apocalypse: Crisis and Recovery in Late Medieval England*. New York: Routledge, 2000.

Apostolopoulos, Yorghos. *Population Mobility and Infectious Disease*. New York: Springer, 2007.

Barroll, John Leeds. *Politics, Plague, and Shakespeare's Theater: The Stuart Years*. Ithaca, NY: Cornell University Press, 1991.

Bewell, Alan. *Romanticism and Colonial Disease*. Baltimore: Johns Hopkins University Press, 1999.

Boeckl, Christine. *Images of Plague and Pestilence: Iconography and Iconology*. Kirksville, MO: Truman State University Press, 2000.

Bolton, James L. "The World Upside Down: Plague as an Agent of Economic and Social Change." In *The Black Death in England*, edited by W. M. Ormrod and P. G. Lindley, pp. 17–77. Stamford: Paul Watkins, 1996.

Brady, Saul Nathaniel. *The Disease of the Soul: Leprosy in Medieval Literature*. Ithaca, NY: Cornell University Press, 1974.

Calvi, Giulia. *Histories of a Plague Year: The Social and the Imaginary in Baroque Florence*. Berkeley: University of California Press, 1989.

Cantor, Norman. *In the Wake of the Plague: The Black Death and the World It Made*. New York: Harper, 2000.

Carlin, Claire L. *Imagining Contagion in Early Modern Europe*. New York: Palgrave, 2005.

Carmichael, Anne G. "Last Past Plague: The Uses of Memory in Renaissance Epidemics." *Journal of the History of Medicine and Allied Sciences* 53 (1998): 132–160.

Cohn, Samuel K., Jr. *The Black Death Transformed: Disease and Culture in Early Renaissance Europe*. Oxford: Oxford University Press, 2002.

Colgrove, James. *State of Immunity: The Politics of Vaccination in Twentieth-Century America*. Berkeley: University of California Presss, 2006.

Conrad, Lawrence I., and Dominik Wujastyk, eds. *Contagion: Perspectives from Pre-Modern Societies*. Burlington, VT: Ashgate, 2000.

Dixon, Laurinda S. *Perilous Chastity: Women and Illness in Pre-Enlightenment Art and Medicine*. Ithaca, NY: Cornell University Press, 1995.

Dohar, William J. *The Black Death and Pastoral Leadership: The Diocese of Hereford in the Fourteenth Century*. Philadelphia: University of Pennsylvania Press, 1995.

Evans, Richard J. *Death in Hamburg: Society and Politics in the Cholera Years, 1830–1910*. New York: Penguin, 2005.

Fairchild, Amy L, Ronald Bayer, and James Colgrove. *Searching Eyes: Privacy, the State, and Disease Surveillance in America*. Berkeley: University of California Press, 2007.

Farmer, Paul. *Infections and Inequalities: The Modern Plagues*. Berkeley: University of California Press, 2001.

———. *Pathologies of Power: Health, Human Rights and the New War on the Poor*. Berkeley: University of California Press, 2005.

Fidler, David P. *International Law and Infectious Diseases*. New York: Oxford University Press, 1999.

Friedman, John B. ""He Hath a Thousand Slayn This Pestilence": Iconography of the Plague in the Late Middle Ages." In *Social Unrest in the Late Middle Ages*, edited by Francis X. Newman, pp. 75–112. Binghamton, New York: Medieval and Renaissance Texts and Studies, 1986.

Gere, David. *How to Make Dances in an Epidemic: Tracking Choreography in the Age of AIDS*. Madison: University of Wisconsin Press, 2004.

Gilman, Sander. *Disease and Representation: Images of Illness from Madness to AIDS*. Ithaca, NY: Cornell University Press, 1988.

Grigsby, Bryon Lee. *Pestilence in Medieval and Early Modern English Literature*. New York: Routledge, 2004.

Guerchberg, Sèraphine. "The Controversy over the Alleged Sowers of the Black Death in the Contemporary Treatises on Plague." In *Change in Medieval Society: Europe North of the Alps, 1050–1500*, edited by Sylvia Thrupp, pp. 208–224. New York: Appleton-Century-Crofts, 1965.

Harrison, Dick. "Plague, Settlement and Structural Change at the Dawn of the Middle Ages." *Scandia: Tidskrift för historisk forskning* 59 (1993): 15–48.

Hatty, Suzanne E., and James Hatty. *The Disordered Body: Epidemic Disease and Cultural Transformation*. New York: State University of New York Press, 1999.

Healy, Margaret. *Fictions of Disease in Early Modern England: Bodies, Plagues and Politics*. New York: Palgrave, 2002.

Herlihy, David. *The Black Death and the Transformation of the West*. Cambridge, MA: Harvard University Press, 1997.

Kimball, Ann Marie. *Risky Trade: Infectious Disease in the Era of Global Trade*. London: Ashgate, 2006.

Kudlick, Catherine J. *Cholera in Post-Revolutionary Paris: A Cultural History*. Berkeley: University of California Press, 1996.

Leavy, Barbara Fass. *To Blight with Plague: Studies in a Literary Theme*. New York: New York University Press, 1992.

Leven, K. H. "*Athumia* and *Philanthropia*: Social Reactions to Plagues in Late Antiquity and Early Byzantine Society." *Clio Medica* 28 (1995): 293–407.

Long, Thomas L. *AIDS and American Apocalypticism: The Cultural Semiotics of an Epidemic*. New York: State University of New York Press, 2005.

Lund R. D. "Infectious Wit: Metaphor, Atheism, and the Plague in Eighteenth-century London." *Literature and Medicine* 22 (2003): 45–64.

Marshall, Louise. "Manipulating the Sacred: Image and Plague in Renaissance Italy." *Renaissance Quarterly* 47 (1994): 485–532.

Meiss, Millard. *Painting in Florence and Siena after the Black Death: The Arts, Religion, and Society in the Mid-fourteenth Century*. Princeton, NJ: Princeton University Press, 1951.

Morris, Robert John. *Cholera, 1832: The Social Response to an Epidemic.* London: Croom Helm, 1976.

Munkhoff, Richelle. "The Interpretation of Plague in England, 1574–1665." *Gender and History* 1 (1999): 1–30.

Norman, Diana. "Change and Continuity: Art and Religion after the Black Death." In *Siena, Florence and Padua, I: Art, Society and Religion 1280–1400,* edited by Diana Norman. Interpretative Essays Series, pp. 177–196. New Haven, CT: Yale University Press, 1995.

O'Conner, Erin. *Raw Material: Producing Pathology in Victorian Culture.* Durham, NC: Duke University Press, 2000.

Ormrod, W. Mark. "The English Government and the Black Death of 1348–1349." In *England in the Fourteenth Century,* edited by W. M. Ormrod, pp. 175–188. Woodbridge, Suffolk: Boydell Press, 1986.

Palmer, R. "The Church, Leprosy and Plague." In *The Church and Healing,* edited by W. J. Scheils, pp. 79–99. New York: Basil Blackwell, 1982.

Palmer, R. C. *English Law in the Age of the Black Death, 1348–1381: A Transformation of Governance and Law.* Chapel Hill: University of North Carolina Press, 1993.

Prinzing, Friedrich. *Epidemics Resulting from Wars.* Oxford: The Clarendon Press, 1916.

Reff, Daniel T. *Plagues, Priests, Demons: Sacred Narratives and the Rise of Christianity in the Old World and the New.* New York: Cambridge University Press, 2005.

Robertson, D. W. "Chaucer and the Economic and Social Consequences of the Plague." In *Social Unrest in the Late Middle Ages,* edited by Francis X. Newman, pp. 49–74, Binghampton: Medieval and Renaissance Texts and Studies, 1986.

Rosenberg, Charles, and Janet Golden, eds. *Framing Disease: Studies in Cultural History.* New Brunswick, NJ: Rutgers University Press, 1992.

San Juan, Rose Marie. *Rome: A City Out of Print.* Minneapolis: University of Minnesota Press, 2001.

Schiferl, Ellen. "Iconography of Plague Saints in Fifteenth-century Italian Painting." *Fifteenth Century Studies* 6 (1983): 205–225.

Selgelid, Michaeal, et al., eds. *Ethics and Infectious Disease.* New York: Blackwell, 2007.

Smith, Raymond. *Encyclopedia of AIDS: A Social, Political, Cultural, and Scientific Record of the HIV Epidemic.* New York: Penguin, 2001.

Steel, David. "Plague Writing: From Boccaccio to Camus." *Journal of European Studies* 11 (1981): 88–110.

Steinhoff, Judith. *Sienese Painting after the Black Death: Artistic Pluralism, Politics, and the New Art Market.* New York: Cambridge University Press, 2006.

Tangherlini, Timothy R. "Ships, Fogs, and Traveling Pairs: Plague Legend Migration in Scandinavia." *Journal of American Folklore* 101 (1988): 176–206.

Totaro, Rebecca. *Suffering in Paradise: The Bubonic Plague in English Literature from More to Milton.* Pittsburg: Duquesnse University Press, 2005.

Treichler, Paula A. *How to Have Theory in an Epidemic: Cultural Chronicles of AIDS.* Durham, NC: Duke University Press, 1999.

Vollmar, L. C., Jr. "The Effect of Epidemics on the Development of English Law from the Black Death through the Industrial Revolution." *Journal of Legal Medicine* 15 (1994): 385–419.

Walter, John. *Famine, Disease and Social Order in Early Modern Society.* New York: Cambridge University Press, 1989.

Watkins, Renee Neu. "Boccaccio as Therapist: Plague Literature and the Soul of the City." *Psychohistory Review* 16 (1988): 173–200.

Williman, Daniel, ed. *The Black Death: The Impact of the Fourteenth-century Plague.* New York: Medieval and Renaissance Texts and Studies, 1982.

About the Editor, Advisory Board Members, and Contributors

About the Editor

JOSEPH P. BYRNE (M.U.P., University of Washington, 1979; Ph.D. in History, Indiana University, 1989) is a cultural and social historian of medieval and early modern Europe and Professor of Honors Humanities at Belmont University in Nashville, Tennessee. He has written extensively for a wide variety of historical reference works and journals and has recently published *The Black Death* (2004) and *Daily Life during the Black Death* (2006) with Greenwood Press. Preparation of these present volumes has taken him to Harvard University, as well as London, Oxford, and Norwich in the UK. He is currently preparing a single-volume, interdisciplinary encyclopedia on plague in the medieval and early modern world.

About the Advisory Board

ANN G. CARMICHAEL possesses M.D. and Ph.D. degrees from Duke University and teaches the history of infectious diseases at Indiana University, Bloomington. One strand of her research publications focuses on plague, pestilence, and underlying health conditions in Renaissance Italian city-states, especially Florence and Milan. The most recent of these is "Universal and Particular: The Language of Plague, 1348–1500" in *Pestilential Complexities: Understanding Medieval Plague* (2008). Within the last decade she has also published several articles on the history of climate and infectious diseases.

KATHARINE DONAHUE heads a special collection focused on the history of medicine and biology with works dating from the fifteenth through twentieth centuries. Previous to her position with UCLA, she was the Museum Librarian of the Natural History Museum of Los Angeles County. She is interested in medical and natural history images and the techniques used to create them as well as the transmission and persistence of images through time.

JOHN PARASCANDOLA retired from the federal government in 2004 after 20 years of service as Chief of the History of Medicine Division of the National Library of Medicine and as Public Health Service Historian. His awards include the Surgeon General's Exemplary Service Award (1989 and 1996). His book *The Development of American Pharmacology: John J. Abel and the Shaping of a Discipline* was awarded the George Urdang Medal (1994) from the American Institute of the History of Pharmacology. His latest research project concerns the history of syphilis in America.

CHRISTOPHER RYLAND is Assistant Director for Special Collections at Vanderbilt University Medical Center's Eskind Library. He received his M.S.I.S. from the University of Tennessee.

WILLIAM C. SUMMERS is Professor of Molecular Biophysics and Biochemistry and of History of Science and Medicine at Yale University. His books include *Felix d'Herelle and the Origins of Molecular Biology*, and he edited the *Encyclopedia of Microbiology*, second edition. His current book manuscript focuses on the geopolitics of epidemic disease in Manchuria in the early twentieth century.

About the Contributors

AVA ALKON holds an M.P.H and is a doctoral candidate in the Sociomedical Sciences Department at the Graduate School of Arts and Sciences and the Mailman School of Public Health at Columbia University. She studies history and public health, with a focus on vulnerable and institutionalized populations.

MARCELLA ALSAN holds an M.D. and an M.P.H. and is a Ph.D. candidate in Economics at Harvard University and a physician in the Howard Hiatt Global Health Equity Program at Brigham's and Women's Hospital, Boston. Her research is focused on the role of health interventions in poverty alleviation and human development.

ROBERT ARNOTT is Professor of the History and Archaeology of Medicine and Director of the Centre for the History of Medicine in the School of Medicine of the University of Birmingham (UK). He is an authority on the history of disease and medicine in the eastern Mediterranean in prehistory and his major work on *Malaria in the Aegean Bronze Age* will appear in 2008.

SUZANNE AUSTIN is Professor of History at the University of Delaware. Her books include *A Pest in the Land: New World Epidemics in a Global Perspective* and *Native Society and Disease in Colonial Ecuador*. She is currently working on a book, *Environment and Empire: European Colonialism and Environmental Change*.

ROBERT BAKER is William D. Williams Professor of Philosophy at Union College and Director of the Union Graduate College-Mount Sinai School of Medicine Bioethics Program. He has coauthored several books including *Ethics and Epidemics*, *The American Medical Ethics Revolution*, and *A History of Medical Ethics*. He is currently conducting research for a documentary history of American medical ethics and is researching the relationship between African American physicians and organized medicine.

RICHARD BARNETT completed his Ph.D. at the Wellcome Trust Centre for the History of Medicine at University College London. His current research focuses on British state medicine in the interwar period and the concept of degeneration in Victorian life science.

ANJA BECKER is a Postdoctoral Fellow at Vanderbilt University funded by the German Academic Exchange Service (DAAD). In her dissertation on Academic Networks of American Students at Leipzig University (1871–1914), she also discussed medical education in nineteenth-century Europe and America. Her current research is on higher education in the American South and West between the Civil War and World War II.

CHARLES V. BENDER earned his M.D. in 1974 from Ohio State University and currently is an Associate Professor of Obstetrics, Gynecology, and Reproductive Sciences at the University of Pittsburgh School of Medicine. He also serves both the Children's Hospital of Pittsburgh and Magee-Womens Hospital as a pediatrician and neonatal specialist.

THOMAS BENEDEK is Professor of Medicine, Emeritus, at the University of Pittsburgh School of Medicine. He is also past president of the American Association for the History of Medicine. His recent publications include "The History of Gold Therapy for Tuberculosis" (2004), "Gonorrhea and the Beginnings of Clinical Research Ethics" (2005), and "The History of Bacteriologic Concepts of Rheumatic Fever and Rheumatoid Arthritis" (2006).

MARK A. BEST holds an M.D. and an M.B.A. from the University of Louisville and an M.P.H. from Case Western Reserve University. He is a former Fellow of the Veterans Administration National Quality Scholars Fellowship Program and is Associate Professor of Pathology. He coauthored *Benjamin Franklin: Verification & Validation of the Scientific Process in Healthcare* and has written numerous articles, book chapters, and book reviews on laboratory medicine, health-care systems, and health-care quality improvement.

SANJOY BHATTACHARYA is a Reader in History at the Wellcome Trust Centre for the History of Medicine at University College London. He specializes in the history of nineteenth- and twentieth-century South Asia, as well as the history of international and global health programs deployed on the subcontinent and beyond. Dr. Bhattacharya's current work examines the structures and workings of health programs sponsored and managed by United Nations' agencies like the World Health Organization; the development of public health and medical institutions at all levels of national and local administration; and the diversity of social and political responses to state– and non-governmental organization–run schemes of preventive and curative medicine. Dr. Bhattacharya is the author of several books and articles dealing with the history of medicine of South Asia and World Health Organization activity in the region.

KARL BIRKELBACH is a Ph.D. candidate in History at the University of Western Australia. His research interests include medieval and early modern plagues. His dissertation, *Plague Debate: A Turning Point in Historiography*, investigates shifting perceptions of plague and its history.

ANNE-EMANUELLE BIRN is Canada Research Chair in International Health at the University of Toronto. Her research explores the history of public health in Latin America and the history and politics of international health. She is the author of *Marriage of Convenience: Rockefeller International Health and Revolutionary Mexico* (2006) and coauthor of the forthcoming *Textbook of International Health* (Oxford University Press). Her current project examines the early twentieth-century international circulation of child health ideologies and policies from the perspective of Uruguay.

DEVON BOAN is Professor of Honors and Director of the Honors Program at Belmont University in Nashville, Tennessee. He has a Ph.D. in Literature from the University of South Carolina and writes on cultural issues, religion, and the arts. His book *The Black "I": Author and Audience in African American Literature* is published by Peter Lang.

KRISTY WILSON BOWERS is Visiting Assistant Professor of History at Northern Illinois University. Her most recent article, "Balancing Individual and Communal Needs: Plague and Public Health in Early Modern Seville," appeared in the *Bulletin of the History of Medicine*. Her current projects include a book manuscript on the impact of plague in sixteenth-century Spain and an article examining debates on surgical methods in seventeenth-century Spain.

LINDSAY BROOCKMAN is a recent graduate of the Development Studies program at Brown University, with a thesis on water sustainability on the U.S.-Mexico border. She has led rural development projects in central Ecuador and Chiapas, Mexico. Currently she is a Manager at the AIDS Action Committee of Massachusetts and has significant experience with nonprofit program coordination and grassroots community organizing.

MARTIN CALLAGHAN, D.Phil., is a research scientist at the University of Oxford Department of Paediatrics where he works within the Oxford Vaccine Group. His current research interests focus on the development of novel vaccines against meningococcal meningitis, and his publications include articles on the molecular evolution of meningococcal adhesins, human genetic susceptibility to meningococcal disease, and the molecular evolution of bacterial restriction-modification systems.

DENNIS GREGORY CARAMENICO studied Italian history (largely that of Renaissance Florence), the history of biology and memory, and medieval Jewish-Islamic philosophy at Vanderbilt University. He received an MA in history from Vanderbilt (2006) with a thesis on Platonic *anamnesis* in Dante's *Paradiso*. He is currently studying the evolutionary psychology of memory.

K. CODELL CARTER is Professor of Philosophy at Brigham Young University. His books include *The Rise of Causal Concepts of Disease* and *Childbed Fever: A Scientific Biography of Ignaz Semmelweis*. He is currently conducting research on the philosophy of Immanuel Kant.

VINCENT J. CIRILLO, Ph.D., an independent scholar in the history of medicine, is past president of the Medical History Society of New Jersey. He is the author of *Bullets and Bacilli: The Spanish-American War and Military Medicine* (2004), published by Rutgers University Press.

ROGER COOTER is a Professorial Fellow at the Wellcome Trust Centre for the History of Medicine at University College London. The author of histories of phrenology, popular science, and orthopedics, and the editor of volumes on child health, war, and medicine; alternative medicine; accidents; and, with John Pickstone, *The Companion to Medicine in the Twentieth Century*, He is currently engaged with Claudia Stein in a study of health posters and health exhibitions in Germany and Britain.

ROHAN DEB-ROY is an M.A in History from the Presidency College Calcutta, India (2004) and holds a Diploma in Academic Research and Training from the Centre for Studies in Social Sciences Calcutta (2005). Currently he is a Doctoral Candidate at the Wellcome Trust Centre for the History of Medicine at University College London. He was awarded a three-year doctoral fellowship from the Centre (2005). His dissertation focuses on certain aspects of pharmaceutical botany, entomology, and knowledge of "malaria" in the nineteenth century. He has been awarded the Ashin Dasgupta Prize (Presidency College, 2004) and the Roy Porter Prize (University College London, 2005).

KLAUDIA DMITRIENKO is a doctoral candidate in the Department of Public Health Sciences at the University of Toronto with a background in health promotion and international relations. Her research interests focus on the political economy of global health; she is currently exploring the history of Canadian international health policy for her dissertation.

BART DREDGE is Associate Professor and Chair of Sociology at Austin College in Sherman, Texas. His research interests include labor in the American South, with special teaching attention to occupational disease and research on human subjects. His dissertation at the University of North Carolina at Chapel Hill was entitled "From Dust to Dust: Byssinosis and the Carolina Brown Lung Association, 1975–1990."

JACALYN DUFFIN is Professor in the Hannah Chair of the History of Medicine at Queen's University in Kingston, Canada. She is a physician, specializing in hematology, as well as a historian. Her books include *To See with a Better Eye: A Life of R. T. H Laennec*, *History of Medicine: A Scandalously Short Introduction*, and *Lovers and Livers: Disease Concepts in History*. Her current research is on medical miracles and medical saints.

ADRIANO DUQUE holds a Ph.D. from the University of North Carolina, Chapel Hill. He is at present Assistant Professor of Spanish at Rider University. Recent articles include "New Visions of the Mongols? Benedict the Pole and the Pian Carpine Mission of 1245" and "Imaginería religiosa in the Poema de Fernán González."

MYRON ECHENBERG is Professor of History at McGill University. His books include *Plague Ports: The Global Urban Impact of Bubonic Plague between 1894 and 1901* (2007) and *Black Death, White Medicine: Bubonic Plague and the Politics of Public Health in Colonial Senegal, 1914–1945* (2001). He is currently writing a work of synthesis on cholera provisionally entitled "'Snake in the Belly': A Global History of Cholera, 1817–2006."

RICHARD EIMAS, B.A., University of Colorado; M.A., University of Denver, is Curator Emeritus of the John Martin Book Room, Hardin Library for the Health Sciences at the University of Iowa. He was editor of *Heirs of Hippocrates: The Development of Medicine in a Catalogue of Historic Books in the Health Sciences Library* (1990), published by University of

Iowa Press, and author of numerous other publications and presentations at national and international meetings.

AMY FAIRCHILD is Associate Professor of Sociomedical Sciences at Columbia University's Mailman School of Public Health. Her book *Science at the Borders: Immigrant Medical Inspection and the Shaping of the Modern Industrial Labor Force, 1891 to 1930* was published by Johns Hopkins University Press in 2003. She is currently working on Hansen's Disease in America and patterns of societal reactions to it.

J. GORDON FRIERSON, M.D., recently retired from private practice in Oakland, California, and as Clinical Professor at the University of California San Francisco, where he was attending at the tropical disesase clinic. He was awarded a Diploma in Clinical Medicine of the Tropics at the London School of Hygiene and Tropical Medicine, has worked in or studied tropical diseases in various areas of the world, and has contributed articles on parasitic diseases to three textbooks. He now devotes time to the history of medicine.

MATTHEW GANDY teaches geography at University College London and has published widely on urban, cultural, and environmental themes. He is author of *Concrete and Clay: Reworking Nature in New York City* and coeditor of *The Return of the White Plague: Global Poverty and the "New" Tuberculosis* and *Hydropolis*.

ALEXANDRA GEUSAU holds a medical degree from the University of Vienna, Austria. She is Associate Professor of Medicine in the Division of Immunodermatology, Allergy, and Infectious Skin Diseases where she established the outpatient department for sexually transmitted diseases. She pursues research and clinical practice with both traditional STDs and with HIV/AIDS, and has published widely in both areas.

FREDERICK W. GIBBS is a Ph.D. candidate at the University of Wisconsin–Madison who studies the intersection of medieval medicine and natural philosophy with attention to how the body interacts with the world around it. His current project investigates the concept and contexts of poison in western medical literature from antiquity to the Renaissance.

PABLO F. GOMEZ is a Ph.D. Candidate in History at Vanderbilt University. Dr. Gomez holds an M.D. from the C.E.S. University in Colombia, holds a degree in orthopedic surgery from Pontificia Universidad Javeriana in Colombia, and has worked as a postdoctoral fellow in genetics and orthopedics oncology at the University of Iowa. His dissertation project *African Slaves' Health Practices in the Nuevo Reino de Granada* explores African influences in sanitary and cultural practices in Latin America.

DONATO GÓMEZ-DÍAZ holds a Doctorate in History from the University of Granada (1991) and served as professor of History and Economic Institutions at Granada; currently he teaches in the Department of Applied Economy at the University of Almería (Spain). He has published over 80 works within his area of specialization, which includes demography, primarily regarding the history of population and diseases (cholera and others), economic history, pedagogy, and new technologies.

CANDACE GREGORY-ABBOTT is an Assistant Professor of History at California State University, Sacramento, where she also teaches in the Humanities and Religious Studies department. Her research and teaching interests include the "other people of the Middle Ages," medieval magic, alchemy, witchcraft, and heresy.

VICTORIA A. HARDEN retired in January 2006 as Director of the Office of NIH History and the Stetten Museum at the National Institutes of Health, an office she created during the 1986–1987 observance of the NIH centennial. She has written and edited several books, including *Rocky Mountain Spotted Fever: History of a Twentieth-Century Disease* and *AIDS and the Public Debate: Historical and Contemporary Perspectives*, and she oversaw an oral history project on the 1960s eradication of smallpox in West Africa.

LESLEY HENDERSON is Lecturer in Sociology and Communications at the Centre for Media and Communications Research, Department of Human Sciences, at Brunel University in London (U.K.), specializing in health and medical issues in mass media—especially television—and their impacts on society and culture. He has recently published "Sad Not Bad: Images of Social Care Professionals in Popular UK Television Drama" in the *Journal of Social Work* (2007).

JOHN HENRY of the University of Edinburgh, Scotland, has published widely on the history of science and medicine from the Renaissance to the nineteenth century. He is the editor, with John M. Forrester, of *Jean Fernel's On the Hidden Causes of Things: Forms, Souls, and Occult Diseases in Renaissance Medicine*.

JUSTO HERNÁNDEZ is Assistant Professor of History of Medicine at the Faculty of Medicine of the University of La Laguna, Tenerife, Canary Islands, Spain, and President of the Canary Society of History of Medicine. His main research deals with Renaissance medicine. His books include *Cristobal de Vega y su Liber de arte medendi (1564)*, *Ciencia y Medicina en la Biblioteca de la Universidad de La Laguna*, and *El enigma de la modorra*. Currently he is working on the development of humanist Galenism in sixteenth-century Spain.

GREGORY J. HIGBY is a third-generation pharmacist. He received his Ph.D. in the history of pharmacy from the University of Wisconsin–Madison in 1984. Since 1986 he has served as the executive director of the American Institute of the History of Pharmacy, located in Madison, Wisconsin. He is the editor of the quarterly journal *Pharmacy in History*.

JULIA F. IRWIN is a Ph.D. candidate in History, with a concentration in the History of Medicine and Science, at Yale University. Her research interests include the histories of public health and U.S. foreign relations. Her dissertation, "Humanitarian Occupations: Disasters, Diplomacy, and the American Red Cross," examines U.S. international relief operations in the wake of war and natural disasters from 1900 to the early 1930s.

TINA JAKOB holds a Ph.D., and her research concentrates on health and disease patterns in archaeological skeletal populations using a bioarchaeological approach. She is currently a Teaching Fellow at the Department of Archaeology, Durham University, UK, and is

Course Director of the M.Sc. in Palaeopathology. Tina has worked on excavations in Germany, Turkey, Britain, Jordan, and the Sudan.

ERIC JARVIS teaches history at King's University College, London, Ontario. He has the article "A Plague in Paradise: Public Health and Public Relations during the 1962 Encephalitis Epidemic in St. Petersburg, Florida" forthcoming in the *Florida Historical Quarterly*.

SUSAN D. JONES is Associate Professor in the Program for the History of Science, Technology and Medicine and the Department of Ecology, Evolution and Behavior at the University of Minnesota. She is the author of *Valuing Animals: Veterinarians and Their Patients in Modern America* and several articles on the history of animal disease.

EZEKIEL KALIPENI is a population, medical, and environmental geographer interested in demographic, health, environmental, and resource issues in Sub-Saharan Africa. He has carried out extensive research on the population dynamics of Malawi and Africa, in general concentrating on fertility, mortality, migration, and health-care issues. He is currently working on HIV/AIDS in Africa and population and environmental issues in Malawi.

TOM KOCH, Ph.D., is Adjunct Professor of Medical Geography at the University of British Columbia and of Gerontology at Simon Fraser University. His books include *Cartographies of Disease: Maps, Mapping, and Medicine*, a survey of the history of medical mapping. He is currently preparing a volume on mapping as a medium for the construction of medical science: *Mapping Medicine, Making Science: Searching for Disease*.

LARA J. KUNSCHNER, M.D., is an Assistant Professor of Neurology at Drexel University College of Medicine and an attending Neurologist and Neurooncologist at Allegheny General Hospital in Pittsburgh, Pennsylvania. Research interests including neurovirology and neurooncology have led to numerous peer-reviewed articles in the medical literature.

WILLIAM LANDON is Assistant Professor of European History at Northern Kentucky University. Currently, he is writing a monograph titled "Patronage and Plague in High Renaissance Florence: Lorenzo di Filippo Strozzi and Niccolò Machiavelli," which includes the first English translation and Italian critical edition of an important, though neglected, plague tract. His first monograph, *Politics, Patriotism and Language*, which focused on Machiavelli, was published in 2005.

LAUREL LENZ is an Assistant Professor in the Department of Immunology at the University of Colorado and the National Jewish Medical and Research Center. His research and teaching focus on understanding basic mechanisms of bacterial pathogenesis and host immunity to microbial pathogens. His publication record includes numerous highly cited publications in microbiological and immunological journals and books.

TERESA LESLIE is a visiting associate professor of history at the University of West Georgia. She earned her doctorate in medieval history at Emory University. Her current research focuses on prayer rituals associated with death in medieval monastic communities.

JEFFREY LEWIS received his Ph.D. in European history from Ohio State University in 2002. His research has focused largely on the history of molecular biology in Germany, but he is also very interested in the importance of science and technology for national security. He has published several articles and book chapters on the history of biology as well as on technology and security issues.

LIEW KAI KHIUN is currently a postdoctoral fellow at the Asia Research Institute, National University of Singapore. His academic research has included the historical involvement of non-government health organizations, infectious diseases such as SARS and influenza, as well as cultural studies. His current project explores the representation of medicine in East Asian films and television dramas.

THOMAS LAWRENCE LONG is professor of English at Thomas Nelson Community College, Hampton, Virginia. He is the author of *AIDS and American Apocalypticism: The Cultural Semiotics of an Epidemic* and of numerous articles on religious discourses in culture.

LOUISE MARSHALL is Senior Lecturer in the Department of Art History and Film Studies at the University of Sydney, where she teaches late medieval and Renaissance art. She is an authority on Renaissance plague images, on which she is preparing a book. Other research interests include Renaissance devotional imagery, the cult of the saints, and representations of purgatory.

ANGELA MATYSIAK is an independent scholar with a Ph.D. in history from George Washington University. Her dissertation, *Albert B. Sabin: The Development of an Oral Vaccine Against Poliomyelitis*, examines the relationship between the science and the scientist in the development of that vaccine. She is expanding it into a full scientific biography of the life and work of Albert Sabin.

ANTHONY McMICHAEL, medical graduate and environmental epidemiologist, was previously Professor of Epidemiology, London School of Hygiene and Tropical Medicine, UK. He has worked with the World Health Organization and IPCC on health risks of climate change, including infectious diseases. His books include: *Human Frontiers, Environments and Disease* (2001), published by Cambridge University Press, and *Climate Change and Human Health: Risks and Responses* (2003), published by WHO.

HENRY MEIER is a final-year doctoral candidate in the history of medicine at the University of Oxford, UK. His thesis examines the history of smallpox in seventeenth-century London, focusing on the epidemiology and various social and economic repercussions of the disease.

LUCY MKANDAWIRE-VALHMU is an Assistant Professor in the College of Nursing at University of Wisconsin–Milwaukee. She received her Ph.D. in nursing from the University of Wisconsin–Madison. Her areas of interest are violence against women in Southern Africa and the intersection of violence and HIV in the lives of women in Southern Africa.

DAVID M. MORENS, M.D., joined U.S. Centers for Disease Control and Prevention (CDC) staff, serving as a medical virologist studying enteroviruses and enteric gastroenteritis viruses, as Chief of CDC's Respiratory & Special Pathogens Branch, and for two years studied Lassa fever in Sierra Leone, West Africa. From 1982 to 1998 he was Professor of Tropical Medicine at the University of Hawaii, and from 1987 to 1998 Professor and Chairman, Epidemiology Department, School of Public Health. Dr. Morens has studied the epidemiology of viral hemorrhagic fevers, viral pathogenesis, and the integration and role of epidemiology in biomedical science and research. His career interest for over 25 years has been in emerging infectious diseases and in diseases of unknown etiology. In the past decade he has published and spoken on numerous aspects of the history of epidemiology and infectious diseases. Currently Dr. Morens is on University leave, working in the Office of the Director, National Institute of Allergy & Infectious Diseases, National Institutes of Health.

HILARY S. MORRIS is a medical historian and Senior Lecturer in the School of Education at the University of Brighton and the Brighton and Sussex Medical School (U.K.). She is also past Deputy President of the Worshipful Society of Apothecaries. Her most recent book is *History of Medicine with Commentaries* (2005), co-authored with Robert Richardson.

SANDRA W. MOSS is a retired internist and clinical professor of medicine with a master's degree in the history of technology, the environment, and medicine. Her publications include many historical papers with a focus on nineteenth-century American medicine. She recently contributed a chapter to *Clio in the Clinic* and regularly presents papers at local, state, and national history meetings.

STEVE MURPHREE is Professor of Biology at Belmont University in Nashville, Tennessee. He is a medical entomologist with broad interests in entomology, ecology, and science education. Dr. Murphree is a native of Tennessee and holds a Ph.D. in Entomology from Auburn University and B.S. and M.S. degrees, both in biology, from Middle Tennessee State University.

ERIC D. NELSON is Assistant Professor of Classics at Pacific Lutheran University. His work includes academic publications on medical history, popular books on Greece and Rome in *The Complete Idiot's Guide* series, and contributions to programs for the History and Discovery channels. He is currently conducting research on the role that facial expressions have played in popular and medical diagnosis of mental states.

QUENTIN OUTRAM is Senior Lecturer in Economics at Leeds University Business School, UK. His interest in the Thirty Years' War arose from studies of warfare and famine in modern Liberia, West Africa.

DANIEL PALAZUELOS holds an M.D. from Brown University and is currently completing his Global Health Equity/Internal Medicine Residency at Brigham and Women's Hospital, Harvard Medical School. He works with the Boston based NGO, Partners in Health, on a project training Community Health Promoters in Chiapas, Mexico.

MELISSA PALMER is an internationally renowned hepatologist and the author of the best-selling book *Dr. Melissa Palmer's Guide to Hepatitis and Liver Disease*. She maintains perhaps the largest private medical practice devoted to liver disease in the United States. Dr. Palmer graduated from Columbia University and was trained in liver disease at the Mount Sinai School of Medicine in New York City.

JOHN PARASCANDOLA retired from the federal government in 2004 after 20 years of service as Chief of the History of Medicine Division of the National Library of Medicine and as Public Health Service Historian. His book *The Development of American Pharmacology: John J. Abel and the Shaping of a Discipline* was awarded the George Urdang Medal. His latest research project concerns the history of syphilis in America.

MARK PARASCANDOLA is an epidemiologist at the U.S. National Cancer Institute. He holds a Ph.D. in philosophy of science from Cambridge University and an M.P.H. in epidemiology from Johns Hopkins University. Dr. Parascandola has published numerous articles on the history of epidemiology and the use of epidemiologic methods in public policy.

KIM PELIS received her Ph.D. in the history of medicine at the Johns Hopkins University. In addition to several articles on the history of bacteriology and of transfusion medicine, she is the author of *Charles Nicolle, Pasteur's Imperial Missionary: Typhus and Tunisia*. Dr. Pelis is currently head speechwriter to the director of the National Institutes of Health in Bethesda, MD.

THOMAS QUINN, D.O., graduated from the Philadelphia College of Osteopathic Medicine and is Board-Certified in Family Practice and Occupational Medicine. He completed his 24-year military career as State Surgeon of the Pennsylvania National Guard. Currently, he is Clinical Associate Professor at Lake Erie College of Osteopathic Medicine-Bradenton and completing *The Feminine Touch: History of Women in Osteopathic Medicine*.

NICK RAGSDALE completed his Ph.D. in Physiology at the University of Tennessee, Memphis. He spent two years investigating antibiotic resistant *Streptococcus pneumoniae* at the St. Jude Children's Research Hospital in Memphis, Tennessee. Currently, he serves as Associate Professor of Biology and Pre-Health Advisor for Belmont University. His current research focuses on environmentally induced Parkinson's Disease.

MRIDULA RAMANNA teaches at the University of Mumbai and researches the history of medicine in India. Her publications include *Western Medicine and Public Health in Colonial Bombay, 1845–1895* (2002), chapters contributed to edited volumes published in the United Kingdom and India, and several articles in refereed research journals. She is currently working on a monograph entitled *Health Care in Bombay, 1896–1930*.

KAREN MEIER REEDS is a Princeton Research Forum, Visiting Scholar, History and Sociology of Science, University of Pennsylvania, formerly Science/Medicine Editor, Rutgers University Press, and independent scholar. Her recent books include *A State of Health: New Jersey's Medical Heritage* and *Visualizing Medieval Medicine and Natural History, 1200–1550* (coeditor). Recent exhibition projects include "Come into a New World: Linnaeus and America" and "Smallpox and the Revolutionary War."

CAROLE REEVES is the Outreach Historian at The Wellcome Trust Centre for the History of Medicine, University College London. She was picture editor and biographer for *The Dictionary of Medical Biography* and is currently researching the history of malaria in eighteenth-century England. Her illustrated articles on medical history, including "Plagues, Pestilence and Public Health," may be read at www.historyworld.net.

JONATHAN REINARZ is a Wellcome Research Lecturer at the Centre for the History of Medicine, University of Birmingham, UK. Between 2000 and 2003 he was the primary research fellow on the University Hospital Birmingham, NHS Trust–funded project, "Healthcare and the Second City: a history of the Birmingham teaching hospitals, 1779–1939." He has published on aspects of medical, labor, brewing, and local history. He is currently writing a Wellcome Trust-funded history of medical education in provincial England, 1800–1948.

HEIDI M. RIMKE is Assistant Professor of Sociology at the University of Winnipeg in Manitoba, Canada. Her doctoral thesis, *Ungovernable Subjects*, documents and analyzes the social history of the doctrine of moral insanity. Currently she is conducting research into the historical relationship between religion, law, and science in nineteenth-century Western medical discourses on dangerousness and immorality.

LISA ROSNER is Professor of History at the Richard Stockton College of New Jersey. She is the author of books and scholarly articles on the history of medical education, including *Medical Education in the Age of Improvement* and *The Most Beautiful Man in Existence*. Currently she is conducting research into the relationship between universities and academies of science during the Enlightenment.

ROBERT SALLARES holds a Ph.D. from the University of Cambridge and is Research Fellow at the University of Manchester Institute of Science and Technology. He is the author of *Malaria and Rome: a History of Malaria in Ancient Italy* (2002), *The Ecology of the Ancient Greek World* (1991), and numerous articles in medical history, ancient history, and biomolecular archeology.

JAMES SCHALLER, M.D. and M.A.R., is the author of 25 books and 25 peer-reviewed journal publications. He is a self-funded full-time researcher and part-time clinician with books and articles in ten areas of medicine, with many focusing on stealth or commonly missed infections. His specialty is patients who fail routine treatments.

JOLE SHACKELFORD is Adjunct Assistant Professor at the University of Minnesota. His books include *A Philosophical Path for Paracelsian Medicine: The Ideas, Intellectual Context, and Influence of Petrus Severinus (1540/2–1602)*. Currently he is researching the history of Paracelsian uroscopy.

DAVID F. SMITH is Senior Lecturer in the History of Medicine in the Schools of Medicine, Divinity, History, and Philosophy, at the University of Aberdeen, Scotland. He is editor of *Nutrition in Britain*, coeditor of *Food, Science, Policy and Regulation in the Twentieth Century*, and principal author of *Food Poisoning, Policy and Politics: Corned Beef and Typhoid in Britain in the 1960s*.

MELISSA SMITH is a postdoctoral fellow at George Washington University. She has published articles on plague and early modern drama and was assistant editor for *Reading Early Modern Women*. She is currently working on a book-length study about the impact of plague and syphilis on early modern drama, as well as a new project about contagious emotions.

DIONYSIOS STATHAKOPOULOS is a Research Fellow at the Department of Byzantine and Modern Greek Studies at King's College London. His book *Famine and Pestilence in the Late Roman and Early Byzantine Empire* was published in 2004. Currently he is conducting research on late Byzantine charity.

JACOB STEERE-WILLIAMS is a Ph.D. student in the History of Medicine and Biological Sciences at the University of Minnesota. His research interests include the history of disease, public health, and epidemiology in nineteenth-century Britain. His dissertation is focused on changes in waterborne disease epidemiology after the investigations of John Snow.

MARTHA STONE is Coordinator for Reference Services, Treadwell Library, Massachusetts General Hospital, Boston, and is a member of the Academy of Health Information Professionals. Her essay on French midwife Marie Boivin (1773–1847) was published in *Notable Women in the Life Sciences*. Her book reviews appear in a wide variety of publications.

MARY SUTPHEN is a Research Scholar at The Carnegie Foundation, working on a study on nursing education. She has also conducted historical research on diversity in U.S. medical schools and the history of public health in Britain's Empire. Sutphen received her B.A. from Brown University, her M.A. from Duke University, and her Ph.D. in history of medicine from Yale University.

VICTORIA SWEET is Associate Clinical Professor of Medicine at the University of California, San Francisco, with an M.D., as well as a Ph.D., in the history of medicine. She is a practicing physician and an active writer and historian. Her books include *Rooted in the Earth, Rooted in the Sky: Hildegard of Bingen and Premodern Medicine* and *God's Hotel: The Last Almshouse in America*, in manuscript.

JOHN M. THEILMANN is Professor of History and Politics at Converse College. He is the author or coauthor of a book and more than 30 articles and book chapters including "A Plague of Plagues: The Problem of Plague Diagnosis in Medieval England," in *Journal of Interdisciplinary History*, and "The Regulation of Public Health in Late Medieval England," in *The Age of Richard II*.

SELMA TIBI-HARB is a community pharmacist, practicing in Oxford, England, where, for the past year, she has run her own pharmacy. Having a strong interest in medieval Islamic medicine, she completed a doctoral thesis on the subject at Oxford University in 2003. This was published by Brill Academic Publishers as *The Medicinal Use of Opium in Ninth-Century Baghdad*.

REBECCA TOTARO is Associate Professor of English at Florida Gulf Coast University and author of *Suffering in Paradise: The Bubonic Plague in English Literature from More to Milton* (2005). A 2006–2007 participant in the Folger Shakespeare Library Year-Long Colloquium on vernacular health and healing and recipient of a short-term fellowship at the Folger for 2007–2008, she is editing an interdisciplinary anthology of early modern responses to plague and completing a monograph on early modern meteorology and physiology.

ALAIN TOUWAIDE is a Historian of Sciences in the Botany Department of the National Museum of Natural History at the Smithsonian Institution. He obtained a Ph.D. in Classics (Belgium) and specialized in the history of medicine and pharmacy in the ancient Mediterranean, working on manuscripts in Greek, Latin and Arabic, as well as on early printed books (fifteenth and sixteenth century). He is an internationally recognized expert in the history of therapeutic uses of plants in Mediterranean cultures. The recipient of many honors and grants, he has extensively published on these topics and lectured worldwide. He is the current president of the International Association for the History of Nephrology; the President-Elect of the Washington Academy of Sciences, and the Secretary of the International Society for the History of Medicine.

TANFER EMIN TUNC is an Assistant Professor of American Culture and Literature at Hacettepe University, Ankara, Turkey. She received her Ph.D. in History from SUNY Stony Brook in 2005, where she specialized in the history of science, medicine, and technology. Her research focuses on the history of women's health; gender, sexuality, and reproduction; and feminist theory. She is currently preparing her manuscript *Technologies of Choice: A History of Abortion Techniques in the United States, 1850–1980* for publication.

NICK TURSE is a recent Ph.D., with a Masters of Public Health, working in the Social Psychiatry Research Unit of the Department of Epidemiology at the Center for the History and Ethics of Public Health in the Mailman School of Public Health at Columbia University.

FRED R. VAN HARTESVELDT is Professor of History and Interim Department Head at Fort Valley State University, Georgia. Among his six books is the edited anthology *The 1918–19 Pandemic of Influenza: The Urban Impact in the Western World*. He is currently researching the role of the Royal Army Medical Corps on the Western Front in World War I.

NÜKHET VARLIK is a Ph.D. candidate in Near Eastern Languages and Civilizations at the University of Chicago. She is interested in the history of diseases and public health in the early modern Mediterranean world. Her dissertation, *Disease and Empire: A Study of Plague Epidemics in the Ottoman World (1453–1600)*, is a study of the relationship between state formation and plague epidemics.

JEFFERSON VAUGHN is currently an Associate Professor of Biology at the University of North Dakota. He began studying arboviruses as a junior researcher at the U.S. Army laoratory at Fort Detrick, MD, and since 2002 has chronicled the spread of West Nile virus into the birds and mosquitoes of eastern North Dakota.

MARK WADDELL is a Visiting Assistant Professor in the Lyman Briggs School of Science at Michigan State University. He has published articles in *Centaurus* and *The Canadian Journal of History* and is currently at work on a book manuscript which explores the links between the meditative and spiritual traditions of the Jesuits on the one hand and, on the other, their attempts to deal with invisible natural phenomena in the seventeenth century.

BARBRA MANN WALL is Associate Professor of Nursing and Associate Director of the Barbara Bates Center for the Study of the History of Nursing at the University of Pennsylvania. She has written numerous articles on nursing history. Her most recent book is *Unlikely Entrepreneurs: Catholic Sisters and the Hospital Marketplace, 1865–1925*. Currently she is conducting research on a second book that extends her analysis of Catholic hospitals into the later twentieth century.

JOHN WALLER is an Assistant Professor in the history of medicine at Michigan State University. His research is focused on ideas of heredity in Western history, and he has also published books on British social history, the advent of the germ theory of disease, and the making of scientific reputations. He is currently completing a book on the dancing mania of Strasbourg in 1518 and a detailed study of Western hereditarian thought since the collapse of the Roman Empire.

ADAM WARREN is an Assistant Professor of history at the University of Washington, Seattle, where he is currently finishing a book project on colonial medical reforms and the politics of disease prevention in eighteenth- and nineteenth-century Lima, Peru. Although his primary training is in Latin American history, most of his research and publications have addressed questions of colonial medical practices.

MARK WHEELIS is Senior Lecturer in Microbiology at the University of California, Davis. For the past 20 years, his research has focused on the history and control of chemical and biological weapons. He is coeditor of *Deadly Cultures: Biological Weapons since 1945*.

STEFAN WÖHRL is Associate Professor for Dermatology and Venerology and Senior Physician for the Division of Immunology, Allergy and Infectious Diseases at the Medical University of Vienna, Austria. He received his medical degree from the University in 1999 and has since presented 45 papers, many internationally, and published 34 coauthored articles, including "A Clinical Update: Syphilis in Adults" with A. Geusau in *Lancet* (2007).

JACQUELINE H. WOLF is Associate Professor of History of Medicine in the Department of Social Medicine at Ohio University where she specializes in the history of women's health, children's health, and public health. She is the author of numerous articles and a book—*Don't Kill Your Baby: Public Health and the Decline of Breastfeeding in the 19th and 20th Centuries* (2001)—on the history of breastfeeding practices in the United States and the effect of those practices on children's health and public health.

WILLIAM H. YORK is Assistant Professor of Interdisciplinary Studies (Humanities) at Portland State University. His dissertation *Experience and Theory in Medical Practice During the Later Middle Ages: Valesco de Tarenta (fl. 1382–1426) at the Court of Foix*, examines the ways in which physicians applied knowledge, garnered from theoretical manuals about disease, in their medical practice. His current research continues to examine these problems.

Index